THE ORIGINS OF SCHIZOPHRENIA

THE ORIGINS
OF SCHIZOPHRENIA

EDITED BY

Alan S. Brown, M.D., M.P.H.

Professor of Clinical Psychiatry and Clinical Epidemiology

Columbia University College of Physicians and Surgeons

Paul H. Patterson, Ph.D.

Anne P. and Benjamin F. Biaggini Professor of Biological Sciences

California Institute of Technology

COLUMBIA UNIVERSITY PRESS New York

Columbia University Press
Publishers Since 1893
New York   Chichester, West Sussex
cup.columbia.edu
Copyright © 2012 Columbia University Press
All rights reserved

Library of Congress Cataloging-in-Publication Data
The origins of schizophrenia / edited by Alan S. Brown and Paul H. Patterson.
    p. ; cm.
    Includes bibliographical references and index.
    ISBN 978-0-231-15124-5 (cloth : alk. paper)—ISBN 978-0-231-52192-5 (e-book)
    1. Schizophrenia—Etiology.   I. Brown, Alan S., M.D.   II. Patterson, Paul H.
    [DNLM: 1. Schizophrenia—etiology.   WM 203]
    RC514.O755   2012
    616.89'8071—dc22   2011012628

Columbia University Press books are printed on permanent and durable acid-free paper.
This book is printed on paper with recycled content.
Printed in the United States of America

c 10 9 8 7 6 5 4 3 2 1

To Anne and Skyler for their support, patience,
and understanding through the long days and late nights
A.S.B.

To Carolyn for her enthusiastic support in all of these efforts.
P.H.P.

CONTENTS

FOREWORD

I know the editors of this important volume, Alan Brown and Paul Patterson, well enough to have a glimmer of insight into how they came together to lead this book. They are both tenacious iconoclasts who have doggedly championed the hypothesis of maternal infection as a risk factor for schizophrenia while the rest of their peers were chasing dopamine and genes. The answer that they arrived at independently, Alan Brown from his tireless and creative work in epidemiology and Paul Patterson from his creative approaches in animal neurobiology, is quite striking because it was entirely unexpected. It is not the infection per se, but rather the reaction of the mother's body to it that seems to affect the fetal development of an individual who only much later in life will become ill with schizophrenia as he or she approaches adulthood. This remarkable story, with converging evidence from two different disciplines, is the cornerstone of the book. It sets the stage for understanding a range of influences on the risk for schizophrenia—genetic variants in the major histocompatability loci, obstetrical complications, and maternal psychological and social stress. All these factors can cause the mother to mount an immune response on the baby or at least its part of the placenta. The effects on fetal development, although subtle, can have ominous consequences. The title, *The Origins of Schizophrenia*, is therefore bold and perhaps off-putting, but the book delivers on its promise.

Furthermore, the book delivers in an exciting and provocative way. Clinical chapters are matched hand in hand with neurobiological models in animals for an astonishing diversity of possible causal factors. As I read each human chapter, I found myself mumbling to the potential animal modeler, "model this!" And yet, there it was: not a promise that there would someday be an animal model, but meaningful research that actually provides the possible if not probable mechanism for an observation in the human population. Of course, Paul Patterson's own work on maternal immune activation as a model for the effects of maternal infection is a prime example.

The book might have begun with the story of how the two of them came together, I suspect at a meeting somewhere when a translational panel was considered. I began to wonder who the other two speakers might have been, if it was the traditional panel of four; who might have organized or chaired it; and if many people were in the audience, or if the panel was held during the last afternoon of the meeting, reserved for the miscellany while the themes currently in vogue grabbed the limelight on the first day.

Why did they do it, and why did they decide to broaden the book beyond their own area of mutual interest? They allude to the reasons in their own introduction. The message, unspoken except in their brief introduction, is that clinical research has advanced to the point to ask many meaningful questions about the pathological mechanisms that cause schizophrenia, and animal neurobiology has responded with answers. These answers carry with them the possibility of new treatments, including new preventive treatment that should begin as early as conception.

This book is a milestone, but I hope that a book on epidemiology and animal models of the relevant mechanisms can be followed soon by a companion book on treatments developed using these animal models and their application to the treatment and ultimately the prevention of schizophrenia in humans. That would indeed be a worthy conclusion to the pioneering efforts of Alan Brown and Paul Patterson and the distinguished cast of contributors who have authored this important volume.

Robert Freedman, M.D.
University of Colorado School of Medicine
Editor-in-Chief, *American Journal of Psychiatry*
Denver, Colorado

ACKNOWLEDGMENTS

In addition to the people and sources of support acknowledged in the dedication and the individual chapters, we are indebted to several individuals who helped make this book possible. First, we wish to thank Patrick Fitzgerald of Columbia University Press for his foresight and unwavering support during the writing, editing, and compilation process. Second, we express our gratitude to Patric Prado, Nicole Stephenson, Jacky Chow, John Donohue, and Bridget Flannery-McCoy for their valuable technical efforts. Finally, we thank all of the individuals who selflessly offered their time as participants in the research studies described herein.

THE ORIGINS OF SCHIZOPHRENIA

INTRODUCTION

ALAN S. BROWN AND PAUL H. PATTERSON

This book was motivated by recent evidence that the origins of schizophrenia almost certainly encompass both environmental and genetic factors, which, through both independent and interactive neurodevelopmental mechanisms, appear to play important roles in this disorder. This theory is based on support from several domains of research. First, many new findings on potential environmental etiologies have emerged from epidemiologic studies. These investigations feature fundamental methodologic improvements over prior work, including birth cohort and other longitudinal approaches, prospective and more precise definitions of exposure status, control of confounding, and addressing bias due to attrition. These developments have markedly improved the validity and interpretability of this body of research and suggest potential novel preventive approaches. Second, rapid advances in molecular genetic and genomic approaches, including genome-wide association studies, and the emerging fields of copy number variation and epigenetics, as well as new statistical methods and bioinformatic strategies, have markedly expanded the power to decipher the genetic variants and modifications that may alter brain development and contribute to susceptibility for schizophrenia. Third, a revolution in preclinical, translational models of schizophrenia has allowed the testing of several environmental and genetic candidates of these disorders, particularly those that act to modify neurodevelopmental processes. This has facilitated validation of clinical findings, enhanced the understanding of etiopathogenic mechanisms, and revealed potential treatment approaches that target the aberrant processes that are triggered by these insults. The reach of these studies has been further enhanced by improvements in behavioral assays, gene expression profiling, laser microdissection–real time polymerase chain reaction, and small-animal magnetic resonance imaging technologies. Finally, further developments in research on the biological basis of schizophrenia have yielded astounding insights into the neurodevelopmental and pathophysiologic basis of schizophrenia. These discoveries are having profound effects on epidemiologic, genetic, and translational approaches to schizophrenia, including the identification of candidate risk factors, the relevant functional effects of putative susceptibility genes, and the molecules, cellular pathways, and neurocircuits to be investigated in preclinical models. Several of these points are further elucidated by John Waddington in the Overview to this book.

This book is divided into two parts. Part 1, "Clinical Research on Risk Factors for Schizophrenia," includes two sections, "Environmental Factors" and "Genetics and Epigenetics." The first section consists of detailed discussion of emerging and prior research on the following putative risk factors: maternal infection, prenatal nutritional factors, obstetric complications, maternal stress, advancing paternal age, and cannabis use. The second section consists of a comprehensive and up-to-date review of the genetics of schizophrenia, including genomewide association studies, copy number variation, and epigenetics. Part 2, "Preclinical Research on Etiologies of Schizophrenia," also contains two sections. In keeping with the translational theme of this volume, the first section, "Animal Models of Environmental Factors and Schizophrenia," focuses on the methods and novel findings from preclinical studies of environmental factors, several of which are included in the first section of Part 1. These include animal models of maternal infection, developmental vitamin D deficiency, prenatal protein malnutrition, and maternal stress. The second section, "Animal Models of Genetic Factors and Schizophrenia," consists of preclinical models of two of the most commonly cited candidate genes for schizophrenia, *DISC1* (Disrupted-in-Schizophrenia 1) and *neuregulin*, which have been investigated extensively.

Although the material presented in this book is the product of several remarkable transformations in research on the epidemiology, genetics, and neurobiology of schizophrenia, and in spite of the high level of collective scientific wisdom that it contains, we must underscore the point that the field is a long way from a complete understanding of this complex and puzzling disorder. Conceivably, some of the findings presented here will fail to be replicated, or will be replaced by more satisfactory explanations, and undoubtedly new environmental risk factors, genes, and pathogenic mechanisms that involve gene-environment interactions will emerge. Moreover, we may not yet have a firm grasp on the pathophysiologic basis of schizophrenia, requiring the development of novel technologies and perhaps radically different approaches to understanding the structure and function of the normal and diseased brain, the relationships of these neurobiological findings to symptoms and behavior, and the developmental trajectories that give rise to this condition. These caveats aside, it is our view that the methods and findings presented here hold great promise toward the ultimate goal of eradicating this devastating illness, providing hope to the millions of afflicted individuals, to society, and to future generations.

OVERVIEW

SCHIZOPHRENIA AND THE LIFETIME TRAJECTORY OF PSYCHOTIC ILLNESS
Developmental Neuroscience and Pathobiology, Redux

JOHN L. WADDINGTON, ROBIN J. HENNESSY,
COLM M. P. O'TUATHAIGH, OLABISI OWOEYE, AND VINCENT RUSSELL

KEY CONCEPTS

- Pathobiology of schizophrenia: There is now voluminous evidence from neuro-imaging, neuropathologic, neurochemical, and neuropsychological studies for the existence of abnormalities of brain structure and function in schizophrenia. These likely reflect dysfunction in one or more neuronal networks that integrate activity across a number of regions to subserve fundamental psychological processes.
- Developmental origins: There is now a wealth of indirect, epidemiologic evidence and increasing "hard" biological evidence that schizophrenia involves disruption to brain development over early gestational life.
- The enigma of "progression": Much current research focuses on whether schizophrenia shows progression—particularly in terms of the emergence of an active, morbid process associated with psychotic ideation—as a component of the disorder's pathobiology. A yet greater challenge is whether this process might be attenuated by early therapeutic interventions.
- The breadth of psychotic illness: We are still seeking to define the boundaries of psychosis and the extent to which those aspects of psychotic illness that we resolve into separate diagnostic categories are actually distinct in any fundamental way.
- Schizophrenia as a "lifetime trajectory" disorder: This schema posits an accumulation of adversities and pathobiology from early gestational life through infancy, childhood, adolescence, early adulthood, and beyond. The result is a cascade of functional sequelae that "sculpt" the overall course of illness, dysfunction, and outcome.

Our understanding of the origins of schizophrenia is a continually evolving tableau that is predicated not just on empirical findings but also on parallel evolution in our underlying concept of the disorder. For example, the impact of advances in epidemiology and clinical science—together with new in vivo imaging, postmortem cytoarchitectural, molecular genetic, and mutant model technologies—continues to be profound. However, these advances are occurring in juxtaposition with a fundamental reevaluation of psychosis. Much contemporary theorizing emphasizes a dimensional rather than a categorical concept of psychotic symptomatology vis-à-vis those other dimensions of psychopathology and dysfunction that we recognize across serious mental illness; thus, what we currently diagnose as schizophrenia may constitute not a discrete entity but rather a domain defined by certain psychopathologic and functional characteristics, the boundaries of which are in fact notional and in continuity with other domains of psychotic illness, through to the limits of "normal" human behavior (Tandon, Nasrallah, & Keshavan, 2009; van Os & Kapur, 2009).

In 1987, the publication of two review articles (Murray & Lewis, 1987; Weinberger, 1987) constituted a point of inflection in the prevailing concept of schizophrenia. Through systematic reevaluation of long-standing notions and appraisal of recent data, they offered a new heuristic for schizophrenia as a neurodevelopmental disorder. Within five years, this heuristic had seeded so extensive a research front as to already justify further review of developmental neuroscience and pathobiology (Waddington, 1993). Thereafter, research advanced so rapidly that these issues are now but one element across the breadth and depth of theorizing on schizophrenia (Waddington et al., 1999; Waddington, 2007; Tandon, Keshavan, & Nasrallah, 2008; Fatemi & Folsom, 2009; van Os & Kapur, 2009). It is on the basis of this background that this overview seeks to reconsider the developmental neuroscience and pathobiology of schizophrenia and further interpret it (redux) within a lifetime trajectory model of psychotic illness.

Pathobiology of Schizophrenia

Structural Brain Abnormalities: Neuroimaging

Recent systematic reviews and meta-analyses have synthesized what is now voluminous evidence from magnetic resonance imaging (MRI) studies for abnormalities of brain structure in schizophrenia that include small volumetric increases in the ventricular system and reductions in overall brain and gray matter volumes, together with subcortical, limbic, and cortical regional changes (Wright et al., 2000; Honea et al., 2005; Keshavan et al., 2008). However, it is important to emphasize that these abnormalities are evident only on a population basis, with measures in patients and controls having clearly overlapping distributions that preclude diagnostic utility on an individual subject basis (Daniel et al., 1991; Vita et al., 2000).

A related issue is whether abnormalities of brain structure are evident in some patients but not others. An all too commonly overlooked implication of this distributional overlap, in the absence of bimodality, is that such abnormalities appear to be present in *all* patients with schizophrenia, even those at the limit of the patient distribution that may be well within the control distribution: for each patient with schizophrenia, brain structure appears abnormal relative to what it would have been had that individual not become ill with schizophrenia (Waddington et al., 1999; Baldwin et al., 2004).

Structural Brain Abnormalities: Neuropathology

These in vivo findings using MRI are, in general, complemented by less voluminous but potentially more incisive evidence from postmortem studies for structural brain pathology in schizophrenia. Although such studies are subject to potential confounds of small numbers of individuals who often are of advanced age, as well as the effects of antemortem circumstances and postmortem delay, the findings sustain and elaborate abnormalities of those subcortical, limbic, and cortical regions implicated on MRI (Harrison, 1999; Keshavan et al., 2008).

Parenthetically, there is now evidence that sustained treatment with antipsychotic drugs can influence brain structure in nonhuman primates (Konopaske et al., 2009) and may do so also in humans (Navari & Dazzan, 2009). The challenge is to distinguish between a "toxic" drug effect that may give rise to adverse sequelae and constitute a potential artifact in studies of brain structure in treated patients, and a "therapeutic" action that is a component of the antipsychotic effect of such medication.

Neuronal Cytoarchitecture

A critical variant of postmortem brain studies goes beyond macroscopic pathology to the microscopic and cellular evaluation of neuronal cytoarchitecture in subcortical, limbic, and cortical regions. For example, it is now possible to begin to resolve and disentangle—at the levels of gene expression, neuronal morphology, and cell biology—abnormalities in the excitatory, inhibitory, and modulatory microcircuitry within regions such as the prefrontal cortex and hippocampus (Harrison, 2004; Benes, 2007; Lewis & Gonzales-Burgos, 2008).

Neurochemical Abnormalities

DOPAMINERGIC SYSTEMS. That the pathobiology of schizophrenia might involve heightened transmission through dopamine (DA) receptors, primarily of the D_2 subtype, derives from the indirect DA-releasing agent amphetamine being psychotomimetic and all known antipsychotic drugs being D_2 receptor antagonists. Putative D_2 DAergic hyperfunction has been given pathophysiologic substance by neuroimaging findings that indicate increased subcortical release of DA onto D_2 receptors in schizophrenia, in proportion with the extent of exacerbation of positive symptoms induced by amphetamine. Aspects of the negative symptom domain and cognitive impairment may additionally reflect associated reduction in release of DA onto D_1 receptors in the prefrontal cortex. It has been suggested that in schizophrenia, inappropriate firing and release of DA in a cue- and context-independent manner results in the misattribution of salience to irrelevant events in the external environment. In essence, this progressive alteration in perception of novelty and salience attribution, accompanied by the disturbance in DA function, results in the misinterpretation of internally generated percepts and memories as externally driven input (Guillin, Abi-Dargham, & Laruelle, 2007; Howes & Kapur, 2009).

GLUTAMATERGIC SYSTEMS. That the pathobiology of schizophrenia might involve reduced transmission through N-methyl-D-aspartate (NMDA)-glutamate receptors has its origins as a corollary to the noncompetitive NMDA antagonist phencyclidine (PCP) being psychotomimetic. This proposition of NMDA-glutamatergic hypofunction has been given pathophysiologic substance by findings of NMDA deficits in postmortem brain in schizophrenia (Coyle, 2006; Stone, Morrison, & Pilowsky, 2007) and recent neuroimaging evidence for an NMDA receptor deficit in living patients (Pilowsky et al., 2006). These may relate to DAergic mechanisms through prominent interactions between NMDA and D_1 receptors in prefrontal cortex (Castner & Williams, 2007; Javitt, 2007).

Neuronal Network Dysfunction Through Disconnectivity

As evidence of schizophrenia pathobiology continues to evolve, the disorder does not appear to involve any unitary brain region. Rather, it seems best accommodated by a model of dysfunction in one or more neuronal networks that integrate activity across a number of regions to subserve fundamental psychological processes. More specifically, synaptic pathology, gene expression, neurophysiology, neuropsychology, neuromotor function, functional magnetic resonance imaging (fMRI), and diffusion tensor imaging combine to implicate disconnectivity as the basis of such dysfunction. For example, candidate systems include fronto-striato-pallido-thalamo-cortical-temporal networks, in which disconnectivity could result in a pattern of dysfunction that integrates our knowledge on the putative roles of DAergic and glutamatergic mechanisms (Ellison-Wright et al., 2008; Glahn et al., 2008; Lisman et al., 2008; Benes, 2009; Ellison-Wright & Bullmore, 2009; Fornito et al., 2009; Howes & Kapur, 2009; Stephan, Friston, & Frith, 2009; Whitty, Owoeye, & Waddington, 2009).

Two Fundamental Questions

At this juncture, two fundamental and related questions must be posed.

First, if brain structure and function can be demonstrated to be abnormal in schizophrenia, is this because (1) a once normal brain was subsequently rendered abnormal by the impact of disease, or (2) the brain has never been normal because of disturbance over an early phase of neurodevelopment?

Second, if (2) were the case, is the emergence of diagnostic, psychotic symptoms accompanied, or actually preceded, by the emergence of some active, morbid process?

Developmental Origins

Indirect Evidence for Early Developmental Disturbance

There is now a wealth of indirect, epidemiologic evidence that environmental adversities acting over early gestational life are associated with increased risk for psychosis in offspring. The extensive literature on infectious and immune factors, prenatal nutrition, obstetric complications, maternal stress, and related factors is considered in Part 1, Section 1 of this book. In a complementary manner, Part 1, Section 2 documents evidence that many of the genetic variations associated with risk for schizophrenia—both common alleles of small effect *and* multiple, individually rare but highly penetrant copy number variations—are expressed in pathways implicated in early brain development.

These lines of indirect, epidemiologic, and genetic evidence for early disruption to brain development are consistent with the neuropathologic signature of schizophrenia, whereby cytoarchitectonic changes have the characteristics of dysplastic processes, in the absence of evidence for any neurodegenerative process as currently conceptualized (Harrison, 1999; Keshavan et al., 2008). Additionally, they are buttressed by evidence that structural brain abnormalities are already present by the first psychotic episode (Steen et al., 2006; Vita et al., 2006) and, even more so, by emerging evidence that structural and neurochemical abnormalities predate the onset of diagnostic symptoms and evolve over a prepsychotic phase, variously described as the "prodrome" or "at-risk mental state," or in "ultrahigh risk groups" (Howes et al., 2009; Sun et al., 2009; Takahashi et al., 2009).

"Hard" Evidence for Early Developmental Disturbance

These issues would be clarified by unambiguous indices of early developmental disturbance that could be accessed directly in living patients and would inform incisively on the nature of any underlying developmental abnormality.

CONGENITAL ANOMALIES. Congenital anomalies constitute hard biological evidence of dysmorphogenic events over embryonic and fetal life that are associated with a variety of early functional impairments. Such anomalies and related functional impairments can be examined prospectively from infancy for their ability to predict adverse adult outcomes, including schizophrenia. Two birth cohort studies (Dalman et al., 1999; Waddington et al., 2008) have now reported the presence of congenital anomalies to be associated with a doubling of risk for schizophrenia.

MINOR PHYSICAL ANOMALIES. Minor physical anomalies are slight anatomic malformations of body regions that share the ectodermal origins of the brain; their presence indicates adverse events acting over the first or second trimester and they occur to excess in most disorders of early neurodevelopmental origin (Waddington et al., 1999). Thus, although found consistently to be overrepresented in schizophrenia (Weinberg et al., 2007; Compton & Walker, 2009), minor physical anomalies constitute a nonspecific, qualitative indicator of early biological adversity.

CRANIOFACIAL DYSMORPHOLOGY. The anterior brain and face evolve in embryologic intimacy. This unity over early fetal life is responsible for facial dysmorphogenesis in disorders of early brain development, ranging from major chromosomal abnormalities such as Down's syndrome to less readily recognizable conditions such as velocardiofacial syndrome (Waddington et al., 1999; Marcucio et al., 2005; Hennessy et al., 2007). Anthropometric techniques have indicated subtle facial dysmorphology also in schizophrenia. We (Lane et al., 1997) and others (McGrath et al., 2002; Donovan-Lepore et al., 2006) have noted altered proportions along the midline together with abnormalities of the eyes and widening of the skull base.

As the developmental biology of facial morphogenesis is considerably better understood than is brain morphogenesis, resolution of the topography of facial dysmorphogenesis in schizophrenia may lead to increased understanding of brain dysmorphogenesis. However, as facial development is an intrinsically three-dimensional process, anthropometry fails to access fundamental, geometric aspects of this process. As an initial approach, we resolved facial dysmorphology and asymmetry in patients with schizophrenia using crude three-dimensional configurations reconstructed from linear measurements (Hennessy et al., 2004). Three-dimensional digitization technologies now allow facial surfaces to be recorded in their entirety and landmark coordinates obtained; in a complementary manner, geometric morphometrics, which analyze three-dimensional landmark coordinates directly, provides the basis for relating shape to other biological variables both statistically and visually (Hennessy et al., 2005).

We have applied portable, hand-held three-dimensional laser surface imaging with a recently implemented algorithm using interpolated landmarks over the entire facial surface (Hennessy et al., 2007). Both male and female patients with schizophrenia evidenced significant facial dysmorphology: narrowing and reduction of the middle and lower face and frontonasal prominences, including reduced width and posterior displacement of the mouth, lips, and chin; increased width of the upper face, mandible, and skull base, with lateral displacement of the cheeks, eyes, and orbits; and anterior displacement of the superior margins of the orbits. In summary, the frontonasal prominences, which enjoy the most intimate embryologic relationship with the anterior brain and also orchestrate aspects of development in maxillary and mandibular domains, evidence a characteristic topography of dysmorphogenesis in schizophrenia.

The Nature of Early Developmental Disturbance

The trajectory of facial-cerebral morphogenesis, primarily a midline process, involves (see Hennessy et al., 2007, and references therein) (1) anterior brain growth with vertical growth and narrowing of the anterior midfacial region, particularly the frontonasal prominences; (2) primary palate formation; (3) dissociation of cranial base width from anterior facial and cerebral changes; and (4) the face growing forward more rapidly than the brain. More specifically, morphogenesis of the frontonasal prominences, forebrain, and anterior midline cerebral regions is intimately regulated via epithelial-mesenchymal signaling interactions: the nascent forebrain, neuroepithelium, neural crest, and facial ectoderm function as a developmental unit in terms of gene expression domains.

The specific dysmorphogenic features encountered in schizophrenia implicate events acting particularly over a time frame whose extreme limits are gestational weeks 6 through 19; more speculatively, they suggest within this time frame a common denominator of weeks 9 or 10 through 14 or 15 of gestation. Additionally, such dysmorphogenesis along the anterior midline would be expected to disrupt neuroectodermal patterning and the critical repulsive and attractive guidance cues that, together with trophic and experiential factors, regulate neuronal connectivity (Chang et al., 2000; Giger & Kolodkin, 2001). This would accord with models of neuronal network disconnectivity in schizophrenia, particularly in fronto-striato-pallido-thalamo-cortical-temporal networks (see "Neuronal Network Dysfunction Through Disconnectivity"). In summary, understanding the genetic, epigenetic, and experiential regulation of midline morphogenesis involving the frontonasal prominences may inform early developmental perturbation in schizophrenia.

The Enigma of "Progression": Antithetical, Complementary, or Integral?

In juxtaposition with such developmental considerations is the controversy as to whether or how schizophrenia might or might not progress over its adult phase and if any such progression would reflect either (1) the passive impact of normal maturational and aging processes on a developmentally compromised brain, in the absence of any active process, or (2) the emergence of an active, morbid process as a component of the pathobiology of the disorder (Waddington et al., 1999; Weinberger & McClure, 2002; Baldwin et al., 2004; McGlashan, 2006).

At a clinical level, one of the most controversial lines of argument involves evidence that the longer psychotic illness runs untreated after onset, before first exposure to antipsychotic medication, the worse is long-term outcome. This could imply that the onset of psychosis has a basis in, or is accompanied by, the onset of some morbid process, the debilitating consequences of which might be ameliorated by early, effective intervention with antipsychotics. The challenge is to disentangle the available relationships (Marshall et al., 2005; Perkins et al., 2005) into an ordered sequence of events. Does increasing duration of untreated psychosis (DUP) reflect increasing duration of a morbid process that mediates poor long-term outcome? Alternatively, do recognized adverse prognosticands such as premorbid functioning or negative symptoms result in longer DUP, as well as predicting poor long-term outcome? If so, would the relationship between DUP and poor long-term outcome be not causal but rather a secondary consequence of their shared relationship to such an adverse prognosticand?

At a biological level, one of the most controversial issues is whether abnormalities of cerebral structure progress over the course of illness. At one level, the challenge would seem straightforward: conduct prospective MRI studies over differing phases of the illness and determine the extent of any longitudinal changes. However, the numerous studies adopting this approach have generated several challenges (Weinberger & McClure, 2002; DeLisi, 2008; Borgwardt et al., 2009):

1. How strong and consistent is the evidence for progressive brain changes?
2. Are they anatomically specific?
3. Are they disease- or subject-specific?
4. What is their time course?
5. What is their underlying pathobiology?
6. Are they central to the disease process?
7. Are they due to treatment with antipsychotic drugs and, if so, as an adverse or a therapeutic effect?
8. Are they epiphenomena, such as physical debilities associated with poor self-care?
9. What is their clinical significance?
10. Are they reversible?
11. What are their implications for treatment?

The available evidence would suggest that subtle, progressive brain changes are apparent over the course of schizophrenia. They may be more prominent over the early phase or phases of illness and may precede the onset of psychosis in those who are at increased symptomatic or genetic risk. They may also be evident over later phases of the illness, but the extent of progression may slowly decline until the emergence of age-related processes. The ventricular system, overall brain and gray matter volumes, and subcortical, limbic, and cortical regions may be affected differentially; their pathobiology, clinical correlates, and treatment implications remain unclear (Waddington, 2007; Arango et al., 2008; DeLisi, 2008; Hulshoff Pol & Kahn, 2008; Lawrie et al., 2008; Wood et al., 2008; Borgwardt et al., 2009).

It should be emphasized that such progressive brain changes are apparent in the absence of pathologic evidence for any neurodegenerative process as currently conceptualized. Thus, it has been suggested that they may involve apoptotic processes (Glantz et al., 2006) or reflect deficits in synaptic plasticity (McGlashan, 2006). It has been argued that developmental pathobiology is primary and disease progression artifactual or an epiphenomenon (Weinberger & McClure, 2002)—i.e., that they are antithetical. However, perhaps the greater challenge is to distinguish between developmental pathobiology and progression as two independent, complementary aspects of the disease processes of schizophrenia, or two interdependent phases that are integral to a unitary disease process. One important prospective study (Cahn et al., 2002) may illustrate the confluence of developmental and progressive processes: the size of the third ventricle was enlarged at the first episode and did not increase further over the one-year period thereafter, as might be expected of an abnormality having its origin in early developmental disruption along the midline; conversely, cortical gray matter volume was unaltered at the first episode but decreased over the subsequent one-year period, as might be expected of an abnormality having its basis in some progressive process associated with the emergence of psychotic symptoms. Provocatively, on extending the follow-up period to five years, loss of gray matter volume was predicted by DUP (Cahn et al., 2009).

Modeling Developmental Events in Mutant Mice

Developmental models of schizophrenia are based on evidence that environmental adversities during early life and genes implicated in neurodevelopment increase risk for psychosis in later life. Thus, new rodent models reviewed in this book reflect increasing understanding of early environmental exposures (see Part 2, Section 1) and genetic risk (see Part 2, Section 2). In particular, construction of mice that are mutant for candidate genes provides a powerful tool for investigating their functional roles. They can be applied to study pathobiological and pharmacological mechanisms thought to be relevant for schizophrenia, from developmental disruption and associated morphologic and functional phenotypes, through to DAergic and glutamatergic dysfunction and response to drugs (Waddington et al., 2007; Desbonnet, Waddington, & Tuathaigh, 2009; Kirby et al., 2010).

An increasingly powerful role for such models is to elaborate a new wave of clinical evidence for gene-environment interactions in schizophrenia (see Part 2, Section 2). Thus, they can now be applied to study how a given risk gene might modify the consequences of a given environmental exposure, as they provide a degree of resolution and control that is not available in clinical studies. For example, our laboratory is currently investigating how the candidate gene *neuregulin 1* might modify the consequences of prenatal immune activation and later exposure to social defeat or the psychotomimetic phencyclidine (O'Tuathaigh et al., 2010) and how the catechol-O-methyltransferase (*COMT*) gene might modify the consequences of adolescent exposure to cannabis (O'Tuathaigh et al., 2009). Similarly, others are investigating how the candidate gene Disrupted-in-Schizophrenia 1 (*DISC1*) might modify the consequences of prenatal immune activation (Ibi et al., 2010).

The Relationship of Schizophrenia to the Breadth of Psychotic Illness

In seeking to understand the origins of schizophrenia, broader challenges must be faced: (1) what are the boundaries of psychotic illness, and (2) to what extent are those components of psychotic illness that we resolve into separate diagnostic categories actually distinct in any fundamental way in terms of their epidemiologic, clinical, and pathobiological "signature"? As a specific example, these challenges have particular currency in continuing reevaluation of the Kraepelinian dichotomy between schizophrenia and bipolar disorder (Jablensky, 1999), where evidence increasingly indicates overlap between these two diagnostic categories in terms of genetics (O'Donovan, Craddock, & Owen, 2009; Moskvina et al., 2010), neuropsychology (Krabbendam et al., 2005; Hill et al., 2008), and pathobiology (Lloyd et al., 2007; Arnone et al., 2009; Fornito, Yucel, & Pantelis, 2009; Tenyi, Trixler, & Csabi, 2009).

Epidemiology and Pathobiology: The Cavan-Monaghan First Episode Psychosis Study

We have advocated and adopted a radical approach in seeking to study the "totality" of psychotic illness naturalistically—to include a first manic episode—in the absence of a priori diagnostic restriction. Subsequent post hoc imposition of contemporary diagnostic criteria then allows the epidemiologic, clinical, and pathobiological characteristics of those categories to be compared systematically. In the Cavan-Monaghan First Episode Psychosis Study (CAMFEPS) (Scully et al., 2002; Baldwin et al., 2005; Owoeye et al., 2010), we have sought, since 1995, the continuing inception of *all* incident cases of psychosis—to include a first manic episode—among a rural region of ethnic and socioeconomic homogeneity.

On post hoc application of *Diagnostic and Statistical Manual of Mental Disorders*, fourth edition (DSM-IV) criteria at six months to all 372 cases of psychosis incepted to date, in the absence of a priori diagnostic restriction it was confirmed, as expected, that schizophrenia and bipolar disorder constitute major diagnostic nodes. Yet these diagnoses each accounted for less than one-fifth of cases. Furthermore, extension to "schizophrenia spectrum" diagnoses (schizophrenia, schizophreniform disorder, schizoaffective disorder) increased the proportion only to less than one-third of cases. One contributory factor was the unexpectedly high incidence of a third major diagnostic node—i.e., a first psychotic episode on a background of major depressive disorder. The remaining diagnoses were delusional disorder, brief psychotic disorder, substance-induced psychosis, substance-induced mood disorder (e.g., selective serotonin reuptake inhibitor-induced mania), psychosis due to a general medical condition, mood disorder (mania) due to a general medical condition, and psychosis not otherwise specified.

Yet varying epidemiologic signatures across the three major diagnostic nodes (Baldwin et al., 2005; Owoeye et al., 2010) must be juxtaposed with substantive homogeneity in terms of indistinguishable overall incidence, presentation throughout the life span, indistinguishable scores for positive symptoms, and substantial stability for up to six years of follow-up. Similarly, dichotomization of bipolar disorder into two subgroups on the basis of the DSM-IV qualifier *with psychotic features* revealed only minimal difference in terms of scores for positive symptoms; psychosis in bipolar disorder appears to be a generic characteristic, most likely evident along a continuum, rather than any basis for arbitrary subtyping of the disorder.

Additionally, we have applied three-dimensional laser surface imaging and geometric morphometrics to identify any domains of craniofacial shape that distinguish bipolar patients from controls and from those with schizophrenia, as already outlined here (see "'Hard' Evidence for Early Developmental Disturbance"). Both male and female bipolar patients had significant facial dysmorphology, as a putative index of brain dysmorphogenesis; furthermore, dysmorphology of the frontonasal prominences and related facial regions in bipolar disorder is more similar to than different from that found in schizophrenia, suggesting some shared dysmorphogenic process (Hennessy et al., 2007, 2010; Owoeye et al., 2010). Schizophrenia and bipolar disorder may reflect similar disturbances acting over slightly differing time frames or slightly differing disturbances acting over a similar time frame.

Refining a Lifetime Trajectory Model for Psychosis

What sort of schema could accommodate what we currently conceptualize and diagnose as schizophrenia within the much broader reality of psychotic disorder among those with serious mental illness and, indeed, of psychotic-like phenomena among the general population? One proposal (Waddington et al., 1999; Baldwin et al., 2004) offers a lifetime trajectory model. We suggest here that psychosis is a continuously distributed phenomenon in the population (van Os et al., 2008), the extent of which is related to variation in the integrity of brain morphogenesis over a period that includes a critical window of weeks 9 or 10 through 14 or 15 of gestation. This nascent brain is then a substrate for the endogenous, programmed processes of later development and maturation, including neuroendocrine processes, myelination, and synaptic pruning (Paus, Keshavan, & Giedd, 2008), with the outcome of these processes variably altered depending on the developmental integrity of the brain on which they act. Additionally, exogenous biological exposures such as prenatal or perinatal infections, nutrition, and other obstetric complications, and environmental exposures such as maternal stress, psychosocial disadvantage (e.g., social defeat or social fragmentation), and substance abuse (Welham et al., 2009) will also have an impact on the development and codification of adult brain integrity and function.

Specifically, this "lifetime trajectory" schema posits the following sequence of events: Individuals having such a developmentally compromised brain subsequently accumulate a diversity of adversities that sculpt, both metaphorically and biologically, later brain development, maturation, and function. The extent to which the resultant brain morphology deviates from what is considered optimal results in neurointegrative, cognitive, and psychosocial deficits over infancy and childhood, as well as the emergence of psychotic ideation. In those whose brain morphology most deviates from what is optimal, the extent of such ideation would cross an arbitrary threshold to qualify for a diagnosis of psychotic illness. Variations in the nature, extent, and timing of these events would influence the quality and overall psychopathologic milieu of psychotic ideation and the arbitrary diagnosis (e.g., schizophrenia, schizoaffective disorder, bipolar disorder, or major depression with psychotic features) assigned to it. The dysfunctional cellular cascade associated with the emergence of psychotic ideation would be a component of some subtle, phasic, and time-limited morbid process associated also with disruption to brain morphology and functional impairment. A major debate endures as to whether any such morbid process might be ameliorated by early, effective intervention with antipsychotic drugs, cognitive therapies, or both so as to improve outcome and, most controversially, to potentially reduce transition to psychotic illness in those having an at-risk mental state (McGorry et al., 2009, 2010).

Acknowledgments

The authors' studies are supported by Science Foundation Ireland (07/IN.1/B960), the Health Research Board (PD/2007/20), the Wellcome Trust [086901/Z/08/Z], the Irish Government's National Development Plan 2007–2013 via HEA PRTLI Cycle 4 under the National Biophotonics and Imaging Platform Ireland, the Stanley Medical Research Institute, and Cavan-Monaghan Mental Health Service. We thank the clinical teams and associated staff of Cavan-Monaghan Mental Health Service for their important contributions.

Selected Readings

Borgwardt, S. J., Dickey, C., Hulshoff Pol, H., Whitford, T. J., & DeLisi, L. E. (2009). Workshop on defining the significance of progressive brain change in schizophrenia: The rapporteurs' report. *Schizophrenia Research* 112(1–3): 32–45.

Hennessy, R. J., Baldwin, P. A., Browne, D. J., Kinsella, A., & Waddington, J. L. (2007). Three-dimensional laser surface imaging and geometric morphometrics resolve frontonasal dysmorphology in schizophrenia. *Biological Psychiatry* 61(10): 1187–1194.

Howes, O. D. & Kapur, S. (2009). The dopamine hypothesis of schizophrenia: Version III—the final common pathway. *Schizophrenia Bulletin* 35(3): 549–562.

Keshavan, M. S., Tandon, R., Boutros, N. N., & Nasrallah, H. A. (2008). Schizophrenia, "just the facts": What we know in 2008, part 3: Neurobiology. *Schizophrenia Research* 106(2–3): 89–107.

Lewis, D. A. & Gonzales-Burgos, G. (2008). Neuroplasticity of neocortical circuits in schizophrenia. *Neuropsychopharmacology* 33(1): 141–165.

Stephan, K. E., Friston, K. J., & Frith, C. D. (2009). Dysconnection in schizophrenia: From abnormal synaptic plasticity to failures of self-monitoring. *Schizophrenia Bulletin* 35(3): 509–527.

van Os, J. & Kapur, S. (2009). Schizophrenia. *Lancet* 374(9690): 635–645.

Waddington, J. L., Corvin, A. P., Donohue, G., O'Tuathaigh, C. M. P., Mitchell, K. J., & Gill, M. (2007). Functional genomics and schizophrenia: Endophenotypes and mutant models. *Psychiatric Clinics of North America* 30(3): 365–399.

Weinberger, D. R. & McClure, R. K. (2002). Neurotoxicity, neuroplasticity, and magnetic resonance imaging morphometry: What is happening in the schizophrenic brain? *Archives of General Psychiatry* 59(6): 553–558.

Welham, J., Isohanni, M., Jones, P., & McGrath, J. (2009). The antecedents of schizophrenia: A review of birth cohort studies. *Schizophrenia Bulletin* 35(3): 603–623.

References

Arango, C., Moreno, C., Martinez, S., Parellada, M., Desco, M., Moreno, D., Fraguas D., Gogtay, N., James, A., & Rapoport, J. (2008). Longitudinal brain changes in early-onset psychosis. *Schizophrenia Bulletin* 34(2): 341–353.

Arnone, D., Cavanagh, J., Gerber, D., Lawrie, S. M., Ebmeier, K. P., & McIntosh, A. M. (2009). Magnetic resonance imaging studies in bipolar disorder and schizophrenia: Meta-analysis. *British Journal of Psychiatry* 195(3): 194–201.

Baldwin, P., Browne, D., Scully, P. J., Quinn, J. F., Morgan, M. G., Kinsella, A., Owens, J. M., Russell, V., O'Callaghan, E., & Waddington, J. L. (2005). Epidemiology of first-episode psychosis: Illustrating the challenges across diagnostic boundaries through the Cavan-Monaghan study at 8 years. *Schizophrenia Bulletin* 31(3): 624–638.

Baldwin, P. A., Hennessy, R. J., Morgan, M. G., Quinn, J. F., Scully, P. J., & Waddington, J. L. (2004). Controversies in schizophrenia research: The "continuum" challenge, heterogeneity vs homogeneity, and the lifetime developmental-"neuroprogresssive" trajectory. In W. Gattaz & H. Hafner (eds.), *Search for the Causes of Schizophrenia* (pp. 394–409). Darmstadt: Steinkopff.

Benes, F. M. (2007). Searching for unique endophenotypes for schizophrenia and bipolar disorder within neural circuits and their molecular regulatory mechanisms. *Schizophrenia Bulletin* 33(4): 932–936.

Benes, F. M. (2009). Neural circuitry models of schizophrenia: Is it dopamine, GABA, glutamate, or something else? *Biological Psychiatry* 65(12): 1003–1005.

Borgwardt, S. J., Dickey, C., Hulshoff Pol, H., Whitford, T. J., & DeLisi, L. E. (2009). Workshop on defining the significance of progressive brain change in schizophrenia: The rapporteurs' report. *Schizophrenia Research* 112(1–3): 32–45.

Cahn, W., Hulshoff Pol, H. E., Lems, E. B., van Haren, N. E., Schnack, H. G., van der Linden, J. A., Schothorst, P. F., van Engeland, H., & Kahn, R. S. (2002). Brain volume changes in first-episode schizophrenia: A 1-year follow-up study. *Archives of General Psychiatry* 59(11): 1002–1010.

Cahn, W., Rais, M., Stigter, F. P., van Haren, N. E. M., Caspers, E., Hulshoff Pol, H. E., & Kahn, R. S. (2009). Psychosis and brain volume changes during the first five years of schizophrenia. *European Neuropsychopharmacology* 19(2): 147–151.

Castner, S. A. & Williams, G. V. (2007). Tuning the engine of cognition: A focus on NMDA/D1 receptor interactions in prefrontal cortex. *Brain and Cognition* 63(2): 94–122.

Chang, J., Kim, O. I., Ahn, J. S., Kwon, J. S., Jeon, S. H., & Kim, S. H. (2000). The CNS midline cells coordinate proper cell cycle progression and identity determination of the drosophila ventral neuroectoderm. *Developmental Biology* 227(2): 307–323.

Compton, M. T. & Walker, E. F. (2009). Physical manifestations of neurodevelopmental disruption: Are minor physical anomalies part of the syndrome of schizophrenia? *Schizophrenia Bulletin* 35(2): 425–436.

Coyle, J. T. (2006). Glutamate and schizophrenia: Beyond the dopamine hypothesis. *Cellular and Molecular Neurobiology* 26(4–6): 365–384.

Dalman, C., Allebeck, P., Cullberg, J., Grunewald, C., & Koster, M. (1999). Obstetric complications and the risk of schizophrenia. *Archives of General Psychiatry* 56(3): 234–240.

Daniel, D. G., Goldberg, T. E., Gibbons, R. D., & Weinberger, D. R. (1991). Lack of a bimodal distribution of ventricular size in schizophrenia. *Biological Psychiatry* 30(9): 887–903.

DeLisi, L. E. (2008). The concept of progressive brain change in schizophrenia: Implications for understanding schizophrenia. *Schizophrenia Bulletin* 34(2): 312–321.

Desbonnet, L., Waddington, J. L., & Tuathaigh, C. M. (2009). Mice mutant for genes associated with schizophrenia: Common phenotype or distinct endophenotypes? *Behavioural Brain Research* 204(2): 258–273.

Donovan-Lepore, A. M., Jaeger, J., Czobor, P., Abdelmessih, S., & Berns, S. M. (2006). Quantitative craniofacial anomalies in a racially mixed schizophrenia sample. *Biological Psychiatry* 59(4): 349–353.

Ellison-Wright, I. & Bullmore, E. (2009). Meta-analysis of diffusion tensor imaging studies in schizophrenia. *Schizophrenia Research* 108(1–3): 3–10.

Ellison-Wright, I., Glahn, D. C., Laird, A. R., Thelen, S. M., & Bullmore, E. (2008). The anatomy of first-episode and chronic schizophrenia: An anatomical likelihood estimation meta-analysis. *American Journal of Psychiatry* 165(8): 1015–1023.

Fatemi, S. H. & Folsom, T. D. (2009). The neurodevelopmental hypothesis of schizophrenia, revisted. *Schizophrenia Bulletin* 35(3): 528–548.

Fornito, A., Yucel, M., & Pantelis, C. (2009). Reconciling neuroimaging and neuropathological findings in schizophrenia and bipolar disorder. *Current Opinion in Psychiatry* 22(3): 312–319.

Fornito, A., Yucel, M., Patti, J., Wood, S. J., & Pantelis, C. (2009). Mapping grey matter reductions in schizophrenia: An anatomical likelihood estimation analysis of voxel-based morphometry studies. *Schizophrenia Research* 108(1–3): 104–113.

Giger, J. M. & Kolodkin, A. L. (2001). Silencing the siren: Guidance cue hierarchies at the CNS midline. *Cell* 105(1): 1–4.

Glahn, D. C., Laird, A. R., Ellison-Wright, I., Thelen, S. M., Robinson, J. L., Lancaster, J. L., Bullmore, E., & Fox, P. T. (2008). Meta-analysis of gray matter anomalies in schizophrenia: Application of anatomic likelihood estimation and network analysis. *Biological Psychiatry* 64(9): 774–781.

Glantz, L. A., Gilmore, J. H., Lieberman, J. A., & Jarskog, L. F. (2006). Apoptotic mechanisms and the synaptic pathology of schizophrenia. *Schizophrenia Research* 81(1): 47–63.

Guillin, O., Abi-Dargham, A., & Laruelle, M. (2007). Neurobiology of dopamine in schizo-phrenia. *International Review of Neurobiology 78*: 1–39.

Harrison, P. J. (1999). The neuropathology of schizophrenia. *Brain 122*(4): 593–624.

Harrison, P. J. (2004). The hippocampus in schizophrenia: A review of the neuropathological evidence and its pathophysiological implications. *Psychopharmacology 174*(1): 151–162.

Hennessy, R. J., Baldwin, P. A., Browne, D. J., Kinsella, A., & Waddington, J. L. (2007). Three-dimensional laser surface imaging and geometric morphometrics resolve frontonasal dys-morphology in schizophrenia. *Biological Psychiatry 61*(10): 1187–1194.

Hennessy, R. J., Baldwin, P. A., Browne, D. J., Kinsella, A., & Waddington, J. L. (2010). Fronto-nasal dysmorphology in bipolar disorder by 3D laser surface imaging and geometric mor-phometrics: Comparisons with schizophrenia. *Schizophrenia Research 122*(1–3): 63–71.

Hennessy, R. J., Lane, A., Kinsella, A., Larkin, C., O'Callaghan, E., & Waddington, J. L. (2004). 3D morphometrics of craniofacial dysmorphology reveals sex-specific asymmetries in schizophrenia. *Schizophrenia Research 67*(2–3): 261–268.

Hennessy, R. J., McLearie, S., Kinsella, A., & Waddington, J. L. (2005). Facial surface analysis by 3D laser scanning and geometric morphometrics in relation to sexual dimorphism in cerebral-craniofacial morphogenesis and cognitive function. *Journal of Anatomy 207*(3): 283–296.

Hill, S. K., Harris, M. S., Herbener, E. S., Pavuluri, M., & Sweeney, J. M. (2008). Neurocogni-tive allied phenotypes for schizophrenia and bipolar disorder. *Schizophrenia Bulletin 34*(4): 743–759.

Honea, R., Crow, T. J., Passingham, D., & Mackay, C. E. (2005). Regional deficits in brain volume in schizophrenia: A meta-analysis of voxel-based morphometry studies. *American Journal of Psychiatry 162*(12): 2233–2245.

Howes, O. D. & Kapur, S. (2009). The dopamine hypothesis of schizophrenia: Version III—The final common pathway. *Schizophrenia Bulletin 35*(3): 549–562.

Howes, O. D., Montgomery, A. J., Asselin, M. C., Murray, R. M., Valli, I., Tabraham, P., Bramon-Bosch, E., Valmaggia, L., Johns, L., Broome, M., et al. (2009). Elevated striatal dopamine function linked to prodromal signs of schizophrenia. *Archives of General Psychiatry 66*(1): 13–20.

Hulshoff Pol, H. E. & Kahn, R. S. (2008). What happens after the first episode? A review of progressive brain changes in chronically ill patients with schizophrenia. *Schizophrenia Bulletin 34*(2): 354–366.

Ibi, D., Nagai, T., Koike, H., Kitahara, Y., Mizoguchi, H., Niwa, M., Jaaro-Peled, H., Nitta, A., Yoneda, Y., Nabeshima, T., et al. (2010). Combined effect of neonatal immune activation and mutant DISC1 on phenotypic changes in adulthood. *Behavioural Brain Research 206*(1): 32–37.

Jablensky, A. (1999). The conflict of the nosologists: Views on schizophrenia and manic-depressive illness in the early part of the 20th century. *Schizophrenia Research 39*(2): 95–100.

Javitt, D. C. (2007). Glutamate and schizophrenia: Phencyclidine, N-methyl-D-aspartate receptors, and dopamine-glutamate interactions. *International Review of Neurobiology 78*: 69–108.

Keshavan, M. S., Tandon, R., Boutros, N. N., & Nasrallah, H. A. (2008). Schizophrenia, "just the facts": What we know in 2008, part 3: Neurobiology. *Schizophrenia Research 106*(2–3): 89–107.

Kirby, B. P., Waddington, J. L., & O'Tuathaigh, C. M. (2010). Advancing a functional genomics for schizophrenia: Psychopathological and cognitive phenotypes in mutants with gene dis-ruption. *Brain Research Bulletin 83*(3–4): 162–176.

Konopaske, G. T., Drorph-Petersen, K. A., Sweet, R. A., Pierri, J. N., Zhang, W., Sampson, A. R., & Lewis, D. A. (2009). Effect of chronic antipsychotic exposure on astrocyte and oligodendrocyte numbers in macaque monkeys. *Biological Psychiatry* 63(8): 759–765.

Krabbendam, L., Arts, B., van Os, J., & Aleman, A. (2005). Cognitive functioning in patients with schizophrenia and bipolar disorder: A quantitative review. *Schizophrenia Research* 80(2–3): 137–149.

Lane, A., Kinsella, A., Murphy, P., Byrne, M., Keenan, J., Colgan, K., Cassidy, B., Sheppard, N., Horgan, R., Waddington, J. L., et al. (1997). The anthropometric assessment of dysmorphic features in schizophrenia as an index of its developmental origins. *Psychological Medicine* 27(5): 1155–1164.

Lawrie, S. M., McIntosh, A. M., Hall, J., Owens, D. G., & Johnstone, E. C. (2008). Brain structure and function changes during the development of schizophrenia: The evidence from studies of subjects at increased genetic risk. *Schizophrenia Bulletin* 34(2): 330–340.

Lewis, D. A. & Gonzales-Burgos, G. (2008). Neuroplasticity of neocortical circuits in schizophrenia. *Neuropsychopharmacology* 33(1): 141–165.

Lisman, J. E., Coyle, J. T., Green, R. W., Javitt, D. C., Benes, F. M., Heckers, S., & Grace, A. A. (2008). Circuit-based framework for understanding neurotransmitter and risk gene interactions in schizophrenia. *Trends in Neurosciences* 31(5): 234–242.

Lloyd, T., Dazzan, P., Dean, K., Park, S. B., Fearon, P., Doody, G. A., Tarrant, J., Morgan, K. D., Morgan, C., Hutchinson, G., et al. (2007). Minor physical anomalies in patients with first-episode psychosis: Their frequency and diagnostic specificity. *Psychological Medicine* 38(1): 71–77.

Marcucio, R. S., Cordero, D. R., Hu, D., & Helms, J. A. (2005). Molecular interactions coordinating the development of the forebrain and face. *Developmental Biology* 284(1): 48–61.

Marshall, M., Lewis, S., Lockwood, A., Drake, R., Jones, P., & Croudace, T. (2005). Association between duration of untreated psychosis and outcome in cohorts of first-episode patients: A systematic review. *Archives of General Psychiatry* 62(9): 975–983.

McGlashan, T. H. (2006). Is active psychosis neurotoxic? *Schizophrenia Bulletin* 32(4): 609–613.

McGorry, P., Johanessen, J. O., Lewis, S., Birchwood, M., Malla, A., Nordentoft, M., Addington, J., & Yung, A. (2010). Early intervention in psychosis: Keeping faith with evidence-based health care. *Psychological Medicine* 40(3): 399–404.

McGorry, P. D., Nelson, B., Amminger, G. P., Bechdolf, A., Francey, S. M., Berger, G., & Yung, A. R. (2009). Intervention in individuals at ultra high risk for psychosis: A review and future directions. *Journal of Clinical Psychiatry* 70(9): 1206–1212.

McGrath, J. C., El-Saadi, O., Grim, V., Cardy, S., Chapple, B., Chant, D., Lieberman, D., & Mowry, B. (2002). Minor physical anomalies and quantitative measures of the head and face in psychosis. *Archives of General Psychiatry* 59(5): 458–464.

Moskvina, V., Craddock, N., Holmans, P., Nikolov, I., Pahwa, P. S., Green, E., Wellcome Trust Case Control Consortium, Owen, M. J., & O'Donovan, M. C. (2010). Gene-wide analyses of genome-wide association data sets: Evidence for multiple common risk alleles for schizophrenia and bipolar disorder and for overlap in genetic risk. *Molecular Psychiatry* 14(3): 252–260.

Murray, R. M. & Lewis, S.W. (1987). Is schizophrenia a neurodevelopment disorder? *British Medical Journal* 295(6600): 681–682.

Navari, S. & Dazzan, P. (2009). Do antipsychotic drugs affect brain structure? A systematic and critical review of MRI findings. *Psychological Medicine* 39(11): 1763–1777.

O'Donovan, M. C., Craddock, N. J., & Owen, M. J. (2009). Genetics of psychosis: Insights from views across the genome. *Human Genetics* 126(1): 3–12.

O'Tuathaigh, C. M., Harte, M., O'Leary, C., O'Sullivan, G. J., Blau, C., Lai, D., Harvey, R. P., Tighe, O., Fagan, A. J., Kerskens, C., et al. (2010). Schizophrenia-related endophenotypes in heterozygous neuregulin-1 "knockout" mice. *European Journal of Neuroscience 31*(2): 349–358.

O'Tuathaigh, C. M., Hryniewiecka, M., Behav, A., Tighe, O., Cannon, M., Karayiorgou, M., Gogos, D. R., Cotter, J. L., & Waddington, J. L. (2009). Chronic adolescent exposure to delta-9-tetrahydrocannabinol in COMT knockout mice: Impact on phenotypes relevant to psychosis. *Program No.248.9.* Abstract viewer/itinerary planner. Chicago: Society for Neuroscience.

Owoeye, O., Kingston, T., Hennessy, R. J., Baldwin, P. A., Browne, D., Scully, P. J., Kinsella, A., Russell, V., O'Callaghan, E., & Waddington, J. L. (2010). The "totality" of psychosis: Epidemiology and developmental pathobiology. In W. Gattaz & G. Busatto (eds.), *Advances in Schizophrenia Research 2009* (pp. 377–385). New York: Springer.

Paus, T., Keshavan, M., & Giedd, J. N. (2008). Why do many psychiatric disorders emerge during adolescence? *Nature Reviews in Neuroscience 9*(12): 947–957.

Perkins, D. O., Gu, H., Boteva, K., & Lieberman, J. A. (2005). Relationship between duration of untreated psychosis and outcome in first-episode schizophrenia: A critical review and meta-analysis. *American Journal of Psychiatry 162*(10): 1785–1804.

Pilowsky, L. S., Bressan, R. A., Stone, J. M., Erlandsson, K., & Mulligan, R. S. (2006). First in vivo evidence of an NMDA receptor deficit in medication-free schizophrenic patients. *Molecular Psychiatry 11*(2): 118–119.

Scully, P. J., Quinn, J. F., Morgan, M. G., Kinsella, A., O'Callaghan, E., Owens, J. M., & Waddington, J. L. (2002). First-episode schizophrenia, bipolar disorder and other psychoses in a rural Irish catchment area: Incidence and gender in the Cavan-Monaghan study at 5 years. *British Journal of Psychiatry, Suppl 43*: s3–s9.

Steen, R. G., Mull, C., McClure, R., Hamer, R. M., & Lieberman, J. A. (2006). Brain volume in first-episode schizophrenia: Systematic review and meta-analysis of magnetic resonance imaging studies. *British Journal of Psychiatry 188*: 510–518.

Stephan, K. E., Friston, K. J., & Frith, C. D. (2009). Dysconnection in schizophrenia: From abnormal synaptic plasticity to failures of self-monitoring. *Schizophrenia Bulletin 35*(3): 509–527.

Stone, J. M., Morrison, P. D., & Pilowsky, L. S. (2007). Glutamate and dopamine dysregulation in schizophrenia—a synthesis and selective review. *Journal of Psychopharmacology 21*(4): 440–452.

Sun, D., Phillips, L., Velakoulis, D., Yung, A., McGorry, D., Wood, S. J., van Erp, T. G., Thompson, P. M., Toga, A. W., Cannon, T. D., et al. (2009). Progressive brain structural changes mapped as psychosis develops in "at risk" individuals. *Schizophrenia Research 108*(1–3): 85–92.

Takahashi, T., Wood, S. J., Yung, A. R., Soulsby, B., McGorry, P. D. Suzuki, M, Kawasaki, Y., Phillips, L. J., Velakoulis, D., & Pantelis, C. (2009). Progressive gray mater reduction of the superior temporal gyrus during transition to psychosis. *Archives of General Psychiatry 66*(4): 366–376.

Tandon, R., Keshavan, M. S., & Nasrallah, H. A. (2008). Schizophrenia, "just the facts": What we know in 2008, part 1: Overview. *Schizophrenia Research 100*(1–3): 4–19.

Tandon, R., Nasrallah, H. A., & Keshavan, M. S. (2009). Schizophrenia, "just the facts" 4. Clinical features and conceptualization. *Schizophrenia Research 110*(1–3): 1–23.

Tenyi, T., Trixler, M., & Csabi, G. (2009). Minor physical anomalies in affective disorders: A review of the literature. *Journal of Affective Disorders 112*(1–3): 11–18.

van Os, J & Kapur, S. (2009). Schizophrenia. *Lancet 374*(9690): 635–645.

van Os, J., Linscott, R. J., Myin-Germeys, I., Delespaul, P., & Krabbendam, L. (2008). A systematic review and meta-analysis of the psychosis continuum: Evidence for a psychosis proneness-persistence-impairment model of psychotic disorder. *Psychological Medicine* 39(2): 179–195.

Vita, A., De Peri, L., Silenzi, C., & Dieci, M. (2006). Brain morphology in first-episode schizophrenia: A meta-analysis of quantitative magnetic resonance imaging studies. *Schizophrenia Research* 82(1): 75–88.

Vita, A., Dieci, M., Silenzi, C., Tenconi, F., Giobbio, G. M., & Invernizzi, G. (2000). Cerebral ventricular enlargement as a generalized feature of schizophrenia: A distribution analysis on 502 subjects. *Schizophrenia Research* 44(1): 25–34.

Waddington, J. L. (1993). Schizophrenia: Developmental neuroscience and pathobiology. *Lancet* 341(8844): 531–536.

Waddington, J. L. (2007). Neuroimaging and other neurobiological indices in schizophrenia: Relationship to measurement of functional outcome. *British Journal of Psychiatry, Suppl* 50: s52–s57.

Waddington, J. L., Brown, A. S., Lane, A., Schaefer, C. A., Goetz, R. R., Bresnahan, M., & Susser, E. S. (2008). Congenital anomalies and early functional impairments in a prospective birth cohort: Risk of schizophrenia-spectrum disorder in adulthood. *British Journal of Psychiatry* 192(4): 264–267.

Waddington, J. L., Corvin, A. P., Donohue, G., O'Tuathaigh, C. M. P., Mitchell, K. J., & Gill, M. (2007). Functional genomics and schizophrenia: Endophenotypes and mutant models. *Psychiatric Clinics of North America* 30(3): 365–399.

Waddington, J. L., Lane, A., Larkin, C., & O'Callaghan, E. (1999). The neurodevelopmental basis of schizophrenia: Clinical clues from cerebro-craniofacial dysmorphogenesis, and the roots of a lifetime trajectory of disease. *Biological Psychiatry* 46(1): 31–39.

Weinberg, S. M., Jenkins, E. A., Marazita, M. L., & Maher, B. S. (2007). Minor physical anomalies in schizophrenia: A meta-analysis. *Schizophrenia Research* 89(1–3): 72–85.

Weinberger, D. R. (1987). Implications of normal brain development for the pathogenesis of schizophrenia. *Archives of General Pychiatry* 44(7): 660–669.

Weinberger, D. R. & McClure, R. K. (2002). Neurotoxicity, neuroplasticity, and magnetic resonance imaging morphometry: What is happening in the schizophrenic brain? *Archives of General Psychiatry* 59(6): 553–558.

Welham, J., Isohanni, M., Jones, P., & McGrath, J. (2009). The antecedents of schizophrenia: A review of birth cohort studies. *Schizophrenia Bulletin* 35(3): 603–623.

Whitty, P. F., Owoeye, O., & Waddington, J. L. (2009). Neurological signs and involuntary movements in schizophrenia: Intrinsic to and informative on systems pathobiology. *Schizophrenia Bulletin* 35(2): 415–424.

Wood, S. J., Pantelis, C., Velakoulis, D., Yucel, M., Fornito, A., & McGorry, P. D. (2008). Progressive changes in the development toward schizophrenia: Studies in subjects at increased symptomatic risk. *Schizophrenia Bulletin* 34(2): 222–229.

Wright, I. C., Rabe-Hesketh, S., Woodruff, P. W., David, A. S., Murray, R. M., & Bullmore, E. T. (2000). Meta-analysis of regional brain volumes in schizophrenia. *American Journal of Psychiatry* 157(1): 16–25.

PART 1

CLINICAL RESEARCH ON RISK FACTORS FOR SCHIZOPHRENIA

SECTION 1
Environmental Factors:
Epidemiologic Studies on the Etiologies of Schizophrenia

CHAPTER 1

MATERNAL INFECTION AND SCHIZOPHRENIA

ALAN S. BROWN

KEY CONCEPTS

- Early studies of the connection between maternal infection and schizophrenia in offspring were limited by relatively imprecise definitions of exposure status.
- Recent studies have capitalized on the use of prospective documentation of exposure using maternal biomarkers of infection and longitudinal follow-up of offspring to provide more definitive evidence of associations between maternal infection and schizophrenia.
- The identification of maternal infectious exposures related to schizophrenia may facilitate the identification of susceptibility genes that interact with these exposures.
- If the findings are replicated, these studies have potentially important implications for prevention given that exposure to infection is relatively common during pregnancy and many practical and inexpensive preventive measures—including vaccination, antibiotics, and hygienic recommendations—already exist.
- Studies of maternal infection and neurobiological outcomes may allow for the possibility of subdividing schizophrenia phenotypes on the basis of a putative etiologic factor.

In recent years, evidence has accumulated in support of a role for neurodevelopmental insults in the etiopathogenesis of schizophrenia (Brown, 2011). The dramatic changes in brain structure and function from conception to birth underscore the particular vulnerability to insults during this stage of development with regard to both short- and long-term disease outcomes (Tau & Peterson, 2010). Hence, the determinants of fetal brain development—both genes and environmental factors— deserve consideration as potential risk factors for schizophrenia. Among many putative environmental risk factors that have been investigated in studies of schizophrenia, infection is generally deemed as one of the most plausible, because microbial pathogens are well-documented causes of congenital brain anomalies and behavioral disorders. For example, prenatal exposure to rubella, toxoplasmosis, herpes simplex virus type 2, and other infections are known causes of developmental disorders that include mental retardation, learning disabilities, sensorineural dysfunction, and several structural brain anomalies (Remington et al., 2006).

Studies of Prenatal Infection and Schizophrenia Based on Ecologic Data

The first clues that fetal infection plays a role in the origins of schizophrenia emerged from studies that utilized ecologic data. The term *ecologic* is used to refer to an event or events that are documented at the level of a population. In the case of a study of in utero infection and a disease outcome, the exposure in an ecologic-based study can be defined as the timing of an epidemic in a population. Among many potential infections, most ecologic studies of schizophrenia examined influenza because of its relatively high prevalence and excellent documentation in many populations, due to extensive surveillance efforts. These investigations assessed whether schizophrenia was more common if an influenza epidemic or epidemics coincided with particular periods of pregnancy in cases and noncases drawn from the population in which the epidemic or epidemics were documented. Two research designs were used in such studies.

The first design focused on a single epidemic, most commonly the 1957 type A2 influenza pandemic. The high morbidity of this epidemic, the circumscribed period of its peak incidence, and the availability of registry-based data on schizophrenia diagnoses among the offspring greatly expedited the ability of investigators to examine this question. The second design consisted of relating the longitudinal variations in influenza epidemics over intervals of many years to births of patients who later developed schizophrenia in the population. Although studies that employed the latter design generally made use of more sophisticated analytic approaches, the basic study aims of the two designs were the same, and both approaches allowed for the assessment of relationships between schizophrenia and the occurrences of epidemics at different periods of gestation.

These studies, conducted in different regions of the world—including Europe, Australia, Japan, and the United States—have been reviewed in a recent publication (Brown & Derkits, 2010). Initial studies yielded significant associations between influenza epidemics during all or part of the second trimester and schizophrenia (Mednick et al., 1988; O'Callaghan et al., 1991). Yet several attempts to replicate these findings in larger studies with more complete case ascertainment yielded negative findings (Erlenmeyer-Kimling et al., 1994; Susser et al., 1994). Ecologic studies of infections other than influenza have also been conducted. Associations between schizophrenia and epidemics of maternal respiratory viral infections (Watson et al., 1984; O'Callaghan et al., 1994), measles, varicella-zoster (Torrey, 1988), mumps (O'Callaghan et al., 1994), and polio (Suvisaari et al., 1999a; Cahill et al., 2002) have been reported.

Although these studies were novel, and the investigations offered approaches that were state-of-the-art at the time, there were a number of methodologic shortcomings that render interpretations difficult. First, studies based on epidemics in populations would undoubtedly misclassify individuals as being exposed who were in fact unexposed. Even during seasons with the highest incidence of influenza, such as the 1957 type A2 epidemic, the prevalence of this infection rarely rises above 30% of the population. Hence, studies that defined individuals as exposed to influenza based on whether they were in utero during the 1957 epidemic would have misclassified approximately 70% of the unexposed population. Influenza is not restricted to epidemic periods or even to the fall and winter months, and some epidemics recur within the same year, as evidenced by the H1N1 epidemic of 2009, which peaked both during the spring and the autumn and winter months. These would result in exposed subjects being incorrectly classified as unexposed. Of note is that none of the ecologic studies of infection and schizophrenia attempted to confirm infection in individual pregnancies.

A second limitation of these studies is that they assumed a full-term pregnancy. The significant number of pregnancies that do not extend to the expected date of birth and the increased rate of preterm and possibly also postterm birth in schizophrenia render estimates of the timing of exposure inaccurate. Each of these two limitations leads to misclassification of exposure. The occurrence of nondifferential misclassification of exposure, defined as no difference in misclassification between the cases and noncases, tends to bias effect sizes toward the null. This may explain some of the failures to replicate these findings.

Birth Cohort Studies of Prenatal Infection and Schizophrenia

To address these limitations, our group, as well as others, initiated birth cohort studies of prenatal infection and schizophrenia (Brown & Derkits, 2010). A birth cohort is a group of individuals born during a specified period and in a specified geographic region. In birth cohort studies, exposures are documented at birth or earlier, the subjects are followed up for an outcome of interest, and relationships between the exposures and the outcomes are examined. Birth cohorts of infection offer numerous advantages over ecologically based studies. First, the birth cohort studies allow for prospective documentation of prenatal infection in individual pregnancies. In some of these studies, this was achieved through obstetric and other medical records that were documented during pregnancy. Second, some existing birth cohorts provide a very valuable resource: archived biological maternal or infant specimens drawn during pregnancy or soon after delivery, which allow for documentation of infection during fetal or infant life using biomarkers such as antibodies to various infectious agents. Third, the longitudinal follow-up afforded by some birth cohort studies offers the potential for survival analytic methods aimed at addressing the effects of loss to followup. Fourth, birth cohort studies generally include access to information on a wide array of potential confounding or interacting influences, such as demographic variables, maternal medical conditions and health habits, other prenatal factors, and characteristics of the infant at birth.

In the case of birth cohort studies of infection and schizophrenia, our group and others documented infections by ascertainment of maternal antibody levels from archived serum specimens acquired in individual pregnancies (Brown et al., 2004a, 2005, 2006; Buka et al., 2001a, 2008) or in blood spots obtained from infants (Mortensen et al., 2007) and related these exposures to risk of schizophrenia following systematic assessment of the offspring later in life. Other studies relied on clinical diagnoses of infection documented during pregnancy (Brown & Derkits, 2010). These studies are reviewed in the sections that follow and the findings are summarized in tables 1.1 and 1.2.

Rubella

One of the first studies of prenatal infection and risk of schizophrenia documented through a birth cohort was based on the Rubella Birth Defects Evaluation Project (RBDEP), which was conducted in New York City following the 1964 rubella pandemic (Brown et al., 2000a, 2001). All mothers were documented as having been exposed to rubella during pregnancy, and offspring were serologically confirmed with infection. Our group demonstrated that exposure to rubella in utero was associated with a greater than fivefold increased risk of nonaffective psychosis (Brown et al., 2000a). In a follow-up study of the cohort in midadulthood, we demonstrated that more than 20% of subjects who were exposed in utero to rubella were diagnosed with schizophrenia or a schizophrenia spectrum disorder based on a structured research interview (Brown et al., 2001). Rubella-exposed subjects who developed schizophrenia had a substantially greater IQ decline than rubella-exposed controls, as well as greater premorbid neuromotor and behavioral anomalies.

Table 1.1 Serologic Studies of Prenatal Infection and Schizophrenia

Authors/ Year	Study Design	Number of Cases	Number of Noncases	Description of Association[a,b,c]	Strengths[d]	Comments Limitations	Other
Child Health and Development Study[e]							
Brown et al., 2004b	Nested case-control study of maternal cytokines and schizophrenia spectrum disorders	N=59 cases N exposed not provided because continuous measure was used	N=105 matched controls N exposed not provided because continuous measure was used	Elevated maternal IL-8: second to early third trimester No statistically significant association for IL-1β, IL-6, or TNF-α		Median TNF-α levels lower than in most studies of this cytokine	
Brown et al., 2004a	Nested case-control study of influenza and schizophrenia spectrum disorders	First half of pregnancy: N=9 exposed cases, 34 unexposed cases Second half of pregnancy: N=13 exposed cases, 51 unexposed cases	First half of pregnancy: N=7 exposed controls, 68 unexposed controls Second half of pregnancy: N=30 exposed controls, 95 unexposed controls	Influenza: First half of pregnancy (OR: 3.0, 95% CI: 0.98–10.1) First trimester (OR: 7.0, 95% CI: .7–75.3)	Influenza exposure was validated in a control sample with sero-conversion data	Exposure based on proxy measure of seroconversion for influenza, but validated Marginally significant findings by standard criterion for significance (p=.052 for first half of pregnancy exposure)	
Brown et al., 2005	Nested case-control study of *Toxoplasma gondii* and schizophrenia spectrum disorders	N=5 cases with "moderate" antibody titer, 13 cases with "high" antibody titer, 45 cases with reference titer (unexposed)	N=9 matched controls with "moderate" antibody titer, 13 controls with "high" antibody titer, 101 controls with reference titer (unexposed)	*Toxoplasma gondii:* High IgG antibody titer (≥1:128) (OR: 2.61, 95% CI: 1.00–6.82) No samples tested positive for IgM-specific		Marginally significant finding by standard criteria (p=.051)	Sera tested from third trimester/ perinatal period

(continued)

Table 1.1 (continued)

Authors/Year	Study Design	Number of Cases	Number of Noncases	Description of Association[a,b,c]	Comments		
					Strengths[d]	Limitations	Other
Brown et al., 2006	Nested case-control study of herpes viruses and schizophrenia spectrum disorders	N=60 cases total Herpes simplex virus type 2 (HSV-2): N=16 exposed cases HSV-1: N=41 exposed cases CMV: N=43 exposed cases	N=110 matched controls total HSV-2: N=24 exposed controls HSV-1: N=70 exposed controls CMV: N=73 exposed controls	No association for IgG antibody level or seroprevalence of HSV-1, HSV-2, or cytomegalovirus (CMV)			Sera tested from third trimester/perinatal period
Collaborative Perinatal Project[f] Buka et al., 2001a	Nested case-control study of numerous maternal infections, Providence, RI cohort from CPP, followed up for psychotic disorders	N=27 cases N exposed not provided because continuous measure of antibody was used	N=54 matched controls N exposed not provided because continuous measure of antibody was used	Elevated total maternal IgG and IgM immunoglobulins and antibodies to HSV-2 No significant associations for IgA class immunoglobulins, IgG antibodies to HSV-1, CMV, *Toxoplasma*	Examined effects of many different infections to assess specificity	Small sample For some subjects, maternal IgG levels included in analysis without documented seropositivity	Broad definition of case sample, including nonaffective and affective psychoses

Toxoplasma gondii antibody, indicating that acute infection was unlikely

Buka et al., 2001b	Nested case-control study of maternal cytokines, Providence, RI cohort from CPP, followed up for psychotic disorders	N=27 cases N exposed not provided because continuous measure was used N=50 matched controls N exposed not provided because continuous measure was used	*gondii,* rubella, human parvovirus B19, *Chlamydia trachomatis,* or human papillomavirus type 16 Elevated maternal TNF-α: third trimester No significant associations for IL-1, IL-2, IL-6, but statistical trend for IL-8	Small sample	Broad definition of case sample, including nonaffective and affective psychoses 7 women were noted as having had an infection during the third trimester and 6 during the first or second trimesters
Buka et al., 2008	Nested case-control study of HSV-2 from three birth cohorts from CPP (Boston, Providence, and Philadelphia), followed up for psychotic disorders	N=62 seropositive cases, 138 unexposed cases N=134 seropositive matched controls, 420 unexposed matched controls	Maternal HSV-2 seropositivity (OR: 1.6; 95% CI: 1.1–2.3) Risk was particularly elevated among women with high rates of sexual activity during pregnancy (OR: 2.6, 95% CI: 1.4–4.6)	Large sample	Broad definition of psychosis, including nonaffective (N=108 cases) and affective psychoses (N=85 cases) Sera tested at the end of pregnancy Diagnosis based on interview for New England cohorts and chart review for Philadelphia cohort

(continued)

Table 1.1 (continued)

[a] P ≤ 0.05 unless otherwise noted.

[b] Measures of effect (relative risks [RR], rate ratios, or odds ratios [OR]) are reported here, if reported in the original paper. CI=confidence intervals.

[c] "Nth month" indicates gestational month of exposure. Rather than estimating gestational age, some studies reported the number of months after the peak of an epidemic during which the number of babies born with schizophrenia increased. This distinction is noted in the table.

[d] All the studies in this table share the following strengths: direct biomarkers of infection obtained from archived maternal sera, population-based birth cohorts, diagnoses based on psychiatric interviews and medical chart reviews, and follow-up for psychosis or schizophrenia using specified protocols. The Child Health and Development Study featured two additional strengths: continuous follow-up and controls who were representative of the source population giving rise to cases.

[e] Child Health and Development Study (CHDS): population-based birth cohort (N=12,094), Alameda County, California, born between 1959 and 1967, followed up for schizophrenia and other schizophrenia spectrum disorders (schizophrenia, schizoaffective disorder, schizotypal personality disorder, delusional disorder, and "other schizophrenia spectrum psychoses") in adulthood. Diagnoses were established using both psychiatric interview (*Diagnostic Interview for Genetic Studies*) and medical chart review. Two types of study designs were used. The first are cohort analytic designs in which classes of infections were defined on the basis of abstracted obstetric records; the second are nested case-control studies of archived maternal serum analyzed for antibodies to infectious exposures.

[f] Collaborative Perinatal Project (CPP): multisite study of population-based birth cohorts throughout the United States. The table includes three CPP population-based birth cohorts, from Boston, Massachusetts; Providence, Rhode Island; and Philadelphia, Pennsylvania, born between 1959 and 1967 (N=25,025 from 19,471 pregnant women for combined cohorts) and followed up for psychotic disorders (schizophrenia, schizophreniform disorder, bipolar disorder with psychotic features, brief cohorts, from Boston, MA, Providence, RI, and Philadelphia, PA, born between 1959 and 1967 (N=25,025 from 19,471 pregnant women for combined cohorts) and followed up for psychotic disorders (schizophrenia, schizophreniform disorder, bipolar disorder with psychotic features, brief psychosis, and psychosis not otherwise specified). Diagnoses were established using psychiatric interview (*Structured Clinical Interview for DSM-IV*), medical chart review, or both. All studies included herein are nested case-control investigations of archived maternal serum analyzed for antibodies to infectious exposures.

SOURCE: Reprinted from Brown and Derkits (2010) with permission from the *American Journal of Psychiatry* (copyright 2010). American Psychiatric Association.

Table 1.2 Other Birth Cohort Studies of Prenatal Infection and Schizophrenia

Authors/Year	Study Design	Number of Cases	Number of Noncases	Description of Association[a,b]	Strengths	Comments Limitations	Other
						Comments	
Crow & Done, 1991	Retrospective assessment for influenza in a birth cohort of subjects born March 3–9, 1958, exposed to the 1957 A2 epidemic in England, Wales, and Scotland Cases identified through record search Diagnoses established by chart review (Present State Examination criteria)	N = 16,268 total cases Exposed in first trimester: N = 231 cases Exposed in second trimester: N = 945 cases Exposed in third trimester: N = 675 cases Number of unexposed cases not reported	Not reported	None	Large national sample Used individual pregnancies to determine exposure	Low statistical power Exposure to influenza determined from retrospective maternal interview	
Cannon et al., 1996	Retrospective assessment for influenza in pregnancies during 1957 A2 influenza epidemic in Ireland and schizophrenia	N = 2 exposed cases, 2 unexposed cases	N = 236 exposed controls, 285 unexposed controls	None	Individual pregnancies	Exposure to influenza determined from retrospective maternal interview Low power due to small number of cases: (2 exposed, 2 unexposed)	Diagnoses made by chart review using the Research Diagnostic Criteria

(continued)

Table 1.2 (continued)

Authors/Year	Study Design	Number of Cases	Number of Noncases	Description of Association[a,b]	Strengths	Limitations	Other
					Comments		
Brown et al., 2000a	Birth cohort study of rubella in Rubella Birth Defects Evaluation Project (RB-DEP), based on physician diagnosis, rubella anti-body titer, or both, followed up for nonaffective psychosis[c]	N = 11 exposed cases with nonaffective psychosis, 18 unexposed cases	N = 42 exposed noncases, 1,526 unexposed noncases	Prenatal rubella exposure associated with increased risk of nonaffective psychosis (RR: 5.2, 95% CI: 1.9–14.3)	Rubella exposure obtained on basis of prospective clinical diagnoses, verification in a subsample by antibody titers, or both Diagnoses based on psychiatric interviews	Lack of unexposed with verified rubella diagnoses; however, prenatal rubella was very rare in the comparison cohorts	
Brown et al., 2000b	Birth cohort analysis of maternal respiratory infection[d] and DSM-IV schizophrenia spectrum disorders[e]	N = 9 exposed cases, 49 unexposed cases	N = 632 exposed noncases, 7,149 unexposed noncases	Maternal respiratory infection: second trimester (rate ratio: 2.13, 95% CI: 1.05–4.35) Strongest association for upper respiratory infections	Physician-based, prospective diagnoses of maternal respiratory infection during pregnancy	Broad measure of respiratory infection	

Study	Description	Cases (N)	Noncases (N)	Findings	Diagnostic basis	Limitations	Cases included
Brown et al., 2001	Birth cohort study of rubella (RBDEP cohort), based on physician diagnosis, rubella antibody titer, or both, followed up for schizophrenia spectrum disorders[e]	N = 11 exposed schizophrenia spectrum disorder cases, no unexposed cases	N = 42 exposed noncases, no unexposed noncases	Prenatal rubella-exposed birth cohort evidenced a markedly high risk of schizophrenia spectrum disorder (20.4% or 11 of 53)	Diagnoses based on psychiatric interviews	No unexposed cohort to calculate effect size, though relative risk estimated at approx. 15-fold based on general population estimates of risk of schizophrenia spectrum disorders. Small sample size	Cases included schizophrenia, schizoaffective disorder, psychotic disorder not otherwise specified (NOS), delusional disorder, schizotypal personality disorder, and paranoid personality disorder
Babulas et al., 2006	Birth cohort study of maternal genital-reproductive infection[f] and schizophrenia spectrum disorders[g]	N = 71 cases	N = 7,723 noncases	Maternal genital-reproductive infections: Periconceptional period (rate ratio: 5.03, 95% CI: 2.00–12.64)	Physician-based, prospective diagnoses of maternal genital-reproductive infections	Small sample of exposed cases (N = 5 exposed)	

(continued)

Table 1.2 (continued)

Authors/Year	Study Design	Number of Cases	Number of Noncases	Description of Association[a,b]	Comments		
					Strengths	Limitations	Other
		Case/noncase status of exposed and unexposed pregnancies not reported	Case/noncase status of exposed and unexposed pregnancies not reported		Genital-reproductive infection diagnoses from preconceptional period		
Mortensen et al., 2007	National cohort-based, case-control study of *Toxoplasma gondii* combining data from national population registers and patient registers and a national neonatal screening biobank of filter paper blood spots in Denmark. Subjects born after 1981 and followed up for schizophrenia through 1999	N = 30 exposed cases, 41 unexposed cases	N = 171 exposed controls, 513 unexposed controls	Elevated *Toxoplasma gondii* IgG antibody (OR: 1.79, 95% CI: 1.01–3.15)	Study compared risks for schizophrenia, schizophrenia-like disorders, and affective disorders Effect was specific to schizophrenia	Diagnoses based on psychiatric registry Partial ascertainment of eligible sample due to missing filter paper blood spots	Blood spots taken from infant Diagnoses based on psychiatric registry

Study	Data source	Sample (cases)	Sample (noncases)	Results	Comments
Sorensen et al., 2009	Data from Copenhagen Perinatal Cohort, born between 1959 and 1961 at Rigshospitalet in Copenhagen, linked with the Danish National Psychiatric Register for diagnoses of schizophrenia	N = 32 cases exposed to any bacterial infection, 121 unexposed cases	N = 1,033 noncases exposed to any bacterial infection, 6,755 unexposed noncases	Maternal bacterial infections:[g] first trimester, for both ICD-8 (OR: 2.53, 95% CI: 1.07–5.96) and broadly defined schizophrenia (ICD-8, ICD-10, or both) (OR: 2.14, 95% CI: 1.06–4.31) Second trimester, for ICD-8 (OR: 2.31, 95% CI: 1.15–4.35) and broadly defined schizophrenia (OR: 1.82, 95% CI: 1.06–3.14), only in unadjusted analysis	Diagnoses based on psychiatric registry Although exposures were based on clinical diagnoses, bacterial infections may have been misclassified Very broad categories of infection (i.e., viral, bacterial) Low statistical power
Clarke et al., 2009	Data from Medical Birth Register linked with Finnish Population Register, to identify women in Helsinki treated during	N = 36 cases exposed prenatally to upper urinary tract infection, 35 unexposed	N = 9,596 noncases exposed prenatally to upper urinary tract infection, 13,808 unexposed noncases	No association with prenatal infection alone, but observed interaction between prenatal exposure to	Large sample size Small number of cases

(continued)

Table 1.2 (continued)

Authors/Year	Study Design	Number of Cases	Number of Noncases	Description of Association[a,b]	Comments		
					Strengths	Limitations	Other
	pregnancy for upper urinary tract infection between 1947 and 1990 Psychiatric outcomes of adult offspring identified through Finnish Hospital Discharge Register	N=12 cases with a family history of psychosis, 59 cases with no family history	N=1,497 noncases with a family history of psychosis, 21,907 noncases with no family history	upper urinary tract infection and family history (Risk Difference: 0.51, 95% CI: 0.06–0.96) 38–46% of cases in sample may have developed schizophrenia as a result of the synergistic action of both risk factors	Used sibling comparison group Hospital-treated infection provided exact information on time of exposure during pregnancy	Statistical power too low to examine each trimester separately	

[a] P≤0.05 unless otherwise noted.

[b] Measures of effect (relative risks [RR], rate ratios, or odds ratios [OR]) are reported here, if reported in the original paper. CI=confidence intervals.

[c] Nonaffective psychosis defined as (1) at least one psychotic symptom (delusions, hallucinations, or both) for a minimum of six months; (2) no evidence of a major affective disorder (bipolar or unipolar) by DSM-III-R criteria concurrent with the psychosis; and (3) no evidence that a medical condition or substance use initiated or maintained the psychosis. Diagnoses established using psychiatric interview (Diagnostic Interview Schedule for Children) and DSM-III-R criteria.

[d] Maternal respiratory infections included tuberculosis, influenza, influenza with pneumonia, bronchopneumonia, atypical pneumonia, pleurisy, emphysema/viral respiratory infections, acute bronchitis, and upper respiratory infections.

[e] Schizophrenia spectrum disorders included schizophrenia, schizoaffective disorder, schizotypal personality disorder, delusional disorder, and "other schizophrenia spectrum psychoses." Diagnoses were established using both psychiatric interview (*Diagnostic Interview for Genetic Studies*) and medical chart review.

[f] Maternal genital-reproductive infection, including endometritis, cervicitis, pelvic inflammatory disease, vaginitis, syphilis, condylomata, "venereal disease," or gonorrhea.

[g] Maternal bacterial infections include sinusitis, tonsillitis, pneumonia, cystitis, pyelonephritis, bacterial venereal infection, and any other bacterial infection.

SOURCE: Reprinted from Brown and Derkits (2010) with permission from the *American Journal of Psychiatry* (Copyright 2010). American Psychiatric Association.

Influenza

In a second birth cohort, our group examined the relationship between serologically documented prenatal influenza infection and schizophrenia in the offspring (Brown et al., 2004a). This study was a follow-up of the Child Health and Development Study (CHDS), a population-based birth cohort born in Alameda County, California, between 1959 and 1967. Maternal sera were drawn prospectively during pregnancy, often at more than one time point, and stored frozen in a central repository. All of the mothers and offspring in this birth cohort were members of the Kaiser Permanente Medical Care Plan (KPMCP), a health maintenance organization that maintained computerized databases on all health visits by members, facilitating identification of offspring with schizophrenia, and diagnoses were confirmed by structured research interviews. In this study, the follow-up took place from 1996 to 1999, a minimum of nearly 30 years from the time of birth; hence, most of the cohort was followed up through the large majority of the period of risk for schizophrenia. Because the dates of membership were known throughout each subject's time in KPMCP, it was possible to adjust for nondifferential loss to follow-up. An additional design advantage is that the membership dates of all the subjects made it possible to identify controls who represented the source population from which the cases were derived. This diminished the potential for bias from loss to follow-up.

For the serologic studies, a nested case-control design was used. In such a study, the cases and matched controls are "nested" within a defined birth cohort. Such a design is especially appropriate for large birth cohorts in which biospecimens are assayed and the costs for assays on the entire cohort are prohibitive.

In this study, our group demonstrated that exposure to influenza during the first half of pregnancy was associated with a threefold increase in risk of schizophrenia (Brown et al., 2004a). The risk of schizophrenia was increased sevenfold for influenza exposure during the first trimester. Influenza exposure during the second half of pregnancy was not related to schizophrenia. Although these findings warrant independent replication, they indicate that early to middle pregnancy may be a period of vulnerability for the development of schizophrenia. Unlike some of the other infections discussed, it is very unlikely that maternal influenza directly infects the fetus. This suggests that fetal infection is not required for an increase in schizophrenia risk.

TOXOPLASMA GONDII (T. GONDII). T. gondii is an intracellular parasite. Numerous studies have documented that this infectious exposure is a cause of central nervous system (CNS) congenital anomalies, and have led to recommendations to minimize exposure among pregnant mothers. Moreover, subtle, delayed neurologic sequelae of T. gondii have been observed (Dukes et al., 1997;

Remington et al., 2006). In the CHDS cohort, prenatal levels of elevated maternal *T. gondii* IgG antibody (titers ≥ 1:128) were associated with a greater than twofold increased risk of schizophrenia (Brown et al., 2005). In a subsequent study, from a sample in Denmark in which *T. gondii* IgG was assayed in filter paper blood spots from the infant taken within the first week of birth, elevated *T. gondii* IgG antibody was also associated with risk of schizophrenia (Mortensen et al., 2007). This finding is essentially a replication of the findings from the study in the CHDS cohort because *T. gondii* IgG antibody in maternal blood crosses the placenta and enters the fetal circulation, and it is very unlikely that infant exposure through a source other than the mother could have occurred in the first week of the infant's life.

HERPES SIMPLEX VIRUS TYPE 2 (HSV-2). HSV-2 is a sexually transmitted disease, and transmission from mother to fetus usually occurs at the time of birth, when the fetus comes into contact with maternal cervicovaginal secretions of the virus, which is shed during primary exposure or reactivation. Like *T. gondii*, neonatal HSV-2 also causes congenital CNS anomalies, including adverse neuropsychiatric outcomes in childhood, such as mental retardation, low-normal IQ, language deficits, and motor disability (Kropp et al., 2006; Engman et al., 2008).

Previous findings from epidemiologic studies of prenatal HSV-2 and schizophrenia are conflicting. Two of these studies were based on selected sites of the Collaborative Perinatal Project (CPP), a multisite population-based study of a birth cohort born between 1959 and 1967 (as in the CHDS). Similar to the CHDS, the cohort featured archived maternal serum samples that were drawn prospectively during pregnancy. An additional strength of the CPP study is that diagnoses were also confirmed by psychiatric interviews and medical record reviews, as in the CHDS follow-up study of schizophrenia.

The first of these studies revealed an association between maternal anti-HSV-2 IgG antibody levels and risk of psychotic disorders among offspring (Buka et al., 2001a). The risk of schizophrenia was increased threefold to fourfold, depending on the antibody cutoff definition for exposure. The investigators followed up this study with a larger sample made up of 200 subjects with a psychotic disorder and more than 500 matched control subjects from the CPP cohort. In that study, a 1.6-fold increase in risk of psychosis was observed among subjects seropositive for HSV-2, based on assays for HSV-2 antibody in the maternal sera. When schizophrenic psychoses were analyzed separately, HSV-2 was related to a 1.8- fold increase in risk (Buka et al., 2008). In the latter study, the finding was isolated to subjects who did not report regular use of contraception and who had frequent intercourse. These findings were not replicated, however, in the CHDS birth cohort study of 60 schizophrenia cases and 120 controls (Brown et al., 2006), with odds ratios close to 1 for all analyses.

Several methodologic explanations might be invoked to explain these discrepant findings. The greater proportion of African Americans in the CPP cohort may have resulted in increased statistical power, given that HSV-2 is more prevalent among African Americans (Buka et al., 2008), and statistical power may have been further enhanced by the larger number of cases with schizophrenic psychoses in the latter CPP study than in the CHDS study. It is therefore conceivable that the lack of association between prenatal HSV-2 and schizophrenia in the latter study may have resulted from a lack of statistical power.

A second issue to be considered regards variations in the way in which exposure status was defined. Different criteria for exposure were applied to the two CPP studies. In the first, exposure was defined on the basis of HSV-2 IgG antibody levels, whereas the primary analysis of the second study was based on HSV-2 seropositivity. The study from the CHDS cohort, which classified HSV-2 with regard to seropositivity and IgG antibody, did not detect an association by either definition of exposure.

A third consideration relates to quantification of loss to follow-up. In both CPP studies, there were no population denominators over the period of follow-up. Consequently, survival analytic methods aimed at mitigating bias from loss to follow-up could not be used in both CPP studies, in contrast to the CHDS study, which offered continuous follow-up of the cohort. If subjects with HSV-2 were more likely to remain in the CPP cohort than controls without HSV-2, a spurious finding may have resulted because of bias.

Other Prenatal Infections Identified from Birth Cohort Studies

Birth cohort studies have also indicated associations between maternal respiratory infection (Brown et al., 2000b), maternal genital-reproductive infection (Babulas et al., 2006), and bacterial infection (Sorensen et al., 2009) and schizophrenia. These studies extend the classes of infections that may increase schizophrenia risk further, suggesting that the type of infection may be less important than common consequences of infectious insults.

In summary, birth cohort studies have provided several key methodologic advantages that have allowed for more rigorous testing of relationships between maternal infection and schizophrenia. These advantages include prospective assessment of infection, maternal biomarkers of infection in individual pregnancies, longitudinal follow-up, and control for confounding influences. Birth cohort studies conducted to date have provided further support for the hypothesis that maternal viral, protozoal, and bacterial infections are related to schizophrenia in adult offspring.

Common Pathways that Mediate Relationships Between Infection and Risk of Schizophrenia

Cytokines

A key question posed by these findings concerns the mechanisms by which maternal infection might alter development of the brain and lead to schizophrenia. As discussed in chapter 10, animal models of maternal immune activation are shedding new light on these pathogenic mechanisms. In this parsimonious model, a wide array of infections is postulated to act through stimulation of the cytokine response (Gilmore & Jarskog, 1997) to alter brain development, resulting in behavioral, neurochemical, neurophysiologic, and neuroanatomic abnormalities similar to those observed in schizophrenia (Patterson, 2009). Cytokines are small proteins that act as the systemic mediators of the host response to infection. These immune factors become markedly elevated both systemically and within the target organs following primary infections, and they are also increased in a number of noninfectious inflammatory conditions (Weizman et al., 1999).

Evidence from clinical studies of neurodevelopmental disorders provides further support for this model (Dammann & Leviton, 1997). Maternal or fetal infection-induced cytokine elevations have been related to an increased occurrence of chorioamnionitis, periventricular leukomalacia, and cerebral palsy. Although the mechanisms are not clearly defined, one potential scenario includes cytokine stimulation of microglia and astroglia in the fetal brain to produce nitric oxide and excitatory amino acids, which are toxic to neurons. A second mechanism could involve disrupted maturation of oligodendrocytes contributing to white matter abnormalities, which have been previously associated with schizophrenia (Davis et al., 2003). A third mechanism involves direct activation of fetal neurons, as cytokines are used for signaling during normal fetal brain development and infection-induced increases can alter developmental processes (Meyer, Feldon, & Yee, 2008; Deverman & Patterson, 2009)). A fourth mechanism could involve activation of cytokine-responsive pathways in the placenta, with consequences for the fetus.

Consistent with a role for cytokines in infection as a risk factor for schizophrenia, the CHDS birth cohort follow-up study revealed that elevated levels of the proinflammatory chemokine interleukin-8 (IL-8) during the second or early third trimester were associated with an increased risk for schizophrenia by a factor of nearly two, in comparison to the risk for matched controls (Brown et al., 2004b). Elevated maternal serum IL-8 levels are also related to histologic chorioamnionitis in term infants (Shimoya et al., 1997). Moreover, maternal and fetal levels of IL-8 have been correlated with one another significantly. IL-8 may be particularly important for neutrophil attraction and for discharge of lysosomal enzymes from neutrophils, the latter of which leads to oxygen-free radicals. In the CPP follow-up study, maternal perinatal levels of tumor necrosis factor-α (TNF-α), another proinflammatory cytokine, were increased in subjects with psychotic disorders (Buka et al., 2001b). Like IL-8, TNF-α has also been associated with chorioamnionitis (Saji et al., 2000; Buka et al., 2001b), and elevated amniotic fluid levels of this cytokine have been related to maternal and fetal infection (Baud et al., 1999; Buka et al., 2001b). Intriguingly, polymorphisms in TNF-α genes have also been associated with schizophrenia (Boin et al., 2001; Buka et al., 2001b).

Individual Effects of Infections

In an alternative scenario, individual prenatal infections act to influence risk of schizophrenia by a variety of effects, rather than by a single common mediator. Infections that have been associated previously with schizophrenia differ significantly from one another with regard to several characteristics, such as duration of symptoms, antigenicity and antibody response, and gestational specificity to known congenital outcomes. In the paragraphs that follow, we consider putative unique mechanisms by which three of the maternal infections already discussed here—influenza, toxoplasmosis, and genital-reproductive infection—may act to increase schizophrenia risk.

INFLUENZA. Influenza is believed to cross the placenta only rarely and largely remains confined to the respiratory tract. Hence, induction of developmental brain changes is more likely to result from the response of the host organism to the infection, which in turn adversely influences fetal brain development, rather than through direct fetal infection. One previously proposed mechanism includes the elicitation of IgG antibodies to the infection and their cross-reaction with fetal brain antigens by molecular mimicry (Wright et al., 1999). Another potential mechanism by which influenza could increase risk of schizophrenia is via nonspecific effects, including hyperthermia, fetal hypoxia, and the use of over-the-counter remedies, such as aspirin.

As reviewed in chapter 10, preclinical studies have suggested that maternal influenza infection leads to neuropathologic alterations of particular relevance to schizophrenia.

TOXOPLASMA GONDII. T. gondii is a microbial pathogen that may exist in an active as well as a latent form. Following primary infection, the parasite may become sequestered as inactive oocysts within the brain and a number of other tissues and become reactivated over the life of the host. Hence, there may be different mechanisms by which *T. gondii* can elevate risk for schizophrenia. Although recommendations to protect against *T. gondii* are aimed at preventing acute infection, it is unlikely that active primary infection by this parasite is by itself sufficient to account for its association with schizophrenia, since the presence of maternal or neonatal anti-*T. gondii* IgM antibodies, a robust marker of recently acquired infection, was not observed in the two studies cited here (Brown et al., 2005; Mortensen et al., 2007). A second possible mechanism consists of reactivation of a previous *T. gondii* infection, leading to an inflammatory response in the developing fetal brain. This inflammatory response is expected to be accompanied by an increase in maternal anti-*T. gondii* IgG antibodies, although to our knowledge these assays have not been conducted in reactivated *T. gondii* infection. In a third scenario, elevated anti-*T. gondii* IgG antibodies—which exist for many years after infection, including the dormant phase—could cause neuropathology, because the IgG antibody is small enough to cross the placenta. It is worth noting in this regard that elevated total IgG antibody is teratogenic in some autoimmune disorders (Nadler et al., 1995).

GENITAL-REPRODUCTIVE INFECTION. Maternal genital-reproductive infections have the potential to disrupt fetal neurodevelopment by direct fetal invasion. These infections are known to infect the fetus by ascending the perineum, vagina, or cervix, and several have been associated with known congenital brain anomalies (Remington et al., 2006).

Implications

Preventive Approaches

One of the most important implications of research on prenatal infections in the etiology of schizophrenia is the potential for preventing this disorder. In this regard, the concept of population-attributable proportion (PAP) offers the potential to estimate the relative importance of preventive efforts. The PAP represents the proportion of cases in a population that would have been prevented if the risk factor was completely removed. This statistic is based on the magnitude of the effect on risk of the outcome and the prevalence of the risk factor in the population studied (Rothman & Greenland, 1998). A number of infections, including influenza, *T. gondii*, and genital-reproductive infections, are highly prevalent in the U.S. and global populations. Moreover, pregnant women are believed to be more vulnerable to these infections than nonpregnant women. We demonstrated that the PAP corresponding to these three maternal infections alone is approximately 30% (Brown & Derkits, 2010), suggesting that if preventive efforts removed these three infections from the pregnant population in our sample, then nearly one-third of schizophrenia cases in the population that we studied would have been eliminated. On the one hand, this may be an over-estimate, because the true effect size could be smaller, and the prevalence of the exposure may vary in other populations. On the other hand, this figure does not take into account the documented risk associated with bacterial infection or the possible risks associated with other microbial infections. This figure nonetheless indicates that greater attention to efforts to prevent infection during pregnancy could play a significant role in reducing the risk of schizophrenia. Further, a more complete estimate of the PAP will need to await studies of the risk of schizophrenia conferred by additional infections, such as other viral and bacte-rial microbes. Confirming these associations would have the effect of increasing the PAP.

Infections are among the most preventable of all risk factors. Vaccination is one of the oldest, safest, and most effective approaches for preventing many in-fections, including some of those associated with schizophrenia. Influenza vac-cination has prevented millions of cases and saved tens of thousands of lives. Because of a process known as *antigenic drift*, in which mutations occur in the strains of influenza, it is necessary to develop new vaccinations each year, requir-ing ongoing surveillance and vigilance on the part of public health administra-tors and experts (Kilbourne, 1987). Occasionally, the subtypes of influenza mu-tate as well, in a process known as *antigenic shift*, which resulted in the H1N1 "swine flu" influenza virus. However, technologic advances to identify the ge-nomic and antigenic sequences of these viruses are hastening the development of new influenza vaccines.

Given the increased vulnerability of pregnant women to influenza, as well as the association between influenza during pregnancy and fetal morbidity and mortality (Zaman et al., 2008), pregnant women are considered to be a high-risk group that should be targeted for influenza vaccination. Clearly, this ap-proach will reduce the adverse effects of influenza during pregnancy to both the mothers and offspring in a significant proportion of the pregnant population. It must also be kept in mind, however, that influenza vaccination will also trigger a cytokine response, which could be detrimental to fetal brain development (Dam-mann & Leviton, 1997). Although more research into the effects of influenza vaccination during pregnancy is necessary, one strategy that might address this issue is to target for vaccination nonpregnant women of reproductive age. Ad-ministering influenza vaccination to this subgroup will provide protection in the event of a pregnancy in the ensuing months, while minimizing the risk of fetal exposure to the release of cytokines during pregnancy, given that the cytokine response ends approximately one week following vaccination.

With regard to the prevention of genital-reproductive infections, there are two approaches that have long been in use: (1) antibiotics, which are highly effective against many bacterial genital-reproductive pathogens, including gonococcus and syphilis, and (2) barrier contraceptives to reduce the transmission of sexually transmitted diseases.

Approaches aimed at the prevention of *T. gondii* represent standard obstetric practices. Because *T. gondii* can be found in cat litter boxes, soil, and uncooked meats and fish, current recommendations during pregnancy are to avoid exposure to these sources of pathogens, to use proper hygienic measures, and to thoroughly cook meats, poultry, and fish to kill *T. gondii* oocysts. The fact that in the cited studies schizophrenia was related to elevated anti-*T. gondii* IgG antibodies (Brown et al., 2005; Mortensen et al., 2007) rather than to the parasite itself suggests that most infections were acquired before pregnancy. Hence, measures to reduce exposure to this infection may need to be initiated long before reproductive age.

In summary, the findings of associations between maternal infectious exposures and schizophrenia have important implications for the prevention of schizophrenia, given that maternal infection occurs commonly during pregnancy, and practical, effective, and relatively inexpensive approaches aimed at reducing or eliminating exposure to these pathogens are already available. Therefore, if the findings reviewed in the previous paragraphs can be replicated in independent cohorts in concert with efforts to identify new, relevant microbial pathogens, these studies may have significant public health implications for reducing the risk of schizophrenia in the global population. In fact, it has been argued previously that the overall decline in bacterial illnesses and initiation of immunization programs may be responsible for the reduction in the incidence of schizophrenia beginning in the 1950s (Suvisaari et al., 1999b).

Relationship Between Infection and Genetic Vulnerability

As discussed in chapters 7 and 8, family, twin, and adoption studies have established a role for genetic vulnerability in the etiology of schizophrenia, and association studies have revealed evidence for individual susceptibility genes and a greater occurrence of copy number variants in this disorder. Given the relatively small effect sizes of individual susceptibility alleles on schizophrenia risk, and the approximately 40–50% discordance rate of schizophrenia in monozygotic twins, it appears likely that a substantial portion of the variance in risk will not be explained solely by genetic effects. Rather, it is now increasingly recognized that most complex disorders, including psychiatric ones, result from an interplay between genetic mutations and environmental exposures (Caspi et al., 2010). This interplay may take several forms, including gene-environment interaction and epigenetic effects, which may include environmental effects on gene expression (see chapter 9, this book). We focus here on gene-environment interaction.

Gene-Environment Interaction

There is increasing evidence that gene-environment interaction may play a significant role in schizophrenia and other neuropsychiatric disorders. Gene-environment interaction is defined as an increase in the effect of an environmental exposure when a susceptibility gene variant is present.

In a recent investigation of a Finnish cohort, prenatal exposure to pyelonephritis had a fivefold greater effect on risk of schizophrenia among subjects with a family history of psychosis than in those with no family history (Clarke et al., 2009). However, there has yet to be a study of interactions between individual susceptibility gene variants and prenatal infections in schizophrenia. In the paragraphs that follow, I discuss strategies that may lead toward the detection of such genes.

GENES THAT PLAY A ROLE IN NEURODEVELOPMENT. Genes involved in neurodevelopmental processes, including those that occur in utero, represent logical candidates to investigate in studies of interactions with prenatal infections. As discussed in more detail in chapters 14 and 15, some of the most important effects of Disrupted-in-Schizophrenia 1 (*DISC1*) and *neuregulin*, two leading susceptibility gene candidates, occur during the prenatal period. Intriguingly, there are a number of compelling similarities between the effects of mutations in these two genes and those of maternal immune activation (Brown & Derkits, 2010).

GENES AND THE IMMUNE RESPONSE. Genes that regulate immune function represent a second class of logical candidates to investigate in studies of gene-infection interactions. The Major Histocompatibility Complex (MHC) Class I proteins, which present antigens to T lymphocytes at the cell surface, are of particular interest in this regard (Boulanger, 2009). In addition to their role in immune regulation, these proteins are critical for brain development and function. These molecules are enriched at the synapse, are essential for normal synaptic function and for synaptic remodeling, and play an especially important role in graded fine-tuning of plasticity. It is also relevant that the expression of MHC Class I proteins is regulated by cytokines (Boulanger & Shatz, 2004). In three of the largest genomewide association studies of schizophrenia, one of the few results to meet statistical significance was that of genetic variants in the extended MHC (Purcell et al., 2009; Shi et al., 2009; Stefansson et al., 2009) (see chapter 7, this book). This finding is particularly striking given that this approach was not hypothesis driven.

GENE IDENTIFICATION. Recent findings from molecular genetic studies of schizophrenia (chapter 7, this book) and from animal models based on mutations of putative susceptibility genes (chapters 14 and 15, this book) offer the promise of discovering the true origins of schizophrenia. Yet, if gene-environment interaction plays a significant role in schizophrenia, strategies that are focused only on the search for genes may be limited in their ability to identify definitive etiologies in the majority of cases. For example, if certain genes produce their effects on the risk of schizophrenia only in the presence of in utero infection, it may be difficult to detect the effects of these genes on risk of the disorder if infection is not measured in these cases. Hence, one strategy that may facilitate gene identification in this scenario is to scan the genome in a subsample of cases whose subjects have been exposed to maternal infection.

This concept also has implications for prevention. If maternal infection and a gene are each necessary but not individually sufficient causes of a hypothetical subset of schizophrenia cases, then it may not be necessary to modify the genetic defect in order to prevent the disorder in this subset of cases. Instead, a much more practical and feasible approach would be the elimination of the environmental factor, such as maternal infection, for which well-known strategies for treatment and prevention exist (see "Implications").

Research on epigenetics and schizophrenia is covered in detail in chapter 9. In this context, an epigenetic approach might involve examining the effects of maternal infection on gene expression. This can occur through different processes, including DNA methylation and histone modifications. These changes represent a mechanism that may lead to lifelong changes in gene expression. In a seminal work on this question, Smith et al. (2007) demonstrated that maternal immune activation in mice leads to dysregulation of gene expression, with overexpression and underexpression of particular subsets of genes that persist in the adult offspring, and virtually all of these changes are mediated by the cytokine interleukin-6 (see chapter 10, this book). These findings suggest that effects of maternal infection might be mediated in part by epigenetic changes in the brain, and that cytokines may play an essential role in infection-induced epigenesis. Although this field is still in its infancy, with no known human studies of infection and epigenetically induced modifications, future birth cohort studies may, at least in theory, have the capacity to test these associations by relating well-documented prenatal infections to epigenetic alterations in offspring with schizophrenia.

Recommendations for Future Epidemiologic Studies of Prenatal Infection and Schizophrenia

Challenges of Previous Research Efforts

In spite of the intriguing findings generated to date from seroepidemiologic studies of prenatal infection and schizophrenia, there have been few attempts to replicate most of these results, and there are numerous additional infectious and immune candidates that have not yet been investigated. This is not surprising given the dearth of opportunities to address these hypotheses. The aforementioned birth cohort studies represent major methodologic advances, including archived prenatal biospecimens, rich data sets to address potential confounders, and follow-up into the age of risk for schizophrenia. Yet, there were also certain limitations to these studies.

First, the sample sizes were small to modest. This may have had several consequences. Statistical power to detect effects of certain exposure variables was somewhat compromised. This may have accounted for the lack of association between some infectious and immune measures and risk of schizophrenia in these studies. A second consequence is that the precision of the observed effects was also less than ideal, as manifested by relatively wide confidence intervals. Third, acute and less common infections were not investigated. It is conceivable that there may be a substantial number of such exposures that in total make an important contribution to the risk of schizophrenia. Fourth, the sample sizes from these studies generally were too small to allow for adequate statistical power to test for gene-environment interaction, which generally requires large sample sizes. Fifth, sample sizes in previous studies also were insufficient to test for interactive and mediating effects of other exposures; for example, power was not adequate to detect maternal cytokines as mediators of the effects of maternal infection on risk of schizophrenia. There are also numerous potential factors, such as sex and race, that may interact with maternal infection to increase schizophrenia risk. Larger sample sizes will be necessary to test for these and other interactive effects. In recent years, new birth cohorts with much larger samples have been established. These include the Finnish Prenatal Studies (FiPS), the Danish National Longitudinal Study (DNLS) (Olsen et al., 2001), and the Mother and Baby Study (MoBA) in Norway (Magnus et al., 2006). The number of births in these cohorts ranges from approximately 100,000 (DNLS, MoBA) to 1.5 million (FiPS).

A second challenge relates to the measurement of infection. As discussed previously, most prior studies assigned exposure status on the basis of whether subjects were in utero at the time of an infection in the population or on records indicating that maternal infection occurred. Studies that classified infection status on the basis of maternal or infant sera frequently used IgG antibody titers rather than direct markers of acute infection. As already noted here, IgG antibody provides evidence that infection occurred in the individual in whom it is measured, but it does not localize the infection to a specified period. It would be preferable to utilize antibody markers, such as IgM, which indicate that infection occurred soon before the time during which the blood sample was drawn; this would allow infection to be diagnosed during pregnancy or infancy. However, acute infection during pregnancy is more difficult to detect than chronic or previous infection, as the corresponding antibody markers are elevated only transiently in active infection. This issue can be surmounted by use of larger sample sizes, which will increase the likelihood of identifying a sufficient number of pregnancies in which the time window of the infection will coincide with the time during which the prenatal serum specimen was drawn.

A third challenge concerns potential biasing effects. First, incomplete ascertainment of cases was a frequent limitation of some cohort studies. In previous birth cohort studies of prenatal infection and schizophrenia, it is likely that a substantial number of cases were missed because of the fact that most ascertainment strategies are based on recruitment of cases from a selected number of facilities rather than from all facilities from which care is received. In this regard, national birth cohorts from countries with universal health insurance—coupled with comprehensive, centralized registries—offer the advantage of more complete case ascertainment. A second issue that can compromise both case and control ascertainment is loss to follow-up, which is more likely to occur when follow-up is conducted over long intervals, such as in disorders with long latency periods, including schizophrenia. Third, nonrepresentative control samples can also contribute to bias. This can occur, for example, when controls are selected from the original birth cohort rather than from the population that would have been identified as cases if they developed schizophrenia. A powerful approach toward addressing these issues is to utilize population registries with systematically collected longitudinal data, including migration.

A fourth limitation is the fact that few studies have adequately examined the specificity of maternal infection for schizophrenia. It is conceivable that this risk factor may be involved in the etiology of a wide range of disorders.

Finally, previous studies of maternal infection and schizophrenia did not consider phenotypes of schizophrenia beyond the presence or absence of diagnosis, which is based only on symptom criteria. In an initial attempt to address this question, we assessed relationships between maternal exposure to influenza and anti-toxoplasma IgG and neuropsychological function in offspring with schizophrenia in the Developmental Insult and Brain Anomaly in Schizophrenia Study (DIBS), which is based on schizophrenia cases in the CHDS birth cohort. We found that maternal exposure to these infections was significantly associated with anomalies in measures of executive function, including the Wisconsin Card Sort Test and the Trails B test, both of which are also specific to cognitive set-shifting (Brown et al., 2009a). These findings suggest that maternal exposure to infection may account for some portion of the neuropsychological disruption in schizophrenia, analogous to findings on genetic variants and neurocognitive anomalies in this disorder (Egan et al., 2001; Hennah et al., 2005). In a second DIBS study, we demonstrated that maternal infection was related to substantially increased volume of the cavum septum pellucidum (CSP), a neuroembryologic anomaly that arises during the prenatal or early postnatal period (Brown et al., 2009b). This provides biologically based evidence in a human study that indicates that prenatal infection disrupts the closure of the CSP, an anomaly that has been repeatedly observed in patients with schizophrenia (Brown et al., 2009a).

Infection and Molecular Genetic Studies

First, as implied from the preceding section, we suggest that future molecular genetic studies, including genomewide association studies, should incorporate prospectively documented, specific, and reliably measured maternal infectious exposures. As already noted here, such studies have the potential to facilitate the identification of susceptibility genes by enriching the sample for maternal infectious exposures.

Translational Studies

As discussed in chapter 10, translational approaches involving maternal immune activation models have helped validate the epidemiologic findings by demonstrating brain and behavioral phenotypes that are consistent with those observed in schizophrenia. These studies are also beginning to suggest potential causal mechanisms by which maternal infection alters brain development and function, most notably by the increase of specific cytokines. Increased interdisciplinary efforts between epidemiologists and molecular and cellular neuroscientists should enhance this work.

Critical Periods of Vulnerability and Developmental Trajectories

As illustrated by this review, the gestational timing of infection appears to be a critical factor that influences vulnerability to schizophrenia. Although initial emphasis was placed on the second trimester as a period of susceptibility, this notion was largely based on ecologic studies. Birth cohort studies, which featured more refined methodologic approaches, have since suggested that, at least for certain infections, exposure earlier in pregnancy, including periconception and the first trimester, may also represent important periods of susceptibility. Hence, it would be of benefit to devote more attention to "windows" of vulnerability to infectious insults. Our understanding of the developmental mechanisms by which these insults increase risk for schizophrenia could also be facilitated by concurrent documentation of the developmental trajectories that potentially mediate the effects of infection on risk of schizophrenia. For this purpose, longitudinal studies on early and later manifestations of schizophrenia in subjects with in utero exposure data who are followed into the age of risk for schizophrenia could begin to address these questions.

Conclusions

In the past two decades, epidemiologic studies of maternal infection and schizophrenia have evolved from work based on ecologic data to sophisticated, longitudinal birth cohort designs that have documented maternal infection by analysis of biomarkers. Most birth cohort studies that have utilized this resource have provided evidence consistent with maternal infection having a role in the etiology of schizophrenia. Although these findings are intriguing, considerable work remains to replicate them and to generate further evidence of a causal association. The study of maternal infection and of other environmental exposures may facilitate the identification of susceptibility genes that interact with these exposures.

These studies offer the potential for the prevention of schizophrenia, which for many infectious exposures can be accomplished through greater implementation of relatively inexpensive and standard interventions, including vaccination, antibiotics, and improved hygiene. Moreover, coupled with translational studies of animal models of infection, this work may elucidate pathogenic mechanisms by which prenatal infection might lead to schizophrenia.

KEY AREAS FOR FUTURE RESEARCH

- Conduct new birth cohort studies with prospective biomarkers of infection that feature significant methodologic advances, including large sample sizes to improve statistical power.
- Address interactions between prenatal infection and other exposures that alter schizophrenia risk.
- Improve methodologies: reduce bias through greater case ascertainment, minimize loss to follow-up, and use representative controls.
- Identify new microbial risk factors, including acute and rare infections.
- Evaluate the specificity of prenatal infection to schizophrenia among other major psychiatric disorders.
- Further assess the relationship between maternal infection and functional or structural phenotypes of schizophrenia, with the goal of parsing phenotypes based on putative etiologic factors.
- Incorporate molecular genetics into birth cohort studies of prenatal exposures and schizophrenia.

- Conduct new translational studies of prenatal infection in animal models and increased interdisciplinary interaction between epidemiologists, clinical researchers, and basic neuroscientists.
- Assess critical periods of vulnerability to prenatal infection and track developmental trajectories that mediate the effects of prenatal infection on risk of schizophrenia.

Acknowledgments

The author wishes to acknowledge National Institute of Mental Health grant 1K02-MH65422 for support of this work, Paul Patterson for his valuable suggestions, and Patric Prado for technical assistance.

Selected Readings

Brown, A. S., Begg, M. D., Gravenstein, S., Schaefer, C. A., Wyatt, R. J., Bresnahan, M. A., Babulas, V., & Susser, E. (2004). Serologic evidence for prenatal influenza in the etiology of schizophrenia. *Archives of General Psychiatry* 61(8): 774–780.

Brown, A. S. & Derkits, E. J. (2010). Prenatal infection and schizophrenia: A review of epidemiologic and translational studies. *American Journal of Psychiatry* 167(3): 261–280.

Buka, S. L., Cannon, T. D., Torrey, E. F., & Yolken, R. H. (2008). Maternal exposure to herpes simplex virus and risk of psychosis among adult offspring. *Biological Psychiatry* 63(8): 809–815.

Meyer, U., Feldon, J., & Yee, B. K. (2008). A review of the fetal brain cytokine imbalance hypothesis of schizophrenia. *Schizophrenia Bulletin* 35(5): 959–972.

Patterson, P. H. (2009). Immune involvement in schizophrenia and autism: Etiology, pathology and animal models. *Behavioural Brain Research* 204(2): 313–321.

Smith, S. E., Li, J., Garbett, K., Mirnics, K., & Patterson, P. H. (2007). Maternal immune activation alters fetal brain development through interleukin-6. *Journal of Neuroscience* 27(40): 10695–10702.

References

Babulas, V., Factor-Litvak, P., Goetz, R., Schaefer, C. A., & Brown, A. S. (2006). Prenatal exposure to maternal genital and reproductive infections and adult schizophrenia. *American Journal of Psychiatry* 163(5): 927–929.

Baud, O., Emilie, D., Pelletier, E., Lacaze-Masmonteil, T., Zupan, V., Fernandez, H., Dehan, M., Frydman, R., & Ville, Y. (1999). Amniotic fluid concentrations of interleukin-1beta, interleukin-6 and TNF-alpha in chorioamnionitis before 32 weeks of gestation: Histological associations and neonatal outcome. *British Journal of Obstetric Gynaecology* 106(1): 72–77.

Boin, F., Zanardini, R., Pioli, R., Altamura, C. A., Maes, M., & Gennarelli, M. (2001). Association between -G308A tumor necrosis factor alpha gene polymorphism and schizophrenia. *Molecular Psychiatry* 6(1): 79–82.

Boulanger, L. M. (2009). Immune proteins in brain development and synaptic plasticity. *Neuron, 64*(1): 93–109.

Boulanger, L. M. & Shatz, C. J. (2004). Immune signalling in neural development, synaptic plasticity and disease. *Nature Reviews Neuroscience 5*(7): 521–531.

Brown, A. S. (2011). The environment and susceptibility to schizophrenia. *Progress in Neurobiology 93*(1): 23–58.

Brown, A. S., Begg, M. D., Gravenstein, S., Schaefer, C. A., Wyatt, R. J., Bresnahan, M. A., Babulas, V., & Susser, E. (2004a). Serologic evidence for prenatal influenza in the etiology of schizophrenia. *Archives of General Psychiatry 61*(8): 774–780.

Brown, A. S., Cohen, P., Greenwald, S., & Susser, E. (2000a). Nonaffective psychosis after prenatal exposure to rubella. *American Journal of Psychiatry 157*(3): 438–443.

Brown, A. S., Cohen, P., Harkavy-Friedman, J., Babulas, V., Malaspina, D., Gorman, J. M., & Susser, E. S. (2001). A. E. Bennett Research Award. Prenatal rubella, premorbid abnormalities, and adult schizophrenia. *Biological Psychiatry 49*(6): 473–486.

Brown, A. S., Deicken, R. F., Vinogradov, S., Kremen, W. S., Poole, J. H., Penner, J. D., Kochetkova, A., Kern, D., & Schaefer, C. A. (2009a). Prenatal infection and cavum septum pellucidum in adult schizophrenia. *Schizophrenia Research 108*(1–3): 285–287.

Brown, A. S. & Derkits, E. J. (2010). Prenatal infection and schizophrenia: A review of epidemiologic and translational studies. *American Journal of Psychiatry 167*(3): 261–280.

Brown, A. S., Hooton, J., Schaefer, C. A., Zhang, H., Petkova, E., Babulas, V., Perrin, M., Gorman, J. M., & Susser, E. S. (2004b). Elevated maternal interleukin-8 levels and risk of schizophrenia in adult offspring. *American Journal of Psychiatry 161*(5): 889–895.

Brown, A. S., Schaefer, C. A., Quesenberry, C. P., Jr., Liu, L., Babulas, V. P., & Susser, E. S. (2005). Maternal exposure to toxoplasmosis and risk of schizophrenia in adult offspring. *American Journal of Psychiatry 162*(4): 767–773.

Brown, A. S., Schaefer, C. A., Quesenberry, C. P., Jr., Shen, L., & Susser, E. S. (2006). No evidence of relation between maternal exposure to herpes simplex virus type 2 and risk of schizophrenia. *American Journal of Psychiatry 163*(12): 2178–2180.

Brown, A. S., Schaefer, C. A., Wyatt, R. J., Goetz, R., Begg, M. D., Gorman, J. M., & Susser, E. S. (2000b). Maternal exposure to respiratory infections and adult schizophrenia spectrum disorders: A prospective birth cohort study. *Schizophrenia Bulletin 26*(2): 287–295.

Brown, A. S., Vinogradov, S., Kremen, W. S., Poole, J. H., Deicken, R. F., Penner, J. D., McKeague, I. W., Kochetkova, A., Kern, D., & Schaefer, C. A. (2009b). Prenatal exposure to maternal infection and executive dysfunction in adult schizophrenia. *American Journal of Psychiatry 166*(6): 683–690.

Buka, S. L., Cannon, T. D., Torrey, E. F., & Yolken, R. H. (2008). Maternal exposure to herpes simplex virus and risk of psychosis among adult offspring. *Biological Psychiatry 63*(8): 809–815.

Buka, S. L., Tsuang, M. T., Torrey, E. F., Klebanoff, M. A., Bernstein, D., & Yolken, R. H. (2001a). Maternal infections and subsequent psychosis among offspring. *Archives of General Psychiatry 58*(11): 1032–1037.

Buka, S. L., Tsuang, M. T., Torrey, E. F., Klebanoff, M. A., Wagner, R. L., & Yolken, R. H. (2001b). Maternal cytokine levels during pregnancy and adult psychosis. *Brain, Behavior, and Immunology 15*(4): 411–420.

Cahill, M., Chant, D., Welham, J., & McGrath, J. (2002). No significant association between prenatal exposure poliovirus epidemics and psychosis. *Australian and New Zealand Journal of Psychiatry 36*(3): 373–375.

Cannon, M., Cotter, D., Coffey, V. P., Sham, P. C., Takei, N., Larkin, C., Murray, R. M., & O'Callaghan, E. (1996). Prenatal exposure to the 1957 influenza epidemic and adult schizophrenia: A follow-up study. *British Journal of Psychiatry 168*(3): 368–371.

Caspi, A., Hariri, A. R., Holmes, A., Uher, R., & Moffitt, T. E. (2010). Genetic sensitivity to the environment: The case of the serotonin transporter gene and its implications for studying complex diseases and traits. *American Journal of Psychiatry* 167(5): 509–527.

Clarke, M. C., Tanskanen, A., Huttunen, M., Whittaker, J. C., & Cannon, M. (2009). Evidence for an interaction between familial liability and prenatal exposure to infection in the causation of schizophrenia. *American Journal of Psychiatry* 166(9): 1025–1030.

Crow, T. J. & Done, D. J. (1991). Schizophrenia and influenza. *Lancet* 338(8759): 116–117.

Dammann, O. & Leviton, A. (1997). Maternal intrauterine infection, cytokines, and brain damage in the preterm newborn. *Pediatric Research* 42(1): 1–8.

Davis, K. L., Stewart, D. G., Friedman, J. I., Buchsbaum, M., Harvey, P. D., Hof, P. R., Buxbaum, J., & Haroutunian, V. (2003). White matter changes in schizophrenia: Evidence for myelin-related dysfunction. *Archives of General Psychiatry* 60(5): 443–456.

Deverman, B. E. & Patterson, P. H. (2009). Cytokines and CNS development. *Neuron* 64(1): 61–78.

Dukes, C. S., Luft, B. J., Durack, D. T., Scheld, W. M., & Whitley, R. J. (1997). *Toxoplasmosis Infections of the Central Nervous System* (vol. 2, pp. 785–806). Philadelphia: Lippincott-Raven.

Egan, M. F., Goldberg, T. E., Kolachana, B. S., Callicott, J. H., Mazzanti, C. M., Straub, R. E., Goldman, D., & Weinberger, D. R. (2001). Effect of COMT Val108/158 Met genotype on frontal lobe function and risk for schizophrenia. *Proceedings of the National Academy of Sciences U.S.A.* 98(12): 6917–6922.

Engman, M. L., Adolfsson, I., Lewensohn-Fuchs, I., Forsgren, M., Mosskin, M., & Malm, G. (2008). Neuropsychologic outcomes in children with neonatal herpes encephalitis. *Pediatric Neurology* 38(6): 398–405.

Erlenmeyer-Kimling, L., Folnegovic, Z., Hrabak-Zerjavic, V., Borcic, B., Folnegovic-Smalc, V., & Susser, E. (1994). Schizophrenia and prenatal exposure to the 1957 A2 influenza epidemic in Croatia. *American Journal of Psychiatry* 151(10): 1496–1498.

Gilmore, J. H. & Jarskog, L. F. (1997). Exposure to infection and brain development: Cytokines in the pathogenesis of schizophrenia. *Schizophrenia Research* 24(3): 365–367.

Hennah, W., Tuulio-Henriksson, A., Paunio, T., Ekelund, J., Varilo, T., Partonen, T., Cannon, T. D., Lonnqvist, J., & Peltonen, L. (2005). A haplotype within the DISC1 gene is associated with visual memory functions in families with a high density of schizophrenia. *Molecular Psychiatry* 10(12): 1097–1103.

Kilbourne, E. D. (1987). *Influenza*. New York: Plenum Medical.

Kropp, R. Y., Wong, T., Cormier, L., Ringrose, A., Burton, S., Embree, J. E., & Steben, M. (2006). Neonatal herpes simplex virus infections in Canada: Results of a 3-year national prospective study. *Pediatrics* 117(6): 1955–1962.

Magnus, P., Irgens, L. M., Haug, K., Nystad, W., Skjaerven, R., & Stoltenberg, C. (2006). Cohort profile: The Norwegian Mother and Child Cohort Study (MoBa). *International Journal of Epidemiology* 35(5): 1146–1150.

Mednick, S. A., Machon, R. A., Huttunen, M. O., & Bonett, D. (1988). Adult schizophrenia following prenatal exposure to an influenza epidemic. *Archives of General Psychiatry* 45(2): 189–192.

Meyer, U., Feldon, J., & Yee, B. K. (2008). A review of the fetal brain cytokine imbalance hypothesis of schizophrenia. *Schizophrenia Bulletin* 35(5): 959–972.

Mortensen, P. B., Norgaard-Pedersen, B., Waltoft, B. L., Sorensen, T. L., Hougaard, D., Torrey, E. F., & Yolken, R. H. (2007). Toxoplasma gondii as a risk factor for early-onset schizophrenia: Analysis of filter paper blood samples obtained at birth. *Biological Psychiatry* 61(5): 688–693.

Nadler, D. M., Klein, N. W., Aramli, L. A., Chambers, B. J., Mayes, M., & Wener, M. H. (1995). The direct embryotoxicity of immunoglobulin-G fractions from patients with systemic lupus-erythematosus. *American Journal of Reproductive Immunology 34*(6): 349–355.

O'Callaghan, E., Gibson, T., Colohan, H. A., Walshe, D., Buckley, P., Larkin, C., & Waddington, J. L. (1991). Season of birth in schizophrenia. Evidence for confinement of an excess of winter births to patients without a family history of mental disorder. *British Journal of Psychiatry 158*(6): 764–769.

O'Callaghan, E., Sham, P. C., Takei, N., Murray, G., Glover, G., Hare, E. H., & Murray, R. M. (1994). The relationship of schizophrenic births to 16 infectious diseases. *British Journal of Psychiatry 165*(3): 353–356.

Olsen, J., Melbye, M., Olsen, S. F., Sorensen, T. I., Aaby, P., Andersen, A. M., Taxbol, D., Hansen, K. D., Juhl, M., Schow, T. B., et al. (2001). The Danish National Birth Cohort—Its background, structure and aim. *Scandavian Journal of Public Health 29*(4): 300–307.

Patterson, P. H. (2009). Immune involvement in schizophrenia and autism: Etiology, pathology and animal models. *Behavioural Brain Research 204*(2): 313–321.

Purcell, S. M., Wray, N. R., Stone, J. L., Visscher, P. M., O'Donovan, M. C., Sullivan, P. F., & Sklar, P. (2009). Common polygenic variation contributes to risk of schizophrenia and bipolar disorder. *Nature 460*(7256): 748–752.

Remington, J. S., Klein, J. O., Wilson, C. B., & Baker, C. J. (2006). *Infectious Diseases of the Fetus and Newborn Infant* (6th ed.). Philadelphia: Elsevier Saunders.

Rothman, K. J. & Greenland, S. (1998). *Modern Epidemiology*. Philadelphia: Lippincott Williams & Wilkins.

Saji, F., Samejima, Y., Kamiura, S., Sawai, K., Shimoya, K., & Kimura, T. (2000). Cytokine production in chorioamnionitis. *Journal of Reproductive Immunology 47*(2): 185–196.

Shi, J., Levinson, D. F., Duan, J., Sanders, A. R., Zheng, Y., Pe'er, I., Dudbridge, F., Holmans, P. A., Whittemore, A. S., Mowry, B. J., et al. (2009). Common variants on chromosome 6p22.1 are associated with schizophrenia. *Nature 460*(7256): 753–757.

Shimoya, K., Matsuzaki, N., Taniguchi, T., Okada, T., Saji, F., & Murata, Y. (1997). Interleukin-8 level in maternal serum as a marker for screening of histological chorioamnionitis at term. *International Journal of Gynaecology and Obstetrics 57*(2): 153–159.

Smith, S. E., Li, J., Garbett, K., Mirnics, K., & Patterson, P. H. (2007). Maternal immune activation alters fetal brain development through interleukin-6. *Journal of Neuroscience 27*(40): 10695–10702.

Sorensen, H. J., Mortensen, E. L., Reinisch, J. M., & Mednick, S. A. (2009). Association between prenatal exposure to bacterial infection and risk of schizophrenia. *Schizophrenia Bulletin 35*(3): 631–637.

Stefansson, H., Ophoff, R. A., Steinberg, S., Andreassen, O. A., Cichon, S., Rujescu, D., Werge, T., Pietilainen, O. P., Mors, O., Mortensen, P. B., et al. (2009). Common variants conferring risk of schizophrenia. *Nature 460*(7256): 744–747.

Susser, E., Lin, S. P., Brown, A. S., Lumey, L. H., & Erlenmeyer-Kimling, L. (1994). No relation between risk of schizophrenia and prenatal exposure to influenza in Holland. *American Journal of Psychiatry 151*(6): 922–924.

Suvisaari, J., Haukka, J., Tanskanen, A., Hovi, T., & Lonnqvist, J. (1999a). Association between prenatal exposure to poliovirus infection and adult schizophrenia. *American Journal of Psychiatry 156*(7): 1100–1102.

Suvisaari, J. M., Haukka, J. K., Tanskanen, A. J., & Lonnqvist, J. K. (1999b). Decline in the incidence of schizophrenia in Finnish cohorts born from 1954 to 1965. *Archives of General Psychiatry 56*(8): 733–740.

Tau, G. Z. & Peterson, B. S. (2010). Normal development of brain circuits. *Neuropsychopharmacology 35*(1): 147–168.

Torrey, E. F. (1988). Stalking the schizovirus. *Schizophrenia Bulletin* 14(2): 223–229.

Watson, C. G., Kucala, T., Tilleskjor, C., & Jacobs, L. (1984). Schizophrenic birth seasonality in relation to the incidence of infectious diseases and temperature extremes. *Archives of General Psychiatry* 41(1): 85–90.

Weizman, R., Bessler, H., Plotnikoff, N. P., Faith, R. E., Murgo, A. J., & Good, R. A. (1999). *Cytokines: Stress and Immunity*. Boca Raton, FL: CRC Press.

Wright, I. C., Sharma, T., Ellison, Z. R., McGuire, P. K., Friston, K. J., Brammer, M. J., Murray, R. M., & Bullmore, E. T. (1999). Supra-regional brain systems and the neuropathology of schizophrenia. *Cerebral Cortex* 9(4): 366–378.

Zaman, K., Roy, E., Arifeen, S. E., Rahman, M., Raqib, R., Wilson, E., Omer, S. B., Shahid, N. S., Breiman, R. F., & Steinhoff, M. C. (2008). Effectiveness of maternal influenza immunization in mothers and infants. *New England Journal of Medicine* 359(15): 1555–1564.

CHAPTER 2

PRENATAL NUTRITION AND THE ETIOLOGY OF SCHIZOPHRENIA

KRISTIN N. HARPER AND ALAN S. BROWN

KEY CONCEPTS

- Studies demonstrating a link between exposure to famine during gestation and elevated risk of developing schizophrenia have drawn attention to the role of prenatal nutrition in the development of this disorder.
- Malnutrition during pregnancy could increase schizophrenia risk through multiple pathways, such as elevated mutation rate, epigenetic alterations, or other types of physiologic changes.
- Epidemiologic associations between a number of prenatal nutrition measures and schizophrenia have been discovered, including low and high maternal body mass index (BMI), low and high birth weight, elevated levels of homocysteine, and low iron levels.
- The case for a biologically plausible role in influencing schizophrenia risk can also be made for a number of other nutrients that have not yet been investigated.

The hypothesis that prenatal nutrition plays an important role in schizophrenia is not a new one. Eighty years ago, Tramer (1929) examined birth data from 3,100 Swiss patients with different types of psychoses. Believing that diet, vitamins, and sunlight were important factors in development, he hypothesized that an individual's month of birth might influence their later risk of developing these disorders. In this study, Tramer found an excess of winter births in the group that later developed schizophrenia. Since then, over 250 studies on birth seasonality and schizophrenia have been published (Torrey et al., 1997). Although many of these studies have had significant limitations, such as lack of controls, small sample sizes, and inaccuracy of birth data, an excess of winter-spring births among individuals with schizophrenia has been consistently demonstrated.

Following Tramer, researchers have hypothesized that a number of nutritional deficiencies could underlie this trend. These include insufficient amounts of vitamin C (De Sauvage Nolting, 1954), vitamin K (Dalén, 1975), protein (Pasamanick, 1961), and vitamin D (McGrath, 1999), among others. In recent years, there is evidence that the seasonal birth effect is becoming less pronounced in high-income countries (Suvisaari et al., 2000). This may be consistent with an improvement in year-round nutrition. Although other explanations for the association between seasonality and schizophrenia births have been proposed—most notably, temporal variations in infectious disease epidemics (Watson et al., 1984)—these data suggest that nutritional deficits represent a viable possible cause.

Nutritional deficiency is common worldwide. It is estimated that maternal and child undernutrition, which includes stunting, wasting, and deficiencies of essential vitamins and minerals, is responsible for 3.5 million deaths every year (Black et al., 2008). Maternal undernutrition, as measured by a BMI of less than $18.5\,kg/m^2$, ranges from 10–19% in most countries but reaches a prevalence of roughly 40% in countries such as India, Bangladesh, and Eritrea (Black et al., 2008). These macronutrient deficiencies are often accompanied by micronutrient deficiencies. For example, it is estimated that over 7.2 million pregnant women in low-income countries are vitamin A deficient (West, 2002). In high-income countries, overnutrition is more common than undernutrition in terms of caloric intake. Micronutrient deficiencies remain common in developed countries, however. An estimated 20% of American women between the ages of 12 and 50 consume less than half of the recommended daily allowance of iron (Ames, 2001).

Because nutritional deficiencies affect such a large segment of the population, including women of reproductive age, a possible role for prenatal nutrition in the development of schizophrenia has been of enduring interest in much of the research community. Progress on definitively linking prenatal nutrition to schizophrenia has been slow, however, because of the difficulty in linking cases of schizophrenia to the prenatal conditions that occurred decades earlier. Recent developments have had appreciable success in overcoming such problems and have led to preliminary evidence supporting this hypothesis. In this chapter, we will begin by describing recent ecologic studies that rekindled interest in prenatal nutrition and schizophrenia, move on to a discussion of the evidence that specific micronutrients play a role, and end with a brief synthesis of current findings and future research directions. Reflecting our own interests, there will be a particular focus on possible genetic and epigenetic pathways through which nutrition could influence risk of schizophrenia. This area of research, although still in its infancy, appears promising and has attracted much attention.

Famine Studies

Studies of children born or conceived during famines, in which periods of maternal nutritional deficiency are well demarcated, have provided a unique opportunity to study the relationship between nutrition and schizophrenia. The first such study involved the Dutch Hunger Winter of 1944–1945, in which a Nazi blockade resulted in severely restricted food rations in the western Netherlands. In the last months of the famine, the daily food ration fell to fewer than 500 calories, and in urban areas alternative food sources that could be used to supplement the diet were very scarce as well (McClellan, Susser, & King, 2006). During the most severe period, mortality doubled and fertility was halved in affected areas. Two unique features of this famine made it ideal for epidemiologic study: (1) the food rations distributed to the population were documented, allowing the caloric content of the rations to be estimated; and (2) the peak period of the famine was of short duration. About 40,000 individuals were exposed to the Hunger Winter at some point in gestation (Hoek, Brown, & Susser, 1997), and a series of studies were performed on what came to be known as the Dutch Famine Birth Cohort. During the initial studies on this cohort, the sole health outcomes that were found to vary in response to severe famine exposure were congenital anomalies of the central nervous system (CNS). This effect was present only when famine was experienced during early gestation, with CNS anomalies peaking during the period in which the famine was at its worst (Susser, Hoek, & Brown, 1998) (figure 2.1). Because schizophrenia is also believed to be a developmental disorder of the CNS, researchers questioned whether a link between gestational exposure to famine and this psychiatric illness might be present. They found that women who had conceived or experienced early pregnancy during the famine had a significantly greater risk of giving birth to a child who would later develop schizophrenia (Susser et al., 1996) (figure 2.1).

More than a decade later, these results were replicated in two studies that examined another disastrous event: the Chinese famine of 1959–1961. During the massive famine that followed Mao's Great Leap Forward, mortality climbed and fertility fell. A study of the famine years in Wuhu (Anhui province), one of the regions most severely affected, found that the average birth rate between 1956 and 1961 was one-third the normal rate and that adults born between 1960 and 1961, who would have been exposed to famine during early gestation, had a significantly higher risk of developing schizophrenia (St Clair et al., 2005). Subsequently, a study in the Liuzhou region of southern China that used a similar design as the Wuhu study found concordant results. The risk of schizophrenia peaked in those annual birth cohorts in which the birth rate dropped (Xu et al., 2009). Although both Chinese studies used similar methods to define famine exposure, they were conducted in two regions that differed dramatically in

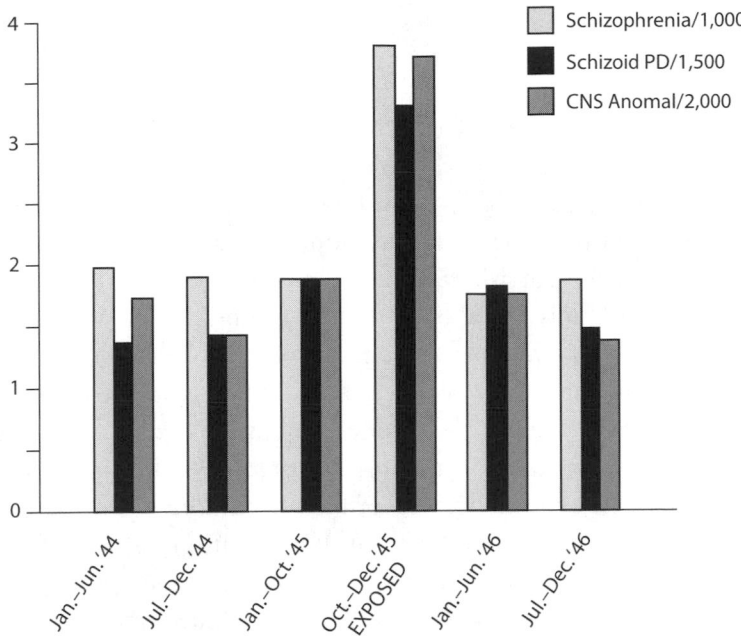

Figure 2.1. Famine during early gestation increases the risk of schizophrenia. Neurodevelopmental disorders and schizophrenia rose in response to early gestational exposure to the Dutch Famine of 1944–1945. CNS Anomal = anomalies of the central nervous system; Schizoid PD = schizoid personality disorders. (Reproduced from Hoek et al. [1997] with the permission of Springer Science + Business Media.)

terms of customs, ethnic diversity, and the experience of the famine. The fact that prenatal exposure to famine was found to result in a higher incidence of schizophrenia in three substantially different locations on two continents and during two time periods creates a solid case for the plausibility of severe maternal nutritional deficiencies in the etiology of this disorder.

Prenatal Nutrition and Schizophrenia: Possible Mechanisms

These results inspired researchers to take a closer look at the link between prenatal nutrition and schizophrenia. Having demonstrated an association between famine during early pregnancy and schizophrenia, investigators focused on the specific factors responsible for this relationship. Here, we focus on biological pathways by which nutritional deficiencies could shape schizophrenia risk. These include genetic changes, epigenetic changes, and direct physiologic consequences, which we define as the direct effects of nutrients on the brain in the absence of genetic or epigenetic mediation.

Genetic Changes

As has been previously hypothesized (McClellan, Susser, & King, 2006), nutritional deficiencies could result in de novo mutations in genes critical for brain development, either in somatic or germ-line cells. Although scientists are now beginning to map out the genes that play important roles during neurodevelopment in animal models (Parrish et al., 2006; Sepp et al., 2008), it seems clear that the genetic loci involved are both numerous and diverse in terms of function. Because of the large number of genes essential for normal brain development and the complex interplay between their translated proteins, it is possible that a relatively high proportion of random mutations could result in the impairment of brain structure and function. Furthermore, during early gestation the embryo or fetus is exquisitely susceptible to mutations because of the high cell division rate during early development. If a mutation occurs before, during, or shortly after conception, the frequency of mutant cells rises rapidly during early fetal growth (Paashuis-Lew & Heddle, 1998). Adequate nutrition plays a vital role in protecting against the DNA damage that results in de novo mutations (Ames, 2001). For example, many micronutrients act as antioxidants, protecting DNA from damage by neutralizing free radicals. Other nutrients function in DNA synthesis and repair. For this reason, exposure to famine and attendant micronutrient deficiencies during early gestation could result in an increased rate of de novo mutation.

The evidence that de novo mutations play an important role in schizophrenia is mounting (International Schizophrenia Consortium, 2008; Stefansson et al., 2008; Vrijenhoek et al., 2008; Walsh et al., 2008; Xu et al., 2008), consistent with the observation that most patients with schizophrenia have no close relatives with the disease (Gottesman & Shields, 1982). The studies cited—which focus on rare copy number variants (CNVs) (see chapter 8, this book), a type of polymorphism that is amenable to whole genome analysis—have established the importance of genetic variants that are individually rare and found in diverse loci (Need et al., 2009; Sebat, Levy, & McCarthy, 2009). Incidentally, these results may provide an explanation for an evolutionary problem that has long puzzled schizophrenia researchers. Individuals with schizophrenia experience a reproductive disadvantage, having fewer children than individuals without the condition (Bassett et al., 1996; Howard et al., 2002). As a result, one would expect the genes that predispose people to schizophrenia to become rarer in each successive generation. How, then, can the disease persist in the population at such a high frequency, generation after generation? A causal role for rare variants, rapidly purged from the population but recurring at high rates, could explain the high prevalence of the disease despite associated fitness costs. In addition, the CNV data dovetail with the finding that schizophrenia is associated with increased paternal age (Malaspina et al., 2001), which itself is associated with increased rates of de novo germ-line mutations (Crow, 2000) (see chapter 5, this book). Given the current evidence suggesting that de novo mutations contribute to schizophrenia risk, the susceptibility of the developing fetus to DNA damage, and the role of micronutrients in guarding against DNA damage, a genetic pathway leading from prenatal famine to increased risk of schizophrenia appears plausible.

Epigenetic Changes

As discussed in chapters 5 and 9, epigenetic changes could also play a role in the etiopathogenesis of schizophrenia (Petronis, 2004; Sharma, 2005). It is known that imprinted genes play important roles in the growth of the fetus and placenta and also in the development of the brain, affecting cognition and behavior long after infancy (Malaspina, 2001). Thus, imprinting errors could increase the risk of schizophrenia by changing the expression of either genes specifically involved in neuropsychiatric pathology or genes related to fetal growth generally. The observation that increased paternal age is linked to schizophrenia could be compatible with increased epigenetic mutation rates as well as genetic mutation rates (Malaspina, 2001) (see chapter 5, this book), and postmortem studies have demonstrated epigenetic alterations in the brains of patients with schizophrenia (see chapter 9, this book). But is there a connection to prenatal nutrition? One recent study found persistent epigenetic changes in the insulin-like growth factor 2 (*igf2*) gene in individuals exposed to the Dutch Hunger Winter during gestation, as opposed to unexposed, same-sex siblings (Heijmans et al., 2008). This result suggests that exposure to famine leads to epigenetic changes in at least one gene important in fetal development. A subsequent study, which examined additional genes in the same cohort, found that persistent epigenetic differences were widespread and that the nature of the changes depended on the timing of gestational exposure (Tobi et al., 2009).

It is well established that various micronutrients play essential roles in maintaining the integrity of the epigenome, as components of enzymes integral in methylation and as methyl-group donors. Although the field of epigenetics is relatively new, it is our view that the possibility that epigenetic differences could mediate the association between prenatal exposure to famine and schizophrenia should be given further attention.

Direct Physiologic Consequences

It is also possible that maternal nutritional deficiencies could result in altered fetal neurodevelopment by depriving cells of the basic substances necessary to divide and differentiate early in development, or by altering gene regulation during critical periods. Indeed, the direct consequences of malnutrition on the developing brain, independent of genetic and epigenetic mechanisms, are well characterized. Macronutrient deficiencies, for example, may result in insufficient energy stores during critical developmental periods, which could alter brain structure and function. For this reason, such deficiencies appear to be a plausible causal factor in the famine studies. Although such deficiencies are rare in high-income countries, the prevalence of schizophrenia does not appear to be less there than in low-income countries (Saha et al., 2009), so it appears unlikely that micronutrient deficiencies account for a large proportion of the variance in risk. In contrast, micronutrient deficiencies are prevalent both in times of famine and in high-income countries. Many micronutrients are essential components of molecules involved in neurodevelopment. For example, iodine is an integral component of the thyroid hormones necessary for normal neurodevelopment; early exposure to iodine deficiency results in irreversible alterations to the brain, illustrated by cretinism (Pharoah, Buttfield, & Hetzel, 1971). Thus, micronutrient deficiency appears to be a plausible risk factor for schizophrenia, based on the results of ecologic studies, their prevalence in affected populations, and what is known about their direct physiologic effects on the developing brain.

Prenatal Nutrition and Schizophrenia: Prospective Birth Cohort Studies

Thus far, our discussion of prenatal nutrition has focused on the results of ecologic studies linking prenatal famine and schizophrenia. Although the results are intriguing, it is important to note that data obtained from such studies are best used to generate hypotheses, as their design is characterized by a limited ability to measure and control for possible confounders. For example, it is possible that nonnutritional factors accompanying famine could have played an important role in increasing schizophrenia risk. Severe maternal stress during early pregnancy has been linked to an increased risk of schizophrenia (van Os & Selten, 1998; Khashan et al., 2008; Malaspina et al., 2008) (see chapter 4, this book), and it is not difficult to imagine that high levels of stress accompanied these famines. In this section, we will discuss results obtained from prospective birth cohort studies, beginning with investigations of general malnutrition, before discussing studies of specific micronutrients. Such studies offer a greater capacity to test specific hypotheses rigorously by allowing investigators to deal better with possible sources of confounding and to characterize risk associated with the factors of interest more accurately. A summary of the studies discussed can be found in table 2.1.

Table 2.1 Epidemiologic Studies of Prenatal Nutrition and Schizophrenia Risk

Exposure	Study Type and Sample	N[a]	Measure of Effect[b]	P-Value	Notes	Source
Prenatal famine	Cohort: Individuals born in western Netherlands, 1944–1946	Birth cohorts in six cities with populations >40,000: Amsterdam, The Hague, Haarlem, Leiden, Rotterdam, and Utrecht	RR: 2.0, 95% CI = 1.2–3.4	p < 0.01	Association between exposure to famine during conception, early gestation, or both, and risk of schizophrenia	Susser et al., 1996
	Cohort: Individuals born in Wuhu region of Anhui, China, 1956–1965	4,397 schizophrenia cases and 561,695 births in reference and treatment groups	RR: 2.30, 95% CI = 1.99–2.65 for 1960 births; RR: 1.93, 95% CI = 1.68–2.23 for 1961 births	Not reported	Association between birth during peak famine years and risk of schizophrenia	St Clair et al., 2005
	Cohort: Individuals born in Liuzhou prefecture of Guangxi, China, 1956–1965	3,223 schizophrenia cases and 823,873 births in reference and treatment groups	RR: 1.50, 95% CI = 1.35–1.68 for 1960 births; RR: 2.05, 95% CI = 1.86–2.27 for 1961 births	Not reported	Association between birth during peak famine years and risk of schizophrenia	Xu et al., 2009
BMI (maternal)	Cohort: Prenatal Determinants of Schizophrenia Study (Alameda County, CA, births 1959–1966)	63 SSD cases, 6,570 unaffected cohort members	RR: 2.9, 95% CI = 1.3–6.6	Not reported	High (≥30.0) but not low (≤19.9) prepregnant maternal BMI associated with increased SSD risk	Schaefer et al., 2000
	Case control: Patients from hospitals in or around Hamamatsu City, Japan. Enrollment period: 1998–2000.	52 schizophrenia cases, 284 healthy subjects	Early pregnancy BMI OR: 1.24; Late pregnancy BMI OR: 1.19	Early pregnancy: p = 0.032; Late pregnancy: p = 0.048	Higher maternal BMI, at the first and last antenatal visits, associated with greater risk of developing schizophrenia in offspring	Kawai et al., 2004
	Cohort: Births at Helsinki University Hospital, 1924–1933	7,086 with 114 schizophrenia cases	OR: 1.09 per kg/m, 95% CI = 1.02–1.17	Not reported	Lower late-pregnancy BMI associated with increased risk of developing schizophrenia in offspring	Wahlbeck et al., 2001

(continued)

Table 2.1 (continued)

Exposure	Study Type and Sample	N^a	Measure of Effect^b	P-Value	Notes	Source
Size at birth	Cohort: Swedish male conscripts born between 1973 and 1980	246,655 with 80 cases of schizophrenia	For <2.5 kg HR: 5.07, 95% CI=1.84–13.95; For >4 kg HR: 3.34, 95% CI=1.77–6.30	Not reported	Both low and high birth weight associated with increased risk of developing schizophrenia in offspring	Gunnell et al., 2003
	Cohort: Births at Helsinki University Hospital, 1924–1933	7,086 with 114 schizophrenia cases	OR: 1.48 per kg, 95% CI=1.03–2.13	Not reported	Low birth weight associated with increased risk of developing schizophrenia in offspring	Wahlbeck et al., 2001
Homocysteine	Nested case control: Prenatal Determinants of Schizophrenia Study (Alameda County, CA, births 1959–1966)	63 SSD cases, 122 controls	OR: 2.39, 95% CI=1.18–4.81	p=0.02	Elevated third-trimester homocysteine levels linked to increased risk of developing schizophrenia in offspring	Brown et al., 2007
Vitamin D	Nested case control: National Collaborative Perinatal Project (Boston, MA, and Providence, RI, births 1959–1966)	26 SSD cases, 51 controls	All subjects: OR: 0.98, 95% CI=0.92–1.05; African American subjects: OR: 0.78, 95% CI=0.55–1.08	African American subjects: p=0.08	Low levels of vitamin D in third-trimester sera found to have a trend-level association with SSD in African American subgroup	McGrath et al., 2003
Iron	Cohort: Prenatal Determinants of Schizophrenia Study (Alameda County, CA, births 1959–1966)	9,917 with 57 SSD cases	RR: 3.73, 95% CI=1.41–9.81	p=0.008	Mean maternal hemoglobin levels of ≤10.0g/dL associated with increased risk of schizophrenia in offspring	Insel et al., 2008

[a] SSD=schizophrenia spectrum disorders.

[b] CI=confidence interval; HR=hazard ratio; OR=odds ratio; RR=relative risk.

SOURCE: Authors.

Protein-Calorie Malnutrition

A number of birth cohort studies have explored the effects of prenatal protein-calorie malnutrition (PCM) on the risk of developing schizophrenia. Such investigations often can be performed in cohorts in which researchers lack the capacity to examine specific micronutrients, as it is possible to make use of maternal and infant weight and height measurements recorded in medical records.

Maternal Body Mass Index (BMI)

If maternal starvation during early pregnancy results in greater risk of schizophrenia, as suggested by the famine studies, then one might expect that low maternal BMI is also a risk factor for this disorder. A study in a Finnish cohort born during the late 1920s and early 1930s found that low maternal BMI resulted in an increased risk of developing schizophrenia. In that study, the odds ratio for schizophrenia increased with every 1.1 decrease in kg/m^2 (Wahlbeck et al., 2001). In contrast, in a Finnish cohort of subjects born in 1966, the relationship was reversed when socioeconomic circumstances had improved. The heaviest fifth percentile of mothers (BMI > 29) had a twofold risk of delivering offspring who later developed schizophrenia, although the finding fell short of statistical significance (Jones et al., 1998). In the Prenatal Determinants of Schizophrenia (PDS) Study, conducted in Alameda County, California, in the 1950s and 1960s, Schaefer et al. (2000) demonstrated that mothers with high maternal BMI were three times more likely to give birth to offspring with schizophrenia, and in this case the results did achieve statistical significance. These findings were replicated in a case-control study based in Hamamutsu City, Japan (Kawai et al., 2004). Considered in aggregate, these findings suggest that although low BMI may increase schizophrenia risk in societies in which nutritional deficits are common, high maternal BMI may represent a more important risk factor in high-income settings. Although the specific factors underlying the increased risk of schizophrenia associated with high BMI are poorly understood, it is possible that obstetric complications such as preeclampsia and delivery by cesarean section—which are more common in pregnant women with both high prepregnant BMI (Crane et al., 1997) and offspring with schizophrenia (Cannon, Jones, & Murray, 2002)—are involved. Gestational diabetes is also correlated with higher BMI (Solomon et al., 1997) and is associated with the types of obstetric complications more common among offspring who develop schizophrenia (McMahon, Ananth, & Liston, 1998).

Size at Birth

In the same early twentieth-century Finnish cohort already described here, Wahlbeck et al. (2001) found that small size at birth was associated with increased risk of schizophrenia; the odds ratio increased by nearly 1.5 for every kilogram decrease in body weight. In a study focusing on a more recent cohort of Swedish male conscripts born between 1973 and 1980, both low (< 2.5 kg) and high (> 4.0 kg) birth weights were associated with an increased risk of developing schizophrenia after controlling for prematurity (Gunnell et al., 2003). The authors hypothesized that gestational diabetes and cerebral anoxia during delivery may have contributed to the observed association between high birth weight and schizophrenia. Other studies have replicated the findings linking low birth weight and schizophrenia risk. Rifkin et al. (1994) found that low birth weight (< 2,500 g) was significantly more common in patients with schizophrenia in a study performed in South London, among patients born between the 1930s and the 1970s. Similar results were found by Smith et al. (2001) in British Columbia when comparing against published norms the prevalence of patients with schizophrenia who were born small for gestational age. Finally, using the Swedish Birth Registry for the years 1973 to 1979, small size for gestational age in males, but not females, was associated with increased risk of schizophrenia (Hultman et al., 1999).

It has been noted that birth weight is a problematic indicator of nutrition during pregnancy. The Dutch famine studies suggest that, to the extent that birth weight does reflect maternal nutrition, it results mainly from nutritional intake during the last trimester of gestation (Stein et al., 1975; Lumey, 1992). On the one hand, the maternal BMI and birth-weight data support the results obtained in the famine studies, pointing toward an increased risk of schizophrenia in the offspring of mothers with low BMI as well as in infants of small size. Intriguingly, however, the data suggest that a shift related to dietary changes may have occurred in high-income nations, in which overnutrition, as well as undernutrition, now represents a risk factor for schizophrenia. Thus, the findings that high BMI and birth weight are also linked to schizophrenia demonstrate that the nutritional state of the population in which the study takes place must be taken into consideration.

It is most likely that prenatal undernutrition could result in increased schizophrenia risk through direct physiologic and, possibly, epigenetic changes. Animal models of prenatal protein deprivation suggest behavioral, neurochemical, and developmental alterations that may correspond to clinical signs and symptoms present in schizophrenia, such as deficits in prepulse inhibition, cognition, and social interaction (see chapter 12, this book). Such changes could be caused by either mechanism. Although little is known about the effects of PCM on the epigenome, one study has demonstrated that calorie restriction in adult rats alters genomic methylation patterns (Hass et al., 1993), illustrating the potential for PCM to work through an epigenetic mechanism. In contrast, a genetic mechanism seems unlikely based on experiments in animal models. Calorie restriction promotes genomic stability in rats by enhancing major DNA repair pathways (Cabelof et al., 2003; Heydari et al., 2007). When rat dams are calorically restricted during the prenatal and lactation periods, protection against mutation induced by environmental stressors during early life has been documented in their pups (Shima, Swiger, & Heddle, 2000). Although the bulk of animal work suggests that prenatal calorie restriction protects against genetic mutations, it is important to note that in most of these studies, caloric intake is reduced by a moderate amount; the effects of severe maternal calorie restriction may be different. Finally, in interpreting the results of the studies discussed here, it is important to consider that the effects of low maternal BMI and small birth size in these studies could be caused by micronutrient deficiencies, which often occur simultaneously with PCM.

The link between schizophrenia and high maternal BMI and large size at birth could result from a number of different mechanisms as well. Overnutrition could lead to an increased induced mutation rate (as already discussed here) and possibly novel methylation patterns or direct physiologic alterations. Studies in animal models indicate that a prenatal diet high in fat results in a number of long-lasting physiologic changes (Armitage et al., 2004; Chang et al., 2008), but the mechanisms by which they occur are unclear. As mentioned, in humans high maternal BMI and large size at birth are also associated with a host of attendant conditions, such as gestational diabetes, which could mediate the observed relationships between these characteristics and schizophrenia.

Micronutrient Deficiency

In recent years, birth cohort studies have capitalized on the availability of archived maternal sera along with the ability to follow participants into adulthood to track the development of schizophrenia. These opportunities have allowed for the testing of hypotheses using prospective assessment of prenatal micronutrient levels and later diagnosis of schizophrenia, as described in this section.

Folate and Homocysteine

As already discussed here (see "Famine Studies"), a sharp increase in both schizophrenia and anomalies of the CNS, including neural tube defects (NTDs), was observed in individuals exposed to the Dutch Hunger Winter during early pregnancy (figure 2.1). Folate deficiency is one of the best known causes of NTDs, leading researchers to speculate that folate deficiency might be responsible for the increase in both conditions (Susser et al., 1998). This suspicion was bolstered by the decades-old findings that L-methionine (figure 2.2), a member of the folate metabolic cycle, can exacerbate psychosis in patients with chronic schizophrenia (Cohen et al., 1974), whereas folate treatment could improve the symptoms of schizophrenia (Godfrey et al., 1990). Folate is a single-carbon donor important in many cellular reactions, including the synthesis of nucleotides, DNA repair, and the methylation of DNA, proteins, lipids, and neurotransmitters. Unfortunately, it is not possible to measure folate in archived serum samples gathered under normal conditions. It is possible, however, to analyze levels of homocysteine, which, like L-methionine, is linked to folate in a metabolic cycle (figure 2.2). Low serum folate levels are typically associated with elevated homocysteine levels, so that the latter can be measured as a proxy for the former. In addition, it appears that high homocysteine levels have deleterious physiologic effects on the developing brain (discussed in the paragraphs that follow) that occur independently of folate deficiency. Thus far, only a single study has examined prenatal levels of homocysteine in patients with schizophrenia (Brown et al., 2007). In this study, which is based on the PDS sample, the investigators found that elevated maternal homocysteine levels in the third trimester were associated with a twofold increase in the risk of schizophrenia.

Additional data that may be relevant to the prenatal environment have been obtained from studies in adults. Susser et al. (1998) found that in individuals with schizophrenia and low folate levels, homocysteine levels were higher than those found in matched controls, suggesting that low folate status may unmask the presence of a defect in homocysteine metabolism that predisposes the carrier to schizophrenia. Other researchers have examined whether methylenetetrahydrofolate reductase (MTHFR) and polymorphisms—which predispose individuals to high homocysteine levels—are associated with schizophrenia. Although one meta-analysis found that individuals who were TT homozygotes at position 677 had an increased risk of schizophrenia (Lewis et al., 2005), a recent family-based study, performed to avoid population stratification, examined the same polymorphism and found no evidence of a higher frequency of this variant in schizophrenic offspring (Muntjewerff et al., 2007). Three case-control studies in Scandinavian countries have also failed to replicate an association between functional MTHFR polymorphisms and schizophrenia (Jönsson et al., 2008). However, Muntjewerff et al. (2007) have cautioned that if schizophrenia is a developmental disorder that starts during gestation, the maternal genotype might be more important than the genotype of the child, which is what has been measured in most studies to date. Although evidence regarding the effect of inherited defects in the folate metabolic cycle on schizophrenia risk appears inconsistent, future work may clarify the veracity of this hypothesis, as

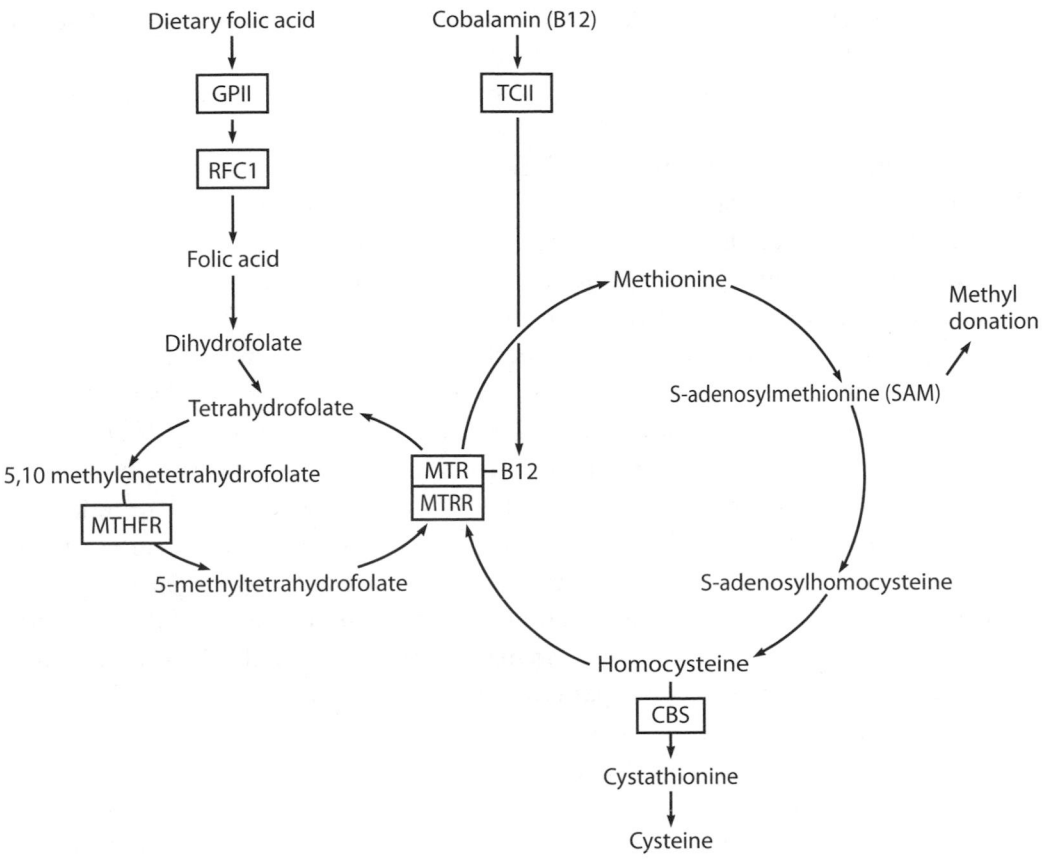

Proteins/Genes		Putative homocysteine-altering polymorphisms
CBS	Cystathionine beta synthase	844ins68, VNTR 18/18
GCPII	Glutamate carboxypeptidase II	1561 C→T
MTHFR	Methylenetetrahydrofolate reductase	677 C− T, 1298 A→ C
MTR	Methionine synthase	2756 A→G
MTRR	Methionine synthase reductase	66 A→G
RFC1	Reduced folate carrier 1	80 G→A
TCII	Transcobalamin II	776 C→G

Figure 2.2. Proteins, genes, and molecules involved in the folate/homocysteine pathways. (Reproduced from Picker & Coyle [2005] with the permission of Informa Healthcare Communications.)

maternal and fetal genotypes could both influence prenatal levels of folate and homocysteine.

Folate deficiency could potentially increase risk of schizophrenia through genetic or epigenetic pathways. Both in vitro and in vivo studies suggest that folate deficiency induces genomic instability (Fenech, 2001; Bagnyukova et al., 2008; Teo & Fenech, 2008), including in spermatozoa (Young et al., 2008; Boxmeer et al., 2009). For this reason, if the genetic pathway is important, it is possible that folate deficiency in the father, as well as the mother, around the time of conception could result in higher schizophrenia risk. An epigenetic mechanism is also plausible. In some of the earliest animal experiments that documented prenatal epigenetic effects, folate and other carbon donors such as methionine and betaine were implicated (Wolff et al., 1998; Cooney, Dave, & Wolff, 2002; Waterland & Jirtle, 2003). Currently, variation in folate intake is one of the best-established sources of epigenetic variation in utero. Because folate influences DNA methylation, which in turn affects gene expression and function (including those genes involved in brain development), folate-induced epigenetic changes could alter the course of neurodevelopment. Thus, prenatal folate deficiency could potentially increase schizophrenia risk by increasing the de novo mutation rate or by altering epigenetic patterns, in addition to altering other cellular processes that could affect neurodevelopment.

Homocysteine, present at high levels during periods of folate deficiency, is linked to a number of additional direct physiologic consequences that could negatively affect brain development. High levels of homocysteine and its derivatives (such as homocysteic acid and homocysteine sulfinic acid) appear to result in neuronal dysfunction (Mattson & Shea, 2003; Görtz et al., 2004). Homocysteine alters the levels of the methyl donor s-adenosylmethionine (SAM), which in turn regulates the expression of a plethora of neurodevelopmental genes (Picker & Coyle, 2005). In addition, elevated homocysteine levels can impair neurotransmitter metabolism (Bottiglieri, 2005) and act as a partial antagonist on the N-methyl-D-aspartate (NMDA) receptor, which is involved in fetal synapse development, plasticity, and neuronal migration (Picker & Coyle, 2005). Homocysteine may also be vasculopathic to the placenta, thereby possibly causing adverse effects on neurodevelopment by disrupting blood flow to the fetal brain (Frankenburg, 2007). Not surprisingly, elevated maternal homocysteine levels are associated with a number of conditions that are detrimental to the fetus, having been documented in preeclampsia (Roberts & Cooper, 2001), defective chorionic villous vascularization (Nelen et al., 2000), and pregnancies that result in NTDs (Mills et al., 1995). Although it is not yet understood whether serum homocysteine levels function simply as a marker of folate levels or whether this amino acid directly causes these conditions, it is clear that high homocysteine levels are associated with physiologic processes that could impair brain development in the growing fetus.

Vitamin D

The seasonality of schizophrenia births described earlier led some researchers to hypothesize that vitamin D deficiency might play a contributory role (Moskovitz, 1978; McGrath, 1999), as levels of this vitamin are lowest in winter and spring (see chapter 11, this book). To date, prenatal vitamin D deficiency, like maternal homocysteine, has been examined in only a single birth cohort. In this study, serum vitamin D levels were assayed in a small number of third-trimester maternal serum samples from pregnancies giving rise to offspring with schizophrenia spectrum disorders and controls in the Providence Cohort of the National Collaborative Perinatal Project (McGrath et al., 2003). No significant difference in maternal vitamin D levels between the two groups was found, although a trend level difference in the predicted direction (p=0.08) was reported among individuals in the African American subgroup. It is possible that the lack of association can be attributed to the low power of this pilot study, which examined only 26 cases and 51 controls.

Two other studies have been performed that, while not focusing on the prenatal environment, may be relevant to our understanding of the role of vitamin D in early development. The first examined the effects of vitamin D supplementation during the first year of life in the Northern Finland 1966 Birth Cohort (McGrath et al., 2004). This study found that, in males, supplementation with at least 2,000 IU of vitamin D was associated with a significantly reduced risk of schizophrenia (RR=0.23, 95% CI 0.06–0.95), suggesting that levels of this vitamin in early life could play an important role in the etiology of this disorder. In the second, Handoko et al. (2006) examined vitamin D receptor polymorphisms in subjects with schizophrenia and in controls, based on the supposition that genetic differences in the ability to utilize the vitamin could be important in the prenatal environment. Although no association was detected in that study, it may be illuminating to characterize the effects of maternal genotype on schizophrenia risk, as with folate and homocysteine.

Vitamin D could act through genetic or direct physiologic consequences to modify schizophrenia risk, as described in chapter 11. Adequate levels of this vitamin may prevent de novo mutations by protecting against oxidative stress that results in DNA damage (Chatterjee, 2001) and functioning in DNA synthesis and repair (Edelson et al., 1994; Ellison et al., 2008). Sufficient levels of vitamin D also play an essential role in neurodevelopmental pathways by modulating blood calcium levels, minimizing inflammation, regulating the expression of various genes, and inducing synthesis of important proteins such as nerve growth factor (NGF) (Musiol & Feldman, 1997). Animal studies examining the effect of vitamin D on the developing brain have demonstrated a number of changes that persist into adulthood, some of which are comparable to those observed in schizophrenia patients. These results are also discussed in detail in chapter 11.

Iron

Iron has attracted the attention of investigators interested in prenatal nutritional deficiencies and schizophrenia because of the pivotal role that this mineral plays in brain development. To date, one study has been performed that specifically aimed to test the hypothesis that maternal iron deficiency, indicated by a decrease in hemoglobin levels, is related to schizophrenia in offspring. The authors examined maternal hemoglobin levels documented in the database of the Child Health and Development Study in pregnancies giving rise to cases and noncases in the cohort (Insel et al., 2008). The results of this study indicated that a mean maternal hemoglobin concentration of 10 g/dL or less was associated with nearly a fourfold increase in risk of developing schizophrenia, adjusting for maternal education and ethnicity.

Iron is essential in a number of processes necessary for proper brain development, playing a role in myelination (Connor & Menzies, 1996) and dopaminergic neurotransmission (Ben-Schachar, Ashkenazi, & Youdim, 1986), among other functions. Intriguingly, myelin deficits have been demonstrated in schizophrenia (Hakak et al., 2001; Flynn et al., 2003), and dopaminergic dysfunction is one of the hallmark features of this disorder (Laruelle et al., 1996; Akil et al., 1999; Meyer-Lindenberg et al., 2002). In addition, maternal iron deficiency can result in anemia, which can cause fetal hypoxia, a complication implicated as a risk factor for schizophrenia (Cannon et al., 2000; Zornberg, Buka, & Tsuang, 2000; Dalman et al., 2001) (see chapter 3, this book). Moreover, iron-deficient children display motor, cognitive, and behavioral deficits (Deinard et al., 1981; Walter et al., 1989; Lozoff et al., 2006) similar to those observed in children who later develop schizophrenia (Jones et al., 1994; Fuller et al., 2002; Schiffman et al., 2009). Iron deficiency may also promote the accumulation of de novo mutations; it has been found that patients with iron deficiency anemia have significantly higher levels of DNA damage (Aslan et al., 2006), probably as a result of oxidative stress (Yoo et al., 2009). Thus, iron could influence schizophrenia risk through a number of direct physiologic mechanisms, and a genetic pathway is also possible.

Additional Prenatal Nutrients

Because the study of prenatal nutrient deficiencies and schizophrenia has only recently emerged, there are many plausible nutrients whose roles in modulating risk for this psychiatric disorder have yet to be studied. In this section, we discuss some promising candidates for study. (For a concise summary, see table 2.2).

n-3 Polyunsaturated Fatty Acids

A considerable body of evidence supports the plausibility of a role for n-3 polyunsaturated fatty acids (PUFAs), such as docosahexaenoic acid (DHA) and eicosapentaenoic acid (EPA), in influencing schizophrenia risk. DHA plays an important structural role in the brain, accounting for one-third of the structural fatty acids found in the gray matter, with particularly high concentrations in the cerebral cortex and synaptic membranes (Svennerholm, 1968; Breckenridge, Gombos, & Morgan, 1971; Bazan & Scott, 1990). PUFAs are incorporated into cellular membranes, where they regulate structure, fluidity, and function. n-3 PUFAs can also act as hormones, controlling the activity of key transcription factors and regulating gene expression (Benatti et al., 2004), which could affect brain development. In addition, animal studies suggest that DHA facilitates serotonin and dopamine neurotransmission and that n-3 PUFA deficiencies during gestation and postnatal life can result in behavioral and neurocognitive disturbances (Greiner et al., 2001; Fedorova & Salem, 2006). Finally, at modest levels, n-3 PUFAs have been shown to reduce oxidative damage in humans (Mori et al., 2003), and maternal supplementation with them has been shown to reduce markers of lipid peroxidation in neonates (Barden et al., 2004). Because lipid peroxidation results in products such as malondialdehyde (MDA), which are mutagenic, it may be expected that, up to a certain point, higher n-3 fatty acid levels as well as lower lipid peroxidation levels would result in lower levels of de novo mutation (Marnett, 2000). Thus, n-3 PUFAs could potentially influence schizophrenia risk through either direct physiologic or genetic pathways.

PUFAs have been the focus of attention in a large number of studies of infant neurodevelopment. Most of these investigations have compared infants fed normal formula with those fed formula supplemented with n-3 PUFAs (Carlson & Neuringer, 1999), and results examining neurocognitive outcomes have yielded mixed results (Scott et al., 1998; Lucas et al., 1999; Birch et al., 2000; O'Connor et al., 2001). Increasingly, however, attention is being paid to the role of fatty acids in prenatal neurodevelopment. Higher maternal fish intake, associated with greater n-3 PUFA intake, is correlated with better performance on tests of cognitive performance and stereoacuity administered to offspring at age three (Williams et al., 2001; Oken et al., 2008), although the same data suggest that this positive relationship is tempered by the high levels of mercury associated with some types of fish consumption. A randomized, double-blind study of maternal supplementation with n-3 or n-6 PUFAs from midpregnancy to three months after delivery found that children born to mothers who had received the

Table 2.2 Plausibility and Potential Importance of Various Prenatal Nutritional Factors in Schizophrenia

Nutrient[a]	How Nutrient Is Obtained	Prevalence of Deficiency in Pregnant Women[b]	Mutations/DNA Damage	Epigenetic Alterations	Brain Development Abnormalities	Ecologic Data Support Role?	No. of Epidemiologic Studies that Have Found Effect
			Evidence for Protection Against:				
Folate[c]	Leafy vegetables; liver; beans and peas; fruits such as bananas, grapefruits, and strawberries; vegetables such as beets, broccoli, and corn; fortified cereals and breads	*Low-income countries:* Sri Lanka: 57% India: 42% Thailand: 15% *Middle-income country:* Venezuela: 36% *High-income country:* Japan: 21%	X	X	X	X	1
Vitamin D[d]	Sun exposure, fish liver oils, fatty fish, eggs, liver, fortified dairy products, breads, and cereals	*Low-income countries:* India: 84% Iran: 46–86% *Middle-income country:* Turkey: 80% *High-income countries:* United States: 5–50% Ireland: 6–44% England: 16–44%	X		X	X	1[e]
Iron[f]	Red meat, fish, poultry, beans and lentils, leafy vegetables, tofu, fortified breads and cereals	*Low-income countries:* India: 49% China: 35% Nigeria: 48% *Middle-income country:* Peru: 65% *High-income country:* Germany: 47%	X		X		1

Nutrient	Food sources	Deficiency prevalence[b]					
n-3 Polyunsaturated fatty acids (PUFAs)	Fish, meats, vegetable oils, grain products, legumes such as soy and pinto beans, nuts and seeds, leeks	N/A				X	X
Zinc[g]	Red meat; crops grown in zinc-rich soil such as wheat, seeds, beans, and nuts	*Low-income countries:* India: 74% Malawi: 37% *Middle-income country:* Peru: 60% *High-income country:* Spain: 35%				X	X
Selenium[h]	Brazil nuts, meat, fish such as tuna and cod, crops grown in selenium-rich soil	*Low-income country:* Ethiopia, HIV–: 19% Ethiopia, HIV+: 45% *Middle-income country:* Russia: 23–50%	X			X	X
Retinoids[i]	Liver; whole milk; vegetables such as carrots, sweet potatoes, kale, spinach, and pumpkin; butter; some fortified foods	*Low-income countries:* Nigeria: 2% Philippines: 18% *Middle-income country:* Mexico: 12% *High-income country:* Canada: 0%				X	

[a] Sources supporting evidence for protection against various conditions as well as epidemiological studies linking specific nutrients to schizophrenia are cited within the body of this chapter. Source for the table as a whole: authors.

[b] Deficiency prevalence was assessed by ecologic methods in the sources cited. National income levels were assigned according to 2009 World Bank (WB) classifications. Low-income countries included those in the low and low-middle income WB categories; middle-income countries included those in the WB upper-middle-income category; and high-income countries included those in the WB high-income category.

[c] Seshadri, 2001; García-Casal et al., 2005; Matsuzaki et al., 2008.

[d] Pehlivan et al., 2003; Sachan et al., 2005; Bodnar et al., 2007; Lee et al., 2007; O'Riordan et al., 2008; Holmes et al., 2009; Kazemi et al., 2009; Saintonge et al., 2009.

[e] Trend level association only.

[f] O'Brien et al., 1999; Seshadri, 2001; Bergmann et al., 2002.

[g] Gibson & Huddle, 1998; Martin-Lagos et al., 1998; Seshadri, 2001; Pathak et al., 2004.

[h] Golubkina & Alfthan, 2002; Kassu et al., 2008.

[i] World Health Organization global database on vitamin A deficiency (WHO 2011).

n-3 supplement scored higher on a test of mental processing than children who had received the n-6 supplement (Helland et al., 2003). Other studies have found no effect of DHA levels at birth (Ghys et al., 2002; Bakker et al., 2003) on cognitive function and visual acuity, however.

Although studies of n-3 PUFAs during pregnancy appear to indicate that adequate levels promote neurodevelopment, there is some evidence that high levels of maternal DHA may have deleterious effects. For example, when rat dams were fed high levels of DHA during pregnancy and gestation, their pups developed the auditory startle reflex significantly later than control pups, and auditory brain stem conduction times were also longer (Stockard et al., 2000; Haubner et al., 2001). The authors hypothesized that these effects may have occurred secondary to abnormal myelination of the auditory brain stem as a result of high DHA levels. Thus, although low prenatal levels of n-3 PUFAS may result in outcomes such as reduced visual acuity and learning ability in rats (Bourre et al., 1989), high levels may also be detrimental. In addition, although modest levels of DHA appear to protect against oxidative damage, high levels may increase susceptibility to this outcome. The six double bonds of the DHA molecule predispose it to attack by oxidants that remove electrons from the molecule. After this occurs, DHA itself can act as an oxidizer, capable of producing a variety of peroxides that damage cellular components. Only one study has examined the effects of DHA levels on oxidative damage in pregnant women. This study found that levels of MDA (a marker of lipid peroxidation) and 8-OHdG (a marker of DNA damage) were no higher in women taking daily doses of 500 mg of DHA supplements than in controls (Shoji et al., 2006). Because this study was limited by a small sample size capable of detecting only large effects, however, the level at which DHA potentially becomes harmful in pregnant women is poorly understood. Collectively, studies of DHA during gestation provide some evidence that moderate levels of n-3 PUFAs promote healthy brain development in utero, although additional investigation is necessary.

Thus far, no human studies on prenatal n-3 PUFA consumption and schizophrenia risk have been published, but the association between breast-feeding and schizophrenia has been examined, providing some insight into early intake of these fatty acids and the risk of developing this disorder. One study in southwest Scotland, based on maternal recall of breast-feeding 40 to 50 years later, found that the incidence of breast-feeding in mothers of schizophrenia patients (N = 45) was lower than that reported for their siblings and in surveys of the general Scottish population during the relevant years (McCreadie, 1997). Subsequently, in a study of the Copenhagen Perinatal Cohort, it was found that both lack of breast-feeding and breast-feeding done for less than two weeks were associated with an elevated risk of schizophrenia (Sørensen et al., 2005). A case-control study in South Africa found that a longer duration of breast-feeding was associated with reduced risk of developing schizophrenia (Hartog, Oosthuizen, & Emsley, 2007). Not all studies have replicated these findings, however. A relatively large study in Japan (Sasaki et al., 2000) and a study of two British national birth cohorts (Leask et al., 2000) found no relationship between breast-feeding and protection against schizophrenia. Finally, a study of schizophrenia cases and controls in Italy reported no association between breast-feeding and protection against schizophrenia, although the evidence did support a correlation between the duration of breast-feeding and delayed onset of the disorder (Amore et al., 2003). Collectively, the evidence linking DHA-rich breast milk and reduced schizophrenia risk is inconsistent. The number of findings suggesting a preventative effect, however, provides some support for the hypothesis that an adequate supply of DHA during early development may protect against development of this disorder.

Trace Metals

ZINC. The hypothesis that prenatal zinc deficiency may play a role in schizophrenia has been proposed (Andrews, 1990, 1992). It is clear that zinc is important in the neurodevelopment of humans, and insufficient zinc levels early in pregnancy can lead to serious deformities, such as anencephaly. In a randomized controlled trial, pregnant women given zinc supplements had babies with improved neurobehavioral development, as measured by fetal heart rate and movement patterns (Merialdi et al., 1999). Studies in animal models are consistent with findings in humans and provide insights into the responsible mechanisms. Embryonic rat neural cells are especially susceptible to zinc deficiency, dying at a higher rate than other types of cells (Harding, Dreosti, & Tulsi, 1988). Not surprisingly, exposure of fetal rats to zinc deficiency results in reduced fetal growth and a lower number of neurons (McKenzie, Fosmire, & Sandstead, 1975). There is also evidence that maternal zinc deficiency in mice suppresses the development of neural stem cells, which could lead to future neuroanatomic and behavioral abnormalities (Wang et al., 2001). In addition to physical changes found in animal models, a number of behavioral sequelae have been noted, which persist into adulthood even after the provision of a normal diet upon weaning (Halas & Hanlon, 1975; Halas & Sandstead, 1975; Halas, Hunt, & Eberhardt, 1986; Bruno et al., 2007).

Low prenatal zinc levels have the potential to result in both increased de novo mutation rates and changes in methylation patterns in the fetus, two mechanisms by which this trace metal could alter schizophrenia risk. First, studies in animal models have demonstrated that zinc guards against DNA damage by reactive oxygen species (Ho & Ames, 2002; Bruno et al., 2007). This metal plays an important role in DNA transcription factor function and in base and nucleotide excision repair, and dietary deficiency can lead to single and double strand breaks in DNA (Castro et al., 1992; Olin et al., 1993). For these reasons, insufficient stores of zinc may facilitate the accumulation of de novo mutations. Second, zinc plays a role in epigenetic regulation. Proteins featuring zinc finger domains establish and maintain methylation patterns (Ohlsson, Renkawitz, & Lobanenkov, 2001) and are associated with epigenetic reprogramming events (Loukinov et al., 2002). Zinc is a cofactor for DNA methyltransferase (Bestor, 1992), and zinc finger domains are found in methyl-DNA-binding proteins (Salozhin, Prokhorchuck, & Georgiev, 2005). Thus, zinc is essential for proper functioning at many levels in the process of epigenetic regulation, and inadequate amounts of this trace metal have the potential to alter methylation patterns.

SELENIUM. It has been proposed previously that selenium deficiency influences schizophrenia risk (Brown & Foster, 1996). Most selenium is ingested through cereal crops, which become enriched with the element through the soil in which they are grown. Ecologic studies have linked selenium-deficient soil with schizophrenia. An analysis of U.S. state and county medical hospital records from 1965 found that of 219 environmental variables, low selenium level in fodder crops was the most strongly correlated with elevated schizophrenia prevalence (Foster, 1998). A subsequent analysis of prevalence data drawn from nine U.S. schizophrenia surveys conducted between 1880 and 1963 also reported a significant correlation between low-selenium soil and increased schizophrenia rates at the state level (Brown, 1994). Although these data suffer from the limitations characteristic of all ecologic studies and could point toward the importance of selenium at any point during the life course, they do provide some rationale for the hypothesis that there is a relationship between prenatal selenium deficiency and schizophrenia.

Laboratory studies further support the plausibility of a role for prenatal selenium levels in schizophrenia. When animals are deprived of selenium, supply to the brain is prioritized (Behne, Hilmert, & Scheid, 1988), indicating that this micronutrient has an important role in brain function (Benton, 2002). In support of this hypothesis, it has been shown that selenite is an essential component of the medium used to culture central neurons (Schweizer & Schomburg, 2006) and that selenoprotein P promotes the survival of cultured neurons (Yan & Barrett, 1998). Selenium has also been shown to protect against neuronal damage and death in response to free radicals (Savaskan et al., 2003). Finally, mRNA levels of brain-derived neurotrophic factor fall in rat pups born to dams fed a selenium-deficient diet, as does the production of selenoenyzymes required for the expression of thyroid enzymes essential for certain stages of normal brain development (Mitchell et al., 1998).

The role of selenium in guarding against oxidative stress, which can result in de novo mutations, and in altering genomic methylation patterns has been well characterized. Selenoenzymes catalyze a number of reactions known to neutralize free radicals (Schweizer & Schomburg, 2006). For example, selenium is an integral component of the enzyme glutathione peroxidase (GPX), which protects against reactive oxygen species. As might be expected, this enzyme's activity is responsive to available selenium, falling with serum levels (Zimmerman et al., 2004). Selenoprotein R and thioredoxin, another selenoprotein, play similar protective roles (Schweizer & Schomburg, 2006). Because oxidative stress increases DNA damage, selenium deficiency could result in a higher mutation rate, increasing the likelihood that the sequence of a schizophrenia-related genetic region will be altered. There is also good evidence that selenium levels influence the methylation of genes and thus affect epigenetic regulation. Selenium can reverse the hypermethylation of genes, such as those coding for tumor suppressors, in human prostate cancer cells (Xiang et al., 2008). Similarly, young rats fed a selenium-rich diet display altered methylation patterns (Davis, Uthus, & Finley, 2000; Uthus, Ross, & Davis, 2006). Thus, prenatal selenium deficiency could potentially influence neurodevelopment via either genetic or epigenetic mechanisms.

RETINOIDS. A role for maternal levels of retinoids in modulating risk of schizophrenia is plausible and has been proposed previously (Goodman, 1995, 1998). Retinol and other retinoids play important roles in basic developmental processes, including signaling pathways (Dräger, 2006), gene expression, and cell differentiation, proliferation, and migration (Omori & Chytil, 1982; Nau & Elmazar, 1999; Maden, 2002). In animal models, prenatal vitamin A deficiency can result in neural crest, ocular, and other nervous system defects (Dickman, Thaller, & Smith, 1997). Conversely, excessive maternal vitamin A can have deleterious effects on neurodevelopment, perhaps through increased oxidative damage. For example, one study found that mothers who consumed more than 15,000 IU of vitamin A had 3.5 times the prevalence of cranial-neural-crest defects than those who consumed 5,000 IU or less (Rothman et al., 1995). There is also evidence that retinoids protect against DNA damage and thus de novo mutations by acting as antioxidants, shielding DNA from free radicals; vitamin A (retinol) deficiency results in oxidative damage in rats (Barber et al., 2000). In vitro studies, however, indicate that high levels of retinol can also cause DNA damage, apparently by generating free radicals and modulating antioxidant enzyme activity (Murata & Kawanishi, 2000; Dal-Pizzol et al., 2001).

Conclusion

In this chapter, we reviewed evidence suggesting that prenatal nutritional factors modify the risk of schizophrenia. This hypothesis, first proposed to account for seasonal birth rate variation in schizophrenia, was strengthened by studies demonstrating the effect of famine during pregnancy on the prevalence of this psychiatric illness. Prospective birth cohort studies have yielded additional evidence for a role of prenatal nutrition in schizophrenia. These findings include significant associations between schizophrenia and both low and high maternal BMI and small and large size at birth, elevated prenatal homocysteine levels, and maternal iron deficiency.

Although most of these results await replication in other samples, it is probable that in the coming years such studies will be performed. We would like to propose a number of additional future directions for research. Studies on n-3 PUFAs, trace elements such as zinc and selenium, and retinoids appear promising in light of the important roles these nutrients play during prenatal brain development. In addition, although investigations thus far have focused primarily on samples in high-income countries, it is our hope that studies in middle- and low-income countries will also become feasible. These would provide insight into the effect of prenatal nutrition on schizophrenia risk in the settings in which many deficiencies are most common. Characterizing the effect of maternal polymorphisms in proteins relevant to prenatal nutrition, such as those participating in the folate cycle or encoding vitamin D receptors, may provide insight into the importance of micronutrients during this period as well. Such studies could potentially be performed using samples from adult subjects and their living parents, circumventing the need for rare and previously banked biological samples drawn during pregnancy or at birth; if the maternal genotype appears to be more important than the offspring genotype in determining risk, nutrition in the prenatal environment would be implicated. Finally, we must remain cognizant of the fact that different micronutrient deficiencies often occur together in individuals. As more is learned about the role of individual micronutrients in the prenatal period, it will be important to contextualize results by characterizing the interactions between them in relation to schizophrenia risk.

One of the most promising implications of these studies is the potential to correct prenatal nutritional imbalances, once they are identified as important risk factors, in order to avert future cases of schizophrenia. The addition of iodine to salt to prevent cretinism and of folate to flour to prevent NTDs are two excellent examples of micronutrient supplementation campaigns factoring among the great public health success stories. These inexpensive interventions are highly cost-effective when one considers the economic impact of the diseases they prevent. They are also relatively easy to administer on a large scale and are able to reach a large fraction of the susceptible population. Schizophrenia is a debilitating disease, estimated to be the eighth leading cause of disability-adjusted life-years (DALYs) lost worldwide (Theodoridou & Watson, 2010). It is our view that pursuing prenatal nutritional interventions could represent an important avenue to alleviating the functional impairments and suffering caused by this disorder and thus could have significant implications for improving public health.

KEY AREAS FOR FUTURE RESEARCH

- Replicate the results of epidemiologic studies demonstrating associations between prenatal nutrient levels and schizophrenia.
- Explore the role of as yet uninvestigated nutrients—such as PUFAs, selenium, zinc, and retinoids—in schizophrenia risk.
- Investigate associations between prenatal malnutrition and schizophrenia in the low-income settings in which they are most common.
- Examine the effect of interactions between multiple micronutrient deficiencies during pregnancy on schizophrenia risk.

Selected Readings

Brown, A., Bottiglieri, T., Schaefer, C., Quesenberry, C., Liu, L., Bresnahan, M., & Susser, E. (2007). Elevated prenatal homocysteine levels as a risk factor for schizophrenia. *Archives of General Psychiatry* 64(1): 31–39.

Gunnell, D., Rasmussen, F., Fouskakis, D., Tynelius, P., & Harrison, G. (2003). Patterns of fetal and childhood growth and the development of psychosis in young males: A cohort study. *American Journal of Epidemiology* 158(4): 291–300.

Hoek, H., Brown, A., & Susser, E. (1997). The Dutch Famine and schizophrenia spectrum disorders. *Social Psychiatry and Psychiatric Epidemiology* 33(8): 373–379.

Insel, B., Schaefer, C., McKeague, I., Susser, E., & Brown, A. (2008). Maternal iron deficiency and the risk of schizophrenia in offspring. *Archives of General Psychiatry* 65(10): 1136–1144.

Kawai, M., Minabe, Y., Takagai, S., Ogai, M., Matsumoto, H., Mori, N., & Takei, V. (2004). Poor maternal care and high maternal body mass index in pregnancy as a risk factor for schizophrenia in offspring. *Acta Psychiatrica Scandinavica* 110(4): 257–263.

McGrath, J., Eyles, D., Mowry, B., Yolken, R., & Buka, S. (2003). Low maternal vitamin D as a risk factor for schizophrenia: A pilot study using banked sera. *Schizophrenia Research* 63(1–2): 73–78.

Schaefer, C., Brown, A., Wyatt, R., Kline, J., Begg, M., Bresnahan, M., & Susser, E. (2000). Maternal prepregnant body mass and risk of schizophrenia in adult offspring. *Schizophrenia Bulletin* 26(2): 275–286.

St Clair, D., Xu, M., Wang, P., Yu, Y., Fang, Y., Zhang, F., Zheng, X., Gu, N., Feng, G., Sham, P., et al. (2005). Rates of adult schizophrenia following prenatal exposure to the Chinese famine of 1959–1961. *Journal of the American Medical Association* 294(5): 557–562.

Wahlbeck, K., Forsén, T., Osmond, C., Barker, D., & Eriksson, J. (2001). Association of schizophrenia with low body mass index, small size at birth, and thinness during childhood. *Archives of General Psychiatry 58*(1): 48–52.

Xu, M., Wen-Sheng, S., Liu, B., Feng, G., Yu, L., Yang, L., He, G., Sham, P., Susser, E., St Clair, D., et al. (2009). Prenatal malnutrition and adult schizophrenia: Further evidence from the 1959–1961 famine. *Schizophrenia Bulletin 35*(3): 568–576.

References

Akil, M., Pierri, J., Whitehead, R., Edgar, C., Mohila, C., Sampson, A., & Lewis, D. (1999). Lamina-specific alterations in the dopamine innervation of the prefrontal cortex in schizophrenic subjects. *American Journal of Psychiatry 156*(10): 1580–1589.

Ames, B. (2001). DNA damage from micronutrient deficiencies is likely to be a major cause of cancer. *Mutation Research 475*(1–2): 7–20.

Amore, M., Balista, C., McCreadie, R., Cimmino, C., Pisani, F., Bevilacqua, G., & Ferrari, G. (2003). Can breast-feeding protect against schizophrenia? *Biology of the Neonate 83*(2): 97–101.

Andrews, R. C. (1990). Unification of the findings in schizophrenia by reference to the effects of gestational zinc deficiency. *Medical Hypotheses 31*(2): 141–153.

Andrews, R. C. (1992). An update of the zinc deficiency theory of schizophrenia. Identification of the sex determining system as the site of action of reproductive zinc deficiency. *Medical Hypotheses 38*(4): 284–291.

Armitage, J., Khan, I., Taylor, P., Nathanielsz, P., & Poston, L. (2004). Developmental programming of the metabolic syndrome by maternal nutritional imbalance: How strong is the evidence from experimental models in mammals? *Journal of Physiology 561*(Pt 2): 355–377.

Aslan, M., Horoz, M., Kocyigit, A., Ozgonül, S., Celik, H., Celik, M., & Erel, O. (2006). Lymphocyte DNA damage and oxidative stress in patients with iron deficiency anemia. *Mutation Research 601*(1–2): 144–149.

Bagnyukova, T., Powell, C., Pavliv, O., Tryndyak, V., & Pogribny, I. (2008). Induction of oxidative stress and DNA damage in rat brain by a folate/methyl-deficient diet. *Brain Research 1237*: 44–51.

Bakker, E., Ghys, A., Kester, A., Vles, J., Dubas, J., Blanco, C., & Hornstra, G. (2003). Long-chain polyunsaturated fatty acids at birth and cognitive function at 7 y of age. *European Journal of Clinical Nutrition 57*(1): 89–95.

Barber, T., Borrás, E., Torres, L., García, C., Cabezuelo, F., Lloret, A., Pallardó, F., & Viña, J. (2000). Vitamin A deficiency causes oxidative damage to liver mitochondria in rats. *Free Radical Biology and Medicine 29*(1): 1–7.

Barden, A., Mori, T., Dunstan, J., Taylor, A., Thornton, C., Croft, K., Beilin, L., & Prescott, S. (2004). Fish oil supplementation in pregnancy lowers F2-ioprostanes in neonates at high risk of atopy. *Free Radical Research 38*(3): 233–239.

Bassett, A., Bury, A., Hodgkinson, K., & Honer, W. (1996). Reproductive fitness in familial schizophrenia. *Schizophrenia Research 21*(3): 151–160.

Bazan, N. & Scott, B. (1990). Dietary omega-3 fatty acids and accumulation of docosahexaenoic acid in rod photoreceptor cells of the retina and at synapses. *Upsala Journal of Medical Sciences Supplement 48*: 97–107.

Behne, D., Hilmert, H., & Scheid, S. (1988). Evidence for specific selenium target tissues and new biologically important selenoproteins. *Biochimica et Biophysica Acta 966*(1): 12–21.

Ben-Schachar, D., Ashkenazi, R., & Youdim, M. (1986). Long-term consequence of early iron-deficiency on dopaminergic neurotransmission in rats. *International Journal of Developmental Neuroscience* 4(1): 81–88.

Benatti, P., Peluso, G., Nicolai, R., & Calvani, M. (2004). Polyunsaturated fatty acids: Biochemical, nutritional and epigenetic properties. *Journal of the American College of Nutrition* 23(4): 281–302.

Benton, D. (2002). Selenium intake, mood, and other aspects of psychological functioning. *Nutritional Neuroscience* 5(6): 363–374.

Bergmann, R., Gravens-Müller, L., Hertwig, K., Hinkel, J., Andres, B., Bergmann, K., & Dudenhausen, J. (2002). Iron deficiency is prevalent in a sample of pregnant women at delivery in Germany. *European Journal of Obstetrics, Gynecology, and Reproductive Biology* 102(2): 155–160.

Bestor, T. (1992). Activation of mammalian DNA methyltransferase by cleavage of a Zn binding regulatory domain. *EMBO Journal* 11(7): 2611–2617.

Birch, E., Garfield, S., Hoffman, D., Uauy, R., & Birch, D. (2000). A randomized controlled trial of early dietary supply of long-chain polyunsaturated fatty acids and mental development in term infants. *Developmental Medicine and Child Neurology* 42(3): 174–181.

Black, R., Allen, L., Bhutta, Z., Caulfield, L., Onis, M. d., Ezzati, M., Mathers, C., & Rivera, J. (2008). Maternal and child undernutrition: Global and regional exposures and health consequenes. *Lancet* 371(9608): 243–260.

Bodnar, L., Simhan, H., Powers, R., Frank, M., Cooperstein, E., & Roberts, J. (2007). High prevalence of vitamin D insufficiency in black and white pregnant women residing in the Northern United States and their neonates. *Journal of Nutrition* 137(2): 447–452.

Bottiglieri, T. (2005). Homocysteine and folate metabolism in depression. *Progress in Neuro-Psychopharmacology and Biological Psychiatry* 29(7): 1103–1112.

Bourre, J., Francois, M., Youyou, A., Dumont, O., Piciotti, M., Pascal, G., & Durand, G. (1989). The effects of dietary alpha-linolenic acid on the composition of nerve membranes, enzymatic activity, amplitude of electrophysiological parameters, resistance to poisons and performance of learning tasks in rats. *Journal of Nutrition* 119(12): 1880–1892.

Boxmeer, J., Smit, M., Utomo, E., Romijn, J., Eijkemans, M., Lindemans, J., Laven, J., Macklon, N., Steegers, E., & Steegers-Theunissen, R. (2009). Low folate in seminal plasma is associated with increased sperm damage. *Fertility and Sterility* 92(2): 548–556.

Breckenridge, W., Gombos, G., & Morgan, I. (1971). The docosahexaenoic acid of the phospholipids of synaptic membranes, vesicles and mitochondria. *Brain Research* 33(2): 581–583.

Brown, A., Bottiglieri, T., Schaefer, C., Quesenberry, C., Liu, L., Bresnahan, M., & Susser, E. (2007). Elevated prenatal homocysteine levels as a risk factor for schizophrenia. *Archives of General Psychiatry* 64(1): 31–39.

Brown, J. (1994). Role of selenium and other trace elements in the geography of schizophrenia. *Schizophrenia Bulletin* 20(2): 387–398.

Brown, J. & Foster, H. (1996). Schizophrenia: An update of the selenium deficiency hypothesis. *Journal of Orthomolecular Medicine* 11(4): 211–222.

Bruno, R., Song, Y., Leonard, S., Mustacich, D., Taylor, A., Traber, M., & Ho, E. (2007). Dietary zinc restriction in rats alters antioxidant status and increases plasma F_2 isoprostanes. *Journal of Nutritional Biochemistry* 18(8): 509–518.

Cabelof, D., Yanamadala, S., Raffoul, J., Guo, Z., Soofi, A., & Heydari, A. (2003). Caloric restriction promotes genomic stability by induction of base excision repair and reversal of its age-related decline. *DNA Repair* 2(3): 295–307.

Cannon, M., Jones, P., & Murray, R. (2002). Obstetric complications and schizophrenia: Historical and meta-analytic review. *American Journal of Psychiatry* 159(7): 1080–1092.

Cannon, T., Rosso, I., Hollister, J., Bearden, C., Sanchez, L., & Hadley, T. (2000). A prospective cohort study of genetic and perinatal influences in the etiology of schizophrenia. *Schizophrenia Bulletin* 26(2): 351–366.

Carlson, S. & Neuringer, M. (1999). Polyunsaturated fatty acid status and neurodevelopment: A summary and critical analysis of the literature. *Lipids* 34(2): 171–178.

Castro, C., Kaspin, L., Chen, S., & Nolker, S. (1992). Zinc deficiency increases the frequency of single-strand DNA breaks in rat liver. *Nutritional Research* 12(6): 721–736.

Chang, G., Gaysinskaya, V., Karatayev, O., & Leibowitz, S. (2008). Maternal high-fat diet and fetal programming: Increased proliferation of hypothalamic peptide-producing neurons that increase risk for overeating and obesity. *Journal of Neuroscience* 28(46): 12107–12119.

Chatterjee, M. (2001). Vitamin D and genomic stability. *Mutation Research* 475(1–2): 69–88.

Cohen, S., Nichols, A., Wyatt, R., & Pollin, W. (1974). The administration of methionine to chronic schizophrenic patients: A review of ten studies. *Biological Psychiatry* 8(2): 209–225.

Connor, J. & Menzies, S. (1996). Relationship of iron to oligodendrocytes and myelination. *Glia* 17(2): 83–93.

Cooney, C., Dave, A., & Wolff, G. (2002). Maternal methyl supplements in mice affect epigenetic variation and DNA methylation of offspring. *Journal of Nutrition* 132(8 Suppl): S2393–2400.

Crane, S., Wojtowycz, M., Dye, T., Aubry, R., & Artal, R. (1997). Association between prepregnancy obesity and the risk of cesarean delivery. *Obstetrics and Gynecology* 89(2): 213–216.

Crow, J. (2000). The origins, patterns and implications of human spontaneous mutation. *Nature Reviews Genetics* 1(1): 40–47.

Dal-Pizzol, F., Klamt, F., Benfato, M., Bernard, E., & Moreira, J. (2001). Retinol supplementation induces oxidative stress and modulates antioxidant enzyme activities in rat Sertoli cells. *Free Radical Research* 34(4): 395–404.

Dalén, P. (1975). *Season of Birth: A Study of Schizophrenia and Other Mental Disorders.* New York: North-Holland/American Elsevier.

Dalman, C., Thomas, H., David, A., Gentz, J., Lewis, G., & Allebeck, P. (2001). Signs of asphyxia at birth and risk of schizophrenia. *British Journal of Psychiatry* 179: 403–408.

Davis, C., Uthus, E., & Finley, J. (2000). Dietary selenium and arsenic affect DNA methylation *in vitro* in Caco-2 cells and *in vivo* in rat liver and colon. *Journal of Nutrition* 130(12): 2903–2909.

De Sauvage Nolting, W. (1954). Vitamin C and the schizophrenic syndrome. *Folia Psychiatrica, Neurologica et Neurochirurgica Neerlandica* 57(3): 347–355.

Deinard, A., Gilbert, A., Dodds, M., & Egeland, B. (1981). Iron deficiency and behavioral deficits. *Pediatrics* 68(6): 828–833.

Dickman, E., Thaller, C., & Smith, S. (1997). Temporally-regulated retinoic acid depletion produces specific neural crest, ocular and nervous system defects. *Development* 124(16): 3111–3121.

Dräger, U. (2006). Retinoic acid signaling in the functioning brain. *Science STKE* 324: pe10.

Edelson, J., Chan, S., Jassal, D., Post, M., & Tanswell, A. (1994). Vitamin D stimulates DNA synthesis in alveolar type-II cells. *Biochimica et Biophysica Acta* 1221(2): 159–166.

Ellison, T., Smith, M., Gilliam, A., & MacDonald, P. (2008). Inactivation of the vitamin D receptor enhances susceptiblity of murine skin to UV-induced tumorigenesis. *Journal of Investigative Dermatology* 128(10): 2508–2517.

Fedorova, I. & Salem, N. (2006). Omega-3 fatty acids and rodent behavior. *Prostaglandins Leukotrienes and Medicine* 75(4–5): 271–289.

Fenech, M. (2001). The role of folic acid and Vitamin B12 in genomic stability of human cells. *Mutation Research* 475(1–2): 57–67.

Flynn, S., Lang, D., Mackay, A., Goghari, V., Vavsour, I., Whittall, K., Smith, G., Arango, V., Mann, J., Dwork, A., et al. (2003). Abnormalities of myelination in schizophrenia detected *in vivo* with MRI, and post-mortem with analysis of oligodendrocyte proteins. *Molecular Psychiatry* 8(9): 811–820.

Foster, H. (1998). The geography of schizophrenia: Possible links with selenium and calcium deficiencies, inadequate exposure to sunlight and industrialization. *Journal of Orthomolecular Medicine* 3(3): 135–140.

Frankenburg, F. (2007). The role of one-carbon metabolism in schizophrenia and depression. *Harvard Review of Psychiatry* 15(4): 146–160.

Fuller, R., Nopoulos, P., Arndt, S., O'Leary, D., Ho, B., & Andreasen, N. (2002). Longitudinal assessment of premorbid cognitive functioning in patients with schizophrenia through examination of standardized scholastic test performance. *American Journal of Psychiatry* 159(7): 1183–1189.

García-Casal, M., Osorio, C., Landaeta, M., Leets, I., Matus, P., Fazzino, F., & Marcos, E. (2005). High prevalence of folic acid and vitamin B12 deficiencies in infants, children, adolescents and pregnant women in Venezuela. *European Journal of Clinical Nutrition* 59(9): 1064–1070.

Ghys, A., Bakker, E., Hornstra, G., & van den Hout, M. (2002). Red blood cell and plasma phospholipid arachidonic and docosahexaenoic acid levels at birth and cognitive development at 4 years of age. *Early Human Development* 69(1–2): 83–90.

Gibson, R. & Huddle, J. (1998). Suboptimal zinc status in pregnant Malawian women: Its association with low intakes of poorly available zinc, frequent reproductive cycling, and malaria. *American Journal of Clinical Nutrition* 67(4): 702–709.

Godfrey, P., Toone, B., Carney, M., Flynn, T., Bottiglieri, T., Laundy, M., Chanarin, I., & Reynolds, E. (1990). Enhancement of recovery from psychiatric illness by methylfolate. *Lancet* 336(8712): 392–395.

Golubkina, N. & Alfthan, G. (2002). Selenium status of pregnant women and newborns in the former Soviet Union. *Biological Trace Element Research* 89(1): 13–23.

Goodman, A. (1995). Chromosomal locations and modes of action of genes of the retinoid (vitamin A) system support their involvement in the etiology of schizophrenia. *American Journal of Medical Genetics* 60(4): 335–348.

Goodman, A. (1998). Three independent lines of evidence suggest retinoids as causal to schizophrenia. *Proceedings of the National Academy of Sciences U.S.A.* 95(13): 7240–7244.

Görtz, P., Hoinkes, A., Fleischer, W., Otto, F., Schwahn, B., Wendel, U., & Siebler, M. (2004). Implications for hyperhomocysteinemia: Not homocysteine but its oxidized forms strongly inhibit neuronal network activity. *Journal of Neuroscience* 218(1–2): 109–114.

Gottesman, I. & Shields, J. (1982). *Schizophrenia: The Epigenetic Puzzle*. Cambridge, UK: Cambridge University Press.

Greiner, R., Moriguchi, T., Slotnick, B., Hutton, A., & Salem, N. (2001). Olfactory discrimination deficits in n-3 fatty acid-deficient rats. *Physiology and Behavior* 72(3): 379–385.

Gunnell, D., Rasmussen, F., Fouskakis, D., Tynelius, P., & Harrison, G. (2003). Patterns of fetal and childhood growth and the development of psychosis in young males: A cohort study. *American Journal of Epidemiology* 158(4): 291–300.

Hakak, Y., Walker, J., Li, C., Wong, W., Davis, K., Buxbaum, J., Haroutunian, V., & Fienberg, A. (2001). Genome-wide expression analysis reveals dysregulation of myelination-related genes in chronic schizophrenia. *Proceedings of the National Academy of Sciences U.S.A.* 98(8): 4746–4751.

Halas, E. & Hanlon, M. (1975). Intrauterine nutrition and aggression. *Nature* 257(5523): 221–222.

Halas, E., Hunt, C., & Eberhardt, M. (1986). Learning and memory disabilities in young adult rats from mildly zinc deficient dams. *Physiology and Behavior* 37(3): 451–458.

Halas, E. & Sandstead, H. (1975). Some effects of prenatal zinc deficiency on behavior of the adult rat. *Pediatric Research* 9(2): 94–97.

Handoko, H., Nancarrow, D., Mowry, B., & McGrath, J. (2006). Polymorphisms in the vitamin D receptor and their associations with risk of schizophrenia and selected anthropometric measures. *American Journal of Human Biology* 18(3): 415–417.

Harding, A., Dreosti, I., & Tulsi, R. (1988). Zinc deficiency in the 11 day rat embryo: A scanning and transmission electron microscope study. *Life Sciences* 42(8): 889–896.

Hartog, M., Oosthuizen, P., & Emsley, R. (2007). Longer duration of breastfeeding associated with reduced risk of developing schizophrenia. *South African Journal of Psychiatry* 13(2): 60–64.

Hass, B., Hart, R., Lu, M., & Lyn-Cook, B. (1993). Effects of caloric restriction in animals on cellular function, oncogene expression, and DNA methylation. *Mutation Research* 295(4–6): 281–289.

Haubner, L., Stockard, J., Saste, M., Benford, V., Phelps, C., Chen, L., Barness, L., Wiener, D., & Carver, J. (2001). Maternal dietary docosahexanoic acid content affects the rat pup auditory system. *Brain Research Bulletin* 58(1): 1–5.

Heijmans, B., Tobi, E., Stein, A., Putter, H., Blauw, G., Susser, E., Slagboom, P., & Lumey, L. (2008). Persistent epigenetic differences associated with prenatal exposure to famine in humans. *Proceedings of the National Academy of Sciences U.S.A.* 105(44): 17046–17049.

Helland, I., Smith, L., Saarem, K., Saugstad, O., & Drevon, C. (2003). Maternal supplementation with very-long-chain n-3 fatty acids during pregnancy and lactation augments children's IQ at 4 years of age. *Pediatrics* 111(1): e39.

Heydari, A., Unnikrishnan, A., Lucente, L., & Richardson, A. (2007). Caloric restriction and genomic stability. *Nucleic Acids Research* 35(22): 7485–7496.

Ho, E. & Ames, B. (2002). Low intracellular zinc induces oxidative DNA damage, disrupts p53, NFκB, and AP1 DNA binding, and affects DNA repair in a rat glioma cell line. *Proceedings of the National Academy of Sciences U.S.A.* 99(26): 16770–16775.

Hoek, H., Brown, A., & Susser, E. (1997). The Dutch Famine and schizophrenia spectrum disorders. *Social Psychiatry and Psyciatric Epidemiology* 33(8): 373–379.

Holmes, V., Barnes, M., Alexander, H., McFaul, P., & Wallace, J. (2009). Vitamin D deficiency and insufficiency in pregnant women: A longitudinal study. *British Journal of Nutrition* 102(6): 876–881.

Howard, L., Kumar, C., Leese, M., & Thornicroft, G. (2002). The general fertility rate in women with psychotic disorders. *American Journal of Psychiatry* 159(6): 991–997.

Hultman, C., Sparén, P., Takei, N., Murray, R., & Cnattingius, S. (1999). Prenatal and perinatal risk factors for schizophrenia, affective psychosis, and reactive psychosis of early onset: Case-control study. *British Medical Journal* 318(7181): 421–426.

Insel, B., Schaefer, C., McKeague, I., Susser, E., & Brown, A. (2008). Maternal iron deficiency and the risk of schizophrenia in offspring. *Archives of General Psychiatry* 65(10): 1136–1144.

International Schizophrenia Consortium. (2008). Rare chromosomal deletions and duplications increase risk of schizophrenia. *Nature* 455(7210): 237–241.

Jones, P., Rantakallio, P., Hartikainen, A., Isohanni, M., & Sipila, P. (1998). Schizophrenia as a long-term outcome of pregnancy, delivery, and perinatal complications: A 28-year follow-up of the 1966 North Finland General Population Birth Cohort. *American Journal of Psychiatry* 155(3): 355–364.

Jones, P., Rodgers, B., Murray, R., & Marmot, M. (1994). Child developmental risk factors for adult schizophrenia in the British 1946 birth cohort. *Lancet* 344(8934): 1398–1402.

Jönsson, E., Larsson, K., Vares, M., Hansen, T., Wang, A., Djurovic, S., Rønningen, K., Andreassen, O., Agartz, I., Werge, T., et al. (2008). Two methylenetetrahydrofolate reductase gene (MTHFR) polymorphisms, schizophrenia ad bipolar disorder: An association study. *American Journal of Medical Genetics B 147B*(6): 976–982.

Kassu, A., Yabutani, T., Mulu, A., Tessema, B., & Ota, F. (2008). Serum zinc, copper, selenium, calcium, and magnesium levels in pregnant and non-pregnant women in Gondar, Northwest Ethiopia. *Biological Trace Element Research 122*(2): 97–106.

Kawai, M., Minabe, Y., Takagai, S., Ogai, M., Matsumoto, H., Mori, N., & Takei, V. (2004). Poor maternal care and high maternal body mass index in pregnancy as a risk factor for schizophrenia in offspring. *Acta Psychiatrica Scandinavica 110*(4): 257–263.

Kazemi, A., Sharifi, F., Jafari, N., & Mousavinasab, N. (2009). High prevalence of vitamin D deficiency among pregnant women and their newborns in an Iranian population. *Journal of Women's Health 18*(6): 835–839.

Khashan, A., Abel, K., McNamee, R., Pedersen, M., Webb, R., Baker, P., Kenny, L., & Mortensen, P. (2008). Higher risk of offspring schizophrenia following antenatal maternal exposure to severe adverse life events. *Archives of General Psychiatry 65*(2): 146–152.

Laruelle, M., Abi-Dargham, A., van Dyck, C. H., Gil, R., D'Souza, C. D., Erdos, J., McCance, E., Rosenblatt, W., Fingado, C., Zoghbi, S. S., et al. (1996). Single photon emission computerized tomography imaging of amphetamine-induced dopamine release in drug-free schizophrenic subjects. *Proceedings of the National Academy of Sciences U.S.A. 93*(17): 9235–9240.

Leask, S., Done, D., Crow, T., Richards, M., & Jones, P. (2000). No association between breast-feeding and adult psychosis in two national birth cohorts. *British Journal of Psychiatry 177*: 218–221.

Lee, J., Smith, J., Philipp, B., Chen, T., Mathieu, J., & Holick, M. (2007). Vitamin D deficiency in a healthy group of mothers and newborn infants. *Clinical Pediatrics 46*(1): 42–44.

Lewis, S., Zammit, S., Gunnell, D., & Smith, G. (2005). A meta-analysis of the MTHFR C677T polymorphism and schizophrenia risk. *American Journal of Medical Genetics B, 135B*(1): 2–4.

Loukinov, D., Pugacheva, E., Vatolin, S., Pack, S., Moon, H., Chernukhin, I., Mannan, P., Larsson, E., Kanduri, C., Vostrov, A., et al. (2002). BORIS, a novel male germ-line-specific protein associated with epigenetic reprogramming events, shares the same 11-zinc-finger domain with CTCF, the insulator protein involved in reading imprinting marks in the soma. *Proceedings of the National Academy of Sciences U.S.A. 99*(10): 6806–6811.

Lozoff, B., Beard, J., Connor, J., Felt, B., Georgieff, M., & Schallert, T. (2006). Long-lasting neural and behavioral effects of iron deficiency in infancy. *Nutrition Reviews 64*(5): S34–43.

Lucas, A., Stafford, M., Morley, R., Abbott, R., Stephenson, T., MacFadyen, U., Ellas-Jones, A., & Clements, H. (1999). Efficacy and safety of long-chain polyunsaturated fatty acid supplementation of infant-formula milk: A randomised trial. *Lancet 354*(9194): 1948–1954.

Lumey, L. (1992). Decreased birthweights in infants after maternal *in utero* exposure to the Dutch famine of 1944–1945. *Paediatric and Perinatal Epidemiology 6*(2): 240–253.

Maden, M. (2002). Retinoid signalling in the development of the central nervous system. *Nature Reviews Neuroscience 3*(11): 843–853.

Malaspina, D. (2001). Paternal factors and schizophrenia risk: *De novo* mutations and imprinting. *Schizophrenia Bulletin 27*(3): 379–393.

Malaspina, D., Corcoran, C., Kleinhaus, K., Perrin, M., Fennig, S., Nahon, D., Friedlander, Y., & Harlap, S. (2008). Acute maternal stress in pregnancy and schizophrenia in offspring: A cohort prospective study. *BMC Psychiatry* 8: 71.

Malaspina, D., Harlap, S., Fennig, S., Heiman, D., Nahon, D., Feldman, D., & Susser, E. (2001). Advancing paternal age and the risk of schizophrenia. *Archives of General Psychiatry* 58(4): 361–367.

Marnett, L. (2000). Oxyradicals and DNA damage. *Carcinogenesis* 21(3): 361–370.

Martín-Lagos, F., Navarro-Alarcón, M., Terrés-Martos, C., Serrana, H. d. l., Pérez-Valero, V., & López-Martínez, M. (1998). Zinc and copper concentrations in serum from Spanish women during pregnancy. *Biological Trace Element Research* 61(1): 61–70.

Matsuzaki, M., Haruna, M., Ota, E., Sasaki, S., Nagai, Y., & Murashima, S. (2008). Dietary folate intake, use of folate supplements, lifestyle factors, and serum folate levels among pregnant women in Tokyo, Japan. *Journal of Obstetrics and Gynaecology Research* 34(6): 971–979.

Mattson, M. & Shea, T. (2003). Folate and homocysteine metabolism in neural plasticity and neurodegenerative disorders. *Trends in Neuroscience* 26(3): 137–146.

McClellan, J., Susser, E., & King, M. (2006). Maternal famine, *de novo* mutations, and schizophrenia. *Journal of the American Medical Association* 296(5): 582–584.

McCreadie, R. (1997). The Nithsdale schizophrenia surveys 16. Breastfeeding and schizophrenia: Preliminary results and hypotheses. *British Journal of Psychiatry* 170(4): 334–337.

McGrath, J. (1999). Hypothesis: Is low prenatal vitamin D a risk-modifying factor for schizophrenia? *Schizophrenia Research* 40(3): 173–177.

McGrath, J., Eyles, D., Mowry, B., Yolken, R., & Buka, S. (2003). Low maternal vitamin D as a risk factor for schizophrenia: A pilot study using banked sera. *Schizophrenia Research* 63(1–2): 73–78.

McGrath, J., Saari, K., Hakko, H., Jokelainen, J., Jones, P., Järvelin, M., Chant, D., & Isohanni, M. (2004). Vitamin D supplementation during the first year of life and risk of schizophrenia: A Finnish birth cohort study. *Schizophrenia Research* 67(2–3): 237–245.

McKenzie, J., Fosmire, G., & Sandstead, H. (1975). Zinc deficiency during the latter third of pregnancy: Effects on fetal rat brain, liver, and placenta. *Journal of Nutrition* 105(11): 1466–1475.

McMahon, M., Ananth, C., & Liston, R. (1998). Gestational diabetes mellitus: Risk factors, obstetric complications and infant outcomes. *Journal of Reproductive Medicine* 43(4): 372–378.

Merialdi, M., Caulfield, L., Zavaleta, N., Figueroa, A., & DiPietro, J. (1999). Adding zinc to prenatal iron and folate tablets improves fetal neurobehavioral development. *American Journal of Obstetrics and Gynecology* 180(2): 483–490.

Meyer-Lindenberg, A., Miletich, R., Kohn, P., Esposito, G., Carson, R., Quarantelli, M., Weinberger, D., & Berman, K. (2002). Reduced prefrontal activity predicts exaggerated striatal dopaminergic function in schizophrenia. *Nature Neuroscience* 5(3): 267–271.

Mills, J., McPartlin, J., Kirke, P., Lee, Y., Conley, M., Weir, D., & Scott, J. (1995). Homocysteine metabolism in pregnancies complicated by neural tube defects. *Lancet* 345(8943): 149–151.

Mitchell, J., Nicol, F., Beckett, G., & Arthur, J. (1998). Selenoprotein expression and brain development in preweanling selenium- and iodine-deficient rats. *Journal of Molecular Endocrinology* 20(2): 203–210.

Mori, T., Woodman, R., Burke, V., Puddey, I., Croft, K., & Beilin, L. (2003). Effect of eicosapentaenoic acid and docosahexaenoic acid on oxidative stress and inflammatory markers in treated-hypertensive type 2 diabetic subjects. *Free Radical Biology and Medicine* 35(7): 772–781.

Moskovitz, R. (1978). Seasonality in schizophrenia. *Lancet 311*(8065): 664.

Muntjewerff, J., Hoogendoorn, M., Aukes, M., Kahn, R., Sinke, R., Blom, H., & Heijer, M. D. (2007). No evidence for a preferential transmission of the methylenetetrahydrofolate reductase 677T allele in families with schizophrenia offspring. *American Journal of Medical Genetics B 144B*(7): 891–894.

Murata, M. & Kawanishi, S. (2000). Oxidative DNA damage by vitamin A and its derivative via superoxide generation. *Journal of Biological Chemistry 275*(3): 2003–2008.

Musiol, I. & Feldman, D. (1997). 1,25-dihydroxyvitamin D3 induction of nerve growth factor in L929 mouse fibroblasts: Effect of vitamin D receptor regulation and potency of vitamin D3 analogs. *Endocrinology 138*(1): 12–18.

Nau, H. & Elmazar, M. (1999). Retinoid receptors, their ligands, and teratogenesis: Synergy and specificity of effects. In H. Nau & W. Blaner (eds.), *Retinoids. The Biochemical and Molecular Basis of Vitamin A and Retinoid Action* (pp. 465–487). New York: Springer-Verlag.

Need, A., Ge, D., Weale, M., Maia, J., Feng, S., Heinzen, E., Shianna, K., Yoon, W., Kasperaviciute, D., Gennarelli, M., et al. (2009). A genome-wide investigation of SNPs and CNVs in schizophrenia. *PLoS Genetics 5*(2): e1000373.

Nelen, W., Bulten, J., Steegers, E., Blom, H., Hanselaar, A., & Eskes, T. (2000). Maternal homocysteine and chorionic vascularization in recurrent early pregnancy loss. *Human Reproduction 15*(4): 954–960.

O'Brien, K., Zavaleta, N., Caulfield, L., Yang, D., & Abrams, S. (1999). Influence of prenatal iron and zinc supplements on supplemental iron absorption, red blood cell iron incorporation, and iron status in pregnant Peruvian women. *American Journal of Clinical Nutrition 69*(3): 509–515.

O'Connor, D., Hall, R., Adamkin, D., Auestad, N., Castillo, M., Connor, W., Connor, S., Fitzgerald, K., Groh-Wargo, S., Hartmann, E., et al. (2001). Growth and development in preterm infants fed long-chain polyunsaturated fatty acids: A prospective, randomized controlled trial. *Pediatrics 108*(2): 359–371.

Ohlsson, R., Renkawitz, R., & Lobanenkov, V. (2001). CTCF is a uniquely versatile transcription regulator linked to epigenetics and disease. *Trends in Genetics 17*(9): 520–527.

Oken, E., Radesky, J., Wright, R., Bellinger, D., Amarasiriwardena, C., Kleinman, K., Hu, H., & Gillman, M. (2008). Maternal fish intake during pregnancy, blood mercury levels, and child cognition at age 3 years in a US cohort. *American Journal of Epidemiology 167*(10): 1171–1181.

Olin, K., Shigenaga, M., Ames, B., Golub, M., Gershwin, M., Hendrickx, A., & Keen, C. (1993). Maternal dietary zinc influences DNA strand break and 8-hydoxy-2'-doxyguanosine levels in infant rhesus monkey liver. *Proceedings of the Society for Experimental Biology and Medicine 203*(4): 461–466.

Omori, M. & Chytil, F. (1982). Mechanism of vitamin A action: Gene expression in retinol-deficient rats. *Journal of Biological Chemistry 257*(23): 14370–14374.

O'Riordan, M., Kiely, M., Higgins, J., & Cashman, K. (2008). Prevalence of suboptimal vitamin D status during pregnancy. *Irish Medical Journal 101*(8): 240–243.

Paashuis-Lew, Y. & Heddle, J. (1998). Spontaneous mutation during fetal development and post-natal growth. *Mutagenesis 13*(6): 613–617.

Parrish, J., Kim, M., Jan, L., & Jan, Y. (2006). Genome-wide analyses identify transcription factors required for proper morphogenesis of *Drosophila* sensory neuron dendrites. *Genes and Development 20*(7): 820–835.

Pasamanick, B. (1961). Epidemiologic investigations of some prenatal factors in the production of neuropsychiatric disorder. In P. Hoch & J. Zubin (eds.), *Comparative Epidemiology of the Mental Disorders* (pp. 260–275). New York: Grune and Stratton.

Pathak, P., Kapil, U., Kapoor, S., Saxena, R., Kumar, A., Gupta, N., Dwivedi, S., Singh, R., & Singh, P. (2004). Prevalence of multiple micronutrient deficiencies amongst pregnant women in a rural area of Haryana. *Indian Journal of Pediatrics 71*(11): 1007–1014.

Pehlivan, I., Hatun, S., Aydogan, M., Babaoglu, K., & Gokalp, A. (2003). Maternal vitamin D deficiency and vitamin D supplementation in healthy infants. *Turkish Journal of Pediatrics 45*(4): 315–320.

Petronis, A. (2004). The origin of schizophrenia: Genetic thesis, epigenetic antithesis, and resolving synthesis. *Biological Psychiatry 55*(10): 965–970.

Pharoah, P., Buttfield, I., & Hetzel, B. (1971). Neurological damage to the fetus resulting from severe iodine deficiency during pregnancy. *Lancet 297*(7694): 308–310.

Picker, J. & Coyle, J. (2005). Do maternal folate and homocysteine levels play a role in neurodevelopmental processes that increase risk for schizophrenia? *Harvard Review of Psychiatry 13*(4): 197–205.

Rifkin, L., Lewis, S., Jones, P., Toone, B., & Murray, R. (1994). Low birth weight and schizophrenia. *British Journal of Psychiatry 165*(3): 357–362.

Roberts, J. & Cooper, D. (2001). Pathogenesis and genetics of pre-eclampsia. *Lancet 357*(9249): 53–56.

Rothman, K., Moore, L., Singer, M., NGuyen, U., Mannino, S., & Milunsky, A. (1995). Teratogeneticity of high vitamin A intake. *New England Journal of Medicine 333*(21): 1369–1373.

Sachan, A., Gupta, R., Das, V., Agarwal, A., Awasthi, P., & Bhatia, V. (2005). High prevalence of vitamin D deficiency among pregnant women and their newborns in northern India. *American Journal of Clinical Nutrition 81*(5): 1060–1064.

Saha, S., Barnett, A. G., Foldi, C., Burne, T. H., Eyles, D. W., Buka, S. L., & McGrath, J. J. (2009). Advanced paternal age is associated with impaired neurocognitive outcomes during infancy and childhood. *PLoS Medicine 6*(3): e40.

Saintonge, S., Bang, H., & Gerber, L. (2009). *Prevalence of vitamin D deficiency in national sample of pregnant women: NHANES 2001–2004.* Paper presented at the American Academy of Pediatrics National Conference. http://aap.confex.com/aap/2009/webprogram/Paper8364.html.

Salozhin, S., Prokhorchuck, E., & Georgiev, G. (2005). Methylation of DNA: One of the major epigenetic markers. *Biochemistry 70*(5): 525–532.

Sasaki, T., Okazaki, Y., Akaho, R., Masui, K., Harada, S., Lee, I., Takazawa, S., Takahashi, S., Iida, S., & Takakuwa, M. (2000). Type of feeding during infancy and later development of schizophrenia. *Schizophrenia Research 42*(1): 79–82.

Savaskan, N., Bräuer, A., Kühbacher, M., Eyüpoglu, I., Kyriakopoulos, A., Ninnemann, O., Behne, D., & Nitsch, R. (2003). Selenium deficiency increases susceptibility to glutamate-induced excitotoxicity. *FASEB Journal 17*(1): 112–114.

Schaefer, C., Brown, A., Wyatt, R., Kline, J., Begg, M., Bresnahan, M., & Susser, E. (2000). Maternal prepregnant body mass and risk of schizophrenia in adult offspring. *Schizophrenia Bulletin 26*(2): 275–286.

Schiffman, J., Sorensen, H., Maeda, J., Mortensen, E., Victoroff, J., Hayashi, K., Michelsen, N., Ekstrom, M., & Mednick, S. (2009). Childhood motor coordination and adult schizophrenia spectrum disorders. *American Journal of Psychiatry 166*(9): 1041–1047.

Schweizer, U. & Schomburg, L. (2006). Selenium, selenoproteins and brain function. In D. Hatfield, M. Berry, & V. Gladyshev (eds.), *Selenium: Its Molecular Biology and Role.* New York: Springer.

Scott, D., Janowsky, J., Carroll, R., Taylor, J., Auestad, N., & Montalto, M. (1998). Formula supplementation with long-chain polyunsaturated fatty acids: Are there developmental benefits? *Pediatrics 102*(5): e59.

Sebat, J., Levy, D., & McCarthy, S. (2009). Rare structural variants in schizophrenia: One disorder, multiple mutations; one mutation, multiple disorders. *Trends in Genetics* 25(12): 528–535.

Sepp, K., Hong, P., Liu, J., Meija, L., Walsh, C., & Perrimon, N. (2008). Identification of neural outgrowth genes using genome-wide RNAi. *PLoS Genetics* 4(7): e1000111.

Seshadri, S. (2001). Prevalence of micronutrient deficiency particularly of iron, zinc and folic acid in pregnant women in South East Asia. *British Journal of Nutrition* 85(S2): S87–92.

Sharma, R. (2005). Schizophrenia, epigenetics and ligand-activated nuclear receptors: A framework for chromatin therapeutics. *Schizophrenia Research* 72(2–3): 79–90.

Shima, N., Swiger, R., & Heddle, J. (2000). Dietary restriction during murine development provides protection against MNU-induced mutations. *Mutation Research* 470(2): 189–200.

Shoji, H., Franke, C., Campoy, C., Rivero, M., Demmelmair, H., & Koletzko, B. (2006). Effect of docosaheaenoic acid and eicosapentaenoic acid supplementation on oxidative stress levels during pregnancy. *Free Radical Research* 40(4): 379–384.

Smith, G., Flynn, S., McCarthy, N., Meistrich, B., Ehmann, T., MacEwan, G., Altman, S., Kopala, L., & Honer, W. (2001). Low birthweight in schizophrenia: Prematurity or poor fetal growth? *Schizophrenia Research* 47(2–3): 177–184.

Solomon, C., Willett, W., Carey, V., Rich-Edwards, J., Hunter, D., Colditz, G., Stampfer, M., Speizer, F., Spiegelman, D., & Manson, J. (1997). A prospective study of pregravid determinants of gestational diabetes mellitus. *Journal of the American Medical Association* 278(13): 1078–1083.

Sørensen, H., Mortensen, E., Reinisch, J., & Mednick, S. (2005). Breastfeeding and risk of schizophrenia in the Copenhagen Perinatal Cohort. *Acta Psychiatrica Scandinavica* 112(1): 26–29.

St Clair, D., Xu, M., Wang, P., Yu, Y., Fang, Y., Zhang, F., Zheng, X., Gu, N., Feng, G., Sham, P., et al. (2005). Rates of adult schizophrenia following prenatal exposure to the Chinese famine of 1959–1961. *Journal of the American Medical Association* 294(5): 557–562.

Stefansson, H., Rujescu, D., Cichon, S., Pietiläinen, O., & Ingason, A. (2008). Large recurrent microdeletions associated with schizophrenia. *Nature* 455(7210): 232–236.

Stein, Z., Susser, M., Saenger, G., & Marolla, F. (1975). *Famine and Human Development: The Dutch Hunger Winter of 1944–1945*. New York: Oxford University Press.

Stockard, J., Saste, M., Benford, V., Barness, L., Auestad, N., & Carver, J. (2000). Effect of docosahexaenoic acid content of maternal diet on auditory brainstem conduction times in rat pups. *Developmental Neuroscience* 22(5–6): 494–499.

Susser, E., Brown, A., Klonowski, E., Allen, R., & Lindenbaum, J. (1998). Schizophrenia and impaired homocysteine metabolism: A possible association. *Biological Psychiatry* 44(2): 141–143.

Susser, E., Hoek, H., & Brown, A. (1998). Neurodevelopmental disorders after prenatal famine: The story of the Dutch Famine Study. *American Journal of Epidemiology* 147(3): 213–216.

Susser, E., Neugebauer, R., Hoek, H., Brown, A., Lin, S., Labovitz, D., & Gorman, J. (1996). Schizophrenia after prenatal famine: Further evidence. *Archives of General Psychiatry* 53(1): 25–31.

Suvisaari, J., Haukka, J., Tanskanen, A., & Lönnqvist, J. (2000). Decreasing seasonal variation of births in schizophrenia. *Psychological Medicine* 30(2): 315–324.

Svennerholm, L. (1968). Distribution and fatty acid composition of phosphoglycerides in normal human brain. *Journal of Lipid Research* 9(5): 570–579.

Teo, T. & Fenech, M. (2008). The interactive effect of alcohol and folic acid on genome stability in human WIL2-NS cells measured using the cytokinesis-block micronucleus cytome assay. *Mutation Research* 657(1): 32–38.

Theodoridou, A. & Watson, R. (2010). Disease burden and disability-adjusted life years due to schizophrenia and psychotic disorders. In V. Preedy & R. Watson (eds.), *Handbook of Disease Burdens and Quality of Life Measures* (pp. 3995–4012). New York: Springer.

Tobi, E., Lumey, L., Talens, R., Kremer, D., Putter, H., Stein, A., Slagboom, P., & Heijmans, B. (2009). DNA methylation differences after exposure to prenatal famine are common and timing- and sex-specific. *Human Molecular Genetics 18*(21): 4046–4053.

Torrey, E., Miller, J., Rawlings, R., & Yolken, R. (1997). Seasonality of births in schizophrenia and bipolar disorder: A review of the literature. *Schizophrenia Research 28*(1): 1–38.

Tramer, M. (1929). Über die biologische Bedeutung des Geburtsmonates, insbesondere für die Psychoseerkrankung. *Schweizer Archiv fur Neurologie und Psychiatrie 24*: 17–24.

Uthus, E., Ross, S., & Davis, C. (2006). Differential effects of dietary selenium (Se) and folate metabolism in liver and colon of rats. *Biological Trace Element Research 109*(3): 201–214.

van Os, J. & Selten, J. P. (1998). Prenatal exposure to maternal stress and subsequent schizophrenia: The May 1940 invasion of the Netherlands. *British Journal of Psychiatry 172*: 324–326.

Vrijenhoek, T., Buizer-Voskamp, J., Stelt, I. V. D., Strengman, E., Consortium, G., & Sabatti, C. (2008). Recurrent CNVs disrupt three candidate genes in schizophrenia patients. *American Journal of Human Genetics 83*(4): 504–510.

Wahlbeck, K., Forsén, T., Osmond, C., Barker, D., & Eriksson, J. (2001). Association of schizophrenia with low body mass index, small size at birth, and thinness during childhood. *Archives of General Psychiatry 58*(1): 48–52.

Walsh, T., McClellan, J., McCarthy, S., Addington, A., Pierce, S., Cooper, G., Nord, A., Kusenda, M., Malhotra, D., Bhandari, A., et al. (2008). Rare structural variants disrupt multiple genes in neurodevelopmental pathways in schizophrenia. *Science 320*(5875): 539–543.

Walter, T., Andraca, I., Chadud, P., & Perales, C. (1989). Iron deficiency anemia: Adverse effects on infant psychomotor development. *Pediatrics 84*(1): 7–17.

Wang, F., Bian, W., Kong, L., Zhao, F., & Guo, J. (2001). Maternal zinc deficiency impairs brain nestin expression in prenatal and postnatal mice. *Cell Research 11*(2): 135–141.

Waterland, R. & Jirtle, R. (2003). Transposable elements: Targets for early nutritional effects on epigenetic gene regulation. *Molecular and Cellular Biology 23*(15): 5293–5300.

Watson, C. G., Kucala, T., Tilleskjor, C., & Jacobs, L. (1984). Schizophrenic birth seasonality in relation to the incidence of infectious diseases and temperature extremes. *Archives of General Psychiatry 41*(1): 85–90.

West, K. (2002). Extent of vitamin A deficiency among preschool children and women of reproductive age. *Journal of Nutrition 132*(9): S2857–2866.

Williams, C., Birch, E., Emmett, P., Northstone, K., & ALSPAC. (2001). Stereoacuity at age 3.5 y in children born full-term is associated with prenatal and postnatal dietary factors: A report from a population-based cohort study. *American Journal of Clinical Nutrition 73*(2): 316–322.

Wolff, G., Kodell, R., Moore, S., & Cooney, C. (1998). Maternal epigenetics and methyl supplements affect agouti gene expression in A^{vy}/a mice. *FASEB Journal 12*(11): 49–57.

World Health Organization. (2011). World Health Global Database on Vitamin A Deficiency. http://www.who.int/vmnis/database/vitamina/en/index.html.

Xiang, N., Zhao, R., Song, G., & Zhong, W. (2008). Selenite reactivates silenced genes by modifying DNA methylation and histones in prostate cancer cells. *Carcinogenesis 29*(11): 2175–2181.

Xu, B., Roos, J., Levy, S., Rensburg, E. v., Gogos, J., & Karayiorgou, M. (2008). Strong association of *de novo* copy number mutations with sporadic schizophrenia. *Nature Genetics 40*(7): 880–885.

Xu, M., Wen-Sheng, S., Liu, B., Feng, G., Yu, L., Yang, L., He, G., Sham, P., Susser, E., St Clair, D., et al. (2009). Prenatal malnutrition and adult schizophrenia: Further evidence from the 1959–1961 famine. *Schizophrenia Bulletin 35*(3): 568–576.

Yan, J. & Barrett, J. (1998). Purification from bovine serum of a survival-promoting factor for cultured neurons and its identification as Selenoprotein-P. *Journal of Neuroscience 18*(21): 8682–8691.

Yoo, J., Maeng, H., Sun, Y., Kim, Y., Park, D., Park, T., Lee, S., & Choi, J. (2009). Oxidative status in iron-deficiency anemia. *Journal of Clinical Laboratory Analysis 23*(50): 319–323.

Young, S., Eskenazi, B., Marchetti, F., Block, G., & Wyrobek, A. (2008). The association of folate, zinc and antioxidant intake with sperm aneuploidy in healthy non-smoking men. *Human Reproduction 23*(5): 1014–1022.

Zimmerman, C., Winnefeld, K., Streck, S., Roskos, M., & Haberl, R. (2004). Antioxidant status in acute stroke patients and patients at stroke risk. *European Neurology 51*(3): 157–161.

Zornberg, G., Buka, S., & Tsuang, M. (2000). Hypoxic-ischemia-related fetal/neonatal complications and risk of schizophrenia and other nonaffective psychoses: A 19-year longitudinal study. *American Journal of Psychiatry 157*(2): 196–202.

CHAPTER 3

OBSTETRIC COMPLICATIONS AND SCHIZOPHRENIA
Historical Overview and New Directions

MARY CLARKE, SARAH RODDY, AND MARY CANNON

KEY CONCEPTS

- The field of obstetric complications has been intensively studied over the last five decades and has evolved over the years from using high-risk designs to case-control designs and finally to population-based studies.
- The population-based design has led to good evidence that there is a small but noteworthy association between obstetric complications and the later development of schizophrenia.
- There are several potential mechanisms that may mediate the relationship between obstetric complications and schizophrenia. There is also evidence that obstetric complications may have synergistic effects with other schizophrenia risk factors.
- Obstetric complications may play an important role in elucidating the etiology of schizophrenia by pointing the way to molecular studies.

Any discussion of the origins of schizophrenia must include a consideration of what is, historically, possibly the most intensively investigated category of environmental risk factor—obstetric complications (OCs). The term *obstetric complications* refers to somatic deviations from the normal course of events over the pregnancy, delivery, and early neonatal periods (McNeil, 1987), and for many years researchers have tried to tease apart the association between OCs and schizophrenia in order to identify the one complication or underlying mechanism that is responsible for the increase in risk. Results from large population-based studies have been pooled to give substantial sample sizes for meta-analysis. Yet no one unifying mechanism has emerged. The most parsimonious approach at present may be to group complications of apparently similar modes of action together. As will be detailed in this chapter, the three "groups" that have emerged from the literature to date are (1) complications of pregnancy, including bleeding, preeclampsia, maternal diabetes, rhesus incompatibility, maternal nonattendance of antenatal appointments, and threatened premature delivery; (2) abnormalities of fetal growth and development, including low birth weight, congenital malformations, small head circumference, and gestational age of less than 37 weeks; and (3) complications of delivery, including asphyxia, uterine atony and emergency cesarean section, manual extraction of the baby, maternal sepsis at childbirth and puerperium, and hemorrhage during delivery (Cannon, Jones, & Murray, 2002; Byrne et al., 2007).

Investigation of these early risk factors has been crucial in promoting awareness of nongenetic etiologic risk factors for schizophrenia and in furthering the idea of gene-environment interaction. This chapter provides a synthesis of the findings from the large number of studies that have been conducted over the last five decades looking at the association between OCs and schizophrenia and an overview of how the findings can be integrated with other developments in the search for the causes of schizophrenia.

A Historical Perspective

The first mention of an association between birth complications and schizophrenia occurred in the *American Journal of Psychiatry* in 1934. Aaron Rosanoff and colleagues (1934) published "The Etiology of So-Called Schizophrenic Psychoses," based on a sample of 142 pairs of twins concordant and discordant for schizophrenia. The authors concluded from their detailed case reports that schizophrenia could be regarded (at least in part) as a "decerebration syndrome which may result from birth trauma." The importance of pregnancy, rather than delivery complications, and the issue of nonspecificity to schizophrenia soon came to the fore. Benjamin Pasamanick and colleagues published "Pregnancy Experience and the Development of Behavior Disorder in Children" in the *American Journal of Psychiatry* in 1956, proposing their now-classic hypothesis of a "continuum of reproductive casualty," whereby pregnancy and birth complications can lead to a gradient of injury that extends from fetal and neonatal death through cerebral palsy, epilepsy, mental deficiency, and behavior disorder. The authors emphasized that "the associations occurred with the prolonged and probably anoxia-producing complications of pregnancy such as toxemias and bleeding . . . rather than the mechanical factors of delivery" (Pasamanick, Rodgers, & Lilienfield, 1956; Pasamanick & Knobloch, 1960).

In 1966 Lane and Albee published an influential paper reporting an association between low birth weight and adult-onset schizophrenia. They reported that the birth weights of 52 hospitalized schizophrenic adults were significantly lower than those of 115 of their siblings, independent of prematurity. Although the results were statistically significant, the difference between the mean birth weight of the schizophrenic subjects and the mean birth weight of the average of the siblings was not great—in the region of 175 g. Few of the subjects actually fell into the low birth weight category (< 2,500 g), but 70% of the subjects weighed less than the average of the other children in the family. Therefore, these results seem to indicate a shift in distribution of birth weight within a population of case subjects as opposed to within a population of noncase subjects, rather than an association between schizophrenia and an arbitrarily defined category of low birth weight. A group of researchers from Hillside Hospital, New York (led by Margaret Woerner and Max Pollack) attempted to replicate the findings of Lane and Albee (1966). However, they used smaller samples, with poorer-quality obstetric data, and on the whole failed to find significant differences (Pollack et al., 1966; Woerner, Pollack, & Klein, 1971, 1973). Although reported as "negative" studies, the magnitude of the difference in birth weight found between case subjects and siblings was very similar to that reported by Lane and Albee (1966).

Two important areas of research that have provided evidence for an association between OCs and schizophrenia are childhood-onset studies and "high-risk" studies looking at the risk of schizophrenia among the offspring of parents with the disease.

Childhood Schizophrenia and Obstetric Complications

A number of studies have examined the association between OCs and childhood schizophrenia (Vorster, 1960; Knobloch & Pasamanick, 1962; Hinton, 1963; Taft & Goldfarb, 1964; Terris, Lapouse, & Monk, 1964). The first review paper on the topic of OCs and schizophrenia (Pollack & Woerner, 1966) compared the results of five studies in the area of childhood psychosis and found consistently significant associations between three complications of pregnancy (toxemia, bleeding, and severe maternal illness) and childhood psychosis. However, the frequent changes in the diagnostic classification of childhood psychosis rendered such research difficult. Torrey, Hersch, & McCabe (1975) reported a positive association between bleeding in early and midpregnancy and childhood psychosis, echoing the earlier conclusions of Pasamanick and Knobloch (1960). Although Nicolson et al. (1999) reported no significant association between any OC and childhood-onset schizophrenia, more than 30 years later the findings of Torrey, Hersch, & McCabe (1975) were replicated by Moreno et al. (2009), who reported that bleeding in pregnancy was noted almost six times more frequently in the obstetric histories of subjects with childhood schizophrenia than in those of controls.

High-Risk Studies

Mednick and colleagues carried out an analysis of OC data from the Copenhagen High Risk Study (Mednick & Schulsinger, 1968; Mednick, 1970) and found that 70% of the high-risk children who were psychiatrically ill by their early twenties had suffered one or more serious pregnancy or birth complications, as opposed to 15% of the high-risk group who remained well and 33% of the control group. He speculated that, given a genetic predisposition, schizophrenia will appear only if the hippocampus is selectively injured by anoxia at birth—a gene-environment interaction. Many interesting findings emerged from other high-risk studies over the next few years. Rieder, Broman, & Rosenthal (1977) reported an excess of bleeding and swelling during high-risk pregnancies. Moreover, a striking excess of unexplained fetal and neonatal deaths among the offspring of schizophrenic parents was reported by a number of investigators (Sobel, 1961; Rieder, Broman, & Rosenthal, 1977; Modrzewska, 1980).

However, a series of largely negative findings from high-risk studies by other groups of investigators (McNeil & Kaij, 1973; Sameroff & Zax, 1973; Mirdal et al., 1974; Cohler et al., 1975; Hanson, Gottesman, & Heston, 1976; Zax, Sameroff, & Babigian, 1977) culminated in a review of the high-risk literature by McNeil and Kaij in 1978, which concluded that there was little evidence for an excess of OCs in births to parents with schizophrenia. This conclusion was challenged two decades later by Sacker, Done, & Crow (1996) and Bennedsen (1998) in further reviews of the literature on OCs among women with schizophrenia. In fact, recent work in large population-based samples from Australia, Sweden, and Denmark show consistently that women with schizophrenia have increased rates of a range of pregnancy, birth, and delivery complications. Jablensky et al. (2005) found increased rates of placental abruption, low birth weight, and cardiovascular congenital anomalies in the obstetric records of women with schizophrenia. Bennedsen et al. (2001) found a higher rate of congenital malformations, stillbirths, and infant deaths among the offspring of women with schizophrenia. A series of studies from a large Danish register-linkage sample showed that many of these complications (in particular stillbirth, neonatal death, and sudden infant death) occur in the birth histories of women with other mental disorders (King-Hele et al., 2009; Webb et al., 2010), although rates of fatal birth defect were highest among women with a diagnosis of schizophrenia (Webb et al., 2008).

Obstetric Complications and the Neurodevelopmental Hypothesis of Schizophrenia

In 1987 a major "paradigm shift" took place in the etiologic thinking on schizophrenia. Two research groups (one from the United States and one from the United Kingdom) set forth similar ideas regarding a "neurodevelopmental hypothesis" of schizophrenia (Murray & Lewis, 1987; Weinberger, 1987). A central tenet of this theory was that schizophrenia can result from a disruption in the normal maturational processes of the brain. This disruption could be caused by a combination of genetic or environmental factors (such as OCs). The association between OCs and later schizophrenia would prove to be a crucial strand of evidence for this theory. In 1987, Lewis and Murray found that patients with schizophrenia had a higher rate of OCs reported in their case notes than patients with other psychiatric disorders. Another profound impact of this study was the introduction of the "Lewis-Murray" scale for rating retrospective information on OCs (Lewis, Owen, & Murray, 1989). This scale was derived from a consensus of six previous scales, three from the obstetric and three from the psychiatric literature. The scale consists of 15 complications, and defined thresholds for rating some complications as "definite" or "equivocal." Ratings from this scale drew on OC information from case notes, birth records, and maternal interview. This user-friendly and atheoretical scale dominated the OC literature for the next decade and formed the basis of three later meta-analyses (Geddes & Lawrie, 1995; Verdoux et al., 1997; Geddes et al., 1999).

The combination of three factors—the theoretical framework provided by the neurodevelopmental hypothesis, the possibility of using maternal recall and case notes as sources of OC information, and the availability of an easy-to-use rating scale—gave a new impetus to research in OCs and schizophrenia. Initially these studies were mostly relatively small case-control studies and therefore prone to the problems associated with that design. There was a significant amount of variability in the findings reported. Some studies found a significant overall effect for OCs (Eagles et al., 1990; O'Callaghan et al., 1992; Verdoux & Bourgeois, 1993; Gunther-Genta, Bovet, & Hohlfield, 1994; Rifkin et al., 1994), whereas others did not (McCreadie et al., 1992; Heun & Maier, 1993). Many variations of the Lewis-Murray scale were used. Some studies had no normal control group (Foerster et al., 1991; Rifkin et al., 1994; Smith et al., 1998), whereas others used sibling controls only (Eagles et al., 1990; McCreadie et al., 1992; Heun & Maier, 1993; Gunther-Genta, Bovet, & Hohlfield, 1994; Willinger, Heiden, & Mesaros, 1996). Although some of the studies clearly attempted to use population-based cases or controls or both (McNeil & Kaij, 1978; Eagles et al., 1990; O'Callaghan et al., 1992; Hultman et al., 1997), the final samples suffered from selection bias (Geddes & Lawrie, 1995). Many studies relied solely on maternal recall as the source of information about the exposure (McCreadie et al., 1992; Verdoux & Bourgeois, 1993; Rifkin et al., 1994). These limitations may have contributed to inconsistencies in the results.

Studies that found no significant overall effect for OCs carried out subgroup analyses: OCs were examined in relation to family history (O'Callaghan et al., 1990; Foerster et al., 1991; McCreadie et al., 1992; McNeil et al., 1993; Kunugi et al., 1996a), premorbid adjustment (Foerster et al., 1991), imaging abnormalities (Owen, Lewis, & Murray, 1988; Smith et al., 1998), age at onset (O'Callaghan, Larkin, & Waddington, 1990; O'Callaghan et al., 1992; Kirov et al., 1996; Nicholson et al., 1999), gender (O'Callaghan et al., 1992; McNeil et al., 1993; Kirov et al., 1996; Kunugi et al., 1996b), neurologic abnormalities (O'Callaghan et al., 1990; McCreadie et al., 1992), ethnicity (Hutchinson et al., 1997), and season of birth (McNeil et al., 1993), among others. Unfortunately there was little consistency in the results from these subgroup analyses.

In 1995, Geddes and Lawrie (1995) carried out a meta-analysis of published results from 16 case-control studies and two cohort studies and reached three important conclusions: (1) a pooled odds ratio of 2.0 (CI 1.6–2.4) suggested that OCs did have a small effect on increasing risk for schizophrenia; (2) there was evidence for selection and publication bias in the OC and schizophrenia literature, with a notable deficit of small negative studies; and (3) there was significant heterogeneity between the results from the case-control studies and the two published birth cohort studies. Hence, this meta-analysis suggested that although there may be an effect of OCs on risk of schizophrenia, this may have been due to selection bias or limitations in the study design. Geddes and Lawrie (1995) concluded their review with the following recommendation: "Future studies should have sample sizes that are large enough to provide sufficient power to quantify risk estimates for individual, rigorously-defined OCs and to be able to adjust the estimates for the effect of potential confounding factors."

Evidence from Population-Based Cohort Studies

These studies have the following characteristics (McNeil, 1995): (1) large and psychiatrically well-defined samples of schizophrenia cases drawn from population-based registers or cohorts; (2) use of standardized, prospectively collected obstetric information from birth records or registers; and (3) control subjects drawn from the general population with OC information from the same source and context. Investigators did not use OC rating scales, usually reported odds ratios for all individual OCs recorded on the birth records, and controlled for demographic confounders by matching or statistical adjustment. However, despite this seemingly optimal methodology, the results from these large population-based studies were far from consistent, leading to another meta-analysis (Cannon,

Jones, & Murray, 2002). This analysis covered population-based studies published up to and including 2001. Eight studies were identified that fulfilled the criteria for an epidemiologic study and were presented in a form suitable for this meta-analysis (Sacker et al., 1995; Jones et al., 1998; Dalman et al., 1999, 2001; Hultman et al., 1999; Byrne et al., 2000; Kendell et al., 2000). Two studies were presented in one paper (Kendell et al., 2000). An additional five studies were identified that fulfilled criteria for epidemiologic studies, but the obstetric data were presented in aggregate form and could not be used in this analysis (Done et al., 1991; Buka, Tsuang, & Lipsitt, 1993; Cannon et al., 2000; Rosso et al., 2000; Zornberg et al., 2000).

The results of the meta-analysis (Cannon, Jones, & Murray, 2002) can be summarized as follows. First, there was no significant heterogeneity between the studies and no evidence for publication bias. Second, the effect sizes for the relationship between obstetric risk factors and later schizophrenia were generally small, with odds ratios of less than two. Specifically, significant differences between cases and controls were found for the following ten variables in order of significance (OR: 95% CI): uterine atony (2.2:1.5–3.5); bleeding in pregnancy (1.7:1.1–2.5); asphyxia (1.7:1.2–2.6); emergency cesarean section (3.2:1.4–7.5); birth weight under 2,000g (3.9:1.4–10.8); birth weight over 2,500g (1.7:1, 2–2.3); congenital malformations (2.3:1.2–4.6); maternal diabetes in pregnancy (7.8:1.4–43.9); rhesus variables (2.0:1.01–3.96) (which includes rhesus incompatibility, rhesus negative mother, rhesus antibodies); and preeclampsia (1.4:0.99–1.85). Two complications nearly missed formal statistical significance: placental abruption (4.02:0.9–18.1) and head circumference less than 32 cm (1.3:0.8–2.06). Cannon, Jones, & Murray (2002) grouped these variables into three categories: complications of pregnancy, abnormal fetal growth and development, and complications of delivery. These effect sizes are similar in magnitude to those reported for the relationship between passive smoking and lung cancer or the risk of breast cancer among users of oral contraceptives. Given these small effects, it would be premature to draw causal inferences. Rather, the study of individual obstetric risk factors for schizophrenia can be conceptualized as the search for uncommon to rare risk factors for a relatively rare disorder, posing challenges for both the case-control and the classical cohort study design.

In the last decade, there have been few studies conducted with a design similar to that in the meta-analysis above. The only comparable study that reports on a broad range of OCs is that of Byrne et al. (2007). This large nested case-control study using Danish register-based data found significant, approximately twofold associations in the rate of schizophrenia among those who had experienced any one of the following complications: maternal nonattendance at antenatal appointments, gestational age of 37 weeks or less, preeclampsia, threatened premature delivery, hemorrhage during delivery, manual extraction of the baby, and maternal sepsis of childbirth and the puerperium. The findings were not appreciably altered by adjustment for the confounding effects of family psychiatric history and socioeconomic and other demographic factors.

As noted above, Cannon, Jones, & Murray (2002) summarized their findings by grouping the variables associated with later schizophrenia into three categories. These categories can be updated by incorporating the results from the Byrne et al. (2007) study (shown in italics): (1) complications of pregnancy: bleeding, preeclampsia, maternal diabetes, rhesus incompatibility, *maternal nonattendance at antenatal appointment, and threatened premature delivery*; (2) abnormalities of fetal growth and development: low birth weight, congenital malformations, small head circumference, and *gestational age less than 37 weeks;* (3) complications of delivery: asphyxia, uterine atony and emergency cesarean section, manual extraction of the baby, maternal sepsis of childbirth and puerperium, and hemorrhage during delivery.

In our view, the Byrne et al. (2007) study marks the end of the first phase of the "Population-Based Studies" Era, because this is the last of the large studies to report on all obstetric variables in the birth records. We have now moved to the second phase of that era, or what we could also call the "Specific Complications Era"—the examination of specific complications using the same population-based methodology, namely the use of population registers to identify the subjects and the use of prospectively collected birth record data.

Investigation of Specific Individual Complications

A number of more recent cohort studies using population-based data have recently been conducted. These studies apply the power of the population-based methods to the more focused examination of certain complications of interest (table 3.1). They do not adopt the "atheoretical" stance of the prior population-based studies; rather, they have aimed to test a priori hypotheses. This approach builds on the findings and the methodologic expertise of the previous eras of OC research documented here but adds something new: a forensic style of investigation and a focus on causative mechanisms.

The advantage of these studies over the work previously described is that the examination of specific "candidate" complications is likely to bring us closer to elucidating causal mechanisms in schizophrenia. For instance, low birth weight and poor fetal growth per se are not causes of schizophrenia but rather general indicators of a deviant neurodevelopmental process caused by other risk factors and genetic mutations that are more proximal to the underlying pathology. Therefore, factors such as maternal iron deficiency, maternal diabetes, or medication use during pregnancy are potentially important in elucidating the underlying causal mechanisms by pointing the way to future molecular studies.

Table 3.1 Recent Population-Based Studies Examining the Association Between Specific Obstetric Complications and Schizophrenia

Risk Factor	Authors/Year	Description
Fetal Growth	Gunnell et al., 2003; Gunnell et al., 2005	Birth weight not associated with schizophrenia when gestational age is taken into account in a cohort of Swedish male conscripts.
Medication		Two studies have examined the association between schizophrenia and medication use during pregnancy using Danish national population–based register data.
	Sørensen et al., 2004	Prenatal exposure to analgesics in the second trimester was associated with an increased risk of schizophrenia (OR: 4.75; 95% CI = 1.9–12.0).
	Sørensen et al., 2003	Prenatal exposure to both hypertension and diuretic treatment in the third trimester conferred a 4-fold (95% CI = 1.41–11.40) increase in risk of developing schizophrenia.
Iron Deficiency	Insel et al., 2008	Maternal mean hemoglobin of 10g/dl or less was associated with an almost 4-fold (RR = 3.7; 95% CI = 1.4–9.8) increase in the rate of schizophrenia spectrum disorders in the Prenatal Determinants of Schizophrenia Study, a U.S. population-based birth cohort study.
	Sørensen et al., 2010	Maternal anemia during pregnancy led to a 1.6-fold (95% CI = 1.2–2.2) increase in risk of schizophrenia in a population-based Danish sample.
Rhesus Incompatibility	Hollister et al., 1996	The rate of schizophrenia was found to be significantly higher in an Rh-incompatible group (2.1%) compared with the Rh-compatible group (0.8%).
	Insel et al., 2005	Maternal-fetal blood incompatibility led to a 2-fold increase in the rate of schizophrenia among exposed offspring in the Prenatal Determinants of Schizophrenia Study. This effect was strongest among male offspring (RR = 2.2; 95% CI = 1.1–4.4).

CI = confidence interval; OR = odds ratio; RR = relative risk.
SOURCE: Authors.

What is the possible mechanism for this association? Given that we have good, consistent evidence for an association between OCs and schizophrenia, we are now in a position to ask a number of questions about the meaning of this association for etiologic theories of schizophrenia. These questions, which we will address in the remainder of the chapter, are as follows:

Are OCs merely markers of genetic risk of schizophrenia or do they exert a truly independent effect? Although some of the studies already reviewed in this chapter had the capacity to adjust for parental psychiatric history, this question was not addressed directly.

If OCs represent independent risk factors for schizophrenia, what are the potential mechanisms of action?

Given the small effect size associated with OCs, it seems both probable and plausible that they combine with other risk factors along the causal pathway to schizophrenia. Do OCs have an additive or an interactive relationship with other schizophrenia risk factors?

How do OCs relate to indicators of neurodevelopmental deviance such as structural brain abnormalities and neurologic soft signs or minor physical anomalies?

Is the risk-increasing effect of OCs specific to schizophrenia or do they also increase risk for other psychotic disorders or psychotic symptoms?

Obstetric Complications and Genetic Risk

Ellman et al. (2007), using Finnish register-based prospective data, have shown that although women with schizophrenia experienced significantly more OCs while pregnant than did both mothers with a first-degree relative who had schizophrenia and controls, there was no difference in the rate of OCs between those with a first-degree relative and controls. The lack of familial liability to OCs in this data indicates that genetic susceptibility to schizophrenia does not underlie the increased incidence of OCs among individuals with schizophrenia. Further evidence that OCs are not a proxy of genetic risk was found in a number of other recent studies (van Erp et al., 2002; Bersani et al., 2003; Jablensky et al., 2005; Nilsson et al., 2005; Boks et al., 2007).

Potential Mechanisms of Action Mediating the Association Between Obstetric Complications and Schizophrenia

An excellent review paper by Schlotz and Phillips (2009) sets forward various models by which prenatal and perinatal complications can give rise to mental and behavioral disorders. They emphasize exposure to fetal adversity during sensitive periods of neurodevelopment and interactions between prenatal and postnatal factors as well as between prenatal and genetic factors as potentially having a causal role in the etiology of mental health outcomes in later life. In figure 3.1, we illustrate potential interrelationships between prenatal and perinatal complications, genetic vulnerability, and environmental adversity and how these interrelationships may ultimately lead to an increased risk of schizophrenia.

It is possible that OCs have a direct effect on fetal neurodevelopment (Boog, 2003). For example, evidence suggests that perinatal hypoxia may have lasting

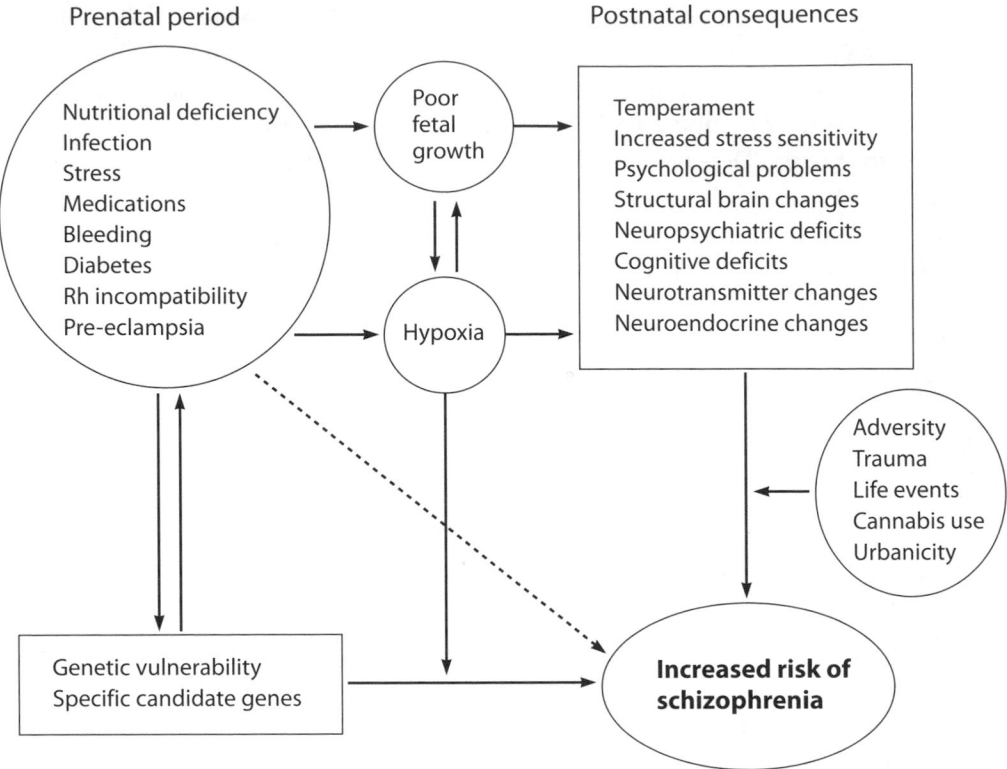

Figure 3.1. Proposed pathways and mechanisms linking obstetric complications and risk of schizophrenia. (Source: Authors.)

effects on dopaminergic function. However, the same data also suggest a further indirect effect of OCs such that birth insults alter the manner in which dopamine function is regulated by stress in adulthood (Boksa & El-Khodor, 2003). Cannon et al. (2008) have recently found that neurotrophic factors, perhaps stimulated in response to fetal distress, may be important in the etiology of schizophrenia. In this nested case-control study, assays from cord and maternal blood samples taken at delivery showed that, among schizophrenia patients, birth hypoxia was associated with a 20% decrease in brain-derived neurotrophic factor (BDNF), whereas among the matched healthy controls birth hypoxia was associated with a 10% increase in BDNF. The deleterious effects of OCs such as hypoxia and hyperbilirubinemia on NMDA receptors have also been proposed as a potential mechanism (Dalman, 2003).

Hypoxia itself has been proposed to mediate the effects of other OCs. Cannon et al. (2000) found a linear relationship between the number of hypoxia-causing OCs, such as abnormal fetal heart rate, third-trimester heart rate, placental hemorrhaging, and risk of schizophrenia, suggesting that any association between these specific OCs and schizophrenia is accounted for by the effect of hypoxia on risk for schizophrenia. These data also suggest that hypoxia interacts with genetic susceptibility to further increase risk. The risk of schizophrenia increased with the number of hypoxia-related OCs within families: given genetic vulnerability to schizophrenia, those who were exposed to hypoxia were more likely to develop schizophrenia than family members not exposed to hypoxia.

The Role of Obstetric Complications in Gene-Environment Interactions

The possibility of OCs interacting with underlying genetic vulnerability has been raised by several other lines of evidence (Mueser & McGurk, 2004; Devlin et al., 2007; Mittal, Ellman, & Canon, 2008; Fatemi & Folsom, 2009). In particular, recent findings show that many of the susceptibility genes identified for schizophrenia are affected by hypoxia (Schmidt-Kastner et al., 2006; Nicodemus et al., 2008). Schmidt-Kastner et al. (2006) have published a thought-provoking discussion of the possible role of hypoxia in gene regulation relevant to schizophrenia. The authors hypothesize that although some genes important for neurodevelopment are influenced by hypoxia in a physiologic manner, excessive hypoxia could result in dysregulation of such genes and an abnormality of gene expression at a critical point of development. The authors propose that, because hypoxia is an element of ischemia and maternal factors may cause circulatory problems, both hypoxia and ischemia should be considered jointly. Schmidt-Kastner et al. (2006) report that about 3.5% of all genes are influenced by hypoxia, have vascular functions, or both, and they devised a simple experiment to investigate the association of such genes with schizophrenia. They searched the literature and devised a list of currently hypothesized candidate genes for schizophrenia. They initially found that 71% of their list of candidate susceptibility genes for schizophrenia was influenced by ischemia-hypoxia, vascular expression, or both. In a more stringent analysis, they examined only those genes that were mentioned in the recent reviews of Harrison and Weinberger (2005) and Kirov, O'Donavan, & Owen (2005). The genes covered in these reviews were only those genes for which there was the most robust evidence. Schmidt-Kastner et al. (2006) found that eight out of 11 of these genes (81%) met their criteria for ischemia-hypoxia regulation, vascular expression, or both. In their discussion the authors note the findings of Prabakaran et al. (2004), in which almost 50% of the altered proteins identified by proteomics in prefrontal postmortem tissue in schizophrenia were associated with mitochondrial function and oxidative stress responses.

Nicodemus et al. (2008) carried out a gene-environment interaction analysis in a family study of schizophrenia probands, siblings, and controls. Data on OCs were obtained by maternal recall, and their severity was classified according to a standardized scale. Psychiatric diagnoses were made using a structured clinical interview. The authors then examined whether a set of schizophrenia candidate genes affected by hypoxia or involved in vascular function in the brain interacted with serious OCs to influence risk for schizophrenia. They found that four of the 13 genes examined showed evidence for significant serious OC-by-gene interaction. All of the OCs rated as serious had the potential to cause hypoxia. The most common effects were bleeding during pregnancy, extended labor, delivery problems, and respiratory distress at birth. The four genes found to interact with these OCs—AKT_1, $BDNF$, $GRM3$, and $DTNBP_1$—showed previous evidence of an association with schizophrenia and were affected by hypoxia. In keeping with the epidemiologic findings already reported here, the OCs identified in this study were diverse and occurred both during the prenatal and perinatal periods. This study provides evidence that serious OCs interact with genetic risk to increase risk for schizophrenia. However, any conclusions from the study must be tempered by the fact that it had limited power to detect interactions, tested a large number of single nucleotide polymorphisms (SNPs) (thereby raising the possibility of false positives due to multiple testing), and used maternal recall of OCs decades after birth. One possibility of furthering this line of investigation is by enriching future samples for OCs (Nicodemus et al., 2008).

Thus evidence is starting to emerge that OCs not only exert an independent effect on schizophrenia risk but also exert a combined effect with underlying genetic vulnerability to schizophrenia. This raises the question of the nature of this combination: Is it merely additive, whereby risk of illness results from a simple addition of accumulated independent risk factors, or is it synergistic, whereby the combined effects of these are greater than the sum of their individual effects on risk for schizophrenia? Current evidence points to both additive and synergistic influences of OCs on schizophrenia risk (Mittal, Ellman, & Cannon, 2008). However, the use of indirect measures of genetic effects, such as family history of schizophrenia, in epidemiologic samples makes finding strong evidence for a particular model of combined risk factor effects very difficult. However, both the additive and the synergistic models predict that a reduction in the incidence of OCs would have the effect of reducing the overall incidence of schizophrenia.

Evidence for Obstetric Complications and Developmental Deviance

The concept of early-life adverse events that affect neurodevelopment and interact with underlying genetic risk is central to the neurodevelopmental hypothesis of the etiology of schizophrenia. If OCs increase risk for schizophrenia by having long-lasting effects on neurodevelopment, perhaps in combination with other risk factors operating at different points during development, then if and how OCs are associated with other markers of suboptimal neurodevelopment is of interest. Two main strands of evidence used in support of the neurodevelopmental hypothesis of schizophrenia are the presence of structural brain abnormalities preceding the onset of schizophrenia and the finding of an increased incidence of minor physical anomalies and neurologic soft signs in childhood in those who later develop schizophrenia. Some, but not all, studies have demonstrated an association between OCs and either structural brain abnormalities or neurologic abnormalities or minor physical anomalies in schizophrenia patients.

STRUCTURAL BRAIN ABNORMALITIES. Cannon et al. (2002) found evidence that fetal hypoxia was associated with cortical gray matter reduction and cerebrospinal fluid increase in both schizophrenia patients and their siblings as opposed to healthy controls who did not have any family history of psychosis. This finding points to a gene-environment interaction in the etiology of schizophrenia. This study also reported evidence of a more complex interaction: the gene-environment effect was three times greater in those who were born small for gestational age, indicating that OCs can interact both with underlying genetic risk and with each other to increase risk for schizophrenia. Cannon et al. also found that fetal hypoxia correlated with ventricular enlargement, but only in subjects with schizophrenia and not in their siblings or controls. Similarly, Falkai et al. (2003) found that neonatal OCs were associated with the size of the ventricle-to-brain ratio in a case-control study of schizophrenia patients, their relatives, and healthy controls with no psychiatric history. Ebner et al. (2008) have found hippocampal volume reduction among schizophrenia patients who had experienced OCs, their first-degree relatives, and healthy controls, suggesting that OCs have an association with structural brain abnormalities that is independent of genetic susceptibility to schizophrenia. This finding replicates that of an association between OCs and hippocampal volume in sporadic schizophrenia (Stefanis et al., 1999). Fearon et al. (2004) have found that adolescents born very preterm or with very low birth weight showed many of the same structural brain abnormalities that are found in schizophrenia patients, such as lateral ventricular enlargement and reduction in hippocampal volume.

MINOR PHYSICAL ANOMALIES. In a case-control study, Bramon et al. (2005) showed that only schizophrenia patients who had a history of OCs had dermatoglyphic abnormalities. Fatjo-Vilas et al. (2008) found in a case-control study that although a main group analysis did not show any differences between schizophrenia patients and controls in the incidence of dermatoglyphic anomalies, patients with a very low birth weight had an increased incidence of such anomalies. Similarly, Rosa et al. (2005) found that among siblings discordant for schizophrenia, the affected siblings had a greater number of dermatoglyphic anomalies.

Are Obstetric Complications Associated with Other Psychotic Disorders or Psychotic Symptoms?

Accumulating evidence suggests that the association between OCs and psychotic disorder is specific to schizophrenia and that no association is present between OCs and bipolar disorder (Murray et al., 2004). Ogendahl et al. (2006), using register-based data on a large Danish cohort, found no evidence that OCs were related to bipolar disorder. Scott et al. (2006) carried out a systematic review and meta-analysis of the effect of exposure to OCs on the risk of later developing bipolar disorder and found a pooled odds ratio of 1.1 (95% 0.76–1.35).

About 5–8% of the general population report nonclinical psychotic symptoms at interview (van Os et al., 2009). Results from three cohort studies (Poulton et al., 2000; Hanssen et al., 2005; Scott et al., 2009) show that these symptoms may lead to risk of clinically meaningful psychotic disorder. Studying these nonclinical psychotic symptoms may therefore increase understanding of how psychotic experiences develop and potentially help elucidate etiologic mechanisms underlying schizophrenia. Three studies have examined associations between adolescent psychotic symptoms and OCs in 6,356 children from the Avon Longitudinal Study of Parents and Children (Thomas et al., 2009; Zammit et al., 2009a, 2009b). The results are remarkably similar to findings for individuals with a diagnosis of schizophrenia. Significant associations were reported between risk of experiencing psychotic symptoms in adolescence and the following obstetric variables: maternal tobacco use and maternal alcohol use (Zammit et al., 2009a); low birth weight and ponderal index (Thomas et al., 2009); maternal infection during pregnancy; maternal diabetes; need for resuscitation; and 5-minute Apgar score (Zammit et al., 2009b). These results indicate that the same prenatal and perinatal complications increase the risk both for schizophrenia and for the risk of experiencing psychotic symptoms in childhood and adolescence. These results also provide further evidence that childhood and adolescent psychotic symptoms may lie on the causal pathway to schizophrenia.

Conclusion

The field of OCs and schizophrenia is moving on from merely documenting the presence of an association between OCs and schizophrenia to a more focused examination of the causal role of this association in the etiology of the disease. Studies are beginning to examine specific complications that might have causal effects and to explore if OCs interact with genetic vulnerability to schizophrenia or with specific candidate genes for schizophrenia. At the same time, more information is emerging about the downstream effects of a range of prenatal and perinatal complications and poor fetal growth and how these risk factors give rise to a range of behavioral, cognitive, and mental health problems in later life, which in turn can increase risk for schizophrenia (Schlotz & Phillips, 2009). The continued study of OCs has the potential to inform us about the neurobiological mechanisms and pathways involved in schizophrenia. It is possible that focusing on those who have notable perinatal insults will help identify etiologic homogeneous subgroups within the heterogeneous schizophrenia phenotype. It also seems likely that the genes influenced by certain OCs are good candidates for the study of gene-environment interactions in schizophrenia. Solely relying on genomewide association studies to identify candidate genes for schizophrenia may not be fruitful because gene-environment interactions may conceal good candidates from these studies. We must also bear in mind the high degree of complexity that is likely to be involved in any pathway to schizophrenia. There is evidence of gene-environment interactions in schizophrenia, but it is also likely that environmental risk factors are either mediated or moderated by each other. For example, it is possible that the reported association between elevated prenatal maternal homocysteine levels and the development of schizophrenia in adult offspring (Brown et al., 2007) is mediated by the induction of fetal hypoxia. Animal models will likely play an increasingly central role in elucidating the role of OCs in the etiology of schizophrenia. These models have the ability to determine precisely both the nature and the timing of exposure to insult. It is only through sharpening measures of environmental insults and through gaining insight into critical windows of vulnerability that the complex etiopathogenesis of schizophrenia can be elucidated.

KEY AREAS FOR FUTURE RESEARCH

- Conduct focused investigation of key prenatal risk factors.
- Collaborate with molecular and cellular science to elucidate pathophysiologic mechanisms underlying key prenatal risk factors.
- Examine the effect of hypoxia or ischemia on gene expression.
- Use animal models to precisely define environment insults and the critical period of exposure to these insults.

Acknowledgments

M. Cannon is supported by a Clinician Scientist Award from the Health Research Board Ireland and an Independent Investigator Award from NARSAD. Drs. Cannon, Clarke, and Roddy are members of the European Network of National Schizophrenia Networks Studying Gene-Environment Interactions (EU-GEI), funded by EU-FP7.

Selected Readings

Cannon, M., Jones, P. B., & Murray, R. M. (2002). Obstetric complications and schizophrenia: Historical and meta-analytic review. *American Journal of Psychiatry 159*(7): 1080–1092.

Clarke, M. C., Harley, M., & Cannon, M. (2006). The role of obstetric events in schizophrenia. *Schizophrenia Bulletin 32*(1): 3–8.

Gilmore, J. H. & Murray, R. M. (2006). Prenatal and perinatal factors. In J. A. Liberman, T. S. Stroup, & D. O. Perkins (eds.), *Textbook of Schizophrenia* (pp. 55–67). Washington, DC: American Psychiatric Publishing.

Schlotz, W. & Philips, D. I. W. (2009). Fetal origins of mental health: Evidence and mechanisms. *Brain, Behavior, and Immunity 23*(7): 905–916.

Schmidt-Kastner, R., van Os, J., Steinbusch, H., & Schmitz, C. (2006). Gene regulation by hypoxia and the neurodevelopmental origin of schizophrenia. *Schizophrenia Research 84*(2–3): 253–271.

References

Bennedsen, B. E. (1998). Adverse pregnancy outcome in schizophrenic women: Occurrence and risk factors. *Schizophrenia Research 33*(1–2): 1–26.

Bennedsen, B. E., Mortensen, P. B., Olesen, A. V., & Henriksen, T. B. (2001). Congenital malformations, stillbirths, and infant deaths among children of women with schizophrenia. *Archives of General Psychiatry 58*(7) ; 674–679.

Bersani, G., Taddei, I., Manuali, G., Ramieri, L., Venturi, P., Osborn, J., & Pancheri, P. (2003). Severity of obstetric complications and risk of adult schizophrenia in male patients: a case-control study. *Journal of Maternal Fetal and Neonatal Medicine 14*(1): 35–38.

Boks, M. P., Selten, J. P., Leask, S., Catelein, S., & van den Bosch, R. J. (2007). Negative association between a history of obstetric complications and the number of neurological soft signs in first-episode schizophrenic disorder. *Psychiatry Research 149*(1–3): 273–277.

Boksa, P. & El-Khodor, B. F. (2003). Birth insult interacts with stress at adulthood to alter dopaminergic function in animal models: Possible implications for schizophrenia and other disorders. *Neuroscience and Biobehavioral Reviews 27*: 91–101.

Boog, G. (2003). Obstetrical complications and further schizophrenia of the infant: A new methodological threat to the obstetrician? *Journal de Gynecologie, Obstetrique et Biologie de la Reproduction 32*: 720–727.

Bramon, E., Walshe, M., McDonald, C., Martin, B., Toulopoulou, T., Wickham, H., van Os, J., Fearon, P., Sham, P. C., Fañanás, L., et al. (2005). Dermatoglyphics and schizophrenia: A meta-analysis and investigation of the impact of obstetric complications upon a-b ridge count. *Schizophrenia Research 75*(2–3): 399–404.

Brown, A. S., Bottiglieri, T., Schaefer, C. A., Quesenberry, C. P., Jr., Liu, L., Bresnahan, M., & Susser, E. S. (2007). Elevated prenatal homocysteine levels as a risk factor for schizophrenia. *Archives of General Psychiatry 64*(1): 31–39.

Buka, S. L., Tsuang, M. T., & Lipsitt, L. P. (1993). Pregnancy/delivery complications and psychiatric diagnosis: A prospective study. *Archives of General Psychiatry 50*(2): 151–156.

Byrne, M., Agerbo, E., Bennedsen, B., Eaton, W. W., & Mortensen, P. B. (2007). Obstetric conditions and risk of first admission with schizophrenia: A Danish national register based study. *Schizophrenia Research 97*(1–3): 51–59.

Byrne, M., Browne, R., Mulryan, N., Scully, A., Morris, M., Kinsella, A., Takei, N., McNeil, T., Walsh, D., & O'Callaghan, E. (2000). Labour and delivery complications and schizophrenia: Case-control study using contemporaneous labour ward records. *British Journal of Psychiatry 176*: 531–536.

Cannon, M., Jones, P. B., & Murray, R. M. (2002). Obstetric complications and schizophrenia: Historical and meta-analytic review. *American Journal of Psychiatry 159*(7): 1080–1092.

Cannon, T. D., Rosso, I. M., Hollister, J. M., Bearden, C. E., & Sanchez, H. T. (2000). A prospective cohort study of genetic and perinatal influences in the etiology of schizophrenia. *Schizophrenia Bulletin 26*(2): 351–366.

Cannon, T. D., van Erp, T. G., Rosso, I. M., Huttunen, M., Lönnqvist, J., Pirkola, T., Salonen, O., Valanne, L., Poutanen, V. P., & Standertskjöld-Nordenstam, C. G. (2002). Fetal hypoxia and structural brain abnormalities in schizophrenic patients, their siblings, and controls. *Archives of General Psychiatry 59*(1): 35–41.

Cannon, T. D., Yolken, R., Buka, S., & Torrey, E. F. (2008). Collaborative study group on the perinatal origins of severe psychiatric D: Decreased neurotrophic response to birth hypoxia in the etiology of schizophrenia. *Biological Psychiatry 64*(9): 797–802.

Cohler, B. J., Gallant, D. H., Grunebaum, H. U., Weiss, J. L., & Gamer, E. (1975). Pregnancy and birth complications among mentally ill and well mothers and their children. *Social Biology 22*(3): 269–278.

Dalman, C. (2003). Obstetric complications and risk of schizophrenia: An association appears undisputed, yet mechanisms are still unknown. *Lakartidningen 100*(22): 1974–1979.

Dalman, C., Allebeck, P., Culberg, J., Grunewald, C., & Köster, M. (1999). Obstetric complications and the risk of schizophrenia: A longitudinal study of a national birth cohort. *Archives of General Psychiatry 56*(3): 234–240.

Dalman, C., Thomas, H. V., David, A. S., Gentz, J., Lewis, G., & Allebeck, P. (2001). Signs of asphyxia at birth increase the risk of schizophrenia: A population based case-control study. *British Journal of Psychiatry 179*: 415–416.

Devlin, B., Klei, L., Myles-Worsely, M., Tiobech, J., Otto, C., Byerley, M., & Roeder, K. (2007). Genetic liability to schizophrenia Oceanic Palau: A search in the affected and maternal generation. *Human Genetics 121*(6): 675–684.

Done, D. J., Johnstone, E. C., Frith, C. D., Golding, J., Shepherd, P. M., & Crow, T. J. (1991). Complications of pregnancy and delivery in relation to psychosis in adult life: Data from the British perinatal mortality survey sample. *British Medical Journal 302*(6792): 1576–1580.

Eagles, J. M., Gibson, I., Bremner, M. H., Clunie, F., Ebmeier, K. P., & Smith, N. C. (1990). Obstetric complications in DSM-III schizophrenics and their siblings. *Lancet 335*(8698): 1139–1141.

Ebner, F., Tepest, R., Dani, I., Pfeiffer, U., Schulze, T. G., Rietschel, M., Maier, W., Träber, F., Block, W., Schild, H. H., et al. (2008). The hippocampus in families with schizophrenia in relation to obstetric complications. *Schizophrenia Research 104*(1–3): 71–78.

Ellman, L. M., Huttunen, M., Lonnqvist, J., & Cannon, T. D. (2007). The effects of genetic liability for schizophrenia and maternal smoking during pregnancy on obstetric complications. *Schizophrenia Research 93*(1–3): 229–236.

Falkai, P., Schneider-Axmann, T., Honer, W. G., Vogeley, K., Schonell, H., Pfeiffer, U., Scherk, H., Block, W., Träber, F., Schild, H. H., et al. (2003). Influence of genetic loading, obstetric complications and premorbid adjustment on brain morphology in schizophrenia: A MRI study. *European Archives of Psychiatry and Clinical Neuroscience 253*(2): 92–99.

Fatemi, S. H. & Folsom, T. D. (2009). The neurodevelopmental hypothesis of schizophrenia, revisited. *Schizophrenia Bulletin 35*(3): 528–548.

Fatjo-Vilas, M., Gourion, D., Campanera, S., Mouaffak, F., Levy-Rueff, M., Navarro, M. E., Chayet, M., Miret, S., Krebs, M. O., & Fañanás, L. (2008). New evidences of gene and environment interactions affecting prenatal neurodevelopment in schizophrenia-spectrum disorders: A family dermatoglyphic study. *Schizophrenia Research 103*(1–3): 209–217.

Fearon, P., O'Connell, P., Frangou, S., Aquino, P., Nosarti, C., Allin, M., Taylor, M., Stewart, A., Rifkin, L., & Murray, R. (2004). Brain volumes in adult survivors of very low birth weight: A sibling-controlled study. *Pediatrics 114*(2): 367–371.

Foerster, A., Lewis, S. W., Owen, M. J., & Murray, R. (1991). Low birth weight and a family history of psychosis predict poor premorbid functioning in psychosis. *Schizophrenia Research 5*(1): 13–20.

Geddes, J. R. & Lawrie, S. M. (1995). Obstetric complications and schizophrenia: A meta-analysis. *British Journal of Psychiatry 167*: 786–793.

Geddes, J. R., Verdoux, H., Takei, N., Lawrie, S. M., Bovet, P., Eagles, J. M., Heun, R., Mc-Creadie, R. G., McNeil, T. F., O'Callaghan, E., et al. (1999). Schizophrenia and complications of pregnancy and labor: An individual-patient data meta-analysis. *Schizophrenia Bulletin 25*(3): 413–423.

Gunnell, D., Harrison, G., Whitley, E., Lewis, G., Tynelius, P., & Rasmussen, F. (2005). The association of fetal and childhood growth with risk of schizophrenia: Cohort study of 720,000 Swedish men and women. *Schizophrenia Research 79*(2–3): 315–322.

Gunnell, D., Rasmussen, F., Fouskakis, D., Tynelius, D., & Harrison, G. (2003). Patterns of fetal and childhood growth and the development of psychosis in young males: A cohort study. *American Journal of Epidemiology 158*(4): 291–300.

Gunther-Genta, F., Bovet, P., & Hohlfeld, P. (1994). Obstetric complications and schizophrenia: A case-control study. *British Journal of Psychiatry 164*: 165–170.

Hanson, D. R., Gottesman, I. I., & Heston, L. C. (1976). Some possible indicators of adult schizophrenia inferred from children of schizophrenics. *British Journal of Psychiatry 129*: 142–154.

Hanssen, M., Bak, M., Bijl, R., Vollebergh, W., & van Os, J. (2005). Incidence and outcome of subclinical psychotic experiences in the general population. *British Journal of Psychiatry 44*: 181–191.

Harrison, P. J. & Weinberger, D. R. (2005). Schizophrenia gene, gene expression, and neuropathology: On the matter of their convergence. *Molecular Psychiatry 10*(1): 40–68.

Heun, R. & Maier, W. (1993). The role of obstetric complications in schizophrenia. *Journal of Nervous and Mental Disease 181*(4): 220–226.

Hinton, G. G. (1963). Childhood psychosis or mental retardation: A diagnostic dilemma II: Paediatric and neurologic aspects. *Canadian Medical Association Journal 89*: 1020–1024.

Hollister, J. M., Laing, P., & Mednick, S. A. (1996). Rhesus incompatibility as a risk factor for schizophrenia in male adults. *Archives of General Psychiatry 53*(1): 19–24.

Hultman, C. M., Öhman, A., Cnattingus, S., Wieselgren, I-M., & Lindström, L. H. (1997). Prenatal and neonatal risk factors for schizophrenia. *British Journal of Psychiatry 170*: 128–133.

Hultman, C. M., Sparen, P., Takei, N., Murray, R. M., & Cnattingius, S. (1999). Prenatal and perinatal risk factors for schizophrenia, affective psychosis and reactive psychosis of early onset: Case-control study. *British Medical Journal 318*(7181): 421–426.

Hutchinson, G., Takei, N., Bhugra, D., Fahy, T. A., Gilvarry, C., Mallett, R., Moran, P., Leff, J., & Murray, R. M. (1997). Increased rate of psychosis among African-Caribbeans in Britain is not due to an excess of pregnancy and birth complications. *British Journal of Psychiatry 171*: 145–147.

Insel, B. J., Brown, A. S., Bresnahan, M. A., Schaefer, C. A., & Susser, E. S. (2005). Maternal-fetal blood incompatibility and the risk of schizophrenia in offspring. *Schizophrenia Research 80*(2–3): 331–342.

Insel, B. J., Schaefer, C. A., McKeague, I. W., Susser, E. S., & Brown, A. S. (2008). Maternal iron deficiency and the risk of schizophrenia in offspring. *Archives of General Psychiatry* 65(10): 1136–1144.

Jablensky, A. V., Morgan, V., Zubrick, S. R., Bower, C., & Yellachich, L. (2005). Pregnancy, delivery, and neonatal complications in a population cohort of women with schizophrenia and major affective disorders. *American Journal of Psychiatry 162*(1): 79–91.

Jones, P. B., Rantakallio, P., Hartikainen, A-L., Isohanni, M., & Sipila, P. (1998). Schizophrenia as a long-term outcome of pregnancy, delivery and perinatal complications: A 28-year follow-up of the 1966 North Finland General Population birth cohort. *American Journal of Psychiatry 155*(3): 355–364.

Kendell, R. E., McInneny, K., Jusczak, E., & Bain, M. (2000). Obstetric complications and schizophrenia: Two case-control studies based on structured obstetric records. *British Journal of Psychiatry 174*: 516–522.

King-Hele, S., Webb, R. T., Mortensen, P. B., Appleby, L., Pickles, A., & Abel, K. M. (2009). Risk of stillbirth and neonatal death linked with maternal mental illness: A national cohort study. *Archives of Disease in Childhood. Fetal and Neonatal Edition* 94(2): F105–110.

Kirov, G., Jones, P. B., Harvey, I., Lewis, S. W., Toone, B. K., Rifkin, L., Sham, P., & Murray, R. M. (1996). Do obstetric complications cause the earlier age at onset in male than female schizophrenics? *Schizophrenia Research* 20(1–2): 117–124.

Kirov, G., O'Donavan, M. C., & Owen, M. J. (2005). Finding schizophrenia genes. *Journal of Clinical Investigation 115*(6): 1440–1448.

Knobloch, H. & Pasamanick, B. (1962) Biological factors in "early infantile autism" and "childhood schizophrenia." Presented at the 10th International Congress of Paediatrics. Lisbon, September 1962.

Kunugi, H., Nanko, S., Takei, N., Saito, K., Murray, R. M, & Hirose, T. (1996a). Perinatal complications and schizophrenia. Data from the Maternal and Child Health Handbook in Japan. *Journal of Nervous and Mental Disease 184*(9): 542–546.

Kunugi, H., Takei, N., Murray, R. M., Saito, K., & Nanko, S. (1996b). Small head circumference at birth in schizophrenia. *Schizophrenia Research* 20(1–2): 165–170.

Lane, E. A. & Albee, G. W. (1966). Comparative birth weights of schizophrenics and their siblings. *Journal of Psychology* 64: 227–231.

Lewis, S. W. & Murray, R. M. (1987). Obstetric complications, neurodevelopmental deviance and risk of schizophrenia. *Journal of Psychiatric Research* 21(4): 413–421.

Lewis, S. W., Owen, M. J., & Murray, R. M. (1989). Obstetric complications and schizophrenia: Methodology and mechanisms. In S. C. Schultz & C. A. Tamminga (eds.), *Schizophrenia: Scientific Progress* (pp. 56–68). New York: Oxford University Press.

McCreadie, R. G., Hall, D. J., Berry, I. J., Robertson, L. J., Ewing, J. I., & Geals, M. F. (1992). The Nithsdale schizophrenia surveys: X. Obstetric complications, family history and abnormal movements. *British Journal of Psychiatry 160*: 799–805.

McNeil, T. (1987). Perinatal influences in the development of schizophrenia. In H. Helmchen & F. A. Henn (eds.), *Biological Perspectives of Schizophrenia* (pp. 125–138). New York: Wiley.

McNeil, T. F. (1995). Perinatal risk factors and schizophrenia: Selective review and methodological concerns. *Epidemiologic Reviews 17*(1): 107–112.

McNeil, T. F., Cantor-Graae, E., Nordstrom, L. G., & Rosenlund, T. (1993). Head circumference in "preschizophrenic" and control neonates. *British Journal of Psychiatry 162*: 517–523.

McNeil, T. F. & Kaij, L. (1973). Obstetric complications and physical size of offspring of schizophrenic, schizophrenic-like and control mothers. *British Journal of Psychiatry 123*: 341–381.

McNeil, T. F. & Kaij, L. (1978). Obstetric factors in the development of schizophrenia: Complications in the births of preschizophrenics and in reproduction by schizophrenic parents.

In L. C. Wynne, R. L. Cromwell, & S. Mathysse (eds.), *The Nature of Schizophrenia: New Approaches to Research and Treatment* (pp. 401–429). New York: Wiley.

Mednick, S. A. (1970). Breakdown in individuals at high risk for schizophrenia: Possible predispositional perinatal factors. *Mental Hygiene 54*: 51–63.

Mednick, S. A. & Schulsinger, F. (1968). Some premorbid characteristics related to breakdown in children with schizophrenic mothers. *Journal of Psychiatric Research 6*: 267–291.

Mirdal, G. K. M., Mednick, S. A., Schulsinger, F., & Fuchs, F. (1974). Perinatal complications in children of schizophrenic mothers. *Acta Psychiatrica Scandinavia 50*(6): 553–568.

Mittal, V. A., Ellman, L. M., & Cannon, T. D. (2008). Gene-environment interaction and covariation in schizophrenia: The role of obstetric complications. *Schizophrenia Bulletin 34*(6): 1083–1094.

Modrzewska, K. (1980). The offspring of schizophrenic parents in a North Swedish isolate. *Clinical Genetics 17*(3): 191–201.

Moreno, D., Moreno-Iniguez, M., Vigil, D., Castro-Fornieles, J., Ortuno, F., González-Pinto, A., Parellada, M., Baeza, I., Otero, S., Graell, M., et al. (2009). Obstetric complications as a risk factor for first psychotic episodes in childhood and adolescence. *European Child and Adolescent Psychiatry 18*(3): 180–184.

Mueser, K. T. & McGurk, S. R. (2004). Schizophrenia. *Lancet 363*(9426): 2063–2072.

Murray, R. M. & Lewis, S. W. (1987). Is schizophrenia a neurodevelopmental disorder? *British Medical Journal 295*(6600): 681–682.

Murray, R. M., Sham, P., van Os, J., Zanelli, J., Cannon, M., & McDonald, C. A. (2004). A developmental model for similarities and dissimilarities between schizophrenia and bipolar disorder. *Schizophrenia Research 71*(2–3): 405–416.

Nicolson, R., Malaspina, D., Giedd, J. N., Hamburger, S., Lenane, M., Bedwell, J., Fernandez, T., Berman, A., Susser, E., & Rapoport, J. L. (1999). Obstetrical complications and childhood-onset schizophrenia. *American Journal of Psychiatry 156*(10): 1650–1652.

Nicodemus, K. K., Marenci, S., Batten, A. J., Vakkalanka, R., Egan, M. F., Straub, R. E., & Weinberger, D. R. (2008). Serious obstetric complications interact with hypoxia-regulated vascular-expression genes to influence schizophrenia risk. *Molecular Psychiatry 18*: 180–184.

Nilsson, E., Stalberg, G., Lichtenstein, P., Cnattingius, S., Olausson, P. O., & Hultman, C. M. (2005). Fetal growth restriction and schizophrenia: A Swedish twin study. *Twin Research and Human Genetics 8*(4): 402–408.

O'Callaghan, E., Gibson, T., Colohan, H. A., Buckely, P., Walshe, D. G., Larkin, C., & Waddington, J. L. (1992). Risk of schizophrenia in adults born after obstetric complications and their association with early onset of illness: A controlled study. *British Medical Journal 305*(6864): 1256–1259.

O'Callaghan, E., Larkin, C., Kinsella, A., & Waddington, J. L. (1990). Obstetric complications, the putative familial-sporadic distinction and tardive dyskinesia in schizophrenia. *British Journal of Psychiatry 157*: 578–584.

O'Callaghan, E., Larkin, C., & Waddington, J. L. (1990). Obstetric complications in schizophrenia and the validity of maternal recall. *Psychological Medicine 20*(1): 89–94.

Ogendahl, B. K., Agerbo, E. M., Byrne, M., Licgt, R. W., Eatin, W. W., & Mortensen, P. B. (2006). Indicators of fetal growth and bipolar disorder: A Danish national register-based study. *Psychological Medicine 36*(9): 1219–1224.

Owen, M. J., Lewis, S. W., & Murray, R. M. (1988). Obstetric complications and schizophrenia: A computed tomographic study. *Psychological Medicine 18*(2): 331–339.

Pasamanick, B. & Knobloch, H. (1960). Brain and Behaviour Symposium, session 2, 1959. Brain damage and reproductive casualty. *American Journal of Orthopsychiatry 30*: 298–305.

Pasamanick, B., Rodgers, M. E., & Lilienfeld, A. M. (1956). Pregnancy experience and the development of behavior disorder in children. *American Journal of Psychiatry* 112(8): 613–618.

Pollack, M. & Woerner, M. G. (1966). Pre- and perinatal complications and "childhood schizophrenia": A comparison of five controlled studies. *Journal of Child Psychology and Psychiatry* 7(3–4): 235–242.

Pollack, M., Woerner, M. G., Goodman, W., & Greenberg I. (1966). Childhood developmental patterns of hospitalized adult schizophrenic patients and non-schizophrenic patients and their siblings. *American Journal of Orthopsychiatry* 36: 510–517.

Poulton, R., Caspi, A., Moffitt, T. E., Cannon, M., Murray, R. M., & Harrington, H-L. (2000). Children's self-reported psychotic symptoms and adult schizophreniform disorder: A 15-year longitudinal study. *Archives of General Psychiatry* 57(11): 1053–1058.

Prabakaran, S., Swatton, J. E., Ryan, M. M., Huffaker, S. J., Hiang, J.T-J., Griffin, J. L., Wayland, M., Freeman, T., Dudbridge, F., Lilley, K. S., et al. (2004). Mitochondrial dysfunction in schizophrenia: Evidence for compromised brain metabolism and oxidative stress. *Molecular Psychiatry* 9(7): 684–697.

Rieder, R. O., Broman, S. H., & Rosenthal, D. (1977). The offspring of schizophrenics 2: Perinatal factors and IQ. *Archives of General Psychiatry* 34(7): 789–799.

Rifkin, L., Lewis, S., Jones, P., Toone, B., & Murray, R. (1994). Low birth weight and schizophrenia. *British Journal of Psychiatry* 165: 357–362.

Rosa, A., Cuesta, M. J., Peralta, V., Zarzuela, A., Serrano, F., Martinez-Larrea, A., & Fañanás, L. (2005). Dermatoglyphic anomalies and neurocognitive deficits in sibling pairs discordant for schizophrenia spectrum disorders. *Psychiatry Research* 137(3): 215–221.

Rosanoff, A. J., Handy, L. M., Plesset, I. R., & Brush, S. (1934). The etiology of so-called schizophrenic psychoses: With special reference to their occurrence in twins. *American Journal of Psychiatry* 91: 247–286.

Rosso, I. M., Cannon, T. D., Huttunen, T., Huttunen, M. O., Lönnqvist, J., & Gasperoni, T. L. (2000). Obstetric risk factors for early-onset schizophrenia in a Finnish birth cohort. *American Journal of Psychiatry* 157(5): 801–807.

Sacker, A., Done, D. J., & Crow, T. J. (1996). Obstetric complications in children born to parents with schizophrenia: A meta-analysis of case-control studies. *Psychological Medicine* 26(2): 279–287.

Sacker, A., Done, D. J., Crow, T. J., & Golding, J. (1995). Antecedents of schizophrenia and affective illness: Obstetric complications. *British Journal of Psychiatry* 166: 734–741.

Sameroff, A. J. & Zax, M. (1973). Perinatal characteristics of the offspring of schizophrenic women. *Journal of Nervous Mental Disease* 157(3): 191–199.

Schlotz, W. & Phillips, D. I. (2009). Fetal origins of mental health: Evidence and mechanisms. *Brain, Behavior, and Immunity* 23(7): 905–916.

Schmidt-Kastner, R., van Os, J., Steinbusch, H., & Schmitz, C. (2006). Gene regulation by hypoxia and the neurodevelopmental origin of schizophrenia. *Schizophrenia Research* 84(2–3): 253–271.

Scott, J., McNeill, Y., Cavanagh, J., Cannon, M., & Murray, R. (2006). Exposure to obstetric complications and subsequent development of bipolar disorder: Systematic review. *British Journal of Psychiatry* 189: 3–11.

Scott, J., Welham, J., Martin, G., Bor, W., Najman, J., O'Callaghan, M., Williams, G., Aird, R., & McGrath, J. (2009). Psychopathology during childhood and adolescence predicts delusional like experiences in adults: A 21-year birth cohort study. *American Journal of Psychiatry* 166(5): 567–574.

Smith, G. N., Kopala, L. C., Lapointe, J. S., MacEwan, G. W., Altman, S., Flynn, S. W., Schneider, T., Falkai, P., & Honer, W. G. (1998). Obstetric complications, treatment response and brain morphology in adult-onset and early-onset males with schizophrenia. *Psychological Medicine* 28(3): 645–653.

Sobel, D. (1961). Infant malformations and mortality in children of schizophrenic parents. *Psychiatric Quarterly* 35: 60–64.

Sørensen, H. J., Mortensen, E. L., Reinisch, J. M., & Mednick, S.A. (2003). Do hypertensions and diuretic treatment in pregnancy increase the risk of schizophrenia in offspring? *American Journal of Psychiatry* 160(3): 464–468.

Sørensen, H. J., Mortensen, E. L., Reinisch, J. M., & Mednick, S. A. (2004). Association between prenatal exposure to analgesics and risk of schizophrenia. *British Journal of Psychiatry* 160: 366–371.

Sørensen, H. J., Nielsen P. R., Pedersen C. B., & Mortensen P. B. (2010). Association between prepartum maternal iron deficiency and offspring risk of schizophrenia: Population-based cohort study with linkage of Danish national registers. *Schizophrenia Bulletin* [epub ahead of print].

Stefanis, N., Frabgou, S., Yakeley, J., Sharma, T., O'Connel, P., Morgan, K., Sigmudsson, T., Taylor, M., & Murray, R. (1999). Hippocampal volume reduction in schizophrenia: Effects of genetic risk and pregnancy and birth complications. *Biological Psychiatry* 46(5): 697–702.

Taft, L. & Goldfarb, W. (1964). Prenatal and perinatal factors in childhood schizophrenia. *Developmental Medicine and Child Neurology* 6: 32–43.

Terris, M., Lapouse, R., & Monk, M. A. (1964). The relations of prematurity and previous fetal loss to childhood schizophrenia. *American Journal of Psychiatry* 121: 476–481.

Thomas, K., Harrison, G., Zammit, S., Lewis, G., Horwood, J., Heron, J., Hollis, C., Wolke, D., Thompson, A., & Gunnell, D. (2009). Association of measures of fetal and childhood growth with non-clinical psychotic symptoms in 12-year-olds: The ALSPAC cohort. *British Journal of Psychiatry* 194: 521–526.

Torrey, E. F., Hersch, S. P., & McCabe, K. D. (1975). Early childhood psychosis and bleeding during pregnancy. *Journal of Autism and Childhood Schizophrenia* 5(4): 287–297.

van Erp, T. G., Saleh, P. A., Rosso, I. M., Huttunen, M., Lonnqvist, J., Pirkola, T., Salonen, O., Valanne, L., Poutanen, V. P., Standertskjöld-Nordenstam, C. G., et al. (2002). Contributions of genetic risk and fetal hypoxia to hippocampal volume in patients with schizophrenia or schizoaffective disorder, their unaffected siblings, and healthy unrelated volunteers. *American Journal of Psychiatry* 159(9): 1514–1520.

van Os, J., Linscott, R. J., Myin-Germeys, I., Delespaul, P., & Krabbendam, L. (2009). A systematic review and meta-analysis of the psychosis continuum: Evidence for a psychosis proneness-persistence-impairment model of psychotic disorder. *Psychological Medicine* 39(2): 179–195.

Verdoux, H. & Bourgeois, M. (1993). A comparative study of obstetric history in schizophrenics, bipolar patients, and normal subjects. *Schizophrenia Research* 9(1): 67–69.

Verdoux, H., Geddes, J. R., Takei, N., Lawrie, S., Bovet, P., Eagles, J. M., Heun, R., McCreadie, R. G., McNeil, T. F., O'Callaghan, E., et al. (1997). Obstetric complications and age at onset of schizophrenia: An international collaborative meta-analysis of individual patient data. *American Journal of Psychiatry* 154(9): 1220–1227.

Vorster, D. (1960). An investigation of the part played by organic factors in childhood schizophrenia. *Journal of Mental Science* 106: 494–522.

Webb, R. T., Pickles, A. R., King-Hele, S. A., Appleby, L., Mortensen, P. B., & Abel, K. M. (2008). Parental mental illness and fatal birth defects in a national birth cohort. *Psychological Medicine* 38(10): 1495–1503.

Webb, R. T., Wicks, S., Dalman, C., Pickles, A. R., Appleby, L., Mortensen, P. B., Haglund, B., & Abel, K. M. (2010). Influence of environmental factors in higher risk of sudden infant death syndrome linked with parental mental illness. *Archives of General Psychiatry* 67(1): 69–77.

Weinberger, D. R. (1987). Implications of normal brain development for the pathogenesis of schizophrenia. *Archives of General Psychiatry* 44(7): 660–669.

Willinger, U., Heiden, A., & Mesaros, K. (1996). Obstetric complications, premorbid and current cognitive functioning in schizophrenics and their same-sex healthy siblings. *Schizophrenia Research* 18: 100.

Woerner, M. G., Pollack, M., & Klein, D. F. (1971). Birth weight and length in schizophrenia, personality disorders and their siblings. *British Journal of Psychiatry* 118: 461–464.

Woerner, M. G., Pollack. M., & Klein D. F. (1973). Pregnancy and birth complications in psychiatric patients: A comparison of schizophrenic and personality disorder patients with their siblings. *Acta Psychiatrica Scandinavica* 49(6): 712–721.

Zammit, S., Odd, D., Horwood, A., Thompson, A., Thomas, K., Menezes, P., Gunnell, D., Hollis, C., Wolke, D., Lewis, G., et al. (2009a). Investigating whether adverse prenatal and perinatal events are associated with non-clinical psychotic symptoms at age 12 years in the ALSPAC birth cohort. *Psychological Medicine* 39: 1457–1467.

Zammit, S., Thomas, K., Thompson, A., Horwood, J., Menezes, P., Gunnell, D., Hollis, C., Wolke, D., Lewis, G., & Harrison, G. (2009b). Maternal tobacco, cannabis, and alcohol use during pregnancy and risk of adolescent psychotic symptoms in offspring. *British Journal of Psychiatry* 195: 294–300.

Zax, M., Sameroff, A. J., & Babigian, H. M. (1977). Birth outcomes in the offspring of mentally disordered women. *American Journal of Orthopsychiatry* 47(2): 218–230.

Zornberg, G. L., Buka, S. L., & Tsuang, M. T. (2000). Hypoxic-ischemia-related fetal/neonatal complications and risk of schizophrenia and other nonaffective psychoses: A 19-year longitudinal study. *American Journal of Psychiatry* 157(2): 196–202.

CHAPTER 4

MATERNAL STRESS DURING PREGNANCY AND SCHIZOPHRENIA

MARY C. IAMPIETRO AND LAUREN M. ELLMAN

KEY CONCEPTS

- The maternal experience of stressful life events during pregnancy is associated with increased risk of schizophrenia in offspring.
- Maternal stress in pregnancy is related to an increased risk of obstetric complications that have been consistently linked with schizophrenia.
- Maternal stress during pregnancy is associated with childhood cognitive, social, and emotional disturbances that commonly occur during the premorbid period of schizophrenia.

Evidence is accumulating that maternal emotional and psychosocial experiences during pregnancy can be communicated to the fetus and influence fetal development and subsequent neurodevelopmental sequelae in offspring. It has been repeatedly documented that mothers who experience certain stressful life events during pregnancy deliver offspring with an increased risk of schizophrenia (e.g., Huttunen & Niskanen, 1978; Malaspina et al., 2008). This chapter will discuss the main research findings linking maternal stress during pregnancy with risk for schizophrenia. We also will discuss research performed in humans exploring how maternal stress during pregnancy is related to a number of obstetric events found in the histories of schizophrenia patients and is related to childhood problems that are frequently found in the premorbid period of schizophrenia. Although there are a number of preclinical studies examining stress during pregnancy and cognitive and brain abnormalities among offspring, we will focus on the primary evidence found in human studies, as these animal studies are extensively discussed in chapter 13 of this book.

Maternal Stress During Pregnancy
and Risk of Schizophrenia in Offspring

The first epidemiologic studies linking maternal stress during pregnancy to increased risk of schizophrenia in offspring were based on evidence from ecologic designs. (For a complete list of studies, see table 4.1.) Although there are some conflicting findings, many of these studies found that mothers who were exposed to a severe life event during pregnancy had offspring with an increased risk for schizophrenia. This association was first noted by Huttunen & Niskanen (1978), who found that mothers whose husbands died during months three to five or nine to ten of gestation had children who were more likely to develop schizophrenia.

Being pregnant during wartime and during natural disasters also has been associated with risk for schizophrenia in a number of studies. Specifically, children of mothers who were in their first and second trimesters of pregnancy during the May 1940 five-day invasion of the Netherlands by German forces were at a significantly increased risk for developing schizophrenia when compared to children of mothers who were pregnant two years before or after the invasion (van Os & Selten, 1998). However, the second-trimester finding appeared to be restricted to males, suggesting that male fetuses may be particularly vulnerable to maternal stress (van Os & Selten, 1998). Similarly, mothers who were in their second month of pregnancy during the 1967 Arab-Israeli War (the "Six Day War") also gave birth to offspring with a heightened risk of schizophrenia (Malaspina et al., 2008). Another study, which examined the effects of prenatal exposure to the 1953 Dutch Flood Disaster, also found an increased risk of schizophrenia in offspring; however, this finding failed to reach statistical significance, possibly because of a limited number of schizophrenia cases in the cohort (Selten et al., 1999).

Although the aforementioned studies suggest an association between maternal stress during pregnancy and increased risk for schizophrenia, ecologic studies are fraught with a number of methodologic concerns. Specifically, in all of these studies, stress was never measured in individuals but rather was assumed on the basis of life events that occurred for an entire population. Further, the aforementioned studies assessed life events that are relatively rare, severe, and likely could be associated with a range of potentially teratogenic conditions, such as malnutrition, increase in substance abuse, or other factors. The question remains as to whether severe life events, such as the ones described above, are measuring stress or other constructs such as fear, trauma, or both.

Nevertheless, three studies have prospectively measured maternal experiences that are presumed to be stressful during individual pregnancies and have linked these experiences with increased risk for schizophrenia in offspring. Khashan et al. (2008a) found that mothers who experienced a death or serious illness of

Table 4.1 Epidemiologic Studies of Stressful Life Events During Pregnancy and Risk for Schizophrenia in Offspring

Authors/Year	Environmental Stressor	Population	Exposed/Unexposed	Main Finding(s)	Statistics
Huttunen & Niskanen, 1978	Loss of husband during pregnancy	Finnish population registers for births 1925–1957	Exposed: 167 persons who lost father before their births (6 developed schizophrenia). Unexposed: 168 controls whose father died during year 1 of life (1 developed schizophrenia).	Loss of husband during months 3–5 and 9–10 of pregnancy increased risk for schizophrenia among offspring more than loss of husband during first year of offspring's life.	$X^2 = 3.87$, $p < .05$
van Os & Selten, 1998	Five-day invasion of the Netherlands by German forces in 1940	Dutch birth cohorts 1938, 1940, and 1942	Exposed: 133,394 pregnant women exposed to the invasion (419 offspring developed schizophrenia). Unexposed: 539,781 controls born during the same period in the previous and subsequent 2 years (1,480 developed schizophrenia).	Offspring whose mothers were pregnant during the invasion (especially in their first trimester) were at greater risk for developing schizophrenia than controls; males whose mothers were in their second trimester were especially affected.	Risk ratio = 1.15 (95% CI = 1.03–1.28)
Selten et al., 1999	Dutch Flood Disaster of February 1953	Dutch birth cohorts 1951 and 1953	Exposed: 1,393 pregnant women exposed to the flood disaster in 1953 between February and October (22 offspring diagnosed with nonaffective psychosis). Unexposed: 7,389 individuals born between the months of February and October in 1951, 1952, 1954, or 1955 (66 diagnosed with nonaffective psychosis).	Offspring of pregnant women exposed to the flood were at greater (nonsignificant) risk of developing nonaffective psychosis than unexposed offspring.	Risk ratio for nonaffective psychosis = 1.8 (95% CI = 0.9–3.5) Risk ratio for schizophrenia = 1.9 (95% CI = 0.6–6.1)

Study	Exposure	Cohort	Sample	Findings	Statistical result
Khashan et al., 2008a	Death or serious illness of 1 or more close maternal relatives	Danish birth cohort 1973–1995	Exposed: 21,987 pregnant women exposed to death or serious illness of close relative during gestation and up to 6 months before pregnancy (80 offspring diagnosed with schizophrenia). Unexposed: 666,159 pregnant women without similar life events (1,813 offspring diagnosed with schizophrenia).	Mothers who experienced a death of 1 or more close relatives during their first trimester of pregnancy gave birth to individuals at an increased risk of developing schizophrenia.	Adjusted relative risk = 1.67 (95% CI = 1.02–2.73) Used log-linear Poisson regression
Malaspina et al., 2008	Arab-Israeli War (Six-Day War) of 1967	Jerusalem birth cohort 1964–1976	Exposed: 4,227 pregnant women during war (37 diagnosed with schizophrenia). Unexposed: 2,922 offspring conceived in 3 months after war or in 3 months before war (20 diagnosed with schizophrenia).	Women pregnant during the second month had offspring at increased risk of developing schizophrenia; the risk was found more in females than males.	Hazard ratio = 2.3 (95% CI = 1.1–4.7)
Myhrman et al., 1996	Unwanted pregnancy	Northern Finland 1966 birth cohort	Exposed: 1,264 individuals from unwanted pregnancies (19 diagnosed with schizophrenia). Unexposed: 9,486 individuals from wanted pregnancies (57 diagnosed with schizophrenia).	Children of unwanted pregnancies were at a significantly greater risk of later developing schizophrenia than the rest of the population.	Odds ratio = 2.5 (95% CI = 1.5–4.2)
Herman et al., 2006	Unwanted pregnancy	Northern California birth cohort 1959–1967	Exposed: 1,499 offspring from unwanted pregnancies (16 diagnosed with SSD). Unexposed: 5,651 offspring from wanted pregnancies (35 diagnosed with SSD).	Unwantedness of pregnancy was related to a nonsignificant increase in risk for SSD in offspring.	Hazard ratio = 1.75 (95% CI = 0.97, 3.17, $p > .05$)

CI = confidence interval; SSD = schizophrenia spectrum disorder.
SOURCE: Authors.

one or more close relatives during the first trimester of pregnancy gave birth to offspring with a significantly increased risk of developing schizophrenia, independent of other factors associated with risk for the disorder, such as the offspring's sex, age, family history of mental illness, place of birth, and maternal age. This is similar to the results of the population-based study by Huttunen & Niskanen (1978), except that the timing of the stressor during pregnancy differed. In a second study, Myhrman and colleagues (1996), in the Northern Finland 1966 birth cohort, found that unwantedness of a pregnancy, as rated by the mothers in the sixth or seventh month of gestation, led to a 2.5-fold increased risk of schizophrenia in offspring. In a replication attempt, Herman et al. (2006), in a birth cohort in northern California, found a similar association (unadjusted hazard ratio = 1.75, 95% CI = 0.97, 3.17) that fell slightly short of statistical significance. It is possible that the latter study failed to detect a significant result because of diminished power. Again, in these studies stress was not directly measured but rather presumed on the basis of an experience, namely unwantedness of the pregnancy, that *could* be associated with stress. Although it is possible that unwantedness of pregnancy is experienced as stressful to most women, it may not be the case for all women. Further, unwantedness of pregnancy also has the potential to be related to other behaviors or emotional states that could cause harm to the fetus, such as depression, substance use, lack of adequate prenatal care, or all of these.

Hence, the existing studies linking stress during pregnancy to risk of psychosis in offspring are suggestive of a relationship, but lack considerable information on intermediate steps, such as maternal interpretation of life events, adequacy of coping resources, biological responses to stress, and engagement in behaviors risky to health. Despite these limitations, there is substantial evidence that fetal exposure to maternal stress is associated with a number of risk factors that have been consistently linked to schizophrenia, including obstetric complications and neurodevelopmental sequelae in offspring. In the remainder of the chapter, we will summarize these findings briefly and provide our views on how future research should proceed in investigating the role of maternal stress during pregnancy in the neurodevelopmental course of schizophrenia.

Maternal Stress During Pregnancy and Fetal Growth

Although there are some conflicting findings, patients with schizophrenia tend to have a history of lower birth weight and fetal growth than nonschizophrenia controls (see chapter 3, this book). Even though many factors can influence the growth of the fetus, it is now clear that maternal psychosocial stress during pregnancy and maternal biological responses to stress can greatly affect the growth of the fetus and result in decreased birth weight and fetal growth restriction. As discussed here, these effects appear to be dependent on the timing during pregnancy and the type of stress experienced by the mothers.

A number of studies have examined the relationship between stressful life events during pregnancy and fetal growth and low birth weight (LBW). Specifically, one study found that objective major life events in the third trimester, such as events considered to be more stressful than a wedding, were significantly associated with LBW (Newton & Hunt, 1984). It is interesting that smoking during pregnancy seemed to mediate this relationship, suggesting that behaviors risky to health may partially account for the relationship between serious life events and damage to the fetus. Similarly, Xiong et al. (2008) examined posttraumatic stress disorder (PTSD) and birth outcomes of women exposed to Hurricane Katrina. The authors found that women who were exposed to three or more severe hurricane-related events, such as feeling that one's life was in danger and walking through flood waters, had a greater than threefold increased risk of delivering LBW infants. Neither general exposure to the hurricane nor the consequent development of PTSD was significantly associated with an increased risk of delivering an LBW infant. In a similar vein, death of a relative during pregnancy or in the six months before pregnancy has been associated with a significantly increased risk of babies weighing below the tenth percentile (Khashan et al., 2008b). Cumulatively, these findings suggest that a number of severe life events are associated with LBW and that smoking may be the link in this relationship for a portion of women. However, it remains unclear whether there are specific periods in gestation that are vulnerable to the effects of stress on LBW, given that there appears to be evidence for both early and late gestational effects of exposure to serious life events during pregnancy on fetal growth.

Another concern with the aforementioned studies is that documentation about maternal emotional responses to stressful life events was not entirely addressed. To this end, Wadhwa et al. (1993) examined the relationship between maternal appraisals of stress associated with life events and risk of LBW in a relatively healthy, nonsmoking pregnant population. It is interesting that maternal subjective reports of stress associated with life events in the first and second trimesters were significantly related to LBW; however, other measures of stress—such as chronic stress, daily hassles, psychological and physical symptom strain, and pregnancy-specific anxiety—were not related to LBW (although pregnancy-specific anxiety was significantly related to decreased gestational length). These results further support the association between maternal stressful life events during pregnancy and risk for decreased fetal growth. Moreover, these findings suggest that maternal appraisals of stress associated with the event may portend deleterious outcomes to the fetus even in the absence of behaviors that are clearly risky to health.

The question arises as to how maternal stress is translated to the fetus, ultimately resulting in disruptions in fetal development, namely fetal growth. One possibility is that fetal exposure to hormones that are associated with stress, such as glucocorticoids (e.g., cortisol), contributes to disruptions in fetal growth. Support for this idea comes from a number of studies that have found that increases in hormones associated with stress during pregnancy are related to decreased fetal growth and LBW. Specifically, one study found a significant association between the number of maternal prenatal corticosteroid administrations and decreased birth weight (French et al., 1999). Similarly, another study found that among women admitted for preterm labor and given a single prenatal treatment of glucocorticoids between 25 and 34 weeks, offspring born at term had significantly reduced length, weight, birth weight percentile, and head circumference, even when compared to offspring of mothers matched for preterm labor admittance and gestational age and sex of infants (Davis et al., 2009). In concert with these findings, elevated levels of placental corticotropin-releasing hormone (CRH) in the thirty-third week of gestation also have been associated with increased rates of small-for-gestational-age (SGA) infants (Wadhwa et al., 2004). Further, offspring of women with high levels of CRH exhibited a 3.7-fold increased risk for fetal growth restriction over women with low CRH levels.

Lastly, it seems as if the timing of exposure to stress hormones and the sex of the fetus are key in determining the consequences to fetal growth and development. Specifically, Ellman et al. (2008) found that increases in maternal cortisol at 15 and 19 weeks gestation were significantly associated with decreases in physical and neuromuscular maturation in the newborn infant. Furthermore, these early cortisol increases were associated with a rise in placental CRH levels at 31 weeks gestation, which also led to decreases in infant physical and neuromuscular maturation, suggesting that early gestational cortisol may prime the placenta to release a surge of CRH later in gestation. In additional analyses that examined males and females separately, the above findings were significant only for males, providing support for the hypothesis that males may be more sensitive to fetal exposure to maternal stress.

Cumulatively, the extant literature suggests that stress hormones are integrally involved in fetal growth and that this involvement may be sex dependent. Altogether, studies indicate that maternal stress hormones during pregnancy may be related to a birth outcome that has been frequently found in the history of schizophrenia patients: decreased fetal growth (French et al., 1999; Wadhwa et al., 2004; Ellman et al., 2008; Davis et al., 2009).

Ethnic and Racial Differences in Responses to Stress During Pregnancy

A number of studies have found that there may be racial and ethnic disparities in schizophrenia (Fearon et al., 2006; Bresnahan et al., 2007). Specifically, individuals from African descent in the United States and the United Kingdom are at significantly increased risk for schizophrenia, even after controlling for a variety of demographic characteristics (Fearon et al., 2006; Bresnahan et al., 2007). Although the causes of this racial disparity remain elusive, there is evidence suggestive of a contribution beginning in utero.

African American women are at substantially increased risk for a variety of poor birth outcomes, such as preterm delivery and LBW (Alexander et al., 2003). However, these racial differences do not seem to be related to socioeconomic status or access to prenatal care (Lu & Halfon, 2003). It has been proposed that racial differences in poor birth outcomes may be attributed, in part, to dissimilar maternal experiences across racial groups. Specifically, one study found that perceived racism significantly predicted birth weight in African Americans but not in other racial or ethnic groups (Dominguez et al., 2008). Moreover, although the number of stressful life events during pregnancy seem to be higher among African American women than among other racial or ethnic groups, their reports of subjective stress and anxiety have been found to be lower, possibly because of underreporting or denial of stressful experiences (Johnson & Crowley, 1996; Dominguez et al., 2005). Nonetheless, these findings suggest that perceived racism and increases in stressful life events may contribute to the racial disparities found in LBW among African Americans and might contribute to the increased risk for schizophrenia.

It also appears as if African Americans exhibit a different profile of stress hormone secretion during pregnancy than other racial and ethnic groups. Specifically, relatively low cortisol levels during the second trimester of pregnancy have been found among African Americans as compared to other racial and ethnic groups (Glynn et al., 2007). This endocrine profile is consistent with a pattern of hypothalamo-pituitary adrenal (HPA) axis dysregulation present in those diagnosed with PTSD. This pattern has been interpreted as being attributable to a lifetime of exposure to increased stress, adverse socioeconomic circumstances, and racial bias (Glynn et al., 2007). Although decreases in cortisol may appear to argue against a direct teratogenic role of this hormone in increasing risk for subsequent neurodevelopmental sequelae, cortisol is essential for fetal growth and development (Welberg, Seckl, & Holmes, 2001; Trainer, 2002; Murphy et al., 2006). Therefore, lower levels of cortisol at key periods of fetal development can result in deleterious birth outcomes as well. It also appears as if African American women may be more sensitive to the effects of stress hormones during pregnancy, whereby smaller increases in stress hormones are more likely to lead to other deleterious birth outcomes, such as preterm delivery (Holzman et al., 2001). Moreover, because cortisol is a potent anti-inflammatory hormone, the damaging effects to the fetus could potentially be a result of relative increases in proinflammatory cytokines among African Americans (Miller, Cohen, & Ritchey, 2002). Taken together, these results support a complex scenario whereby fetal exposure to both decreased and increased levels of cortisol can lead to deleterious effects on birth outcomes (such as LBW) and potentially to risk for schizophrenia in adulthood. Although this latter relationship has not been tested, it is clear that issues of timing of exposure to stress, fetal sex, and maternal race or ethnicity are key factors that should be explored in future investigations.

Maternal Stress During Pregnancy and Immune Functioning

As discussed in chapters 1 and 10 of this book, a number of maternal infections during pregnancy (e.g., influenza, upper respiratory infections, and *toxoplasma gondii*) have been repeatedly linked to increased risk of schizophrenia through a series of ecologic and, more recently, serologic studies (Brown & Derkits, 2010). Nevertheless, many infections do not appear to cross the placenta; therefore, the deleterious influences to fetal brain development seem related to maternal antiviral responses to infection, such as increases in proinflammatory cytokines (Patterson, 2009). Two studies have found that elevations in proinflammatory cytokines during pregnancy result in an increased risk of schizophrenia in offspring (Buka et al., 2001; Brown et al., 2004).

There is a preponderance of evidence that both psychological stress and neuroendocrine markers of stress affect immune functioning and susceptibility to infection, depending on the duration and severity of the stressor. Sympathetic neuronal fibers directly innervate both primary (bone marrow and thymus) and secondary (spleen and lymph nodes) lymphoid tissues, releasing hormones that bind to receptors on leukocytes, leading to multiple changes in their distribution and function (Felten & Felten, 1994; Ader, Felten, & Cohen, 2001). Similarly, multiple studies have demonstrated direct interactions between inflammatory mediators and the HPA axis. Both animal and human studies have linked multiple proinflammatory cytokines, such as interleukin-1 (IL-1), tumor necrosis factor- α (TNF-α), interleukin-8 (IL-8), and interleukin-6 (IL-6) with activation of the HPA axis, including direct activation of CRH production by the hypothalamus (Cupps & Fauci, 1982; Fontana, Weber, & Dayer, 1984; Sapolsky et al., 1987; Bernardini et al., 1990; Buckingham et al., 1994; Farina & Winkelman, 2005). Although glucocorticoids act in certain circumstances as potent anti-inflammatory agents, numerous studies suggest that exposure to stressors can lead to relative increases in inflammatory cytokines, likely due to an inflammatory rebound that occurs once the stressor has ceased (Miller, Cohen, & Ritchey, 2002). This assertion is supported by a number of studies (Segerstrom & Miller, 2004). Consistent with these findings, stress has been shown to exacerbate the consequences of influenza infections in humans and alter cytokine production in respiratory infections (Cohen, Doyle, & Skoner, 1999).

Despite consistently documented relationships between stress and immune functioning, very few studies have examined this association in pregnant populations, although the results of available studies are consistent with those from studies of nonpregnant populations. Specifically, one study found that maternal self-reported elevations in stress during pregnancy were positively correlated with higher levels of the proinflammatory cytokines IL-6 and TNF-α and with low levels of the anti-inflammatory cytokine IL-10 (Coussons-Read et al., 2005). Furthermore, increases in cortisol during weeks 19 through 21, 23 through 26, and 31 through 35 of gestation have been associated with greater prevalence of genitourinary infection (Ruiz et al., 2001).

Altogether, the aforementioned studies suggest that maternal stress during pregnancy may contribute to the previously observed relationship between maternal infection during pregnancy and risk for schizophrenia. Specifically, maternal stress during pregnancy could result in increased susceptibility to infection, more severe infections, and larger inflammatory responses to infection. Further, maternal stress during pregnancy has been found to lead to increases in inflammation in the absence of known infections (Coussons-Read et al., 2005), suggesting that the previously observed associations between increases in proinflammatory cytokines during pregnancy and risk for schizophrenia may be partially accounted for by maternal stress during pregnancy.

Maternal Stress During Pregnancy and Hypoxia-Associated Obstetric Complications

Some evidence suggests that maternal stress during pregnancy is associated with fetal hypoxia (reduced oxygen delivery to the fetus) and hypoxia-associated obstetric complications. Specifically, studies have investigated the relationship between stress and pregnancy-induced hypertension, a maternal health complication commonly associated with fetal hypoxia (Sharma, Norris, & Kalkunte, 2010). These studies are particularly relevant to schizophrenia research, as hypoxia-associated obstetric complications have been consistently linked to an increased risk of schizophrenia, an earlier age of onset for the disorder, and more severe brain abnormalities among patients (Cannon, 1997; McGorry et al., 2001; Cannon et al., 2002; Van Erp et al., 2002; McGorry et al., 2008; McGrath, 2008) (see chapter 3, this book). Specifically, in an examination of psychosocial work stress and pregnancy-induced hypertension, Landsbergis and Hatch (1996) found that women working outside of the home had a significantly increased incidence of pregnancy-induced hypertension than did unemployed pregnant women. However, this increased incidence was explained partly by confounding variables, and the mechanisms driving this finding were not elucidated. Similarly, Vollebregt and colleagues (2008) also discovered that working was associated with approximately twice the risk for development of preeclampsia and gestational hypertension than was not working. A more in-depth analysis revealed that this risk was explained significantly by having perceived control at work, as high or moderate work control reduced the discrepancy of these outcomes between the working and not working groups, whereas low work control increased the risks of developing preeclampsia and gestational hypertension considerably; job strain also resulted in approximately twice the risk. Notably, all of these associations were no longer significant after controlling for medical and socioeconomic covariates, again bringing the direct relationship of work stress and preeclampsia into question.

Other maternal stressors during pregnancy also have been studied in relation to hypoxia-associated obstetric complications. Specifically, in a population of black African women in Nigeria, Anorlu, Iwuala, & Odum (2005) found that a stressful home environment and stressful work during pregnancy (defined by a 5-level activity score) both were significantly associated with increased risk for developing preeclampsia. As the aforementioned studies attributed working outside the home, low work control, and high job strain to increased risk of this outcome, this study found that work per se during pregnancy was not significantly associated with preeclampsia, suggesting that specific types of stress associated with work may be involved in the development of the condition. In contrast, Sikkema and colleagues (2001) studied white women who developed preeclampsia after 33 weeks of gestation and found no significantly increased levels of cortisol, state or trait anxiety scores, or pregnancy-specific anxiety over those of normotensive control women. These apparent discrepancies may be related to racial differences in responses to stress during pregnancy, as one study found that maternal stress during pregnancy was related to elevated blood pressure in African Americans but not whites (Hilmert et al., 2008). Lastly, one study found that elevated levels of the stress hormone CRH led to restricted blood flow to the fetus, measured through ultrasonography (Harville et al., 2008).

In sum, it remains unclear whether maternal stress during pregnancy is related to increased risk for hypoxia-associated obstetric complications. There is some evidence that maternal stress during pregnancy may place individuals of African descent at increased risk for hypoxia-associated obstetric complications, namely through increases in blood pressure. In addition, there is preliminary evidence that elevations in maternal stress hormones during pregnancy lead to restricted blood flow and oxygen to the fetus. These data suggest a possible relationship between fetal hypoxia and maternal stress during pregnancy, although this question warrants further investigation.

Maternal Stress During Pregnancy and Eating Behaviors

As other chapters in this book describe in detail (chapters 2 and 12), there is growing support for a relationship between maternal nutrition and risk for schizophrenia in offspring. Specifically, both prenatal famine and increased pre-pregnancy body mass index (BMI) have been associated with an increased risk for schizophrenia, implicating nutritional factors in the pathogenesis of the disorder (Schaefer et al., 2000; Brown & Susser, 2008). Further, elevated homocysteine levels, which occur secondary to folate deficiency during pregnancy, also have been associated with increased risk for schizophrenia (Brown et al., 2007). It is becoming increasingly clear that stress affects eating behaviors in a variety of ways. Specifically, stress has been associated with changes in the amount of food consumed, and it influences food preference and choices. In both laboratory and naturalistic environments, studies have consistently demonstrated that people exposed to stressful situations prefer sweeter foods and foods with a higher fat content (Oliver, Wardle, & Gibson, 2000; Epel et al., 2001). Although stress also has been associated with dietary restriction, this finding may be limited to normal-weight women (Epel et al., 2001; Newman, O'Connor, & Conner, 2007; Habhab, Sheldon, & Loeb, 2009; Rutters et al., 2009a, 2009b). These studies raise the possibility that the relationship between maternal nutrition during pregnancy and risk for schizophrenia likely operates within a context of maternal experiences and, potentially, stress-related behaviors that should be considered in investigations that explore the long-term sequelae of nutrients during pregnancy.

Maternal Stress During Pregnancy and Childhood Outcomes

Maternal stress during pregnancy also has been associated with a range of childhood disturbances—including cognitive, social, and emotional difficulties—that commonly occur during the premorbid period of schizophrenia (Jones et al., 1994; Cannon et al., 1997; Cannon et al., 1999; Bearden et al., 2000; Niendam et al., 2003). Specifically, multiple types of stressors during pregnancy (e.g., life events, pregnancy anxiety, daily hassles) have been associated with a range of cognitive problems in offspring, including decreased IQ, decreased language functioning, poor attention regulation, and difficulties adapting to new situations (Buitelaar et al., 2003; Huizink et al., 2003; Slykerman et al., 2005; Laplante et al., 2008). Stress during pregnancy and elevations in stress hormones have also been linked to changes in offspring behavior, such as displaying a fearful temperament (de Weerth, van Hees, & Buitelaar, 2003; Davis et al., 2005). Moreover, in an examination of children six to nine years of age, Buss and colleagues

(2010) found that maternal self-report of pregnancy anxiety at 19 weeks gestation was associated with gray matter volume reductions specifically in six distinct brain regions, including the prefrontal cortex and the medial temporal lobe, abnormalities of which have been consistently implicated in volumetric brain imaging studies in schizophrenia (Wright et al., 2000; Gur, Keshavan, & Lawrie, 2007). Cumulatively, these studies lend support to the putative role of maternal stress during pregnancy in neurodevelopmental precursors of schizophrenia; however, there still is a paucity of long-term follow-up studies to confirm these associations.

Discussion and Future Directions

There is emerging evidence of an association between maternal stress during pregnancy and increased risk for schizophrenia. This evidence derives from multiple lines of investigation, including the relationship between severe stressful life events and schizophrenia in ecologic studies, between maternal stress during pregnancy and obstetric complications that are found in the histories of schizophrenia patients, and between maternal stress during pregnancy and childhood disturbances that occur more commonly in the premorbid period of individuals diagnosed with schizophrenia as opposed to controls.

There are, however, a number of limitations in previous studies that should be investigated in future work. Specifically, no study, to our knowledge, has prospectively examined different types of maternal stress during pregnancy, such as perceived stress and appraisals of life events, in relation to risk for the subsequent development of schizophrenia in offspring. These studies are necessary, as only rare and severe stressful life events during pregnancy (e.g., death of a spouse or exposure to war) have been examined thus far in relation to schizophrenia with no information on maternal cognitive or emotional responses to these events (Huttunen & Niskanen, 1978; Malaspina et al., 2008). Therefore, it is possible that the findings from existing studies may not generalize to most pregnant populations. Moreover, no study has determined whether maternal neuroendocrine responses to stress during pregnancy are related to the development of schizophrenia in offspring. This is necessary for us to begin to understand how maternal subjective experiences of stress during pregnancy are translated to the fetus, subsequently leading to risk for future developmental disruptions.

The role of ethnic and racial differences in relation to maternal stress during pregnancy and subsequent risk for schizophrenia also should be considered in future investigations. As reviewed earlier in this chapter (see "Ethnic and Racial Differences in Responses to Stress During Pregnancy"), there are differences in the number of life events, appraisals of life events, and endocrine responses to stress in African American populations (Dominguez et al., 2005; Glynn et al.,

2007; Dominguez et al., 2008). Given these differences, it is clear that future studies would benefit by incorporating race and ethnicity into explanatory models of the relationship between prenatal stress and schizophrenia.

As discussed previously in this chapter (see "Maternal Stress During Pregnancy and Fetal Growth"), there also are findings suggesting that the timing of exposure to stress and the sex of the fetus may be important in determining the future outcomes of offspring (e.g., Ellman et al., 2008). Although this area has been relatively understudied, there is evidence for both late and early effects of stress on detrimental outcomes to offspring. Consequently, we believe that this line of research is an important next step for future work.

It also is clear that maternal behaviors during pregnancy can be affected by stress and other emotional states, some of which can have damaging influences on fetal development. In this chapter, we discussed the relationship between stress and eating (see "Maternal Stress During Pregnancy and Eating Behaviors"); however, it is clear that stress can influence rates of substance abuse and smoking, as well as cause disruptions in sleep, all of which have the potential to induce teratogenic effects (Oliver, Wardle, & Gibson, 2000; Repetti, Taylor, & Seeman, 2002; Irwin et al., 2008; Rutters et al., 2009b; Chang et al., 2010). Incorporating into future studies information on behaviors during pregnancy that are risky to maternal health may be critical in understanding important intermediate steps between prenatal stress and subsequent risk for schizophrenia.

Lastly, we discussed how maternal stress during pregnancy has been associated with a number of obstetric events that have been consistently linked to schizophrenia (see "Maternal Stress During Pregnancy and Hypoxia-Associated Obstetric Complications"). Determining whether maternal stress during pregnancy acts as an antecedent to other obstetric risk factors observed in the etiology of schizophrenia has not only the potential to elucidate important causal pathways in the development of the disorder but also the potential to influence both primary prevention strategies and potential interventions in pregnant populations.

KEY AREAS FOR FUTURE RESEARCH

- Prospectively collect information on different types of stressors, maternal appraisals of stress, and neuroendocrine response to stress.
- Investigate racial and ethnic differences in baseline stress hormones and responses to stress.
- Examine the relations between maternal stress during pregnancy and behavior risky to health.
- Analyze the timing of fetal exposure to stress.
- Evaluate the relations between maternal stress and obstetric complications found in the histories of schizophrenia patients.

Acknowledgments

Mary Iampietro was supported by a Temple University start-up award to Dr. Ellman. The authors also would like to thank Alan Brown for his helpful edits.

Selected Readings

Cohen, S., Kessler, R. C., & Gordon, L. U. (1997). *Measuring Stress: A Guide for Health and Social Scientists.* New York: Oxford University Press.

Dunkel Schetter, C. (2011). Psychological science on pregnancy: Stress processes, biopsychosocial models, and emerging research issues. *Annual Review of Psychology 62*: 531–558.

Ellman, L. M. & Susser, E. S. (2009). The promise of epidemiologic studies: Neuroimmune mechanisms in the etiologies of brain disorders. *Neuron 64*(1): 25–27.

Felten, S. Y. & Felten, D. (1994). Neural-immune interaction. *Progress in Brain Research 100*: 157–162.

Kinsella, M. T. & Monk, C. (2009). Impact of maternal stress, depression and anxiety on fetal neurobehavioral development. *Clinical Obstetrics and Gynecology 52*(3): 425–440.

Miller, G. E., Cohen, S., & Ritchey, A. K. (2002). Chronic psychological stress and the regulation of pro-inflammatory cytokines: A glucocorticoid-resistance model. *Health Psychology 21*(6): 531–541.

Segerstrom, S. C. & Miller, G. E. (2004). Psychological stress and the human immune system: A meta-analytic study of 30 years of inquiry. *Psychological Bulletin 130*(4): 601–630.

Talge, N. M., Neal, C., & Glover, V. (2007). Antenatal maternal stress and long-term effects on child neurodevelopment: How and why? *Journal of Child Psychology and Psychiatry 48*(3–4): 245–261.

Wadhwa, P. D., Buss, C., Entringer, S., & Swanson, J. M. (2009). Developmental origins of health and disease: Brief history of the approach and current focus on epigenetic mechanisms. *Seminars in Reproductive Medicine 27*(5): 358–368.

Weinstock, M. (2008). The long-term behavioural consequences of prenatal stress. *Neuroscience and Biobehavioral Reviews 32*(6): 1073–1086.

References

Ader, R., Felten, D. L., & Cohen, N. (2001). *Psychoneuroimmunology* (3rd ed.). San Diego: Academic.

Alexander, G. R., Kogan, M., Bader, D., Carlo, W., Allen, M., & Mor, J. (2003). US birth weight/gestational age-specific neonatal mortality: 1995–1997 rates for whites, Hispanics, and blacks. *Pediatrics 111*(1): e61–e66.

Anorlu, R. I., Iwuala, N. C., & Odum, C. U. (2005). Risk factors for pre-eclampsia in Lagos, Nigeria. *Australian and New Zealand Journal of Psychiatry 45*(4): 278–282.

Bearden, C. E., Rosso, I. M., Hollister, J. M., Sanchez, L. E., Hadley, T., & Cannon, T. D. (2000). A prospective cohort study of childhood behavioral deviance and language abnormalities as predictors of adult schizophrenia. *Schizophrenia Bulletin 26*(2): 395–410.

Bernardini, R., Kamilaris, T. C., Calogero, A. E., Johnson, E. O., Gomez, M. T., Gold, P. W., & Chrousos, G. P. (1990). Interactions between tumor necrosis factor-alpha, hypothalamic corticotropin-releasing hormone, and adrenocorticotropin secretion in the rat. *Endocrinology* 126(6): 2876–2881.

Bresnahan, M., Begg, M. D., Brown, A., Schaefer, C., Sohler, N., Insel, B., Vella, L., & Susser, E. (2007). Race and risk of schizophrenia in a US birth cohort: Another example of health disparity? *International Journal of Epidemiology* 36(4): 751–758.

Brown, A. S., Bottiglieri, T., Schaefer, C. A., Quesenberry, C. P., Jr., Liu, L., Bresnahan, M., & Susser, E. S. (2007). Elevated prenatal homocysteine levels as a risk factor for schizophrenia. *Archives of General Psychiatry* 64(1): 31–39.

Brown, A. S. & Derkits, E. J. (2010). Prenatal infection and schizophrenia: A review of epidemiologic and translational studies. *American Journal of Psychiatry* 167(3): 261–280.

Brown, A. S., Hooton, J., Schaefer, C. A., Zhang, H., Petkova, E., Babulas, V., Perrin, M., Gorman, J. M., & Susser, E. S. (2004). Elevated maternal interleukin-8 levels and risk of schizophrenia in adult offspring. *American Journal of Psychiatry* 161(5): 889–895.

Brown, A. S. & Susser, E. S. (2008). Prenatal nutritional deficiency and risk of adult schizophrenia. *Schizophrenia Bulletin* 34(6): 1054–1063.

Buckingham, J. C., Loxley, H. D., Taylor, A. D., & Flower, R. J. (1994). Cytokines, glucocorticoids and neuroendocrine function. *Pharmacological Research* 30(1): 35–42.

Buitelaar, J. K., Huizink, A. C., Mulder, E. J., de Medina, P. G., & Visser, G. H. (2003). Prenatal stress and cognitive development and temperament in infants. *Neurobiology of Aging* 24(Suppl 1): S53–S60; discussion S67–S68.

Buka, S. L., Tsuang, M. T., Torrey, E. F., Klebanoff, M. A., Wagner, R. L., & Yolken, R. H. (2001). Maternal cytokine levels during pregnancy and adult psychosis. *Brain, Behavior, and Immunology* 15(4): 411–420.

Buss, C., Davis, E. P., Muftuler, L. T., Head, K., & Sandman, C. A. (2010). High pregnancy anxiety during mid-gestation is associated with decreased gray matter density in 6–9-year-old children. *Psychoneuroendocrinology* 35(1): 141–153.

Cannon, M., Jones, P., Gilvarry, C., Rifkin, L., McKenzie, K., Foerster, A., & Murray, R. M. (1997). Premorbid social functioning in schizophrenia and bipolar disorder: Similarities and differences. *American Journal of Psychiatry* 154(11): 1544–1550.

Cannon, M., Jones, P., Huttunen, M. O., Tanskanen, A., Huttunen, T., Rabe-Hesketh, S., & Murray, R. M. (1999). School performance in Finnish children and later development of schizophrenia: A population-based longitudinal study. *Archives of General Psychiatry* 56(5): 457–463.

Cannon, T. D. (1997). On the nature and mechanisms of obstetric influences in schizophrenia: A review and synthesis of epidemilogic studies. *International Review of Psychiatry* 9: 387–397.

Cannon, T. D., van Erp, T. G., Rosso, I. M., Huttunen, M., Lonnqvist, J., Pirkola, T., Salonen, O., Valanne, L., Poutanen, V. P., & Standertskjold-Nordenstam, C. G. (2002). Fetal hypoxia and structural brain abnormalities in schizophrenic patients, their siblings, and controls. *Archives of General Psychiatry* 59(1): 35–41.

Chang, J. J., Pien, G. W., Duntley, S. P., & Macones, G. A. (2010). Sleep deprivation during pregnancy and maternal and fetal outcomes: Is there a relationship? *Sleep Medicine Reviews* 14(2): 107–114.

Cohen, S., Doyle, W. J., & Skoner, D. P. (1999). Psychological stress, cytokine production, and severity of upper respiratory illness. *Psychosomatic Medicine* 61(2): 175–180.

Coussons-Read, M. E., Okun, M. L., Schmitt, M. P., & Giese, S. (2005). Prenatal stress alters cytokine levels in a manner that may endanger human pregnancy. *Psychosomatic Medicine* 67(4): 625–631.

Cupps, T. R. & Fauci, A. S. (1982). Corticosteroid-mediated immunoregulation in man. *Immunological Reviews 65*: 133–155.

Davis, E. P., Glynn, L. M., Dunkel Schetter, C., Hobel, C., Chicz-Demet, A., & Sandman, C. A. (2005). Corticotropin-releasing hormone during pregnancy is associated with infant temperament. *Developmental Neuroscience 27*(5): 299–305.

Davis, E. P., Waffarn, F., Uy, C., Hobel, C. J., Glynn, L. M., & Sandman, C. A. (2009). Effect of prenatal glucocorticoid treatment on size at birth among infants born at term gestation. *Journal of Perinatology 29*(11): 731–737.

de Weerth, C., van Hees, Y., & Buitelaar, J. K. (2003). Prenatal maternal cortisol levels and infant behavior during the first 5 months. *Early Human Development 74*(2): 139–151.

Dominguez, T. P., Dunkel-Schetter, C., Glynn, L. M., Hobel, C., & Sandman, C. A. (2008). Racial differences in birth outcomes: The role of general, pregnancy, and racism stress. *Health Psychology 27*(2): 194–203.

Dominguez, T. P., Schetter, C. D., Mancuso, R., Rini, C. M., & Hobel, C. (2005). Stress in African American pregnancies: Testing the roles of various stress concepts in prediction of birth outcomes. *Annals of Behavioral Medicine 29*(1): 12–21.

Ellman, L. M., Schetter, C. D., Hobel, C. J., Chicz-Demet, A., Glynn, L. M., & Sandman, C. A. (2008). Timing of fetal exposure to stress hormones: Effects on newborn physical and neuromuscular maturation. *Developmental Psychobiology 50*(3): 232–241.

Epel, E., Lapidus, R., McEwen, B., & Brownell, K. (2001). Stress may add bite to appetite in women: A laboratory study of stress-induced cortisol and eating behavior. *Psychoneuroendocrinology 26*(1): 37–49.

Farina, L. & Winkelman, C. (2005). A review of the role of proinflammatory cytokines in labor and noninfectious preterm labor. *Biological Research for Nursing 6*(3): 230–238.

Fearon, P., Kirkbride, J. B., Morgan, C., Dazzan, P., Morgan, K., Lloyd, T., Hutchinson, G., Tarrant, J., Fung, W. L., Holloway, J., et al. (2006). Incidence of schizophrenia and other psychoses in ethnic minority groups: Results from the MRC AESOP Study. *Psychological Medicine 36*(11): 1541–1550.

Felten, S. Y. & Felten, D. (1994). Neural-immune interaction. *Progress in Brain Research 100*: 157–162.

Fontana, A., Weber, E., & Dayer, J. M. (1984). Synthesis of interleukin 1/endogenous pyrogen in the brain of endotoxin-treated mice: A step in fever induction? *Journal of Immunology 133*(4): 1696–1698.

French, N. P., Hagan, R., Evans, S. F., Godfrey, M., & Newnham, J. P. (1999). Repeated antenatal corticosteroids: Size at birth and subsequent development. *American Journal of Obstetrics and Gynecology 180*(1 Pt 1): 114–121.

Glynn, L. M., Schetter, C. D., Chicz-DeMet, A., Hobel, C. J., & Sandman, C. A. (2007). Ethnic differences in adrenocorticotropic hormone, cortisol and corticotropin-releasing hormone during pregnancy. *Peptides 28*(6): 1155–1161.

Gur, R. E., Keshavan, M. S., & Lawrie, S. M. (2007). Deconstructing psychosis with human brain imaging. *Schizophrenia Bulletin 33*(4): 921–931.

Habhab, S., Sheldon, J. P., & Loeb, R. C. (2009). The relationship between stress, dietary restraint, and food preferences in women. *Appetite 52*(2): 437–444.

Harville, E. W., Savitz, D. A., Dole, N., Herring, A. H., Thorp, J. M., & Light, K. C. (2008). Stress and placental resistance measured by Doppler ultrasound in early and mid-pregnancy. *Ultrasound in Obstetrics and Gynecology 32*(1): 23–30.

Herman, D. B., Brown, A. S., Opler, M. G., Desai, M., Malaspina, D., Bresnahan, M., Schaefer, C. A., & Susser, E. S. (2006). Does unwantedness of pregnancy predict schizophrenia in the offspring? Findings from a prospective birth cohort study. *Social Psychiatry and Psychiatric Epidemiology 41*(8): 605–610.

Hilmert, C. J., Schetter, C. D., Dominguez, T. P., Abdou, C., Hobel, C. J., Glynn, L., & Sandman, C. (2008). Stress and blood pressure during pregnancy: Racial differences and associations with birthweight. *Psychosomatic Medicine* 70(1): 57–64.

Holzman, C., Jetton, J., Siler-Khodr, T., Fisher, R., & Rip, T. (2001). Second trimester corticotropin-releasing hormone levels in relation to preterm delivery and ethnicity. *Obstetrics and Gynecology* 97(5 Pt 1): 657–663.

Huizink, A. C., Robles de Medina, P. G., Mulder, E. J., Visser, G. H., & Buitelaar, J. K. (2003). Stress during pregnancy is associated with developmental outcome in infancy. *Journal of Child Psychology and Psychiatry* 44(6): 810–818.

Huttunen, M. O. & Niskanen, P. (1978). Prenatal loss of father and psychiatric disorders. *Archives of General Psychiatry* 35(4): 429–431.

Irwin, M. R., Wang, M., Ribeiro, D., Cho, H. J., Olmstead, R., Breen, E. C., Martinez-Maza, O., & Cole, S. (2008). Sleep loss activates cellular inflammatory signaling. *Biological Psychiatry* 64(6): 538–540.

Johnson, R. & Crowley, J. (1996). An analysis of stress denial. In H. Neighbors & J. Jackson (eds.), *Mental Health in Black America* (pp. 62–76). Thousand Oaks: Sage.

Jones, P., Rodgers, B., Murray, R., & Marmot, M. (1994). Child development risk factors for adult schizophrenia in the British 1946 birth cohort. *Lancet* 344(8934): 1398–1402.

Khashan, A. S., Abel, K. M., McNamee, R., Pedersen, M. G., Webb, R. T., Baker, P. N., Kenny, L. C., & Mortensen, P. B. (2008a). Higher risk of offspring schizophrenia following antenatal maternal exposure to severe adverse life events. *Archives of General Psychiatry* 65(2): 146–152.

Khashan, A. S., McNamee, R., Abel, K. M., Pedersen, M. G., Webb, R. T., Kenny, L. C., Mortensen, P. B., & Baker, P. N. (2008b). Reduced infant birthweight consequent upon maternal exposure to severe life events. *Psychosomatic Medicine* 70(6): 688–694.

Landsbergis, P. A. & Hatch, M. C. (1996). Psychosocial work stress and pregnancy-induced hypertension. *Epidemiology* 7(4): 346–351.

Laplante, D. P., Brunet, A., Schmitz, N., Ciampi, A., & King, S. (2008). Project Ice Storm: Prenatal maternal stress affects cognitive and linguistic functioning in 5 1/2-year-old children. *Journal of the American Academy of Child and Adolescent Psychiatry* 47(9): 1063–1072.

Lu, M. C. & Halfon, N. (2003). Racial and ethnic disparities in birth outcomes: A life-course perspective. *Maternal and Child Health Journal* 7(1): 13–30.

Malaspina, D., Corcoran, C., Kleinhaus, K. R., Perrin, M. C., Fennig, S., Nahon, D., Friedlander, Y., & Harlap, S. (2008). Acute maternal stress in pregnancy and schizophrenia in offspring: A cohort prospective study. *BMC Psychiatry* 8(71).

McGorry, P. D., Yung, A. R., Bechdolf, A., & Amminger, P. (2008). Back to the future: Predicting and reshaping the course of psychotic disorder. *Archives of General Psychiatry* 65(1): 25–27.

McGorry, P. D., Yung, A. R., & Phillips, L. J. (2001). "Closing In": What features predict the onset of first-episode psychosis within an ultra-high-risk group? In C. Schulz & R. B. Zipursky (eds.), *The Early Stages of Schizophrenia* (pp. 3–32). Washington, DC: American Psychiatric Press.

McGrath, J. (2008). Hypotheses desert us, while data defend us. *Schizophrenia Research* 102(1–3): 27–28.

Miller, G. E., Cohen, S., & Ritchey, A. K. (2002). Chronic psychological stress and the regulation of pro-inflammatory cytokines: A glucocorticoid-resistance model. *Health Psychology* 21(6): 531–541.

Murphy, V. E., Smith, R., Giles, W. B., & Clifton, V. L. (2006). Endocrine regulation of human fetal growth: The role of the mother, placenta, and fetus. *Endocrine Reviews* 27(2): 141–169.

Myhrman, A., Rantakallio, P., Isohanni, M., Jones, P., & Partanen, U. (1996). Unwanted-ness of a pregnancy and schizophrenia in the child. *British Journal of Psychiatry* 169(5): 637–640.

Newman, E., O'Connor, D. B., & Conner, M. (2007). Daily hassles and eating behaviour: The role of cortisol reactivity status. *Psychoneuroendocrinology* 32(2): 125–132.

Newton, R. W. & Hunt, L. P. (1984). Psychosocial stress in pregnancy and its relation to low birth weight. *British Medical Journal (Clinical Research Ed)* 288(6425): 1191–1194.

Niendam, T. A., Bearden, C. E., Rosso, I. M., Sanchez, L. E., Hadley, T., Nuechterlein, K. H., & Cannon, T. D. (2003). A prospective study of childhood neurocognitive functioning in schizophrenic patients and their siblings. *American Journal of Psychiatry* 160(11): 2060–2062.

Oliver, G., Wardle, J., & Gibson, E. L. (2000). Stress and food choice: A laboratory study. *Psychosomatic Medicine* 62(6): 853–865.

Patterson, P. H. (2009). Immune involvement in schizophrenia and autism: Etiology, pathol-ogy and animal models. *Behavioural Brain Research* 204(2): 313–321.

Repetti, R. L., Taylor, S. E., & Seeman, T. E. (2002). Risky families: Family social environ-ments and the mental and physical health of offspring. *Psychological Bulletin* 128(2): 330–366.

Ruiz, R. J., Fullerton, J., Brown, C. E., & Schoolfield, J. (2001). Relationships of cortisol, per-ceived stress, genitourinary infections, and fetal fibronectin to gestational age at birth. *Bio-logical Research for Nursing* 3(1): 39–48.

Rutters, F., Nieuwenhuizen, A. G., Lemmens, S. G., Born, J. M., & Westerterp-Plantenga, M. S. (2009a). Acute stress-related changes in eating in the absence of hunger. *Obesity (Silver Spring)* 17(1): 72–77.

Rutters, F., Nieuwenhuizen, A. G., Lemmens, S. G., Born, J. M., & Westerterp-Plantenga, M. S. (2009b). Hyperactivity of the HPA axis is related to dietary restraint in normal weight women. *Physiology and Behavior* 96(2): 315–319.

Sapolsky, R., Rivier, C., Yamamoto, G., Plotsky, P., & Vale, W. (1987). Interleukin-1 stimulates the secretion of hypothalamic corticotropin-releasing factor. *Science* 238(4826): 522–524.

Schaefer, C. A., Brown, A. S., Wyatt, R. J., Kline, J., Begg, M. D., Bresnahan, M. A., & Susser, E. S. (2000). Maternal prepregnant body mass and risk of schizophrenia in adult offspring. *Schizophrenia Bulletin* 26(2): 275–286.

Segerstrom, S. C. & Miller, G. E. (2004). Psychological stress and the human immune system: A meta-analytic study of 30 years of inquiry. *Psychological Bulletin* 130(4): 601–630.

Selten, J. P., van der Graaf, Y., van Duursen, R., Gispen-de Wied, C. C., & Kahn, R. S. (1999). Psychotic illness after prenatal exposure to the 1953 Dutch Flood Disaster. *Schizophrenia Research* 35(3): 243–245.

Sharma, S., Norris, W. E., & Kalkunte, S. (2010). Beyond the threshold: An etiological bridge between hypoxia and immunity in preeclampsia. *Journal of Reproductive Immunology* 85: 112–116.

Sikkema, J. M., Robles de Medina, P. G., Schaad, R. R., Mulder, E. J., Bruinse, H. W., Buite-laar, J. K., Visser, G. H., & Franx, A. (2001). Salivary cortisol levels and anxiety are not increased in women destined to develop preeclampsia. *Journal of Psychosomatic Research* 50(1): 45–49.

Slykerman, R. F., Thompson, J. M., Pryor, J. E., Becroft, D. M., Robinson, E., Clark, P. M., Wild, C. J., & Mitchell, E. A. (2005). Maternal stress, social support and preschool chil-dren's intelligence. *Early Human Development* 81(10): 815–821.

Trainer, P. J. (2002). Corticosteroids and pregnancy. *Seminars in Reproductive Medicine* 20(4): 375–380.

Van Erp, T. G., Saleh, P. A., Rosso, I. M., Huttunen, M., Lonnqvist, J., Pirkola, T., Salonen, O., Valanne, L., Poutanen, V. P., Standertskjold-Nordenstam, C. G., et al. (2002). Contributions of genetic risk and fetal hypoxia to hippocampal volume in patients with schizophrenia or schizoaffective disorder, their unaffected siblings, and healthy unrelated volunteers. *American Journal of Psychiatry 159*(9): 1514–1520.

van Os, J. & Selten, J. P. (1998). Prenatal exposure to maternal stress and subsequent schizophrenia: The May 1940 invasion of The Netherlands. *British Journal of Psychiatry 172*: 324–326.

Vollebregt, K. C., van der Wal, M. F., Wolf, H., Vrijkotte, T. G., Boer, K., & Bonsel, G. J. (2008). Is psychosocial stress in first ongoing pregnancies associated with pre-eclampsia and gestational hypertension? *Bjog 115*(5): 607–615.

Wadhwa, P. D., Garite, T. J., Porto, M., Glynn, L., Chicz-DeMet, A., Dunkel-Schetter, C., & Sandman, C. A. (2004). Placental corticotropin-releasing hormone (CRH), spontaneous preterm birth, and fetal growth restriction: A prospective investigation. *American Journal of Obstetrics and Gynecology 191*(4): 1063–1069.

Wadhwa, P. D., Sandman, C. A., Porto, M., Dunkel-Schetter, C., & Garite, T. J. (1993). The association between prenatal stress and infant birth weight and gestational age at birth: A prospective investigation. *American Journal of Obstetrics and Gynecology 169*(4): 858–865.

Welberg, L. A., Seckl, J. R., & Holmes, M. C. (2001). Prenatal glucocorticoid programming of brain corticosteroid receptors and corticotrophin-releasing hormone: Possible implications for behaviour. *Neuroscience 104*(1): 71–79.

Wright, I. C., Rabe-Hesketh, S., Woodruff, P. W., David, A. S., Murray, R. M., & Bullmore, E. T. (2000). Meta-analysis of regional brain volumes in schizophrenia. *American Journal of Psychiatry 157*(1): 16–25.

Xiong, X., Harville, E. W., Mattison, D. R., Elkind-Hirsch, K., Pridjian, G., & Buekens, P. (2008). Exposure to Hurricane Katrina, post-traumatic stress disorder and birth outcomes. *American Journal of Medical Sciences 336*(2): 111–115.

CHAPTER 5

ADVANCING PATERNAL AGE AND THE RISK FOR SCHIZOPHRENIA

SARAH CRYSTAL, KARINE KLEINHAUS, MARY PERRIN, AND DOLORES MALASPINA

KEY CONCEPTS

- Epidemiologic evidence has established the relationship between advanced paternal age and schizophrenia.
- Animal models and epidemiologic research have described effects of paternal age on learning and cognition.
- Paternal age-related schizophrenia may be a variant of schizophrenia.
- Genetic mechanisms may underlie the relation between paternal age and schizophrenia.
- Epigenetics may partially explain the finding that advanced paternal age is associated with schizophrenia.

An increasing risk of schizophrenia with advancing paternal age has been demonstrated through epidemiologic studies during the past decade. Before 2001, the results of research studying paternal age and schizophrenia were inconsistent with regard to risk of schizophrenia and advancing paternal age (Granville-Grossman, 1966; Hare & Moran, 1979; Kinnell, 1983; Malama et al., 1988; Bertranpetit & Fananas, 1993). However, in a large prospective cohort study in Jerusalem, Malaspina et al. (2001) reported that the risk of schizophrenia doubled with each 10-year increment of paternal age. Other studies confirmed that older paternal age is a risk factor for schizophrenia (Brown et al., 2002; Dalman & Allebeck, 2002; Byrne et al., 2003; Zammit et al., 2003; El-Saadi et al., 2004; Sipos et al., 2004; Tsuchiya et al., 2005), although two others did not find an association (El-Saadi et al., 2004; Pulver et al., 2004). Collectively, these studies strengthened the evidence that paternal age at birth is an important risk factor for schizophrenia.

In this chapter we will outline (1) the epidemiologic evidence supporting the relationship between advanced paternal age and schizophrenia; (2) animal and human models pointing to a role for paternal age in learning and cognition; and (3) genetic and epigenetic mechanisms that may underlie the relationship between advanced paternal age and schizophrenia.

Seminal Findings

The maintenance of schizophrenia in the population despite the reduced fecundity of affected individuals has been one of the enigmatic features of the disease. One possible explanation could be the replenishment of disease genes through new mutations. Paternal age is reported to be the major source of de novo mutations in humans and other mammals, likely due to the constant cell replication cycles that occur in spermatogenesis. Following puberty, spermatogonia undergo some 23 divisions per year. At ages 20 and 40, a man's germ cell precursors will have undergone about 200 and 660 such divisions, respectively. During a man's life, the spermatogonia are vulnerable to DNA damage, and mutations may accumulate in clones of spermatogonia as men age (Crow, 1999). We hypothesize, therefore, that advanced paternal age might increase the risk of schizophrenia in the offspring through de novo genetic changes.

The Jerusalem Perinatal Study (JPS) is a population-based cohort that contains information on all 92,408 individuals born in West Jerusalem between 1964 and 1976. Information on maternal conditions, obstetric complications and interventions during labor and delivery, parental ages, immigration status, ethnicity, and occupation was recorded at birth. Postpartum and antepartum interviews of the mothers occurred from 1965 to 1968 and 1974 to 1976, respectively. Staff from the Israeli Ministry of the Interior linked the JPS data to the Israeli Psychiatric Case Registry in order to identify subjects with psychiatric diagnoses and maintain full confidentiality. In 2001, Malaspina and colleagues reported a monotonic increase in the risk of schizophrenia as paternal age increased (Malaspina et al., 2001).

Epidemiologic Evidence

Malaspina's finding was replicated in numerous studies in the United States (Malaspina et al., 2001; Brown et al., 2002), Europe (Dalman & Allebeck, 2002; Byrne et al., 2003; Zammit et al., 2003; El-Saadi et al., 2004; Sipos et al., 2004), Australia (El-Saadi et al., 2004), and Japan (Tsuchiya et al., 2005). Many studies used a cohort design (Malaspina et al., 2001; Brown et al., 2002; Zammit et al., 2003;

El-Saadi et al., 2004; Sipos et al., 2004), but others employed a case-control design in a large population data set (Dalman & Allebeck, 2002; Byrne et al., 2003; El-Saadi et al., 2004; Pulver et al., 2004; Tsuchiya et al., 2005; St Clair, 2009). Details of these studies are provided in tables 5.1 and 5.2.

Collectively, the studies showed a tripling of risk for schizophrenia in the offspring of the oldest group of fathers, in comparison with the risk from younger fathers. Furthermore, the research demonstrated that the paternal age effect is not explained by other factors, including family history of psychosis, maternal age, parental education and social ability, family social integration, social class, birth order, birth weight, or birth complications.

Biological Plausibility

Several approaches have been employed to examine the biological plausibility of paternal age as a risk factor for schizophrenia. First, animal models were used to examine whether paternal age is related to specific outcomes that are relevant to schizophrenia. A translational approach using an animal model offers the opportunity to identify candidate genes, epigenetic mechanisms, or both that may explain the association of cognitive functioning with advancing paternal age. Second, epidemiologic studies have examined whether advanced paternal age is related to specific cognitive or social deficits in offspring.

Animal Models of Paternal Age Effects

Auroux was the first scientist to report that paternal age could negatively affect the learning capacity of Wistar rats sired by aged males (Auroux, 1983). Between 10 and 13 weeks of age, rat offspring were evaluated for learning capacity with an avoidance conditioning test. The results demonstrated that offspring of aged fathers had less spontaneous activity and worse learning capacity than those of mature rodents, despite having no noticeable physical anomalies.

In the laboratory of Jay Gingrich, this effect was replicated in inbred mice: the behavioral performance of progeny of 18- to 24-month-old sires was inferior to the performance of progeny of 4-month-old sires (Bradley-Moore et al., 2002). This study demonstrated significantly decreased learning in an active avoidance test, less exploration in the open field, and a number of other behavioral decrements in the offspring of older sires. Other investigations showed that offspring of 10-month-old sires had significantly fewer social and exploratory behaviors than offspring of two-month-old sires (Smith et al., 2009) and that aged rats sired offspring with a reduced capacity for passive-avoidance learning (Garcia-Palomares et al., 2009). Male progeny of older rats are also reported to have alterations

Table 5.1 Results of Cohort Studies Examining the Association Between Paternal Age and Schizophrenia, Schizophrenia Spectrum Disorders, or Psychosis

Authors/Year	Paternal Age Categories	Cohort No.	Case No.	RR	95% CI	p-value
Malaspina et al., 2001						
United States, schizophrenia spectrum disorders						
Adjusted for maternal age. < 20 included with 20–24; ≥ 55 included with 50–54						
	<20	227	3	. . .		
	20–24	11,497	58	1.00	Reference	
	25–29	28,145	167	1.14	0.84–1.53	
	30–34	22,212	169	1.42	1.03–1.96	
	35–39	14,457	126	1.64	1.13–2.38	
	40–44	7,424	67	1.73	1.11–2.70	
	45–49	2,626	28	2.02	1.17–3.51	
	50–54	794	14	2.96	1.60–5.47	
	≥55	435	6	. . .	. . .	
Brown et al., 2002						
United States, schizophrenia spectrum disorders						
Adjusted for maternal age, paternal education, paternal race, and parity						
	15–24			1.0	Reference	
	25–34			1.6	0.6–4.1	
	35–44			2.2	0.7–7.1	
	45–68			2.7	0.6–13.4	
Zammit et al., 2003						
Sweden, schizophrenia and other psychoses						
Adjusted for maternal age, drug use, IQ score, poor social integration, and place of upbringing						
	15–24	6,139	36	1.0	Reference	
	25–34	25,159	157	1.2	0.8–1.8	
	35–44	13,403	118	1.6	1.0–2.6	
	45–54	2,405	22	1.6	0.8–3.1	
	≥55	187	4	3.8	1.3–11.8	
	Test for trend			1.3	1.0–1.5	.02
Sipos et al., 2004						
Sweden, schizophrenia and nonaffective psychosis						
Adjusted for sex, age, maternal age, birth weight, birth length, gestational age, place of birth, season, Apgar score at one and five minutes, parity, multiple birth, parental death, family history of schizophrenia, and socioeconomic variables						
	<21		15	1.31	0.73–2.36	
	21–24		72	1.00	Reference	
	25–29		204	1.26	0.93–1.69	
	30–34		194	1.66	1.18–2.34	
	35–39		103	2.32	1.56–3.44	
	40–44		32	2.08	1.25–3.46	
	45–49		7	1.30	0.56–3.06	
	≥50		12	4.62	2.28–9.36	
	For each 10-year increase in paternal age			1.47	1.23–1.76	
El-Saadi et al., 2004						
Denmark study, psychosis						
Adjusted for maternal age for psychotic disorder						
	<20			1.10	0.96–1.26	
	20–24			1.00	Reference	
	25–29			0.97	0.92–1.03	
	30–34			1.04	0.97–1.11	
	35–39			1.14	1.05–1.24	
	40–44			1.26	1.13–1.40	
	45–49			1.34	1.16–1.56	
	50–54			1.62	1.30–2.02	
	≥55			1.84	1.33–2.53	

CI = confidence interval; RR = relative risk.
SOURCE: Authors.

Table 5.2 Results of Case Control Studies Examining the Association Between Paternal Age and Schizophrenia, Psychosis, Schizoaffective Disorder, Affective Psychosis, and Nonaffective Psychosis

Authors/Year	Paternal Age Categories	Cases	Controls	OR	95% CI	p-value
Dalman & Allebeck, 2002						
Sweden, broad schizophrenia						
Adjusted for maternal age, socioeconomic status, parity, maternal psychosis, marital status, and obstetric complications						
	<20	2	4	1.2	0.2–7.0	
	20–24	63	142	1.0	Reference	
	25–34	242	516	1.2	0.8–1.9	
	35–44	94	174	1.5	0.9–2.6	
	≥45	19	21	2.8	1.3–6.3	
Byrne et al., 2003						
Denmark, schizophrenia						
Adjusted for family psychiatric history socioeconomic factors, parental education, wealth, marital status, death before case admission (not by suicide), history of suicide in parent or sibling, reference to father, place of birth, and sibship size						
	<20	177	3,394	1.04	0.88–1.23	
	20–24	1,424	37,867	1.00	Referent	
	25–29	2,257	62,305	0.99	0.92–1.07	
	30–34	1,654	43,125	1.04	0.95–1.13	
	35–39	870	22,546	1.02	0.91–1.13	
	40–44	449	10,052	1.15	1.00–1.31	
	45–49	169	3,794	1.09	0.90–1.31	
	50–54	61	1,153	1.22	0.92–1.62	
	≥55	36	319	2.45	1.69–3.54	
Pulver et al., 2004						
United States, schizophrenia and schizoaffective disorder						
Adjusted for illness in paternal relatives of schizophrenic subjects, given paternal age at birth, sex of subject, and socioeconomic status						
	15–25			1.00	Referent	
	26–30			0.48	0.12–1.93	
	31–35			0.63	0.18–2.30	
	36+			0.90	0.29–2.86	
El-Saadi et al., 2004						
Australia, nonaffective psychosis, affective psychosis						
Adjusted for maternal age						
	<20	6	2	1.83	0.29–11.56	
	20–24	24	27	1.00	Referent	
	25–29	48	56	0.96	0.47–1.97	
	30–34	27	33	0.88	0.36–2.14	
	>35	14	23	0.77	0.24–2.46	
El-Saadi et al., 2004						
Sweden, psychosis						
Adjusted for maternal age						
	<20	2	78	1.32	0.70–2.47	
	20–24	13	1,266	1.00	Referent	
	25–29	32	2,778	1.13	0.59–2.18	
	30–34	35	2,381	1.47	0.75–2.87	
	>35	52	2,184	2.42	1.19–4.89	

Tsuchiya et al., 2005
Japan, schizophrenia
Adjusted for age and gender of the subject, parity, family history, and age of the other parent

≤28	22	138	1.00	Referent
29–31	36	120	2.08	1.12–3.86
≥32	41	123	3.00	1.49–6.04
			Test for trend	.002

CI = confidence interval; OR = odds ratio.
SOURCE: Authors.

in cortical growth, which are perhaps relevant to the behavioral findings (Foldi et al., 2010). These studies strongly indicate that advancing paternal age is related to cognitive, social, and anatomic changes in offspring.

Paternal Age and Intelligence

A relationship between cognitive function and later paternal age in humans was explored by Auroux and colleagues, following their discovery of paternal age effects in rodents. The authors demonstrated a "U shaped" relationship between paternal age and cognition in a study of 1,700 male military recruits in Nancy, France, in 1985, wherein sons of very young fathers and of much older fathers did less well on psychometric tests without significant maternal age effects (Auroux et al., 1989).

Another study showed that higher paternal age (35 years or older) was associated with decreased reading ability in girls, although not in boys (St Sauver et al., 2001). A study that included more than 44,000 of the offspring from the JPS population-based cohort showed that maternal and paternal age exerted independent effects on intelligence in late adolescence (Malaspina et al., 2005). These results were adjusted for parental education, social class, sex, birth order, birth weight, and birth complications. They showed reductions in performance intelligence only for the offspring of the oldest fathers, whereas later maternal age comparably lowered verbal and nonverbal intelligence.

An effect of later paternal age on cognition in children was demonstrated in a sample of 33,437 offspring from the U.S. Collaborative Perinatal Project (CPP). In models that adjusted for potential confounders (including maternal age), they reported that children of older fathers were more likely to be cognitively impaired. Later paternal age was associated with worse performance in five out of six cognitive measures, whereas later maternal age was linked with better performance on intelligence tests (Saha et al., 2009).

The pathophysiology linking paternal age to intelligence is yet to be elucidated. Numerous genes participate in determining intelligence, and any of these might undergo mutations. As described here, paternal age is the most robust factor in determining the human spontaneous mutation rate (Crow, 1993). Both schizophrenia and autism entail reduced learning ability, so these findings may be relevant to the mechanism linking later paternal age to these conditions (Reichenberg et al., 2006; Corbett et al., 2009; Koenen et al., 2009; Mesholam-Gately et al., 2009).

This work is still nascent, and many explanations remain to be proposed and tested to explain the linkage of paternal age to intelligence and learning. For example, cigarette smoking can damage DNA in germ cells (Zenzes, 2000), and there may be higher rates of smoking in older cohorts. As detailed later in this chapter, changes may occur in the epigenetic processes in sperm cells with male aging. Epigenetic mechanisms are heritable regulators of gene expression that are independent of DNA sequence (Oakes et al., 2003) (see chapter 9 in this book). Socioeconomic status is also related to cognition in offspring (Turkheimer et al., 2003; Lawlor et al., 2006). In the study of paternal age and cognition in the CPP that was mentioned here, adjustment for socioeconomic status reduced the difference in intelligence scores for offspring of older and younger fathers, although it did not account for the paternal age effect (Saha et al., 2009). Additional large studies are needed to elucidate better the relationship between advanced paternal age and cognition. As childbearing is increasingly delayed, this association, if confirmed, could have important public health implications.

A Variant of Schizophrenia

A persistent question is whether the association of paternal age and schizophrenia could be explained by psychiatric problems in the parents—problems that both delay childbearing and are heritable by their offspring. If so, then advanced paternal age would be more common among familial cases than sporadic cases; however, this is not so (Sipos et al., 2004). It is also possible that de novo genetic events in the paternal germ line are affecting the same genes that influence the risk in familial cases. Available evidence suggests this is not the case. The few genetic studies that examined familial and sporadic cases separately found that the "at-risk haplotypes" linked to familial schizophrenia were not associated with sporadic cases, including dystrobrevin-binding protein (Van Den Bogaert et al., 2003) and neuregulin (Williams et al., 2003). Segregating sporadic cases from the analyses actually strengthened the magnitude of the genetic association in the familial cases, consistent with etiologic heterogeneity between familial and sporadic groups. Furthermore, sporadic cases have more de novo copy number variants (CNVs) than do familial cases in which CNVs are more likely to be inherited (Xu et al., 2008.).

Individuals with schizophrenia who have no family history of psychosis may have different phenotypes than familial cases. For example, only sporadic subjects showed a significant improvement in negative symptoms after changing from a "medication-free" condition to one where they received antipsychotic treatment (Malaspina et al., 2000). Sporadic subjects also have significantly more disruptions in their smooth pursuit eye movement quality (Malaspina et al., 1998) and have distinct intelligence test profiles (Wolitzky et al., 2006). The sporadic group of subjects had greater hypofrontality, with increased medial temporal lobe activity (frontotemporal imbalance), whereas the familial group had left lateralized temporoparietal hypoperfusion along with widespread regional cerebral blood flow (rCBF) changes in cortico-striato-thalamo-cortical regions (Malaspina et al., 2004). These findings support the hypothesis that familial and sporadic cases of schizophrenia may have distinct neural underpinnings.

Genetic Mechanisms

Several genetic mechanisms might explain the relationship between paternal age and the risk for schizophrenia. Spermatagonial stem cells divide constantly, undergoing hundreds of replications throughout a lifetime. Males have a higher frequency of point mutations, and the frequency increases with age and higher rates of de novo genetic disorders and birth defects in offspring (Crow, 1999).There are other possible explanations for the paternal age effects, as described in the sections that follow.

De Novo Mutations

Approximately 20% of birth defects are attributed to new mutations (Nelson & Holmes, 1989; Crow, 1997). Single base pair changes are the most frequently occurring mutations in paternal gametes. These may be random events or they may occur in certain "hot spots." Achondroplastic dwarfism is an example of a "hot spot" mutation (Wilkin et al., 1998), wherein 90% of cases have a de novo mutation at the same single codon, leading to a missense mutation in the fibroblast growth factor 3 gene (Orioli et al., 1995; Yu et al., 2000).

Trinucleotide Repeat Expansions

Trinucleotide repeat disorders are caused by multiple insertions of three specific nucleotides in certain genes. An example is the $(CAG)_n$ repeat in the androgen receptor gene. Multiple insertions of a repeat sequence in genes may lead to repeat sizes that are above the normal threshold. These larger-than-normal repeat lengths may often result in a defective protein or no protein. These disorders are characterized by an autosomal dominant mode of inheritance, a progressive course, and anticipation—i.e., an earlier age of onset and an increasing severity of disease from one generation to the next. Anticipation has been reported in several neuropsychiatric disorders including myotonic dystrophy, spinocerebellar ataxias, and Huntington's disease. For a detailed review of trinucleotide repeat disorders, see Orr and Zoghbi (2007).

The sex of the transmitting parent may influence anticipation (Telenius et al., 1993); many disorders show greater trinucleotide repeat expansion with paternal inheritance than with maternal inheritance (Duyao et al., 1993; Lindblad & Schalling, 1999; Schols et al., 2004). Consistent with anticipation, onset of schizophrenia may occur earlier in successive generations of multiply affected pedigrees (Gorwood et al., 1995; Petronis et al., 1995; Heiden et al., 1999).

It is not known if anticipation in schizophrenia is more likely for paternal or maternal transmission of the trinucleotide repeats, and the results of studies have been mixed (Gorwood et al., 1997; Johnson et al., 1997; Husted, Scutt, & Bassett, 1998; Imamura et al., 1998). Not all studies find longer trinucleotide repeats in family members with schizophrenia who have an earlier onset than the preceding generation (Morris et al., 1995; O'Donovan et al., 1996; O'Donovan & Owen, 1999; Bowen et al., 2000; Vincent et al., 2000).

Copy Number Variation

Over the last decade there has been an upsurge of interest in the possible role of CNVs in certain genes or regions of the genome in the etiology of schizophrenia, autism, mental retardation, and other neuropsychiatric disorders (St Clair, 2009). Copy number variation refers to a segment of DNA that can be from 1 kilobase to 1 or more megabases (Cook & Scherer, 2008) and that can include one or more genes, copy duplications, copy deletions, or multiallelic or complex rearrangements. A significant number of CNVs are over 50 kilobases in size and are recurrent. They have an increased mutation rate and are located in unstable parts of the genome. CNVs are discussed in more detail in chapter 8.

A difference between the rare inherited variants within some familial cases and de novo variants in sporadic cases of schizophrenia may be related to paternal age, given that the genetic variation is introduced through the paternal line.

Epigenetics and Advanced Paternal Age

Epigenetic phenomena are defined as heritable changes in the genome that are unrelated to the DNA sequence (Feinberg, 2004). Epigenetic mechanisms regulate the expression of genes and include methylation, acetylation, alterations in chromatin structure, and RNAi. Epigenetic changes occur in somatic cells with aging more frequently than mutations do (Bennett-Baker, Wilkowski, & Burke, 2003; Fraga et al., 2005). Epigenetics is described in detail in chapter 9.

A number of genes are imprinted in that they are only expressed from the paternal or maternal allele. Imprinting errors could increase with advancing paternal age through a number of pathways, including environmental exposures. In a recent study, it was reported that paternal occupation as a dry cleaner significantly increased the risk of schizophrenia in the offspring, an effect possibly due to chronic exposure to perchlorethylene, a common dry-cleaning solvent (Perrin et al., 2007).

X-Chromosome Inactivation

The association between advancing paternal age and schizophrenia among women may result at least in part from imprinting errors in the paternal X-chromosome of older fathers. X-chromosome inactivation is typically a random process in which 50% of cells have a paternal X-chromosome activated and maternal X-chromosome inactivated and 50% of cells have the maternal X-chromosome activated and the paternal X-chromosome inactivated, resulting in dosage compensation between males and females. A significant number of females have skewed X-chromosome inactivation—i.e., deviating from the 50:50 ratio just described. In females, only one allele is expressed on the X-chromosome and, in combination with skewed X-inactivation, results in a functional loss of heterozygosity (LOH) (Buller et al., 1999). This functional LOH may render women more susceptible to cognitive and neuropsychiatric disorders.

The hypothesis that imprinting errors on the X-chromosome may explain some of the risk in women associated with paternal age is supported by studies in women with Turner's syndrome (45, X). It has been reported in some but not all studies that among women with Turner's syndrome there are differences between those women whose X-chromosome has been transmitted through the maternal line (X_M) and those whose X-chromosome has been transmitted through the paternal line (X_P). Some studies have noted differences in social skills and executive function and arithmetic ability between 45, X_P and 45, X_M women (Skuse et al., 1997; Chong et al., 2000). Others have noted that there is strong correlation with cardiovascular disease in X_M women but not X_P women (Chu et al., 1994). Another more recent study reported that X_M and X_P women differed in superior temporal gyrus gray matter but not in white matter (Kesler et al., 2003). On the basis of these and other studies, imprinted genes are expected to be identified on the X-chromosome. Imprinting errors associated with advanced paternal age, coupled with skewed X-chromosome inactivation, could result in partial or complete loss of protein from a paternally expressed allele, increasing the risk of schizophrenia in females.

Failures to Replicate

Among all the epidemiologic evidence examining paternal age in relation to schizophrenia, there have been few failures to replicate either the paternal age effect or its approximate magnitude (El-Saadi et al., 2004; Pulver et al., 2004). The uniformity of the results across different cultures lends further credence to the robust relationship between advanced paternal age and schizophrenia. This relation is likely to reflect an innate human biological phenomenon that progresses over aging in the male germ line, independent of regional environmental risk factors for schizophrenia. The most plausible explanation is that the relation between advanced paternal age and schizophrenia is mediated through de novo genetic mechanisms and alterations in the epigenetic profile of different alleles.

Conclusion

Current findings on the relationship between paternal age and schizophrenia suggest new directions for research into the etiology of the disease. The studies linking advanced paternal age to the risk of schizophrenia indicate that we should expand this event horizon to consider the effects of environmental exposures on the fidelity of the male germ cell line over the life span of the father. The mutational stigmata of an exposure may remain in spermatogonial cells and be manifested in the clones of spermatozoa that it will subsequently generate over a man's reproductive life.

KEY AREAS FOR FUTURE RESEARCH

- To further investigate the biological basis of the association between advancing paternal age and schizophrenia, we need to employ a translational approach. Animal models need to be developed to determine those genetic and epigenetic processes that are aberrant in older male animals but not in younger male animals.
- We need to assess the errors in imprinting, methylation, acetylation, and X-chromosome inactivation that may be increased in offspring of older fathers compared to offspring of younger fathers.

Acknowledgments

Dr. Malaspina is supported by the following grants: National Institute of Mental Health (NIMH) 5K24 MH01699-11 and NIMH 5R01 MH59114-09. M. Perrin is supported by the following grants: National Institutes of Health (NIH) 5K07 CA131094-03, NIH 3K07 CA131094-02S1, and a National Alliance for Research on Schizophrenia and Depression Young Investigator Award. K. Kleinhaus is supported by NIH K08 MH085807.

Selected Readings

Harlap, S., Davies, A. M., Deutsch, L., Calderon-Margalit, R., Manor, O., Paltiel, O., Tiram, E., Yanetz, R., Perrin, M. C., Terry, M. B., et al. (2007). The Jerusalem Perinatal Cohort, 1964–2005: Methods and a review of the main results. *Paediatric and Perinatal Epidemiology* 21(3): 256–273.

Midgeon, B. R. (2007). *Females Are Mosaics*. New York: Oxford University Press.

Perrin, M., Brown, A. S., & Malaspina, D. (2007). Aberrant epigenetic regulation could explain the relationship of paternal age to schizophrenia. *Schizophrenia Bulletin* 33(6): 1270–1273.

Roth, T. L. & Lubin, F. D. (2009). Lasting epigenetic influence of early-life adversity on the BDNF gene. *Biological Psychiatry* 65(9): 760–769.

Rutten, B. P. F. & Mill, J. (2009). Epigenetic mediation of environmental influences in major psychotic disorders. *Schizophrenia Bulletin* 35(6): 1045–1056.

References

Auroux, M. (1983). Decrease of learning capacity in offspring with increasing paternal age in the rat. *Teratology* 27(2): 141–148.

Auroux, M. R., Mayaux, M. J., Guihard-Moscato, M. L., Fromantin, M., Barthe, J., & Schwartz, D. (1989). Paternal age and mental functions of progeny in man. *Human Reproduction* 4(7): 794–797.

Bennett-Baker, P., Wilkowski, J., & Burke, D. (2003). Age-associated activation of epigenetically repressed genes in the mouse. *Genetics* 165: 2055–2062.

Bertranpetit, J. & Fananas, L. (1993). Parental age in schizophrenia in a case-controlled study. *British Journal of Psychiatry* 162: 574.

Bowen, T., Guy, C. A., Cardno, A. G., Vincent, J. B., Kennedy, J. L., Jones, L. A., Gray, M., Sanders, R. D., McCarthy, G., Murphy, K. C., et al. (2000). Repeat sizes at CAG/CTG loci CTG18.1, ERDA1 and TGC13-7a in schizophrenia. *Psychiatric Genetics* 10(1): 33–37.

Bradley-Moore, M., Abner, R., Edwards, T., Lira, J., Lira, A., Mullen, T., Paul, S., Malaspina, D., Brunner, D., & Gingrich, J. A. (2002). Modeling the effect of advanced paternal age on progeny behavior in mice. *Developmental Psychobiology* 41(3): 230.

Brown, A. S., Schaefer, C. A., Wyatt, R. J., Begg, M. D., Goetz, R., Bresnahan, M. A., Harkavy-Friedman, J., Gorman, J. M., Malaspina, D., & Susser, E. S. (2002). Paternal age and risk of schizophrenia in adult offspring. *American Journal of Psychiatry* 159(9): 1528–1533.

Buller, R. E., Sood, A. K., Lallas, T., Buekers, T., & Skilling, J. S. (1999). Association between nonrandom X-chromosome inactivation and BRCA1 mutation in germline DNA of patients with ovarian cancer. *Journal of the National Cancer Institute* 91(4): 339–346.

Byrne, M., Agerbo, E., Ewald, H., Eaton, W. W., & Mortensen, P. B. (2003). Parental age and risk of schizophrenia: A case-control study. *Archives of General Psychiatry* 60(7): 673–678.

Chong, E. Y. Y., Pang, J. C. S., Ko, C. W., Poon, W. S., & Ng, H. K. (2000). Telomere length and telomerase catalytic subunit expression in non-astrocytic gliomas. *Pathology, Research and Practice* 196(10): 691–699.

Chu, C. E., Donaldson, M. D., Kelnar, C. J., Smail, P. J., Greene, S. A., Paterson, W. F., & Connor, J. M. (1994). Possible role of imprinting in the Turner phenotype. *Journal of Medical Genetics* 31(11): 840–842.

Cook, E. & Scherer, S. (2008). Copy-number variations associated with neuropsychiatric conditions. *Nature* 455: 919–923.

Corbett, B. A., Constantine, L. J., Hendren, R., Rocke, D., & Ozonoff, S. (2009). Examining executive functioning in children with autism spectrum disorder, attention deficit hyperactivity disorder and typical development. *Psychiatry Research* 166(2–3): 210–222.

Crow, J. F. (1993). How much do we know about spontaneous human mutation rates? *Environmental and Molecular Mutagenesis* 21(2): 122–129.

Crow, J. F. (1997). The high spontaneous mutation rate: Is it a health risk? *Proceedings of the National Academy of Sciences U.S.A.* 94(16): 8380–8386.

Crow, J. F. (1999). Spontaneous mutation in man. *Mutation Research* 437(1): 5–9.

Dalman, C. & Allebeck, P. (2002). Paternal age and schizophrenia: Further support for an association. *American Journal of Psychiatry* 159(9): 1591–1592.

Duyao, M., Ambrose, C., Myers, R., Novelletto, A., Persichetti, F., Frontali, M., Folstein, S., Ross, C., Franz, M., Abbott, M., et al. (1993). Trinucleotide repeat length instability and age of onset in Huntington's disease. *Nature Genetics* 4(4): 387–392.

El-Saadi, O., Pedersen, C. B., McNeil, T. F., Saha, S., Welham, J., O'Callaghan, E., Cantor-Graae, E., Chant, D., Mortensen, P. B., & McGrath, J. (2004). Paternal and maternal age as risk factors for psychosis: Findings from Denmark, Sweden and Australia. *Schizophrenia Research* 67(2–3): 227–236.

Feinberg, A. P. (2004). The epigenetics of cancer etiology. *Seminars in Cancer Biology* 14(6): 427–432.

Foldi, C. J., Eyles, D. W., McGrath, J. J., & Burne, T. H. (2010). Advanced paternal age is associated with alterations in discrete behavioural domains and cortical neuroanatomy of C57BL/6J mice. *European Journal of Neuroscience* 31(3): 556–564.

Fraga, M., Ballestar, E., Paz, M., Ropero, S., Setien, F., Ballestar, M., Heine-Suñer, D., Cigudosa, J., Urioste, M., Benitez, J., et al. (2005). Epigenetic differences arise during the lifetime of monozygotic twins. *Proceedings of the National Academy of Sciences U.S.A.* 102(30): 10604–10609.

Garcia-Palomares, S., Pertusa, J. F., Minarro, J., Garcia-Perez, M. A., Hermenegildo, C., Rausell, F., Cano, A., & Tarin, J. J. (2009). Long-term effects of delayed fatherhood in mice on postnatal development and behavioral traits of offspring. *Biology of Reproduction* 80(2): 337–342.

Gorwood, P., Leboyer, M., Falissard, B., Rouillon, F., Jay, M., & Feingold, J. (1997). Further epidemiological evidence for anticipation in schizophrenia. *Biomedicine and Pharmacotherapy* 51(9): 376–380.

Gorwood, P., Leboyer, M., Jay, M., Payan, C., & Feingold, J. (1995). Gender and age at onset in schizophrenia: Impact of family history. *American Journal of Psychiatry* 152(2): 208–212.

Granville-Grossman, K. L. (1966). Parental age and schizophrenia. *British Journal of Psychiatry* 112(490): 899–905.

Hare, E. H. & Moran, P. A. (1979). Parental age and birth order in homosexual patients: A replication of Slater's study. *British Journal of Psychiatry* 134: 178–182.

Heiden, A., Willinger, U., Scharfetter, J., Meszaros, K., Kasper, S., & Aschauer, H. N. (1999). Anticipation in schizophrenia. *Schizophrenia Research* 35(1): 25–32.

Husted, J., Scutt, L. E., & Bassett, A. S. (1998). Paternal transmission and anticipation in schizophrenia. *American Journal of Medical Genetics 81*(2): 156–162.

Imamura, A., Honda, S., Nakane, Y., & Okazaki, Y. (1998). Anticipation in Japanese families with schizophrenia. *Journal of Human Genetics 43*(4): 217–223.

Johnson, J. E., Cleary, J., Ahsan, H., Harkavy Friedman, J., Malaspina, D., Cloninger, C. R., Faraone, S. V., Tsuang, M. T., & Kaufmann, C. A. (1997). Anticipation in schizophrenia: Biology or bias? *American Journal of Medical Genetics 74*(3): 275–280.

Kesler, S. R., Blasey, C., Brown, W. E., Yankowitz, J., Zeng, S. M., Bender, B. G., & Reiss, A. L. (2003). Effects of X-monosomy and X-linked imprinting on superior temporal gyrus morphology in Turner Syndrome. *Biological Psychiatry 54*(6): 636–646.

Kinnell, H. G. (1983). Parental age in schizophrenia. *British Journal of Psychiatry 142*: 204.

Koenen, K. C., Moffitt, T. E., Roberts, A. L., Martin, L. T., Kubzansky, L., Harrington, H., Poulton, R., & Caspi, A. (2009). Childhood IQ and adult mental disorders: A test of the cognitive reserve hypothesis. *American Journal of Psychiatry 166*(1): 50–57.

Lawlor, D. A., Najman, J. M., Batty, G. D., O'Callaghan, M. J., Williams, G. M., & Bor, W. (2006). Early life predictors of childhood intelligence: Findings from the Mater-University study of pregnancy and its outcomes. *Paediatric and Perinatal Epidemiology 20*(2): 148–162.

Lindblad, K. & Schalling, M. (1999). Expanded repeat sequences and disease. *Seminars in Neurology 19*(3): 289–299.

Malama, I. M., Papaioannou, D. J., Kaklamani, E. P., Katsouyanni, K. M., Koumantaki, I. G., & Trichopoulos, D. V. (1988). Birth order sibship size and socio-economic factors in risk of schizophrenia in Greece. *British Journal of Psychiatry 152*: 482–486.

Malaspina, D., Friedman, J. H., Kaufmann, C., Bruder, G., Amador, X., Strauss, D., Clark, S., Yale, S., Lukens, E., Thorning, H., et al. (1998). Psychobiological heterogeneity of familial and sporadic schizophrenia. *Biological Psychiatry 43*(7): 489–496.

Malaspina, D., Goetz, R. R., Yale, S., Berman, A., Friedman, J. H., Tremeau, F., Printz, D., Amador, X., Johnson, J., Brown, A., et al. (2000). Relation of familial schizophrenia to negative symptoms but not to the deficit syndrome. *American Journal of Psychiatry 157*(6): 994–1003.

Malaspina, D., Harkavy-Friedman, J., Corcoran, C., Mujica-Parodi, L., Printz, D., Gorman, J. M., & Van Heertum, R. (2004). Resting neural activity distinguishes subgroups of schizophrenia patients. *Biological Psychiatry 56*(12): 931–937.

Malaspina, D., Harlap, S., Fennig, S., Heiman, D., Nahon, D., Feldman, D., & Susser, E. S. (2001). Advancing paternal age and the risk of schizophrenia. *Archives of General Psychiatry 58*(4): 361–367.

Malaspina, D., Reichenberg, A., Weiser, M., Fennig, S., Davidson, M., Harlap, S., Wolitzky, R., Rabinowitz, J., Susser, E., & Knobler, H. Y. (2005). Paternal age and intelligence: Implications for age-related genomic changes in male germ cells. *Psychiatric Genetics 15*(2): 117–125.

Mesholam-Gately, R. I., Giuliano, A. J., Goff, K. P., Faraone, S. V., & Seidman, L. J. (2009). Neurocognition in first-episode schizophrenia: A meta-analytic review. *Neuropsychology 23*(3): 315–336.

Morris, A. G., Gaitonde, E., McKenna, P. J., Mollon, J. D., & Hunt, D. M. (1995). CAG repeat expansions and schizophrenia: Association with disease in females and with early age-at-onset. *Human Molecular Genetics 4*(10): 1957–1961.

Nelson, K. & Holmes, L. B. (1989). Malformations due to presumed spontaneous mutations in newborn infants. *New England Journal of Medicine 320*(1): 19–23.

O'Donovan, M. C., Guy, C., Craddock, N., Bowen, T., McKeon, P., Macedo, A., Maier, W., Wildenauer, D., Aschauer, H. N., Sorbi, S., et al. (1996). Confirmation of association between expanded CAG/CTG repeats and both schizophrenia and bipolar disorder. *Psychological Medicine* 26(6): 1145–1153.

O'Donovan, M. C. & Owen, M. J. (1999). Candidate-gene association studies of schizophrenia. *American Journal of Human Genetics* 65(3): 587–592.

Oakes, C. C., Smiraglia, D. J., Plass, C., Trasler, J. M., & Robaire, B. (2003). Aging results in hypermethylation of ribosomal DNA in sperm and liver of male rats. *Proceedings of the National Academy of Sciences U.S.A.* 100(4): 1775–1780.

Orioli, I. M., Castilla, E. E., Scarano, G., & Mastroiacovo, P. (1995). Effect of paternal age in achondroplasia, thanatophoric dysplasia, and osteogenesis imperfecta. *American Journal of Human Genetics* 59(2): 209–217.

Orr, H. T. & Zoghbi, H. Y. (2007). Trinucleotide repeat disorders. *Annual Review of Neuroscience 30*: 575–621.

Perrin, M. C., Opler, M. G., Harlap, S., Harkavy-Friedman, J., Kleinhaus, K., Nahon, D., Fennig, S., Susser, E. S., & Malaspina, D. (2007). Tetrachloroethylene exposure and risk of schizophrenia: Offspring of dry cleaners in a population birth cohort, preliminary findings. *Schizophrenia Research* 90(1–3): 251–254.

Petronis, A., Sherrington, R. P., Paterson, A. D., & Kennedy, J. L. (1995). Genetic anticipation in schizophrenia: Pro and con. *Journal of Clinical Neuroscience* 3(2): 76–80.

Pulver, A. E., McGrath, J. A., Liang, K. Y., Lasseter, V. K., Nestadt, G., & Wolyniec, P. S. (2004). An indirect test of the new mutation hypothesis associating advanced paternal age with the etiology of schizophrenia. *American Journal of Medical Genetics Part B: Neuropsychiatric Genetics 124*(1): 6–9.

Reichenberg, A., Gross, R., Weiser, M., Bresnahan, M., Silverman, J., Harlap, S., Rabinowitz, J., Shulman, C., Malaspina, D., Lubin, G., et al. (2006). Advancing paternal age and autism. *Archives of General Psychiatry* 63(9): 1026–1032.

Saha, S., Barnett, A. G., Foldi, C., Burne, T. H., Eyles, D. W., Buka, S. L., & McGrath, J. J. (2009). Advanced paternal age is associated with impaired neurocognitive outcomes during infancy and childhood. *PLoS Medicine* 6(3): e40.

Schols, L., Bauer, P., Schmidt, T., Schulte, T., & Riess, O. (2004). Autosomal dominant cerebellar ataxias: Clinical features, genetics, and pathogenesis. *Lancet Neurology* 3(5): 291–304.

Sipos, A., Rasmussen, F., Harrison, G., Tynelius, P., Lewis, G., Leon, D. A., & Gunnell, D. (2004). Paternal age and schizophrenia: A population based cohort study. *British Medical Journal* 329(7474): 1070.

Skuse, D. H., James, R. S., Bishop, D. V., Coppin, B., Dalton, P., Aamodt-Leeper, G., Bacarese-Hamilton, M., Creswell, C., McGurk, R., & Jacobs, P. A. (1997). Evidence from Turner's syndrome of an imprinted X-linked locus affecting cognitive function. *Nature 387*(6634): 705–708.

Smith, R. G., Kember, R. L., Mill, J., Fernandes, C., Schalkwyk, L. C., Buxbaum, J. D., & Reichenberg, A. (2009). Advancing paternal age is associated with deficits in social and exploratory behaviors in the offspring: A mouse model. *PLoS One* 4(12): e8456.

St Clair, D. (2009). Copy number variation and schizophrenia. *Schizophrenia Bulletin* 35(1): 9–12.

St Sauver, J. L., Katusic, S. K., Barbaresi, W. J., Colligan, R. C., & Jacobsen, S. J. (2001). Boy/girl differences in risk for reading disability: Potential clues? *American Journal of Epidemiology* 154(9): 787–794.

Telenius, H., Kremer, H. P., Theilmann, J., Andrew, S. E., Almqvist, E., Anvret, M., Greenberg, C., Greenberg, J., Lucotte, G., Squitieri, F., et al. (1993). Molecular analysis of juvenile Huntington disease: The major influence on (CAG)n repeat length is the sex of the affected parent. *Human Molecular Genetics* 2(10): 1535–1540.

Tsuchiya, K. J., Takagai, S., Kawai, M., Matsumoto, H., Nakamura, K., Minabe, Y., Mori, N., & Takei, N. (2005). Advanced paternal age associated with an elevated risk for schizophrenia in offspring in a Japanese population. *Schizophrenia Research 76*(2–3): 337–342.

Turkheimer, E., Haley, A., Waldron, M., D'Onofrio, B., & Gottesman, I. I. (2003). Socioeconomic status modifies heritability of IQ in young children. *Psychological Science 14*(6): 623–628.

Van Den Bogaert, A., Schumacher, J., Schulze, T. G., Otte, A. C., Ohlraun, S., Kovalenko, S., Becker, T., Freudenberg, J., Jonsson, E. G., Mattila-Evenden, M., et al. (2003). The DTNBP1 (dysbindin) gene contributes to schizophrenia, depending on family history of the disease. *American Journal of Human Genetics 73*(6): 1438–1443.

Vincent, J. B., Paterson, A. D., Strong, E., Petronis, A., & Kennedy, J. L. (2000). The unstable trinucleotide repeat story of major psychosis. *American Journal of Medical Genetics 97*(1): 77–97.

Wilkin, D. J., Szabo, J. K., Cameron, R., Henderson, S., Bellus, G. A., Mack, M. L., Kaitila, I., Loughlin, J., Munnich, A., Sykes, B., et al. (1998). Mutations in fibroblast growth-factor receptor 3 in sporadic cases of achondroplasia occur exclusively on the paternally derived chromosome. *American Journal of Human Genetics 63*(3): 711–716.

Williams, N. M., Preece, A., Spurlock, G., Norton, N., Williams, H. J., Zammit, S., O'Donovan, M. C., & Owen, M. J. (2003). Support for genetic variation in neuregulin 1 and susceptibility to schizophrenia. *Molecular Psychiatry 8*(5): 485–487.

Wolitzky, R., Goudsmit, N., Goetz, R. R., Printz, D., Gil, R., Harkavy-Friedman, J., & Malaspina, D. (2006). Etiological heterogeneity and intelligence test scores in patients with schizophrenia. *Journal of Clinical and Experimental Neuropsychology 28*(2): 167–177.

Xu, B., Roos, J., Levy, S., van Rensburg, E., Gogos, J., & Karayiorgou, M. (2008). Strong association of de novo copy number mutations with sporadic schizophrenia. *Nature Genetics 40*(7): 880–885.

Yu, K., Herr, A. B., Waksman, G., & Ornitz, D. M. (2000). Loss of fibroblast growth factor receptor 2 ligand-binding specificity in Apert syndrome. *Proceedings of the National Academy of Sciences U.S.A. 97*(26): 14536–14541.

Zammit, S., Allebeck, P., Dalman, C., Lundberg, I., Hemmingson, T., Owen, M. J., & Lewis, G. (2003). Paternal age and risk for schizophrenia. *British Journal of Psychiatry 183*: 405–408.

Zenzes, M. T. (2000). Smoking and reproduction: Gene damage to human gametes and embryos. *Human Reproduction Update 6*(2): 122–131.

CHAPTER 6

CANNABIS USE AS A COMPONENT CAUSE OF SCHIZOPHRENIA

PAOLA CASADIO, MARTA DI FORTI, AND ROBIN M. MURRAY

KEY CONCEPTS

- Cannabis is the most popular illicit drug in the world. Epidemiologic studies have reported consistently that cannabis use is associated with later schizophrenia, even after controlling for several confounding factors. Those studies that collected data on the extent of cannabis use also reported a dose-response effect.
- Experimental studies confirm that administration of Δ_9-tetrahydrocannabinol (Δ_9-THC), the main psychoactive ingredient of cannabis, can induce psychosis.
- Only a minority of cannabis users develop psychosis. This can be explained in part by the amount and duration of the consumption of cannabis. Individual genetic vulnerability may also play a role.
- There exists a plausible biological explanation for the cannabis-psychosis interaction. Repeated or high exposure to Δ_9-THC produces a prolonged and excessive stimulation of cannabinoid CB1 receptors, which overwhelms the system. This overstimulation of CB1 receptors on GABAergic (transmitting or secreting gamma-aminobutyric acid) and glutamatergic terminals, which modulate dopaminergic projection firing from the brain stem to the striatum, has been shown to play an important role in the genesis of Δ_9-THC-induced psychosis.
- Recent neuroimaging studies suggest that heavy cannabis use may (1) modify brain structure and (2) induce dopamine release in the striatum.

Introduction

Cannabis is the most popular illicit drug in the world. The World Drug Report 2009, published by the United Nations, estimates that the number of people globally who used cannabis at least once in 2007 was between 143 million and

190 million. The highest levels of use remain in the established markets of North America, Western Europe, West and Central Africa, and Oceania (United Nations Office on Drugs and Crime, 2009).

The term *Cannabis* refers to different types of preparations derived from the plant *Cannabis sativa*, all of which contain chemical substances called *cannabinoids*. Until recently, the main types of cannabis available on the "street" consisted of marijuana (grass) and resin (hash), but in recent years a more potent variant termed *sinsemilla* or "skunk" has become available in many countries. The psychoactive ingredient of cannabis is Δ_9-THC; marijuana and resin have traditionally contained about 4% Δ_9-THC, but the concentration of Δ_9-THC in skunk in countries such as Holland and England has increased to between 16 and 22% (Potter, Clark, & Brown, 2008; Hardwick & King, 2008). This increase is partly because of selective breeding and partly because of the use of intensive indoor cultivation methods (King, Carpentier, & Griffiths, 2004). Of the other constituents of cannabis, cannabidiol (CBD) has aroused the most interest. It is not hallucinogenic, and in contrast to Δ_9-THC it appears to have anxiolytic properties. Surprisingly, it has even been suggested to have antipsychotic effects (Murray et al., 2007).

Epidemiology of Cannabis and Psychosis

It has long been accepted that cannabis intoxication can lead to acute psychotic episodes (Negrete et al., 1986; Thornicroft, 1990; Mathers & Ghodse, 1992). However, starting in the 1990s, reports have appeared stating that patients suffering from schizophrenia are more likely to use cannabis than the general population (Thornicroft, 1990) and that continued cannabis use is associated with poor outcome in those with existing psychotic illness (Linszen, Dingemans, & Lenior, 1994). Of course, such reports cannot answer the question of whether cannabis use caused the psychosis in the first place.

Such a question can be addressed only by longitudinal studies in the general population. The first of these was a cohort study of 45,570 Swedish conscripts who were followed up after 15 years (Andreasson et al., 1987; Zammit et al., 2002). Those who had smoked cannabis by the age of conscription had double the risk of developing schizophrenia in the ensuing 15 years (adjusted OR = 2.3, 95% CI = 1.0–5.3). These findings were confirmed in a further follow-up of the cohort after 27 years. Moreover, a dose-response relationship was observed: heavy cannabis users were six times more likely than nonusers to later receive a diagnosis of schizophrenia (Zammit et al., 2002).

Between 2002 and 2007, more studies were published that essentially substantiated the findings of the Swedish Army Study. For instance, in the Netherlands (van Os et al., 2002), a population-based prospective study examined the effect of cannabis use on self-reported psychotic symptoms among 4,045 psychosis-free persons who were assessed at baseline and were then followed up one year later and again three years after the baseline assessment. Individuals using cannabis at baseline were nearly three times (adjusted OR = 2.8, 95% CI = 1.2–6.5) more likely to manifest psychotic symptoms at follow-up, and there was a dose-response relationship between exposure load and psychosis outcome. A baseline lifetime history of cannabis use was a stronger predictor of psychosis outcome than was use over the follow-up period or use of other drugs. Moreover, the difference in risk of psychosis at follow-up between those who did and did not use cannabis was much stronger for those with an established vulnerability to psychosis at baseline than for those without one.

Two birth cohort studies from New Zealand on cannabis use and psychotic symptoms were also reported. The Christchurch study (Fergusson, Horwood, & Swain-Campbell, 2003), which examined the development of its participants for more than two decades, showed that individuals with cannabis dependence disorder at age 18 years had a twofold (adjusted OR = 1.8, 95% CI = 1.2–2.6) increased risk of developing psychotic symptoms than those without cannabis dependence. Statistical control for previous psychotic symptoms clarified the temporal sequence, ruling out the alternative explanation that psychotic symptoms induce cannabis use.

The Dunedin study (Arseneault et al., 2002) showed that individuals using cannabis at the age of 15 years reported significantly more schizophreniform disorder at age 26 than did nonusers (OR = 4.50, 95% CI = 1.11–18.21). This was the only study to take into account childhood psychotic symptoms antedating cannabis use (self-reported psychotic symptoms at age 11 years). Cannabis use was associated with an increased risk of schizophreniform disorder even after these psychotic symptoms preceding the onset of cannabis use were controlled for (OR = 3.12, 95% CI = 0.73–13.29), although the result failed to reach statistical significance, possibly because of lack of statistical power. Moreover, cannabis use by age 15 did not predict depressive outcome at age 26, indicating specificity of the outcome. Similarly, the use of other illicit drugs in adolescence did not predict schizophrenia outcomes over and above the effect of cannabis use, indicating specificity of the exposure.

Henquet et al. (2005a) carried out a prospective study of 2,437 young Germans with a four-year follow-up. Cannabis use moderately increased the risk of psychotic symptoms in these young people (OR = 1.7, 95% CI = 1.1–1.5), and again there was a dose-response relationship with increasing frequency of cannabis use. The authors also reported that cannabis use had a much stronger effect in those with psychosis vulnerability at baseline, but predisposition for psychosis at baseline did not significantly predict cannabis use at follow-up, thus refuting the self-medication hypothesis. Data from these and other studies are shown in table 6.1.

Table 6.1 Epidemiology of Cannabis and Psychosis

Country Where Study Was Conducted (Citation)	Study Design	No. of Participants	Follow-up	Odds Ratio (95% CI) (Adjusted Risk)
United States (Tien & Anthony, 1990)	Population based	4,494	NA	2.4 (1.2–7.1)
Sweden (Andreasson et al., 1987; Zammit et al., 2002)	Conscript cohort	50,053	15 years 27 years	2.3 (1.0–5.3) 3.1 (1.7–5.5)
The Netherlands (NEMESIS) (van Os et al., 2002)	Population based	4,045	3 years	2.8 (1.2–6.5)
Israel (Weiser et al., 2002)	Population based	9,724	4–15 years	2.0 (1.3–3.1)
New Zealand (Christchurch) (Fergusson, Horwood, & Swain-Campbell, 2003)	Birth cohort	1,265	3 years	1.8 (1.2–2.6)
New Zealand (Dunedin) (Arseneault et al., 2002)	Birth cohort	1,034	15 years	3.1 (0.7–13.3)
The Netherlands (Ferdinand et al., 2005)	Population based	1,580	14 years	2.8 (1.79–4.43)
Germany (EDSP) (Henquet et al., 2005a)	Population based	2,437	4 years	1.7 (1.1–1.5)
United Kingdom (Wiles et al., 2006)	Population based	8,580	18 months	1.5 (0.55–3.94)
Greece (Stefanis et al., 2004)	Birth cohort	3,500	NA	4.3 (1.0–17.9)

CI = Confidence interval.
SOURCE: Authors.

Meta-analyses of these prospective studies were carried out by Henquet et al. (2005b) finding a pooled adjusted OR = 2.1 (95% CI = 1.7-2.5) and by Moore et al. (2007), finding a pooled OR = 1.41 (95% CI = 1.20–1.65).

Experimental Studies

Other researchers have explored the effects of the constituents of cannabis through experimental studies. The first of these was carried out by D'Souza et al. (2004): 22 healthy individuals, who had been exposed to cannabis but had never been diagnosed with a cannabis abuse disorder, were assessed for a range of symptoms associated with schizophrenia after the intravenous administration of 0 mg, 2.5 mg, and 5 mg of Δ_9-THC. The Δ_9-THC produced transient effects, including positive symptoms, negative symptoms, perceptual alterations, euphoria, anxiety, and deficits in working memory and verbal recall. The observed positive symptoms (rated with the Positive and Negative Syndrome Scale, or PANSS) were suspiciousness, paranoid and grandiose delusions, illusions, depersonalization and derealization, feelings of unreality, and extreme slowing of time. The peak of these symptoms induced by Δ_9-THC occurred 10 minutes after drug administration and returned to baseline levels within 200 minutes.

Similar effects were observed by Morrison et al. (2009), who—using the PANSS and the Community Assessment of Psychic Experiences (CAPE)—assessed the effect of the intravenous administration of 2.5 mg Δ_9-THC versus placebo in normal individuals. Δ_9-THC induced psychotic symptoms and impaired neuropsychological performance, the most commonly observed positive symptom, concerned ideas of reference. Moreover, the participants' CAPE and investigators' PANSS scores were highly correlated, so that the subjective feelings of the volunteers were comparable with the observer ratings. Furthermore, the psychotic symptoms did not correlate with Δ_9-THC-elicited anxiety, suggesting that these are separable psychological effects.

D'Souza et al. (2005) conducted a further study, in which they gave intravenous Δ_9-THC to patients with schizophrenia who were clinically stable. Δ_9-THC administration was again associated with transient positive symptoms, and the schizophrenic patients showed significant enhanced sensitivity for cognitive effects compared with normal individuals. The increases in positive symptoms were brief and modest but occurred even if patients were receiving antipsychotic drugs. This exacerbation in symptoms despite treatment with dopamine antagonists raises the possibility that dopaminergic systems might not play a significant role in the psychotic symptoms induced by Δ_9-THC.

Another study carried out by D'Souza et al. (2008) compared the effects of Δ_9-THC in frequent users of cannabis (at least 10 exposures to cannabis within the past month) (N = 30) against those same measures in healthy nonusing controls (N = 22). In frequent users, Δ_9-THC-induced perceptual alterations, psychotomimetic effects, anxiety, and recall impairments were all blunted, and increased scores on several measures resolved faster than in the nonusing control group. This did not happen for the "desirable" effects of cannabis like feeling "high," calm, and relaxed. This suggests that frequent users either develop tolerance to the "adverse psychological" effects of Δ_9-THC or alternatively are less susceptible to these adverse effects.

Henquet et al. (2006) compared the effects of smoked Δ_9-THC in patients with psychotic disorders (N = 30), relatives of patients with psychotic disorders (N = 12), and healthy controls (N = 32). They replicated the evidence of Δ_9-THC-induced effects on psychosis and cognition, but hypothesized that it was conditioned by other variables such as genetic susceptibility and psychosis liability.

What Determines Who Will Develop Psychosis?

It is clear from the epidemiologic studies already discussed here that only a minority of cannabis users develop psychosis; for example, in the Swedish Army study only 3% of heavy cannabis users went on to develop schizophrenia. This can be explained in part by the amount and duration of the consumption of cannabis (Arseneault et al., 2002; Henquet et al., 2005b). The most clear-cut demonstration of this comes from Di Forti et al. (2009), who found that cannabis users suffering their first episode of psychosis were more likely to have taken cannabis for a longer period of time and on a daily basis than were control users from the general population. They also noted that the psychotic patients were much more likely to have used the high-potency cannabis variety, skunk (OR = 6.8, 95% CI 2.6–25.4), which has three or four times more Δ_9-THC than traditional marijuana or resin.

It may also be that individual genetic vulnerability plays a significant role. Caspi and colleagues (2005) reported an interaction between cannabis use and variation in the gene that encodes catecholamine-O-methyl transferase (COMT) in the Dunedin study that was discussed earlier in this chapter. COMT is the key enzyme involved in the prefrontal cortex metabolism of dopamine released into synapses, and it contains a G to A missense mutation that generates a valine (Val) to methionine (Met) substitution at codon 158 (Val[158]Met). The Met variant produces less enzymatic activity and consequently a slower breakdown of dopamine. The Val variant corresponds to the high-activity enzyme, resulting in a combination of reduced dopamine neurotransmission in the prefrontal cortex and increased levels of mesolimbic dopamine. Caspi et al. (2005) found that adolescent cannabis use was associated with the greatest increase in the risk of subsequent schizophreniform disorder among Val/Val individuals, a lesser increase among Val/Met individuals, and no increase in Met/Met individuals.

This interaction between cannabis and the COMT Val[158]Met polymorphism gene was investigated experimentally by Henquet et al. (2006), who gave 300 µg of Δ_9-THC per kg of body weight or a placebo to patients with psychotic disorders, relatives of patients with a psychotic disorder, and healthy controls. Those with the homozygous Val genotype were more likely to develop Δ_9-THC-induced psychotic symptoms, but this was conditional on prior evidence of psychosis liability. Psychosis liability was defined as a "psychometric measure of liability for psychosis" (using the CAPE) and as "illness risk" (a variable indicating progressively increasing risk from healthy controls to relatives of patients with a psychotic disorder to patients with a psychotic disorder).

In a subsequent study, Henquet et al. (2009) used the experience sampling method to collect data on cannabis use and the occurrence of psychotic symptoms in daily life. Use of cannabis significantly increased hallucinatory experiences only in those individuals who were carriers of the Val allele and had high levels of psychometric psychosis liability; this suggests that the COMT Val[158]Met genotype moderates the association between cannabis and psychotic symptoms in the flow of daily life in psychosis-prone people. In contrast, in a study of psychotic patients, Zammit et al. (2007) found no evidence for a differential effect of cannabis use on psychosis risk according to variation in COMT Val[158]Met.

In short, there is intriguing evidence suggesting an interaction between cannabis consumption and the COMT genotype in provoking psychosis. However, the hypothesis remains to be adequately confirmed or refuted, and individual response to cannabis use is likely to be moderated by a number of genes rather than a single polymorphism.

How Does Δ$_9$-THC Produce Its Effects?

Δ$_9$-THC acts on the cannabinoid receptor 1 (CB1), which is one of the most abundant G-protein-coupled receptors in the brain (see figure 6.1). Consequently, the

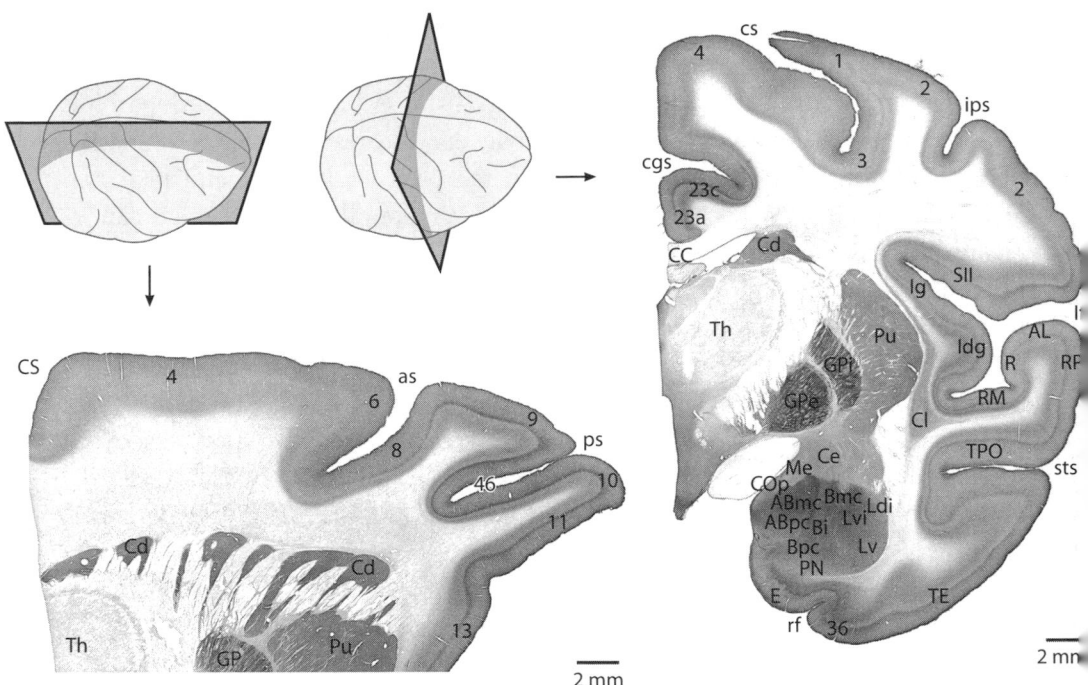

Figure 6.1. Distribution of the Cannabinoid CB1 Receptor in the Primate Neocortex.
(A) Photomicrograph of a parasagittal section through a macaque monkey frontal lobe processed fo CB1 immunoreactivity. (B) Photomicrograph of a coronal section through macaque monkey brain illustrating the distribution of CB1-IR axons. Association areas such as the cingulate cortex (area 23), insul. (Ig, Idg), auditory association cortex (RP), and the entorhinal cortex (EI) had an overall higher density o CB1-IR axons than primary somatosensory areas (areas 3, 1, 2) and the primary motor cortex (area 4) In subcortical structures, the intensity of CB1 immunoreactivity was high in the claustrum (Cl), the basa and lateral nuclei of the amygdala, and globus pallidus (GP); intermediate to low in the caudate (Cd) an putamen (Pu) and the central and medial nuclei of the amygdala; and not detectable in the thalamus (Th (Reprinted from Eggan & Lewis [2007] by permission of Oxford University Press.)

effects of Δ_9-THC are best understood in terms of the functions of the endocannabinoid system.

The physiologic endogenous agonists of the CB1 (and CB2) receptors, N-arachidonoylethanolamine (anandamide) and 2-arachidonoylglycerol (2-AG) (Di Marzo, Bifulco, & De, 2004) are synthesized "on demand" from membrane phospholipids and act as local mediators in an autocrine and paracrine manner (Di Marzo, Bifulco, & De, 2004). In binding to CB1, they further the closure of Ca^{2+} channels, the opening of K^+ channels, inhibition of adenylyl cyclase activity, and stimulation of kinases (Piomelli, 2003).

Endocannabinoids act presynaptically to inhibit the release of amino acid neurotransmitters on the terminals of neighboring GABAergic and glutamatergic neurons (see figure 6.2). They are synthesized by principal output neurons, such as Purkinje cells in the cerebellum, pyramidal neurons in the hippocampus and cortex, medium spiny neurons in the striatum, and dopaminergic neurons in the midbrain (Freund, Katona, & Piomelli, 2003). Thus, these neurons regulate their excitatory and inhibitory inputs by releasing endocannabinoids that intervene in both short-term and long-term forms of synaptic plasticity.

The endocannabinoids are involved in regulating cognitive functions in neuronal circuits of the cortex, memory in neurons of the hippocampus, and emotions in neurons of the amygdala. The terminal fields of striatal projection neurons contain the highest densities of CB1 receptors, implying an important modulation of motor activity. Cannabinoid agonists also influence the central processing of pain by interacting with CB1 receptors in periaqueductal gray matter, the medulla, and the spinal trigeminal nucleus. Moreover, they are involved in the reinforcing effects of substances of abuse in the mesolimbic system (Piomelli, 2003; Di Marzo, Bifulco, & De, 2004).

Δ_9-THC is a powerful cannabinoid agonist, and consequently repeated or high exposure to it produces a prolonged and excessive stimulation of the CB1 receptor that overwhelms the system. This overstimulation of the CB1 receptor in the hippocampus, the cerebellum, the basal ganglia, and the neocortex is responsible for many of the cognitive and motor effects of Δ_9-THC, while its stimulation in peripheral nerve fibers, the dorsal root ganglion, the spinal dorsal horn, and the periaqueductal gray matter accounts for its analgesic properties (Di Marzo, Bifulco, & De, 2004; Murray et al., 2007). It is postulated that overstimulation of CB1 receptors on GABAergic and glutamatergic terminals modulating dopaminergic projection firing from the brain stem to the striatum may play an important role in the genesis of Δ_9-THC-induced psychosis (Morrison & Murray, 2009).

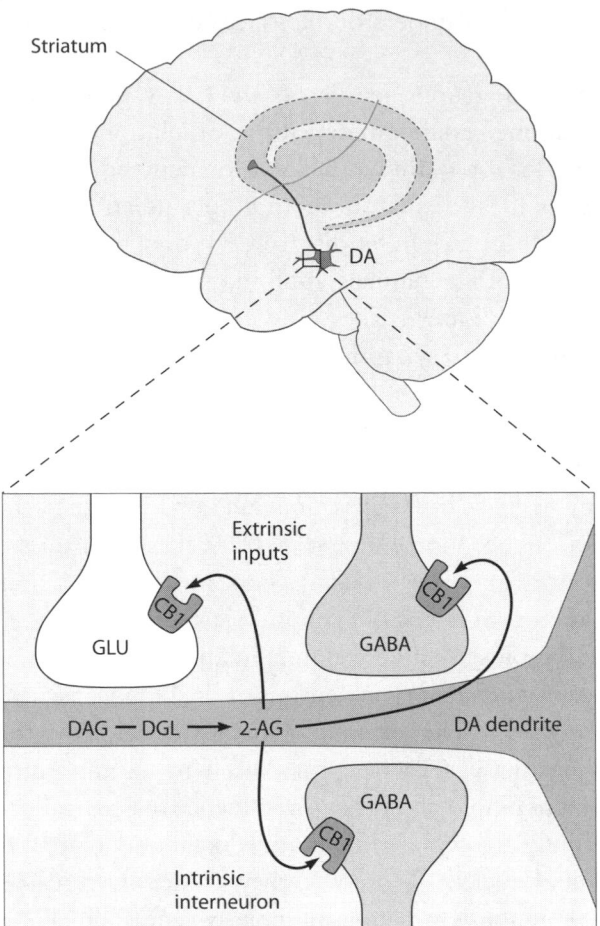

Figure 6.2. The endocannabinoids "fine-tune" synaptic signaling.
GABA and glutamate modulate the excitability of midbrain dopamine neurons and prefrontal cortical pyramidal cells. These are influenced by endocannabinoids by way of CB1 receptors. THC is the most potent CB1 agonist and appears to switch off inhibitory inputs to dopamine neurons. DAG = Diacylglycerol; DGL = Diacylglycerol Lipase; 2-AG = 2-Arachidonoylglycerol. (Source: Authors.)

Why Do Patients Persist in Cannabis Use to Their Detriment?

When patients with psychosis are asked why they use cannabis, they give reasons that are very similar to those of users in the population as a whole: they enjoy the "high," feelings of calmness, and mild perceptual changes. However, clinicians have been puzzled as to why cannabis users who develop psychotic symptoms or even schizophrenia persist in using the drug in spite of advice—borne out by their own experience—that taking cannabis exacerbates their psychosis. It could be because the patients still enjoy the relief from anxiety and other positive effects even when they know these will be followed by increased paranoia. But it might also be because of dependence on the drug.

Controlled studies have demonstrated abstinence symptoms following cessation of cannabis. Haney and colleagues (1999a) gave 12 heavy marijuana smokers placebo pills on study days 1–3, 8–11, and 16–19; 20 mg of oral Δ_9-THC on days 4–7; and 30 mg of oral Δ_9-THC on days 12–15. Abstinence from Δ_9-THC was associated with increased anxiety, depression and irritability, decreased sleep, and decreased food intake. Similar results were found in an analogous study conducted with marijuana cigarettes (Haney et al., 1999b).

A study of marijuana smokers in their homes (Budney et al., 2001) showed that withdrawal discomfort increased significantly during a three-day abstinence period and returned to baseline only when cannabis smoking resumed. Craving for marijuana, decreased appetite, sleep difficulty, and weight loss were observed. Subsequently Budney and colleagues (2003) conducted a study with a five-day smoking-as-usual phase followed by a 45-day abstinence phase. Onset of withdrawal symptoms typically occurred between days 1 and 3, peaked between days 2 and 6, and began to wear off over days 4 to 14. Sleep problems, including particularly unusual dreams, however, did not return to baseline by the end of the 45-day abstinence period.

Thus, it seems that Δ_9-THC can cause dependence but that withdrawal symptoms are subtle, with the long half-life of cannabis probably preventing profound physical withdrawal. But the reports just cited show that dependence does exist, and animal studies have shown that administration of a CB1 receptor antagonist precipitates acute withdrawal symptoms. This does not happen in CB1 receptor knockout mice, suggesting pharmacological specificity of a cannabinoid abstinence effect (Gonzalez et al., 2004). To our knowledge there has not been adequate investigation of the role of dependence on cannabis in those psychotic patients who persist in taking the drug. Such studies are urgently needed.

Effects of Cannabis on Brain Structure and Function

Recent studies conducted with magnetic resonance imaging (Arnone et al., 2008; Rais et al., 2008; Yucel et al., 2008; Mata et al., 2009) have raised the question of whether heavy cannabis use may modify brain structure. Yucel et al. (2008) compared nonusers against users who had used more than five joints daily for more than 10 years. The heavy cannabis users had bilaterally reduced hippocampal and amygdala volumes, with a greater effect in the former. Left-hemisphere hippocampal volume was inversely associated with cumulative exposure to cannabis and with subthreshold positive psychotic symptoms. Hippocampal abnormalities in schizophrenia are more prominent in the left hemisphere (Petty, 1999).

Rais and colleagues (2008) examined the effects of cannabis use on brain structure in a follow-up of first-episode patients with schizophrenia. Those who continued to use cannabis showed a more pronounced gray matter loss together with greater lateral and third ventricle enlargement over the five-year follow-up period than both healthy subjects and nonusing patients with schizophrenia.

Arnone et al. (2008) examined the effects of prolonged heavy cannabis use in 11 subjects and a similar number of nonusers, using diffusion tensor imaging, which can examine white matter tracts. They observed a significant increase in diffusivity in cannabis users relative to controls in that region of the corpus callosum where white matter passes between the prefrontal lobes. This could indicate that cannabis exercises an effect on white matter structural integrity.

Mata and colleagues (2009) investigated the influence of cannabis use on cortical brain gyrification in 30 cannabis users and 44 nonusers. Cannabis users had bilaterally decreased concavity of the sulci and thinner sulci in the right frontal lobe. Among nonusers, age was significantly correlated with decreased gyrification and cortical thickness loss. However, in the group of cannabis users these modifications were not dependent on age and were present even in young subjects. The researchers questioned whether chronic exposure to cannabinoids during adolescence may alter normal brain neurodevelopment, leading to a pattern of decreased gyrification with less concave and thinner sulci similar to that in aging subjects.

Functional neuroimaging studies suggest that resting global, prefrontal, and anterior cingulate cortex blood flow are lower in cannabis users than in controls (Martin-Santos et al., 2009). Evidence of effects of Δ_9-THC on activity in these areas is consistent with the relatively high concentration of CB1 receptors in the prefrontal and cingulate cortex. Moreover, functional imaging studies that examined brain activity after the acute experimental administration of Δ_9-THC or marijuana cigarettes showed increased prefrontal, insular, and anterior cingulate activity both during the resting state and during cognitive tasks.

In one functional magnetic resonance imaging (fMRI) study, Bhattacharyya and colleagues (2009) investigated the effect of Δ_9-THC on brain function as the subjects performed various verbal learning tasks. Δ_9-THC modulated mediotemporal and anterocingulate as well as medioprefrontal cortex function in the context of learning, and induced psychotic symptoms by modulating ventrostriatal activity. The effect on hippocampal activation is consistent with the evidence that the CB1 receptor is highly expressed there and with the well-known detrimental effect of cannabis on memory function.

Evidence that Δ_9-THC influences activation in the striatum (Bhattacharyya et al., 2009) is consistent with a study by Bossong and colleagues (2009), who used a dopamine D_2/D_3 receptor tracer (raclopride) and positron emission tomography to examine striatal synaptic dopamine release. The tracer binding was significantly reduced in the ventral striatum and the precommisural dorsal putamen after inhalation of Δ_9-THC compared to placebo, implying an increased release of endogenous dopamine in these regions. The ability of Δ_9-THC to induce dopamine release in the striatum suggests that Δ_9-THC shares properties with other drugs of abuse, as dopamine has a central role in their rewarding effects, but the increase was modest over that obtained with other drugs like cocaine, nicotine, or alcohol. This modest effect on dopamine release in the striatum might be explained by the indirect effects of Δ_9-THC through cannabinoid CB1 receptors on glutamate and GABA (gamma-aminobutyric acid) neurons in the nucleus accumbens and the ventral tegmental area.

This finding of Δ_9-THC-induced release of dopamine in the striatum suggests that human striatal dopamine release is partly under the control of the endogenous cannabinoid system, and could explain how cannabis use contributes to the development and pathophysiology of schizophrenia (Bossong et al., 2009). However, another positron emission tomography (PET) study, this time using FluroDopa, by Stokes et al. (2009), failed to find a significant increase in presynaptic dopamine synthesis in the striatum following oral Δ_9-THC. Hence, whether Δ_9-THC provokes a modest alteration in the striatal dopamine system remains unclear.

Conclusion

The classic approach to determining the role of a risk factor in a disease is to assess whether it meets the Bradford Hill criteria for causality (Hill, 1965), which are: (1) strength, (2) consistency, (3) specificity of association, (4) temporality, (5) dose response, (6) biological plausibility and coherence, and (7) availability of experimental data. Does the cannabis-psychosis relationship measure up to these criteria?

The epidemiologic studies reviewed here have consistently found that cannabis use is associated with later schizophrenia outcomes, even after controlling for several confounding factors. The association is generally moderate in strength when the exposure to cannabis has been measured as "ever used." The Dunedin and Christchurch studies clearly demonstrated the temporal relationship (i.e., cannabis before psychosis), which casts doubt on a reverse causality explanation. All the studies that collected data on the degree of exposure to cannabis use reported a dose-response effect (Andreasson et al., 1987; van Os et al., 2002; Zammit et al., 2002; Henquet et al., 2005a), most clearly with regard to the evidence for the impact of cannabis potency on magnitude of risk for psychosis in the study of Di Forti et al. (2009). Furthermore, the Dunedin study has also indicated how cannabis use seems to increase the risk for psychosis but not for depression, suggesting a specificity of effect.

The experimental data we have reviewed confirm the existence of acute Δ_9-THC-induced psychosis, and there exists a possible biological explanation for the cannabis-psychosis interaction in that one study claims that cannabis use can induce dopamine release in the striatum; however, this remains controversial (D'Souza et al., 2004, 2005, 2008; Howes et al., 2004; Henquet et al., 2005b; D'Souza, Sewell, & Ranganathan, 2009; Morrison et al., 2009).

On balance, the evidence suggests that cannabis use does play a causal role in the etiology of schizophrenia-like illnesses. However, it is clearly neither a necessary cause (not all those with schizophrenia have used cannabis) nor a sufficient cause (the majority of cannabis users do not develop schizophrenia). Cannabis use is best considered as one of a number of component causes in the development of psychosis. Its use may confer only a modest increase in relative risk for schizophrenia in the individual, but its use is so widespread in the general population as to have significant public health implications. The proportion of schizophrenia attributed to cannabis use in different countries has varied from 8–15% (Henquet et al., 2005b; Moore et al., 2007), indicating the potential for preventive measures. Education concerning the risks of frequent heavy use of potent varieties of cannabis such as skunk may well be more useful than attempts to prohibit use by severe legal sanctions. The evidence that some individuals may be particularly vulnerable could in the future allow the targeting of preventive and treatment efforts onto such individuals. However, in our view, the evidence is not yet well enough established to merit these interventions.

KEY AREAS FOR FUTURE RESEARCH

- Elucidate the genetic and personality predisposition to develop psychosis following cannabis use.
- Establish the pathogenic mechanism whereby Δ_9-THC produces its propsychotic effects.
- Replicate studies suggesting that heavy cannabis use decreases the volumes of certain brain regions.
- Undertake further studies to confirm whether cannabidiol, another constituent of cannabis, has a moderating effect on the propsychotic effects of Δ_9-THC.

Selected Readings

Bhattacharyya, S., Fusar-Poli, P., Borgwardt, S., Martin-Santos, R., Nosarti, C., O'Carroll, C., Allen, P., Seal, M. L., Fletcher, P. C., Crippa, J. A., et al. (2009). Modulation of mediotemporal and ventrostriatal function in humans by Delta9-tetrahydrocannabinol: A neural basis for the effects of *Cannabis sativa* on learning and psychosis. *Archives of General Psychiatry* 66(4): 442–451.

Caspi, A., Moffitt, T. E., Cannon, M., McClay, J., Murray, R., Harrington, H., Taylor, A., Arseneault, L., Williams, B., Braithwaite, A., et al. (2005). Moderation of the effect of adolescent-onset cannabis use on adult psychosis by a functional polymorphism in the catechol-O-methyltransferase gene: Longitudinal evidence of a gene X environment interaction. *Biological Psychiatry* 57(10): 1117–1127.

Di Forti, M., Morgan, C., Dazzan, P., Pariante, C., Mondelli, V., Marques, T. R., Handley, R., Luzi, S., Russo, M., Paparelli, A., et al. (2009). High-potency cannabis and the risk of psychosis. *British Journal of Psychiatry* 195: 488–491.

Morrison, P. D., Zois, V., McKeown, D. A., Lee, T. D., Holt, D. W., Powell, J. F., Kapur, S., & Murray, R. M. (2009). The acute effects of synthetic intravenous Delta9-tetrahydrocannabinol on psychosis, mood and cognitive functioning. *Psychological Medicine* 39: 1607–1616.

Murray, R. M., Morrison, P. D., Henquet, C., & Di, F. M. (2007). Cannabis, the mind and society: The hash realities. *Nature Reviews Neuroscience* 8: 885–895.

Zammit, S., Allebeck, P., Andreasson, S., Lundberg, I., & Lewis, G. (2002). Self reported cannabis use as a risk factor for schizophrenia in Swedish conscripts of 1969: Historical cohort study. *British Medical Journal* 325: 1199.

References

Andreasson, S., Allebeck, P., Engstrom, A., & Rydberg, U. (1987). Cannabis and schizophrenia: A longitudinal study of Swedish conscripts. *Lancet* 2: 1483–1486.

Arnone, D., Barrick, T. R., Chengappa, S., Mackay, C. E., Clark, C. A., & Bou-Saleh, M. T. (2008). Corpus callosum damage in heavy marijuana use: Preliminary evidence from diffusion tensor tractography and tract-based spatial statistics. *Neuroimage* 41: 1067–1074.

Arseneault, L., Cannon, M., Poulton, R., Murray, R., Caspi, A., & Moffitt, T. E. (2002). Cannabis use in adolescence and risk for adult psychosis: Longitudinal prospective study. *British Medical Journal* 325: 1212–1213.

Bhattacharyya, S., Fusar-Poli, P., Borgwardt, S., Martin-Santos, R., Nosarti, C., O'Carroll, C., Allen, P., Seal, M. L., Fletcher, P. C., Crippa, J. A., et al. (2009). Modulation of mediotemporal and ventrostriatal function in humans by Delta9-tetrahydrocannabinol: A neural basis for the effects of *Cannabis sativa* on learning and psychosis. *Archives of General Psychiatry* 66(4): 442–451.

Bossong, M. G., van Berckel, B. N., Boellaard, R., Zuurman, L., Schuit, R. C., Windhorst, A. D., van Gerven, J. M., Ramsey, N. F., Lammertsma, A. A., & Kahn, R. (2009). Delta 9-tetrahydrocannabinol induces dopamine release in the human striatum. *Neuropsychopharmacology* 34: 759–766.

Budney, A. J., Hughes, J. R., Moore, B. A., & Novy, P. L. (2001). Marijuana abstinence effects in marijuana smokers maintained in their home environment. *Archives of General Psychiatry* 58: 917–924.

Budney, A. J., Moore, B. A., Vandrey, R. G., & Hughes, J. R. (2003). The time course and significance of cannabis withdrawal. *Journal of Abnormal Psychology* 112: 393–402.

Caspi, A., Moffitt, T. E., Cannon, M., McClay, J., Murray, R., Harrington, H., Taylor, A., Arseneault, L., Williams, B., Braithwaite, A., et al. (2005). Moderation of the effect of adolescent-onset cannabis use on adult psychosis by a functional polymorphism in the catechol-O-methyltransferase gene: Longitudinal evidence of a gene X environment interaction. *Biological Psychiatry* 57: 1117–1127.

D'Souza, D. C., Abi-Saab, W. M., Madonick, S., Forselius-Bielen, K., Doersch, A., Braley, G., Gueorguieva, R., Cooper, T. B., & Krystal, J. H. (2005). Delta-9-tetrahydrocannabinol effects in schizophrenia: Implications for cognition, psychosis, and addiction. *Biological Psychiatry* 57: 594–608.

D'Souza, D. C., Perry, E., MacDougall, L., Ammerman, Y., Cooper, T., Wu, Y. T. Braley, G., Gueorguieva, R., & Krystal, J. H. (2004). The psychotomimetic effects of intravenous delta-9-tetrahydrocannabinol in healthy individuals: Implications for psychosis. *Neuropsychopharmacology* 29: 1558–1572.

D'Souza, D. C., Ranganathan, M., Braley, G., Gueorguieva, R., Zimolo, Z., Cooper, T., Perry, E., & Krystal, J. (2008). Blunted psychotomimetic and amnestic effects of delta-9-tetrahydrocannabinol in frequent users of cannabis. *Neuropsychopharmacology* 33: 2505–2516.

D'Souza, D. C., Sewell, R. A., & Ranganathan, M. (2009). Cannabis and psychosis/schizophrenia: Human studies. *European Archives of Psychiatry and Clinical Neuroscience* 7: 413–431.

Di Forti, M., Morgan, C., Dazzan, P., Pariante, C., Mondelli, V., Marques, T. R., Handley, R., Luzi, S., Russo, M., Paparelli, A., et al. (2009). High-potency cannabis and the risk of psychosis. *British Journal of Psychiatry* 195: 488–491.

Di Marzo V, Bifulco, M., & De, P. L. (2004). The endocannabinoid system and its therapeutic exploitation. *Nature Reviews Drug Discovery* 3: 771–784.

Eggan, S. M. & Lewis, D. A. (2007). Immunocytochemical distribution of the cannabinoid CB1 receptor in the primate neocortex: A regional and laminar analysis. *Cerebral Cortex* 17(1): 175–191.

Ferdinand, R. F., Sondeijker, F., van der, E. J., Selten, J. P., Huizink, A., & Verhulst, F. C. (2005). Cannabis use predicts future psychotic symptoms, and vice versa. *Addiction* 100: 612–618.

Fergusson, D. M., Horwood, L. J., & Swain-Campbell, N. R. (2003). Cannabis dependence and psychotic symptoms in young people. *Psychological Medicine* 33: 15–21.

Freund, T. F., Katona, I., & Piomelli, D. (2003). Role of endogenous cannabinoids in synaptic signaling. *Physiological Reviews* 83: 1017–1066.

Gonzalez, S., Fernandez-Ruiz, J., Di, M.V., Hernandez, M., Arevalo, C., Nicanor, C. Cascio, M. G., Ambrosio, E., & Ramos, J. A. (2004). Behavioral and molecular changes elicited by acute administration of SR141716 to Delta9-tetrahydrocannabinol-tolerant rats: An experimental model of cannabinoid abstinence. *Drug and Alcohol Dependence* 74: 159–170.

Haney, M., Ward, A. S., Comer, S. D., Foltin, R. W., & Fischman, M. W. (1999a). Abstinence symptoms following oral THC administration to humans. *Psychopharmacology (Berl)* 141: 385–394.

Haney, M., Ward, A. S., Comer, S. D., Foltin, R. W., & Fischman, M. W. (1999b). Abstinence symptoms following smoked marijuana in humans. *Psychopharmacology (Berl)* 141: 395–404.

Hardwick, S. & King, L. (2008). *Cannabis Potency Study 2008*. London: Home Office Scientific Development Branch.

Henquet, C., Krabbendam, L., Spauwen, J., Kaplan, C., Lieb, R., Wittchen, H. U., & van Os, J. (2005a). Prospective cohort study of cannabis use, predisposition for psychosis, and psychotic symptoms in young people. *British Medical Journal* 330: 11.

Henquet, C., Murray, R., Linszen, D., & van Os, J. (2005b). The environment and schizophrenia: The role of cannabis use. *Schizophrenia Bulletin* 31: 608–612.

Henquet, C., Rosa, A., Delespaul, P., Papiol, S., Fananas, L., van Os, J., & Myin-Germeys, I. (2009). COMT ValMet moderation of cannabis-induced psychosis: A momentary assessment study of "switching on" hallucinations in the flow of daily life. *Acta Psychiatrica Scandinavica* 119: 156–160.

Henquet, C., Rosa, A., Krabbendam, L., Papiol, S., Fananas, L., Drukker, M. Ramaekers, J. G., & van Os, J. (2006). An experimental study of catechol-o-methyltransferase Val158Met moderation of delta-9-tetrahydrocannabinol-induced effects on psychosis and cognition. *Neuropsychopharmacology* 31: 2748–2757.

Hill, A. B. (1965). The environment and disease: Association or causation? *Proceedings of the Royal Society of Medicine 58*: 295–300.

Howes, O. D., McDonald, C., Cannon, M., Arseneault, L., Boydell, J., & Murray, R. M. (2004). Pathways to schizophrenia: The impact of environmental factors. *International Journal of Neuropsychopharmacology 7*(Suppl 1): S7–S13.

King, L. A., Carpentier, C., & Griffiths, P. (2004). *An Overview of Cannabis Potency in Europe*. Insights no. 6. Lisbon: European Monitoring Centre for Drugs and Drug Addiction.

Linszen, D. H., Dingemans, P. M., & Lenior, M. E. (1994). Cannabis abuse and the course of recent-onset schizophrenic disorders. *Archives of General Psychiatry 51*: 273–279.

Martin-Santos, R., Fagundo, A. B., Crippa, J. A., Atakan, Z., Bhattacharyya, S., Allen, P., Fusar-Poli, P., Borgwardt, S., Seal, M., Busatto, G. F., et al. (2009). Neuroimaging in cannabis use: A systematic review of the literature. *Psychological Medicine 40*(3): 383–398.

Mata, I., Perez-Iglesias, R., Roiz-Santianez, R., Tordesillas-Gutierrez, D., Pazos, A., Gutierrez, A., Vazquez-Barquero, J. L., & Crespo-Facorro, B. (2009). Gyrification brain abnormalities associated with adolescence and early-adulthood cannabis use. *Brain Research 1317*: 297–304.

Mathers, D. C. & Ghodse, A.H. (1992). Cannabis and psychotic illness. *British Journal of Psychiatry 161*: 648–653.

Moore, T. H., Zammit, S., Lingford-Hughes, A., Barnes, T. R., Jones, P. B., Burke, M., & Lewis, G. (2007). Cannabis use and risk of psychotic or affective mental health outcomes: A systematic review. *Lancet 370*: 319–328.

Morrison, P. D. & Murray, R. M. (2009). From real-world events to psychosis: The emerging neuropharmacology of delusions. *Schizophrenia Bulletin 35*: 668–674.

Morrison, P. D., Zois, V., McKeown, D. A., Lee, T. D., Holt, D. W., Powell, J. F., Kapur, S., & Murray, R.M. (2009). The acute effects of synthetic intravenous Delta9-tetrahydrocannabinol on psychosis, mood and cognitive functioning. *Psychological Medicine 39*: 1607–1616.

Murray, R. M., Morrison, P. D., Henquet, C., & Di, F. M. (2007). Cannabis, the mind and society: The hash realities. *Nature Reviews Neuroscience 8*: 885–895.

Negrete, J. C., Knapp, W. P., Douglas, D. E., & Smith, W. B. (1986). Cannabis affects the severity of schizophrenic symptoms: Results of a clinical survey. *Psychological Medicine 16*: 515–520.

Petty, R. G. (1999). Structural asymmetries of the human brain and their disturbance in schizophrenia. *Schizophrenia Bulletin 25*: 121–139.

Piomelli, D. (2003). The molecular logic of endocannabinoid signalling. *Nature Reviews Neuroscience 4*: 873–884.

Potter, D. J., Clark, P., & Brown, M. B. (2008). Potency of delta 9-THC and other cannabinoids in cannabis in England in 2005: Implications for psychoactivity and pharmacology. *Journal of Forensic Science 53*: 90–94.

Rais, M., Cahn, W., Van, H. N., Schnack, H., Caspers, E., Hulshoff, P. H, & Kahn, R. (2008). Excessive brain volume loss over time in cannabis-using first-episode schizophrenia patients. *American Journal of Psychiatry 165*: 490–496.

Stefanis, N. C., Delespaul, P., Henquet, C., Bakoula, C., Stefanis, C. N., & van Os, J. (2004). Early adolescent cannabis exposure and positive and negative dimensions of psychosis. *Addiction 99*: 1333–1341.

Stokes, P. R. A., Mehta, M. A., Curran, H. V., Breen, G., & Grasby, P. M. (2009). Can recreational doses of THC produce significant dopamine release in the human striatum? *NeuroImage 48*: 186–190.

Thornicroft, G. (1990). Cannabis and psychosis: Is there epidemiological evidence for an association? *British Journal of Psychiatry 157*: 25–33.

Tien, A. Y. & Anthony, J. C. (1990). Epidemiological analysis of alcohol and drug use as risk factors for psychotic experiences. *Journal of Nervous and Mental Disease 178*: 473–480.

United Nations Office on Drugs and Crime. (2009). *UNODC World Drug Report 2009.* New York: United Nations.

van Os, J., Bak, M., Hanssen, M., Bijl, R. V., de Graaf, R., & Verdoux, H. (2002). Cannabis use and psychosis: A longitudinal population-based study. *American Journal of Epidemiology 156*: 319–327.

Weiser, M., Knobler, H. Y., Noy, S., & Kaplan, Z. (2002). Clinical characteristics of adolescents later hospitalized for schizophrenia. *American Journal of Medical Genetics 114*: 949–955.

Wiles, N. J., Zammit, S., Bebbington, P., Singleton, N., Meltzer, H., & Lewis, G. (2006). Self-reported psychotic symptoms in the general population: Results from the longitudinal study of the British National Psychiatric Morbidity Survey. *British Journal of Psychiatry 188*: 519–526.

Yucel, M., Solowij, N., Respondek, C., Whittle, S., Fornito, A., Pantelis, C., & Lubman, D. I. (2008). Regional brain abnormalities associated with long-term heavy cannabis use. *Archives of General Psychiatry 65*: 694–701.

Zammit, S., Allebeck, P., Andreasson, S., Lundberg, I., & Lewis, G. (2002). Self reported cannabis use as a risk factor for schizophrenia in Swedish conscripts of 1969: Historical cohort study. *British Medical Journal 325*: 1199.

Zammit, S., Spurlock, G., Williams, H., Norton, N., Williams, N., O'Donovan, M. C., & Owen, M. J. (2007). Genotype effects of CHRNA7, CNR1 and COMT in schizophrenia: Interactions with tobacco and cannabis use. *British Journal of Psychiatry 191*: 402–407.

SECTION 2
Genetics and Epigenetics

CHAPTER 7

SCHIZOPHRENIA GENETICS
What Have We Learned from Genomewide Association Studies?

ALAN R. SANDERS, JUBAO DUAN, AND PABLO V. GEJMAN

KEY CONCEPTS

- Genomewide experiments are bringing about major conceptual changes in our understanding of the genetics of schizophrenia.
- Uncommon copy number variations (mainly deletions—see chapter 8, this book) and common single nucleotide polymorphism alleles have been reliably demonstrated to be associated with schizophrenia.
- A polygenic model is plausible.
- Partial genetic overlap of schizophrenia with autism and with bipolar disorder is supported.

The first family studies of schizophrenia were conducted in the early twentieth century, but only recently, myriad genomic, bioinformatic, and analytic tools have made possible an incipient understanding of the molecular genetics of schizophrenia. We review here the status of the field and its main developments.

Schizophrenia is typically a chronic and severe psychotic disorder with a median lifetime prevalence of 4.0 per 1,000 and a morbid risk of 7.2 per 1,000 (McGrath et al., 2008). As there are no diagnostic laboratory tests, the diagnosis of schizophrenia relies on clinical observations and on information gathered from informants—relatives and various health care providers. Although ascertainment and assessment methods have been quite variable, the large majority of epidemiologic studies of the clinical phenotype have pointed consistently to the importance of genetic factors in schizophrenia.

From the very beginning, much effort focused on the characterization of schizophrenia as an individual diagnostic entity with a unified pathophysiology. Emil Kraepelin grouped periodic and circular insanity, simple mania, and melancholia under the term *manic-depressive psychoses*, which he thought did not result in deterioration, and defined *dementia praecox* (later called *schizophrenia*) as having a tendency toward poor prognosis (Kraepelin, 1899). However, schizoaffective disorder (Kasanin, 1933), considered intermediate between schizophrenia and bipolar disorder, is a relatively common clinical phenotype characterized by a mixture of psychotic and severe mood symptoms and episodes. The existence of schizoaffective disorder makes it difficult to reconcile the diagnostic categories with a pure dichotomous model, where schizophrenia and bipolar disorder would be at each end, with no clinical entities in between. Family studies show that schizoaffective disorder is present in excess in families ascertained from probands with schizophrenia and in families ascertained from probands with bipolar disorder (Gershon et al., 1982; Gershon et al., 1988; Kendler et al., 1993; Maier et al., 1993; Valles et al., 2000; Maier et al., 2002). However, the clinical separation of schizophrenia and schizoaffective disorder is reliable only after careful clinical training (Spitzer, Endicott, & Robins, 1978; Nurnberger et al., 1994; Suarez et al., 2006; Heckers, 2009). One continuing major complication is that the specific time criterion for affective symptoms relative to the schizophrenic symptoms is arbitrary (and sometimes ambiguous or simply unspecified), varying in different modern classifications. Also, clinical records frequently are insufficiently detailed with regard to temporal overlap of psychotic and affective symptoms. The possibility of shared family history of schizophrenia and other severe non-mood-related mental disorders has been less investigated, but the existing evidence suggests a relationship with autism is plausible (Stahlberg et al., 2004; Larsson et al., 2005; Daniels et al., 2008; Mouridsen et al., 2008; see the section "Pleiotropy and Overlap with Bipolar Disorder, Autism, and Other Disorders" in this chapter).

A Landscape of Extreme Complexity

The complexity of schizophrenia genetics is at this point unsurprising, because despite a century of biological research, our knowledge of the specific molecular mechanisms underlying schizophrenia remains at a very tentative level; some main reasons include the following. First, the absence of well-defined, specific, or focal neuropathology, and specific symptoms, diminishes the number of research approaches, in contrast with the relatively well-characterized brain abnormalities in Parkinson's and Alzheimer's disease that have enabled their respective fields to move faster. Second, the immense number of neuronal interconnections and permutations (approximately 2×10^{10} neocortical neurons and approximately 10^{14} synapses) (Drachman, 2005; Sporns, Tononi, & Kotter, 2005) and extreme redundancy (Morris, Nevet, & Bergman, 2003; Bastian, Chacron, & Maler, 2004; Chechik et al., 2006) make the brain disproportionately more complicated than any other human organ; consequently, our knowledge of the physiologic basis of higher brain functions (and of schizophrenia) is still very incomplete.

Schizophrenia is conceptualized as a complex disorder. Genomewide association studies (GWAS) (see the section on them later in this chapter) show that many genes are involved in complex disorders, with each gene conferring only a small effect on the phenotype (a polygenic model being the logical extreme). Individual genetic variants do not predict risk well. It has also been proposed that complex disorders are "system disorders" that result from dysfunction of entire molecular networks (as opposed to arising from abnormal function of individual genes); this is being tested (Schadt, 2009). Epistasis (i.e., nonadditive interactions between these genes or their protein products) and interactions between genes and environmental risk factors are also assumed. However, the study of genetic interactions remains largely unexplored because of the need to correct for a large number of statistical comparisons, although approaches continue to develop (Cornelis et al., 2010). GWAS data suggest a frequency spectrum with many common and rare mutations (Purcell et al., 2009; Shi et al., 2009; Stefansson et al., 2009).

Twin studies show incomplete concordance for schizophrenia in monozygotic twins, making conceivable an epigenetic mechanism whereby changes in phenotype not explained by DNA sequence may contribute to the transmission of schizophrenia (see chapter 9, this book). Few studies have tested this hypothesis, however, because of methodologic difficulties (Roth et al., 2009).

Evidence for Environmental Factors

As reviewed elsewhere in this book, multiple environmental risk factors increase risk for schizophrenia—namely, various obstetric complications (Cannon, Jones, & Murray, 2002; Byrne et al., 2007; Mittal, Ellman, & Cannon, 2008) (see chapter 3, this book), urban birth or residence, famines and micronutrient deficiencies (Susser & Lin, 1992; St Clair et al., 2005; Brown et al., 2007) (see chapter 2, this book), migrant status, seasonal effects (possibly by way of prenatal infections, including influenza) (McGrath et al., 2008; Brown & Derkits, 2010) (see chapters 1 and 10, this book), advanced paternal age (Malaspina et al., 2001; Torrey et al., 2009) (see chapter 5, this book), and maternal stress (see chapter 4, this book).

Evidence for Genetic Factors

Three epidemiologic sources have underscored the importance of genetic factors in schizophrenia and to the apportioning of environmental and genetic risks: family studies, twin studies, and adoption studies.

Family Studies

Family studies have consistently shown that the child of a parent with schizophrenia has a risk about tenfold over the general population and that the risk for schizophrenia to a relative decays much more rapidly than the proportion of shared genes, which is inconsistent with a simple Mendelian model. It is interesting that most cases of schizophrenia in the general population are sporadic (Kendler, 1987; Yang, Visscher, & Wray, 2009). Although surprising at first glance for such a familial disorder, assuming polygenic inheritance, many more sporadic (approximately 80–90%) than familial cases are expected via simulations (Yang, Visscher, & Wray, 2009) that match well with family study data (Lichtenstein et al., 2006; Lichtenstein et al., 2009).

Twin Studies

Differences between monozygotic (identical) twins are attributed to the environment, and differences between dizygotic (fraternal) twins are attributed to both hereditary and environmental factors. Contrasting findings for each twin type enables estimations of the proportion of variance explained by genetic factors, or heritability. The concordance (diagnostic agreement) rates of schizophrenia for monozygotic twins have been found to be about 40–50% both in older and in more recent population or hospital registry-based studies (Klaning, Mortensen, & Kyvik, 1996; Cannon et al., 1998; Franzek & Beckmann, 1998; Cardno et al., 1999), and heritability estimates are around 80% (Cardno & Gottesman, 2000; Sullivan, Kendler, & Neale, 2003). Notably, the risk of schizophrenia and schizophrenia-related disorders seems similar for the offspring of both the unaffected and the affected monozygotic twins (Gottesman & Bertelsen, 1989; Kringlen & Cramer, 1989), which suggests that the unaffected twins do carry a heritable genetic risk for schizophrenia without expressing the disease, supporting either or both epigenetic factors and nonshared environments (although the data are from only about 20 reproducing monozygotic twin pairs from each study). It has recently been proposed that DNA methylation differences might be the cause of monozygotic twin discordance (Mill et al., 2008).

Adoption Studies

Adoption studies allow further dissection of genetics, from environmental contributions to a disorder. Key findings from many studies (see the review by Ingraham & Kety, 2000) include the following: (1) the risk for schizophrenia is conferred by (i.e., travels with) the biological relationship, not the adoptive relationship; (2) the risk is conferred regardless of when a schizophrenic parent experiences the onset of illness; and (3) risk is conferred independently of rearing environment (foster parents or institutional).

Darwinian Paradox

Schizophrenia is associated with decreased fertility, particularly in males (Rüdin, 1916; Kallmann, 1938; Haukka, Suvisaari, & Lonnqvist, 2003; Svensson et al., 2007). Although natural selection should decrease the population frequencies of genes that diminish fertility, the prevalence of schizophrenia, which is highly heritable, has not markedly diminished in the global population. Multiple hypotheses have been proposed for the "Darwinian paradox" of how schizophrenia seemingly circumvents the effect of natural selection (see the review by Keller & Miller, 2006). Earlier evidence for balancing selection—that relatives of schizophrenia patients might have a compensatory increase in fertility (Fananas & Bertranpetit, 1995)— did not replicate in larger samples (Haukka, Suvisaari, & Lonnqvist, 2003; Svensson et al., 2007; MacCabe et al., 2009). Potential explanations for balancing selection include (1) heterozygote advantage, in which either homozygote shows reduced fitness compared to the heterozygote (such as in sickle cell anemia [Allison, 1954], where heterozygotes have less susceptibility to malaria than do major allele homozygotes, and less burden of sickle cell anemia than do minor allele homozygotes); and (2) antagonist pleiotropy, where an allele might reduce fitness for one trait while increasing fitness for a related trait. Both of these explanations are weakened by the lack of evidence for increased fertility in relatives of schizophrenia patients (Keller & Miller, 2006).

The clinical schizophrenia phenotype might also have poor correlation with its underlying genetic susceptibility (i.e., genotype). It has been suggested that endophenotypic variables (sometimes called *intermediate phenotypes*) such as structural and functional neuroimaging characteristics may constitute a better index of the underlying gene effects than does the clinical phenotype (Gottesman & Gould, 2003). However, a large body of genetic epidemiology is based on the clinical phenotype, and none of the proposed endophenotypes has been proved yet to be more heritable than the aggregate clinical phenotype (Greenwood et al., 2007; see also the recent review for other limitations of the endophenotype approach by Kendler & Neale, 2010).

A high mutation rate might maintain schizophrenia susceptibility alleles in the population even against negative selection (Book, 1953), although, as noted (Malaspina et al., 2001), this idea was largely abandoned because it was thought that such mutation rates would be unsustainably high (Huxley et al., 1964). However, more recently it was shown that humans (and other hominids) have substantial new deleterious mutation rates (e.g., 1.6 such mutations per diploid genome per generation [Eyre-Walker & Keightley, 1999], renewing interest in the area [Malaspina et al., 2001]). One should keep in mind, though, that the more mildly deleterious a mutation is the longer it will persist before elimination from the gene pool, so much of the mutational burden is not from new mutations (Keller & Miller, 2006). Nevertheless, as reviewed in chapter 5, advanced paternal age could be a putative risk factor as spermatogonia replicate many more times over life than oocytes and the age of fathers is greater than expected for some autosomal dominant diseases that are due to new mutations (Friedman, 1981). In a study on the Jerusalem Perinatal Cohort, an epidemiologic sample, the relative risk of schizophrenia increased continuously with the age of the fathers (adjusting for maternal age) to a maximum of 2.96 in offspring of fathers age 50 and 54 years, but there were no maternal age effects after adjusting for paternal age (Malaspina et al., 2001) (see chapter 5, this book). This finding has been replicated in larger samples from different populations, especially for older fathers (see the review by Torrey et al., 2009), and the effect was found to be stronger in sporadic (family history negative) cases (Sipos et al., 2004), as would be predicted for de novo mutations. As reviewed (Keller & Miller, 2006), paternal age effects are expected under a mutation-selection model (Crow, 2000). This is due to mutations accumulating much more rapidly in male than in female gametes because of the much greater number of cell divisions, leaving most other schizophrenia cases resulting from milder, older, and more numerous mutations (Keller & Miller, 2006). Polygenic mutation-selection balance (with many new rare alleles at many loci, which in the aggregate form a large pool) can preserve genetic variation in spite of stabilizing selection, and it is consistent with the prevalence and reproductive fitness costs of schizophrenia (Keller & Miller, 2006), as well as with recent GWAS findings (see the section "Genomewide Association Studies" in this chapter).

Linkage

During meiotic recombination, or crossing over between homologous chromosomes, adjacent loci are unlikely to be separated and are thus likely to be inherited together. The hypothesis that one or a few common major gene effects can explain schizophrenia in the general population was tested in genomewide linkage scans, but results mostly fell short of genomewide significance. However, similar (or overlapping) regions on chromosome 8p have been implicated (suggestive, i.e., expected to occur about once per genome scan just by chance) in previous linkage studies (e.g., Blouin et al., 1998; Stefansson et al., 2002; Suarez et al., 2006), in meta-analyses (Badner & Gershon, 2002; Lewis et al., 2003), and in a combined genomewide linkage scan, which consists of multiple clinical samples jointly genotyped rather than only a joint statistical analysis (Holmans et al., 2009). For example, the maximum evidence for linkage (multipoint Z_{lr} of 3.25) in a sample of schizophrenia-affected sibling pairs from 409 pedigrees was in this chromosome 8p region (1-LOD 18.4-32.1 Mb) (Suarez et al., 2006). Note that there is overlap between some of the above samples—for example, with regard to earlier versus later meta-analyses and individual linkage studies included in the meta-analyses. The clearest and most inclusive study, in our view, is the most recent genomewide linkage study meta-analysis of 22 European ancestry (EA) samples (1,813 pedigrees, 4,094 genotyped cases, including samples from most of the other studies). In this study, the strongest linkage region, which was genomewide-significant, resided on chromosome 8p (15.7–32.7 Mb) (Ng et al., 2009), a region of continuing interest in schizophrenia genetics, given that it contains NRG1 (Stefansson et al., 2002) and PPP3CC (Gerber et al., 2003).

First Modern Association Studies

Association studies are based on linkage disequilibrium (LD), a nonrandom statistical association of alleles at two or more loci, characteristically correlated with short physical distance between genetic markers. The effect size can be conceptualized as the strength of the association between a marker and the disorder, and it can be expressed as the odds ratio (OR), which is the odds for an event (in this instance, the odds for possession of a risk allele) in cases, divided by the odds in controls. Before the availability of GWAS, most gene association studies consisted of tests of candidate gene involvement. Close to 800 genes have been tested for association (see www.schizophreniaforum.org/res/sczgene; Allen et al., 2008), making schizophrenia one of the most studied disorders through a candidate gene approach. Unfortunately, none of these candidate genes can be considered established. Given that samples in previous candidate gene association studies frequently lacked sufficient statistical power, the problem of nonreplication has been far from trivial. In a comprehensive study of some of the most cited candidate genes (e.g., DISC1, DTNBP1, NRG1, DRD2, HTR2A, and COMT), 14 genes were each tested by genotyping an EA sample of 1,870 cases and 2,002 screened controls (Sanders et al., 2008). A total of 789 single nucleotide polymorphisms (SNPs), including tags for common variation in each gene (tag SNPs are SNPs that are correlated with many other nearby SNPs, for which they are proxies), SNPs previously reported as associated, and SNPs located in functional domains of genes were genotyped, but no association was found (figure 7.1). These findings contradict the relatively large ORs that would be predicted from association observed in small samples.

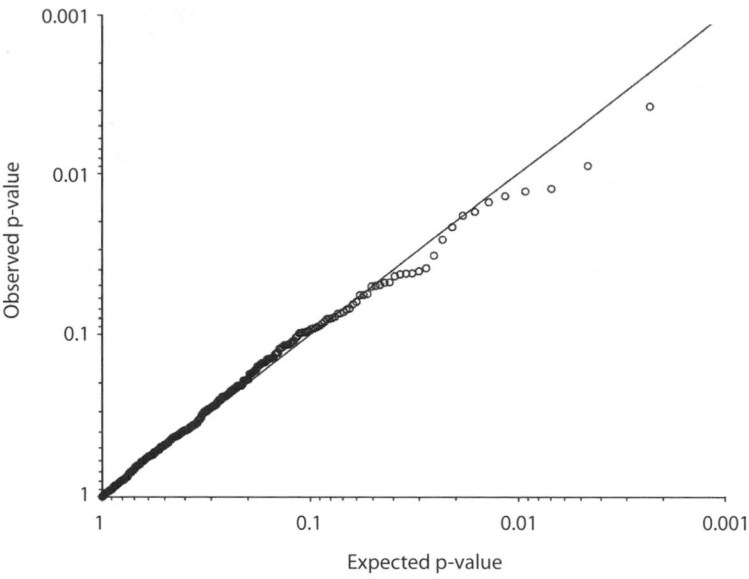

Figure 7.1. Quantile-quantile plot of observed vs. expected *p*-values for tag SNPs for 14 schizophrenia candidate genes.
Open circles represent the relationship between the expected (*x*-axis) and observed (*y*-axis) *p*-values for pointwise nominal Armitage trend tests for the 433 SNPs that represent tags (at $r^2 > 0.8$) for common SNPs in each of 14 tested genes (*RGS4, DISC1, DTNBP1, STX7, TAAR6, PPP3CC, NRG1, DRD2, HTR2A, DAOA, AKT1, CHRNA7, COMT,* and *ARVCF*). The solid line represents the null expectation. The observed distribution is within the 95% confidence interval of the null expectation, consistent with a lack of evidence in the tested sample for association with schizophrenia in the tested candidate genes. The lowest *p*-values are slightly below the line (less significant than expected), but still within the confidence interval. (Reprinted from Sanders et al. [2008] with permission from the American Journal of Psychiatry [Copyright 2008]. American Psychiatric Association.)

There are an abundance of positive and negative associations between candidate genes and schizophrenia. It is likely that the use of small sample sizes and inadequate or loose statistical thresholds accounts for many of the unreplicated observations. Other potential causes of false positive findings are multiple analyses and selective reporting (Ioannidis, 2008). It is possible that genetic heterogeneity in some specific cases would preclude a replication, but it would seem unlikely that this would be a robust general argument. (For a detailed discussion of heterogeneity, see McCarthy et al., 2008). Multiplicative epistasis (where the individual gene effects might not be detectable but the product of the individual effects might become detectable) is another largely unexplored possibility that could in principle explain nonreplication. Another source of heterogeneity is environmental variation. Furthermore, very provocative work (Richter, Garner, & Wurbel, 2009) suggests that increased standardization—such as in experiments designed to decrease

Table 7.1 Top Genes or Genomic Regions Identified in Recent Schizophrenia GWAS

First Author and Year	Sample (Case/Control)	Gene or Region	Lowest p-Values	OR	Reference
Lencz, 2007	178/144 (EA)	CSF2RA, SHOX	3.7×10^{-7}	3.23	Lencz et al., 2007
Sullivan, 2008	738/733 (EA)	AGBL1	1.71×10^{-6}	6.01	Sullivan et al., 2008
O'Donovan, 2008	Discovery: 479/2,937 (EA) Follow-up: 6,829/9,897 (EA)	ZNF804A	1.61×10^{-7}	1.12	O'Donovan et al., 2008
Need, 2009	Discovery: 871/863 (EA) Follow-up: 1,460/12,995 (EA)	ADAMTSL3	1.35×10^{-7}	0.68	Need et al., 2009
Purcell, 2009 (ISC)	3,322/3,587 (EA)	MHC region[a]	9.5×10^{-9}	0.82	Purcell et al., 2009
		MYO18B	3.4×10^{-7}		
Stefansson, 2009 (SGENE)	Discovery: 2,663/13,498 (EA)	MHC region[b]	1.4×10^{-12}	1.16[c]	Stefansson et al., 2009
	Follow-up: 4,999/15,555 (EA)	NRGN[b] TCF4[b]	2.4×10^{-9} 4.1×10^{-9}	1.15 1.23	
Shi, 2009 (MGS)	2,681/2,653 (EA) 1,286/973 (AA)	MHC region[a] CENTG2 (in EA only) ERBB4 (in AA only)	9.5×10^{-9} 4.59×10^{-7} 2.14×10^{-6}	0.88 1.23 0.73	Shi et al., 2009

[a] Combined analysis of ISC, SGENE-plus (GWAS set), and MGS.
[b] Combined analysis of ISC and MGS, along with SGENE-plus and follow-up samples.
[c] or (odds ratio) is for common allele of the associated SNP, which is different from that in ISC and MGS.
SOURCE: Reprinted from Gejman, Sanders, & Duan (2010) with permission from *Psychiatric Clinics of North America* (copyright Elsevier).

heterogeneity—that allows and frequently requires smaller sample sizes can actually decrease reproducibility in animal behavioral experiments. This finding challenges long held ideas and might be important for the design of association studies. In the aggregate, recent schizophrenia GWAS results (in which each candidate gene is covered with more SNPs than in most candidate gene experiments) have not supported most associations to classical candidate genes (table 7.1; see supplementary data file 3 from Hindorff et al., 2009; Shi et al., 2009; this is a pattern consistent with the general results of GWAS in complex disorders, www.genome.gov/gwastudies). Most associations discovered from GWAS for complex disorders have been either in genes that were not previously suspected to be involved in the disease, or in regions of the genome with no obvious genes. Additional research and the analysis of cumulative data, with particular attention to both quality control and statistical rigor, will be required for definitive conclusions.

Genomewide Association Studies

Genomewide studies, in combination with other fields in systems biology, yield comprehensive information and have been demonstrated to be more useful in dealing with complex phenotypes. Systems biology is a biology-based interdisciplinary approach focusing on complex interactions in biological systems—i.e., the "-omics" strategies. The main assumption under GWAS is the common disease/common variant hypothesis (Pritchard, 2001; Reich & Lander, 2001). Thus, GWAS interrogate common SNPs across the human genome, investigating all genes and the majority of the nongenic regions, whether they were previously implicated by pathophysiologic hypotheses or not. The Human Genome Project (see www.ornl .gov/sci/techresources/Human_Genome/home.shtml), to a large extent, made GWAS possible. Major improvements in SNP genotyping and DNA sequencing were spin-offs from the Human Genome Project, and microarrays made possible rapid and accurate genomewide genotyping that resulted in a map of common genetic variation in a reference set of individuals of European, Asian, and African descent (the HapMap project). The majority of the markers used for GWAS are tag SNPs; thus the most significant associated SNP in a GWAS may reflect an indirect association (i.e., be in LD with a causative variant). The Affymetrix 6.0 and Illumina 1M SNP arrays include approximately 1 million common SNPs and probes for analysis of copy number variants (CNVs), with their SNPs assaying about 80% of the common variation in the genome for EA samples (Li, Li, & Guan, 2008). However, the estimated number of common (minor allele frequency, MAF > 1%) SNPs is approximately 10 million, but our genotyping capabilities are not sufficiently developed yet to genotype every SNP in a very large clinical sample, although deep resequencing technology and new arrays may soon overcome this difficulty. In the meantime, imputation—the computational prediction of genotypes from nongenotyped SNPs—is used to extend GWAS map coverage (Halperin & Stephan, 2009; Nothnagel et al., 2009).

The large number of SNPs makes GWAS highly susceptible to false positives; therefore, the estimation of an appropriate genomewide significance threshold is fundamental. The genomewide significance threshold, for a value of 5% significance assuming tests for all common SNPs, has been estimated to be around $p < 5 \times 10^{-8}$ (Dudbridge & Gusnanto, 2008; Hoggart et al., 2008; Pe'er et al., 2008). GWAS have been more successful than any previous approach to find new susceptibility loci for complex disorders. According to www.genome.gov/gwastudies (as of September 20, 2009), 732 genes were reported to be associated to one or more complex disease phenotypes at genomewide significant levels $(p < 5 \times 10^{-8})$ (Hindorff et al., 2009; Manolio et al., 2009), and many of these associations have already been replicated. (Small individual ORs do not permit prediction of "caseness" from specific individual susceptibility loci.)

Recent GWAS of complex disorders show two main characteristics. First, common loci with small effects are typically reported (ORs = 1.1–1.5); these are an empirical confirmation that a large body of epidemiologic studies predicting multiple small common genetic effects for complex disorders was correct, including for schizophrenia (Gottesman & Shields, 1967; Risch, 1990), because loci with larger effects are eliminated rapidly from the population through selection. Second, most studies have tended to detect new susceptibility loci, and only very large samples obtained from combining studies are powered to show robust replication. This is because the power to detect one out of many possible risk loci is much larger than the power to detect specific disorder alleles (Kraft & Hunter, 2009). Furthermore, if only small effects are found, many genes would be predicted to underlie the pathophysiology of most complex genetic disorders. On the other hand, it is important to also emphasize some main GWAS limitations. The statistical power of GWAS to detect an association with rare alleles (MAF < 1%) is very limited. Resequencing is more useful than GWAS in the study of rare variants. The study of gene-gene interactions (epistasis), although widely expected to be a significant source of heritability, is strictly limited by the statistical power of currently existing samples due to the large number of such tests.

GWAS have already yielded genomewide significant results for schizophrenia, which we will now discuss in more detail. Seven GWAS for schizophrenia have been published (table 7.1). The sizes of the investigated discovery samples have ranged from 322 to more than 16,161, but even the largest studies did not yield a genomewide significant result before combined testing of independent samples. This was not unexpected. A typical susceptibility locus has an OR of 1.1–1.3, which often necessitates extremely large samples for detection. A sample with a total N of 5,334, such as the Molecular Genetics of Schizophrenia (MGS) EA sample (most investigated samples have been smaller), has adequate statistical power only to detect very common risk alleles (30–60% frequency, log additive effects) with genotypic relative risks of about 1.3 (Shi et al., 2009). To reach sufficient statistical power, the combined analysis of independent data sets is useful. Although the diagnostic spectrum of the final combined sample is naturally wider than for the component data sets, combining data sets has been remarkably successful for a variety of complex disorders including schizophrenia (Purcell et al., 2009; Shi et al., 2009; Stefansson et al., 2009) (see the section immediately following in this chapter). Different samples often were typed with different platforms, but imputation largely overcomes the limitation of many nonoverlapping SNPs. These results suggest that schizophrenia, despite its very high reported heritability, is among the most complex of human genetic disorders. An additional analysis of the International Schizophrenia Consortium (ISC) and MGS samples (Purcell et al., 2009) supported a polygenic model for schizophrenia susceptibility, involving a set of hundreds of genes, each with unquantified but very small individual effects (Gottesman & Shields, 1967). (See the section

"Polygenic Contributions to Schizophrenia" in this chapter.) Finally, rapidly mounting evidence shows that cases have more rare (< 1%) and large (> 100 kb) CNVs than do controls (chapter 8, this book).

Meta-analysis of Genomewide Association Studies Data and the Major Histocompatibility Complex Locus

The initial attempts to map schizophrenia to the major histocompatibility complex (MHC) started in the 1970s (Worden et al., 1976), only a few years after the discovery of the human leukocyte antigen (HLA) system (Bach, Bach, & Poo, 1969). Many attempts have been made since then, and some yielded suggestive evidence (Wei & Hemmings, 2000), but compelling evidence of MHC involvement was only recently obtained from a combined analysis of GWAS data. Three GWAS studies published jointly in 2009 (ISC, MGS, and the Schizophrenia Genetics Consortium, or SGENE), reaching a total EA sample of 8,008 cases and 19,077 controls, performed a meta-analysis of schizophrenia GWAS for the first time (Purcell et al., 2009; Shi et al., 2009; Stefansson et al., 2009). The meta-analysis combined the p-values for all imputed and genotyped SNPs from the most significant regions of each study. This analysis generated a genomewide significant association at the MHC region on chromosome 6.

The MHC signal extends over much of the MHC region, from approximately 26 Mb to approximately 33 Mb (figure 7.2). The strongest evidence (rs13194053, $p = 9.54 \times 10^{-9}$) for association from the meta-analysis was near a cluster of histone genes and several immune-related genes, including *butyrophilin subfamily 3 member A2* and *A1* (*BTN3A2* and *BTN3A1*) and *protease serine 16* (*PRSS16*), but each individual data set has a different location for its strongest association. The MHC region has a very high gene density and long-range LD blocks (Traherne, 2008)—the human genome is structured in many "blocklike" islands of LD generated by a great variation of recombination rates. Blocks from regions of low recombination are long and interspersed with interblock regions of higher recombination (Daly et al., 2001; Gabriel et al., 2002). The location of the causative variation remains indeterminate, but it could be in one or more genes or a nongenic region within the MHC. In the MGS sample, about 50% of the 1,000 highest-ranking GWAS SNPs were intergenic, located outside the 10 kb region on either side of a gene, although many of these may represent a genic region signal because of LD. Even at the MHC locus, rs13194053—the SNP with the most significant association from the meta-analysis—is roughly 29 kb away from its closest gene, *HIST1H2AH* (*histone cluster 1, H2ah*) (Purcell et al., 2009; Shi et al., 2009; Stefansson et al., 2009). A functional role for many intergenic regions would not be surprising, as they might contain highly conserved sequences, which are believed to have a regulatory function (Kleinjan & van Heyningen, 2005). The associated vari-

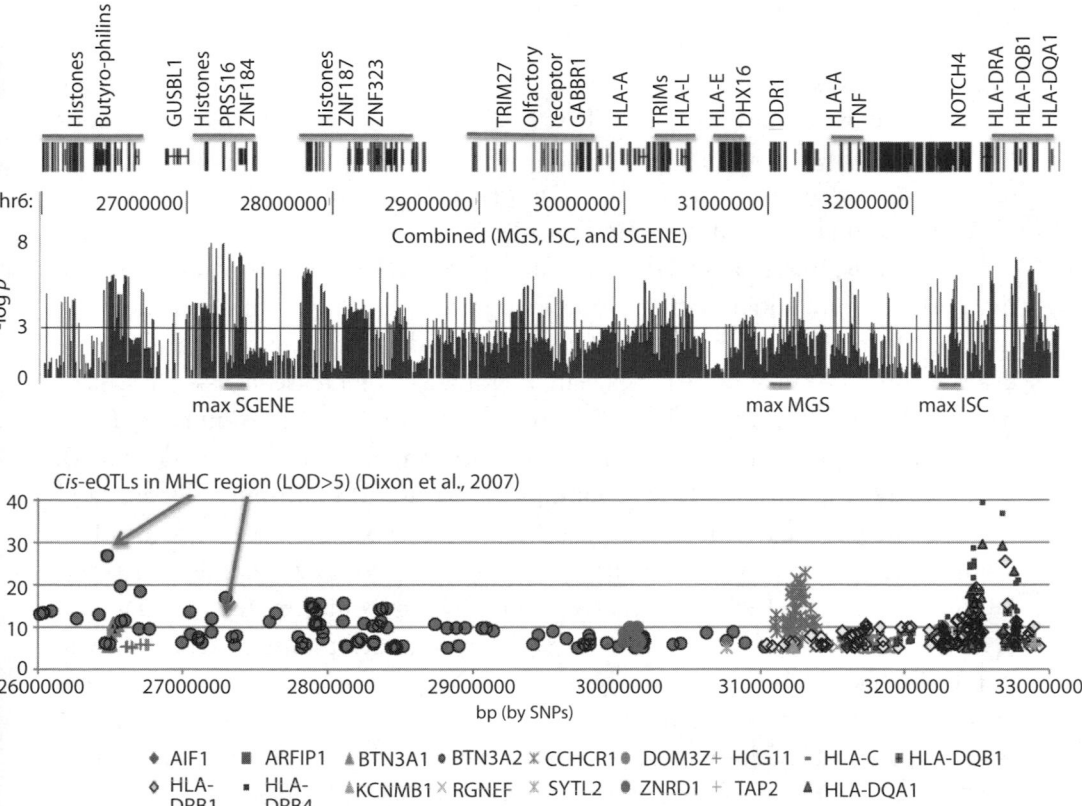

Figure 7.2. Combined *p*-values of three data sets (MGS, ISC, and SGENE) at the MHC region (approx. 26–33 Mb).
The positions of the three histone gene clusters and *NOTCH4* are indicated in the RefSeq track (top of the graph). The relative location of the maximum peak in each data set is indicated by a line below the *p*-value peaks. *Cis*-eQTLs (with LOD > 5; Dixon et al., 2007), calculated on the basis of the average of expression probes for each gene, are shown below the graph with association -log *p*-values. LOD = logarithm of the odds. (Reprinted from Gejman, Sanders, & Duan [2010] with permission from *Psychiatric Clinics of North America* [copyright Elsevier].)

ants, or variants in LD with them, in intergenic regions may then alter expression of upstream or downstream genes. Moreover, most of the human genome is transcribed, with some transcripts serving as regulatory RNAs, but the function of most human transcripts is still undefined (Birney et al., 2007).

The genes in the MHC region have many different biological functions, but genes with an immune function predominate. Histones regulate DNA transcription by chromatin modification through histone methylation or acetylation (Costa et al., 2007; Shi, 2007; Adegbola et al., 2008) (see chapter 9, this book), and have a role as antimicrobial agents by disrupting the bacterial cell membrane and interfering with microbial gene expression (Kawasaki & Iwamuro, 2008). In human placenta, histones (H2A and H2B) neutralize bacterial endotoxins (Kim et al., 2002). This raises the possibility that genetic variation in histones underlies variation in placental susceptibility to infections, and thus genetic variation may increase the susceptibility to schizophrenia. These findings are also consistent with previous studies indicating associations between in utero exposure to infection and risk of schizophrenia (see chapter 1, this book, as well as Brown & Derkits, 2010).

A Danish registry study reported an increased risk of autoimmune disorders (thyrotoxicosis, intestinal malabsorption, acquired hemolytic anemia, chronic active hepatitis, interstitial cystitis, alopecia areata, myositis, polymyalgia rheumatica, and Sjögren's syndrome) for schizophrenia, and a history of any autoimmune disorder (of 29 evaluated) was associated with a 45% increase in risk for schizophrenia (Eaton et al., 2006). The MHC region has been implicated in many genetic disorders with immune-related abnormalities (Shiina, Inoko, & Kulski, 2004), including type 1 diabetes (T1D), multiple sclerosis (MS), Crohn's disease, and rheumatoid arthritis, among many others (see www.genome.gov/gwastudies; Hindorff et al., 2009). It is noteworthy that rs3800307 (found on the DRB1*03-DQA1*0501-DQB1*0201 haplotype)—an SNP in complete LD ($r^2 = 1$) with rs13194053 that reached genomewide significant association with schizophrenia in the combined GWAS meta-analysis (Purcell et al., 2009; Shi et al., 2009; Stefansson et al., 2009)—is associated with T1D (Viken et al., 2009). In addition, rs3131296 at *NOTCH4* is in strong LD ($r^2 > 0.73$) with the classical HLA allele DRB1*03 and other SNPs that are associated with several autoimmune disorders (T1D, celiac disease, systemic lupus erythematosus, and so forth), albeit with opposite alleles (Stefansson et al., 2009). Finally, the MGS GWAS showed some evidence, with $p = 3.5 \times 10^{-5}$ in the EA data set and $p = 1.9 \times 10^{-6}$ in the EA plus African American (AA) data set, for association with schizophrenia at the chromosome 1p22.1 *FAM69A-EVI-RPL5* gene cluster (Shi et al., 2009), which has been implicated in MS (Oksenberg et al., 2008).

Other genes in the same region are involved in chromatin structure (*high mobility group nucleosomal binding domain 4, HMGN4*); transcriptional regulation (*activator of basal transcription 1, ABT1; zinc finger protein 322A, ZNF322A; zinc finger protein 184, ZNF184*); G-protein-coupled receptor signaling (*FKSG83*); and the nuclear pore complex (*nuclear pore membrane protein 121-like 2, POM121L2*). The SGENE-plus (their GWAS set) and follow-up samples (i.e., an extended SGENE data set that added a follow-up EA sample of 4,999 cases and 15,555 controls) analysis reported an independent association (i.e., in weak LD with rs13194053 at the histone gene cluster) at *NOTCH4* (*Notch homolog 4 [Drosophila]*, rs3131296, $p = 2 \times 10^{-8}$), located at 32.28 Mb on chromosome 6, and the combined meta-analysis of SGENE-plus and follow-up samples, along with MGS and ISC samples, gave a $p = 2.3 \times 10^{-10}$ there (Stefansson et al., 2009). For a list of genes mentioned in the text and their functions, see table 7.2.

Table 7.2 Genes Mentioned in Review, and Their Functions

Gene Symbol	Gene Description	Chromosome	Function
ABT1	*Activator of basal transcription 1*	6	Transcriptional regulation
APOE	*Apolipoprotein E*	19	A main apoprotein of the chylomicron; E4 allele is an established risk factor for Alzheimer's disease
AKT1	*V-akt murine thymoma viral oncogene Homolog 1*	14	Critical mediator of growth factor-induced neuronal survival
ARVCF	*Armadillo repeat gene deletes in VCFS*	22	Catenin family member (adherens junction complex formation)
BTN3A1	*Butyrophilin subfamily 3 member A1*	6	Immunoglobulin superfamily
BTN3A2	*Butyrophilin subfamily 3 member A2*	6	Immunoglobulin superfamily
CACNA1C	*Calcium channel, voltage-dependent, L type, Alpha 1C subunit*	12	Regulates muscle contraction, hormone or neurotransmitter release, cell cycle
CENTG2	*Centaurin gamma 2*	2	Protein trafficking in the endosomal-lysosomal system
CHRNA7	*Cholinergic receptor, nicotinic, alpha 7*	15	Ligand-gated ion channel mediating synaptic transmission
CNTNAP2	*Contactin associated protein-like 2*	7	A member of the neurexin family that functions in the vertebrate nervous system as cell adhesion molecules and receptors
COMT	*Catechol-O-methyltransferase*	22	Catecholamine neurotransmitter metabolism; VCFS region (22q deletion syndrome)
DAOA	*D-amino acid oxidase activator*	13	Activator of the enzyme DAAO, which degrades D-serine
DISC1	*Disrupted in schizophrenia 1*	1	Neurite outgrowth and cortical development; disrupted in t(1;11)(q42.1;q14.3)
DRD2	*Dopamine receptor D2*	11	G-protein coupled receptor for dopamine; inhibits adenylyl cyclase
DTNBP1	*Dystrobrevin binding protein 1*	6	Component of the biogenesis of lysosome-related organelles complex 1
ERBB4	*V-erb-a erythroblastic leukemia viral Oncogene*	2	Receptors for neuregulins; cell differentiation
EVI	*Ecotropic viral integration site 5*	1	Cell cycle progression
FAM69A	*Family with sequence similarity 69, member A*	1	Unknown; implicated in MS (multiple sclerosis)
FKSG83	*Hypothetical protein*	6	G-protein-coupled receptor signaling
FMR1	*Fragile X mental retardation 1*	23	may be involved in nucleus→cytoplasm mRNA trafficking
FXR1	*Fragile X mental retardation, autosomal Homolog 1*	3	RNA-binding protein; embryonic and postnatal development of muscle tissue
HIST1H2AH	*Histone cluster 1, H2ah*	6	Chromatin modification, transcription regulation, host defense

(continued)

Table 7.2 (continued)

Gene Symbol	Gene Description	Chromosome	Function
HTR2A	5-hydroxytryptamine (serotonin) receptor 2A	13	G-protein coupled receptor for serotonin; activates phosphoinositide hydrolysis
HMGN4	High mobility group nucleosomal binding Domain 4	6	Involved in chromatin structure
MYO18B	Myosin XVIIIB	22	Regulate muscle-specific genes; intracellular trafficking
NOTCH4	Notch homolog 4 (Drosophila)	6	Receptor for Jagged1, Jagged2, and Delta1; cell-fate determination
NRG1	Neuregulin 1	8	Signaling protein that mediates cell-cell interactions; roles in growth and development
NRGN	Neurogranin	11	Postsynaptic protein kinase substrate; learning and memory; glutamate signaling
POM121L2	Nuclear pore membrane protein 121-like 2	6	Nuclear pore complex
PPP3CC	Protein phosphatase 3 (formerly 2B), catalytic Subunit, gamma isoform	8	Ca^{++}-dependent modifier of phosphorylation status
PRSS16	Protease serine 16	6	Alternative antigen presenting
RGS4	Regulator of G-protein signaling 4	1	GTPase activating protein for G alpha subunits of G proteins
RPL5	Ribosomal protein L5	1	rRNA maturation and formation of the 60S ribosomal subunits
STX7	Syntaxin 7	6	Endosomal soluble N-ethylmaleimide-sensitive factor attachment protein receptors (SNARE)
TAAR6	Trace amine associated receptor 6	6	Trace amines are endogenous amine compounds, chemically similar to classic biogenic amines like dopamine
TCF4	Transcription factor 4	18	Neuronal transcriptional factor; neurogenesis
ZNF184	Zinc finger protein 18	6	Transcriptional regulation
ZNF322A	Zinc finger protein 322A	6	Transcriptional regulation
ZNF804A	Zinc finger protein 804A	2	Transcription factor; neuronal connectivity in the dorsolateral prefrontal cortex

NOTES: Genes are listed alphabetically by symbol. All chromosome 6 genes are in the MHC except *DTNBP1*.
SOURCE: Reprinted from Gejman, Sanders, & Duan (2010) with permission from *Psychiatric Clinics of North America* (copyright Elsevier).

Non-Major Histocompatibility Complex Loci that Have Also Achieved Genomewide Significance

The combined analysis of SGENE-plus GWAS samples and replication samples uncovered associations with *neurogranin* (*NRGN*) and with *transcription factor 4* (*TCF4*) that subsequently reached genomewide significance in the combined analysis of SGENE-plus and replication samples along with ISC and MGS samples (table 7.1) (see Stefansson et al., 2009). *NRGN* encodes a postsynaptic protein kinase substrate that binds calmodulin, mediating N-methyl-d-aspartate (NMDA) receptor signaling that is important for learning and memory and also relevant to the proposed glutamate pathophysiology of schizophrenia (Harrison & Weinberger, 2005; Wang et al., 2008). *TCF4* is a neuronal transcriptional factor essential for brain development, specifically neurogenesis (Gulacsi & Anderson, 2008). Mutations in *TCF4* cause Pitt–Hopkins syndrome, a neurodevelopmental disorder characterized by severe motor and mental retardation, including absence of language development, microcephaly, epilepsy, and facial dysmorphisms (Brockschmidt et al., 2007; Flora et al., 2007; Kalscheuer et al., 2008). It is also of interest that homozygous and compound-heterozygote deletions and mutations in *CNTNAP2* and *NRXN1* can symptomatically resemble Pitt–Hopkins syndrome along with autistic behavior (Zweier et al., 2009), and both *NRXN1* (via the 2p16.3 CNV) and *CNTNAP2* (a rarer CNV) (Friedman et al., 2008) have previously been implicated in schizophrenia (and also autism spectrum disorders and epilepsy, as reviewed in Zweier et al., 2009). Another new schizophrenia susceptibility gene from schizophrenia GWAS is *zinc finger protein 804A* (*ZNF804A*), which was identified by a two-stage study, with a GWAS discovery phase using 479 cases and 2,937 controls, followed with 6,829 cases and 9,897 controls for loci with a discovery $p < 10^{-5}$ (O'Donovan et al., 2008). A combined $p = 1.61 \times 10^{-7}$ was obtained for SNP rs1344706 in the initial report, and the association evidence was supported in a later large GWAS of schizophrenia (Purcell et al., 2009; Shi et al., 2009; Stefansson et al., 2009). Subsequently, rs1344706 in *ZNF804A* was reported to be associated with altered neuronal connectivity in the dorsolateral prefrontal cortex in a functional magnetic resonance imaging study of healthy controls (Esslinger et al., 2009).

Polygenic Contributions to Schizophrenia

Many genetic variants with very small effects, combined together, can increase risk substantially under a polygenic model, first hypothesized for schizophrenia four decades ago (Gottesman & Shields, 1967). Simulations show that even a disorder with 1,000 risk loci with low mean relative risks (RR = 1.04), when evaluated on a large scale (10 K cases and 10 K controls), GWAS would still allow prediction of individual disorder risk with an accuracy greater than 0.75 by using 75 loci explaining approximately 50% of the risk variance (Wray, Goddard, & Visscher, 2007). ISC used their GWAS (discovery data set) to define a large set of very small effect common variants as "score" alleles with increasingly liberal association significance thresholds (Purcell et al., 2009). ISC then generated an aggregate risk score for each individual in independent target GWAS data sets, using the MGS EA and AA data sets as well as a U.K. sample (O'Donovan et al., 2008; Shi et al., 2009). Aggregate risk scores in cases were found to be higher than in controls in each of the GWAS data sets of schizophrenia, and also in GWAS data sets of bipolar disorder (WTCCC, 2007; Sklar et al., 2008), but not in control GWAS data sets of nonpsychiatric disorders (WTCCC, 2007; Purcell et al., 2009). They concluded that thousands of common polygenic variants with very small individual effects explain about one-third of the total variation in genetic liability to schizophrenia (Purcell et al., 2009). In an independent bioinformatics-based study (Sun et al., 2009), candidate genes selected from literature mining were found to be enriched in the list of genes with small p-values from schizophrenia GWAS data sets (the Clinical Antipsychotic Trials of Intervention Effectiveness [CATIE] study [Sullivan et al., 2008] and the Genetic Association Information Network [GAIN] portion of MGS [Shi et al., 2009]). A polygenic model with less common causal alleles (MAF < 5%) did not fit the data as well (Purcell et al., 2009). Simulated and empirical data indicate that the spectrum of risk alleles for common disorders includes both common and rare variants (Pritchard, 2001; Kathiresan et al., 2009). The problem of how to explain the substantial missing heritability remains fundamental. Missing heritability here refers to heritability that is unexplained after well-powered GWAS have been conducted. Although it has been argued that the heritability of some behavioral traits and disorders may have been overestimated (Kamin & Goldberger, 2002), this seems unlikely for schizophrenia given the large body of high-quality evidence that is available, and other reasons seem more plausible (see an excellent review on the topic by Herold et al., 2009).

Pleiotropy and Overlap with Bipolar Disorder, Autism, and Other Disorders

Pleiotropy refers to the common phenomenon of variation in a gene simultaneously affecting different phenotypes. It has been found in humans for genes for body weight and height (Weedon et al., 2008) and also for disorders such as type 2 diabetes (T2D) (Zeggini et al., 2008) and prostate cancer (Thomas et al., 2008). The molecular genetic overlaps between schizophrenia and bipolar disorder, and between schizophrenia and autism, are consistent with pleiotropy, but shared genetic loci may actually determine an aspect (somewhat in isolation from the overall phenotype) shared by two disorders such as psychosis in schizophrenia and in bipolar disorder (Schulze et al., 2006).

Overlap with Bipolar Disorder

Schizophrenia and bipolar disorder share several characteristics: peak onset in early adulthood, similar prevalence, psychotic symptoms in more than half of bipolar disorder type 1 subjects, response to antipsychotic medications, substance use comorbidity, increased suicide risk, and severe mood episodes (often present in schizophrenia). Family studies have shown that schizoaffective disorder is more common in families—as ascertained from probands with schizophrenia or with bipolar disorder type 1—than in the general population (Gershon et al., 1982; Gershon et al., 1988; Kendler et al., 1993; Maier et al., 1993; Valles et al., 2000; Maier et al., 2002). A recent meta-analysis of family studies found familial coaggregation of schizophrenia and bipolar disorder (Van Snellenberg & de Candia, 2009). The largest family study (Sweden; schizophrenia N approximately 36,000 and bipolar disorder N approximately 40,000 probands) found familial coaggregation between schizophrenia and bipolar disorder to be roughly 63% because of additive genetic effects common to both disorders (Lichtenstein et al., 2009).

Overlap of susceptibility genes has been postulated (Berrettini, 2000; Craddock & Owen, 2007; van Os & Kapur, 2009), including for more circumscribed aspects such as psychosis proneness (Schulze et al., 2006; Goes et al., 2007). An overlapping CNV for schizophrenia and bipolar disorder has been reported for the 16p11.2 duplication in a meta-analysis with an association $p = 4.8 \times 10^{-7}$ for schizophrenia and $p = 0.017$ for bipolar disorder (McCarthy et al., 2009). GWAS SNP data suggest a genetic overlap between schizophrenia and bipolar disorder, clinical entities shown to share polygenic common variants with very small effect sizes (Purcell et al., 2009). A genewide analysis found a significant excess of genes showing associations with both disorders (Moskvina et al., 2009). ZNF804A and CACNA1C (*calcium channel, voltage-dependent, L type, alpha 1C subunit*) are two such genes that are shared by both disorders: ZNF804A was identified initially as a schizophrenia susceptibility gene, and CACNA1C was identified initially as a bipolar disorder susceptibility gene, in respective GWAS (O'Donovan et al., 2008; Green et al., 2009).

Overlap with Autism

Schizophrenia and autism also share a few clinical features such as social interaction and communication impairments, and some negative or deficit symptoms

(Konstantareas & Hewitt, 2001). This is more noticeable for childhood-onset schizophrenia, where developmental delays may be more marked, than in adult-onset schizophrenia, in which such findings are subtler (Rapoport et al., 2009). However, autism remains an exclusion criterion for schizophrenia in the DSM-IV unless prominent hallucinations and delusions are present for at least a month (APA, 1994). A study of 129 adults with autism spectrum disorders (ASD) found that 7% had psychotic bipolar disorder and 8% had schizophrenia or other psychotic disorders (Stahlberg et al., 2004). The current diagnostic hierarchy, which largely treats ASD and schizophrenia as mutually exclusive, could mask some ASD-schizophrenia comorbidity because an autism case might be less likely to be diagnosed with schizophrenia in adulthood (Rapoport et al., 2009), even in the presence of overt and chronic psychosis. A twofold increase of schizophrenia in the parents of individuals with autism (Daniels et al., 2008), a risk ratio of 3.44 for autism when prenatal parental history of a schizophrenia-like psychosis was present in a nationwide Danish study (Larsson et al., 2005), and an increased risk of schizophrenia in autism patients (Stahlberg et al., 2004; Mouridsen et al., 2008) suggest overlapping risk factors between schizophrenia and autism.

It is interesting that the strongest SNP association of $p = 4.6 \times 10^{-7}$ in the MGS GWAS EA data set was found with *centaurin gamma 2* (*CENTG2*, also known as *AGAP1*), a gene that has been implicated in autism (Wassink et al., 2005). It is also noteworthy that our exploratory analysis of MGS GWAS data combining both EA and AA (3,967 cases and 3,626 controls) showed a $p = 1.9 \times 10^{-6}$ association with *fragile X mental retardation, autosomal homolog 1* (*FXR1*; see Shi et al., 2009), and the association reached genomewide significance when the ISC and SGENE-plus GWAS data sets were included in the analysis along with MGS EA and AA (data not shown). *FXR1* is a paralog of *fragile X mental retardation 1* (*FMR1*), dysfunction of which causes the FMR syndrome that includes autism as a common feature (Bassell & Warren, 2008). CNV loci common to autism and schizophrenia have also been reported (see the next section and chapter 8).

Overlap with Other Conditions

The idea that there is genetic overlap between schizophrenia and autism (and other conditions) has recently received indirect support because a number of individuals with schizophrenia carrying rare and large CNVs have comorbidities such as learning disabilities, mental retardation, autism and autism spectrum disorders, and seizures or epilepsy, and because such disorders' own CNV scans have implicated the same CNV loci (Sebat et al., 2007; Brunetti-Pierri et al., 2008; Christian et al., 2008; Kumar et al., 2008; Marshall et al., 2008; Mefford et al., 2008; Sharp et al., 2008; Weiss et al., 2008; de Kovel et al., 2009; Dibbens et al., 2009; Helbig et al., 2009; McCarthy et al., 2009). Seizures are also overrepresented in schizophrenia (Hyde & Weinberger, 1997; Cascella, Schretlan, & Sawa, 2009). Finally, evidence for pleiotropy from model organisms (Griswold & Whitlock, 2003) suggests that pleiotropic genes might not be selectively neutral: the "unintended" effect (e.g., conferring susceptibility to a common disorder) may be overshadowed by the "intended effect" (e.g., protecting against another disorder, such as one that is more lethal or that has similar lethality but earlier expression [see also Cheverud, 2007]). The recent observation that somatic mutations in *PARK2*, a gene with an established role in Parkinson's disease, are associated with glioblastoma and other human malignancies also suggests a pleotropic effect (Veeriah et al., 2010). If a gene (pleiotropically) increases the risk for schizophrenia through two unrelated mechanisms, one independent (i.e., directly affecting the risk for schizophrenia) and another one through an association with a secondary associated phenotype (e.g., mood disorder or nicotine addiction, which are both associated with schizophrenia), it may induce bias in association analyses, depending on the specific ascertainment rules and their effect on recruitment of subjects with the secondary phenotype (Monsees, Tamimi, & Kraft, 2009).

The New Reality and Challenges for the Field of Schizophrenia Genetics

The GWAS experiments have defined multiple chromosomal regions of high interest, in addition to 6p21.3-p22.1, and several have already surpassed the genomewide significance threshold. Ongoing larger multisample combined GWAS (e.g., the Psychiatric GWAS Consortium [PGC]) for schizophrenia [Gejman, 2009], with a sample N > 21,000) and large-scale replication studies (e.g., the PGC combined schizophrenia replication with a sample N > 30,000) are very likely to expand the number of chromosomal regions that attain genomewide significance and the number of other regions of high interest that also merit further laboratory efforts. As additional large samples are studied, the number of regions that reach genomewide significance is expected to increase, a general trend for complex genetics (albeit the gene effects become progressively smaller because the larger-effect size loci are found first). Therefore it is reasonable to conclude that GWAS-enabled discoveries in the schizophrenia genetics field reflect incremental progress. However, it is also clear that we have not yet identified the DNA loci associated with the bulk of the transmission of schizophrenia in the general population, or the biological mechanisms for any of the confirmed associations. In GWAS, SNPs that constitute a genomewide genotyping array typically are selected because they are common and are informative of many other SNPs, not because of their functional properties. This method of SNP selection tends to yield results where the large majority of associated alleles are unlikely to be causative. Furthermore, the associated SNPs typically are not in coding sequences where a signal would be easier to interpret, but in intergenic and intronic regions for which the function of most associated variation remains unknown. The planning of follow-up resequencing experiments is not simple, either. The association signals frequently are from regions with an extended LD block that spans many genes, an extreme example being the MHC locus implicated in schizophrenia where it is challenging to disentangle which of the several hundred genes in the region is or are likely to be causal. The causative variants may be close to the associated locus but may also be farther removed, even on a different chromosome (as could happen with a *trans*-acting gene expression factor). The extent of rare variation involvement in schizophrenia in the general population remains unknown. This includes CNVs within risk loci already detected as being associated by GWAS, or in other regions of the genome for which there is no evidence of association, although genomewide resequencing will empirically address this question. In the context of our still incipient knowledge of the genome and of the genetics of complex disorders, it is important to avoid trying to fit our hypotheses to a Procrustean bed and instead keep an open mind to a variety of approaches. From the collective experience of model organisms (Mackay, 2009), it is unlikely that explanations relying only on single genes will capture the fundamental complexity of most human complex traits. All associated genetic variation needs to be pursued, and their effects integrated, to understand the pathophysiology of a complex disorder. There are a few issues of momentous importance, which we have selected for brief discussion.

Replication and Fine Mapping of Genomewide Association Studies Associations

This includes the location and boundaries of each locus and is best done by analyzing, in the aggregate and separately, a large combined sample. (Single samples lack the necessary size or power.) The follow-up experiments to replicate GWAS results need to be thorough and systematic. It is essential to predefine the statistical thresholds of loci that are to be included in replication experiments. These do not necessarily need to be only genomewide significant loci, because the combination of GWAS and new replication samples may establish new risk loci (e.g., among SNPs that were strongly associated but did not fulfill GWAS criteria for genomewide significance previously). Replication is one of the main aims of the PGC. The preferred approach is to combine GWAS data from independent samples, but for those samples that lack GWAS data, focused genotyping is still useful, although less informative. Non-EA populations might have some non-overlapping susceptibility loci; thus, it is fundamental to investigate for these differences because they are potentially informative for both genetic and environmental risk factors. An important characteristic of African populations (e.g., AA) is reduced LD, which helps in narrowing the associated genomic intervals;

existing limitations of CNV and SNP map coverage and imputation of AA data sets are currently being addressed (for examples, see Hao et al., 2009; McElroy et al., 2009). The new data-sharing policy (see gwas.nih.gov) has strongly stimulated collaboration, including follow-up replication studies.

Large-Scale Functional Approaches

The integration of GWAS data with measures of gene expression regulation is fundamental. The combined study of genomewide transcription and GWAS association data may generate mechanistic explanations for formerly purely statistical GWAS associations. It is important that such studies be sufficiently powered to allow for the detection of small effects. The approach has proved successful in asthma (Moffatt et al., 2007). It is interesting that within the MHC region implicated in schizophrenia, there are more than 10 *cis*-expression QTL (*cis*-eQTL, *cis* meaning nearby on the same chromosome) (figure 7.2) (see Dixon et al., 2007), and the SNP showing the most significant association with schizophrenia, rs13194053 with $p=9.54\times10^{-9}$, is in LD ($r^2=0.43$) with an SNP showing the strongest association with *BTN3A2* expression (figure 7.2). It is noteworthy that, in the absence of buffering effects of entire multiorgan physiologic systems, simple in vitro models offer the advantage of allowing the observation of smaller effects, particularly when the system of interest can be stimulated (perturbed to further expose variation) in pharmacogenetic experiments.

Basic genomics research has produced major breakthroughs during recent years. Examples are the discovery of microRNAs, long-range promoters, epigenetic factors, and variable CNVs. Many more will probably be made as our knowledge of the genome rapidly increases. It should not be surprising if still unknown genetic mechanisms will, in the end, explain a substantial proportion of the heritability of schizophrenia. Nonetheless, the task of defining the spectrum of molecular genetic mechanisms in schizophrenia is now at the forefront of our field. Rapid progress in biotechnology (Mardis, 2009) is making the study of rare variants in many genes or in large genomic regions in large samples increasingly feasible (see chapter 8, this book). Proof of principle is provided by the 1,000 genomes project (see www.1000genomes.org), which is designed to build a deep catalog of human genetic variation. The design of experiments aimed at fine mapping of regions of association and the precision of imputation will both benefit from this project.

It is anticipated that as genetic discoveries accumulate, the application of myriad tools from systems biology (e.g., genomics, transcriptomics, proteomics, and so forth) will lead to a delineation of biological pathways involved in the pathophysiology of schizophrenia, and eventually to new therapies. Developments in treatment still lag behind discoveries of new genetic associations for complex disorders (see O'Rahilly, 2009), but this situation is expected to change as biological research makes inroads into still purely statistical associations. A long-term aim, and a task of utmost importance, is the integration of the spectrum of mutations found in schizophrenia into explanations that take into account constantly changing environments and evolutionary forces.

KEY AREAS FOR FUTURE RESEARCH

- Conduct GWAS replication and fine mapping.
- Pursue deep re-sequencing—first likely exomic and then genomewide.
- Apply functional systems biology approaches—genomics, transcriptomics, and proteomics.
- Expand studied samples, especially non-EA groups (i.e., AA, Asian).
- Integrate the myriad data generated by these studies
- Reduce the "missing heritability."

Acknowledgments

This review was supported by funding from National Institutes of Health grant U01MH79469 to Pablo V. Gejman and by the Paul Michael Donovan Charitable Foundation.

Selected Readings

Daly, M. J., Rioux, J. D., Schaffner, S. F., Hudson, T. J., & Lander, E. S. (2001). High-resolution haplotype structure in the human genome. *Nature Genetics* 29(2): 229–232.

Gottesman, I. I. & Shields, J. (1967). A polygenic theory of schizophrenia. *Proceedings of the National Academy of Sciences U.S.A.* 58(1): 199–205.

Ioannidis, J. P. (2008). Why most discovered true associations are inflated. *Epidemiology* 19(5): 640–648.

Keller, M. C. & Miller, G. (2006). Resolving the paradox of common, harmful, heritable mental disorders: Which evolutionary genetic models work best? *Behavioral Brain Science* 29(4): 385–404.

Ng, M. Y., Levinson, D. F., Faraone, S. V., Suarez, B. K., DeLisi, L. E., Arinami, T., Riley, B., Paunio, T., Pulver, A. E., Irmansyah, Holmans, P. A., et al. (2009). Meta-analysis of 32 genome-wide linkage studies of schizophrenia. *Molecular Psychiatry* 14(8): 774–785.

Purcell, S. M., Wray, N. R., Stone, J. L., Visscher, P. M., O'Donovan, M. C., Sullivan, P. F., & Sklar, P. (2009). Common polygenic variation contributes to risk of schizophrenia and bipolar disorder. *Nature* 460(7256): 748–752.

Sanders, A. R., Duan, J., Levinson, D. F., Shi, J., He, D., Hou, C., Burrell, G. J., Rice, J. P., Nertney, D. A., Olincy, A., et al. (2008). No significant association of 14 candidate genes with schizophrenia in a large European ancestry sample: Implications for psychiatric genetics. *American Journal of Psychiatry* 165(4): 497–506.

Shi, J., Levinson, D. F., Duan, J., Sanders, A. R., Zheng, Y., Pe'er, I., Dudbridge, F., Holmans, P. A., Whittemore, A. S., Mowry, B. J., et al. (2009). Common variants on chromosome 6p22.1 are associated with schizophrenia. *Nature* 460(7256): 753–757.

Suarez, B. K., Duan, J., Sanders, A. R., Hinrichs, A. L., Jin, C. H., Hou, C., Buccola, N. G., Hale, N., Weilbaecher, A. N., Nertney, D. A., et al. (2006). Genomewide linkage scan of 409 European-ancestry and African American families with schizophrenia: Suggestive evidence of linkage at 8p23.3–p21.2 and 11p13.1–q14.1 in the combined sample. *American Journal of Human Genetics* 78(2): 315–333.

Wray, N. R., Goddard, M. E., & Visscher, P. M. (2007). Prediction of individual genetic risk to disease from genome-wide association studies. *Genome Research* 17(10): 1520–1528.

References

Adegbola, A., Gao, H., Sommer, S., & Browning, M. (2008). A novel mutation in JARID1C/SMCX in a patient with autism spectrum disorder (ASD). *American Journal of Medical Genetics A* 146A(4): 505–511.

Allen, N. C., Bagade, S., McQueen, M. B., Ioannidis, J. P., Kavvoura, F. K., Khoury, M. J., Tanzi, R. E., & Bertram, L. (2008). Systematic meta-analyses and field synopsis of genetic association studies in schizophrenia: The SzGene database. *Nature Genetics* 40(7): 827–834.

Allison, A. C. (1954). Notes on sickle-cell polymorphism. *Annals of Human Genetics* 19(1): 39–51.

APA. (1994). *Diagnostic and Statistical Manual of Mental Disorders* (4th ed.). Washington, DC: American Psychiatric Association.

Bach, M. L., Bach, F. H., & Joo, P. (1969). Leukemia-associated antigens in the mixed leukocyte culture test. *Science* 166(3912): 1520–1522.

Badner, J. A. & Gershon, E. S. (2002). Meta-analysis of whole-genome linkage scans of bipolar disorder and schizophrenia. *Molecular Psychiatry* 7(4): 405–411.

Bassell, G. J. & Warren, S. T. (2008). Fragile X syndrome: Loss of local mRNA regulation alters synaptic development and function. *Neuron* 60(2): 201–214.

Bastian, J., Chacron, M. J., & Maler, L. (2004). Plastic and nonplastic pyramidal cells perform unique roles in a network capable of adaptive redundancy reduction. *Neuron* 41(5): 767–779.

Berrettini, W. H. (2000). Are schizophrenic and bipolar disorders related? A review of family and molecular studies. *Biological Psychiatry* 48(6): 531–538.

Birney, E., Stamatoyannopoulos, J. A., Dutta, A., Guigo, R., Gingeras, T. R., Margulies, E. H., Weng, Z., Snyder, M., Dermitzakis, E. T., Thurman, R. E., et al. (2007). Identification and analysis of functional elements in 1% of the human genome by the ENCODE pilot project. *Nature* 447(7146): 799–816.

Blouin, J. L., Dombroski, B. A., Nath, S. K., Lasseter, V. K., Wolyniec, P. S., Nestadt, G., Thornquist, M., Ullrich, G., McGrath, J., Kasch, L., et al. (1998). Schizophrenia susceptibility loci on chromosomes 13q32 and 8p21. *Nature Genetics* 20(1): 70–73.

Book, J. A. (1953). Schizophrenia as a gene mutation. *Acta Genetica et Statistica Medica* 4(2–3): 133–139.

Brockschmidt, A., Todt, U., Ryu, S., Hoischen, A., Landwehr, C., Birnbaum, S., Frenck, W., Radlwimmer, B., Lichter, P., Engels, H., et al. (2007). Severe mental retardation with breathing abnormalities (Pitt-Hopkins syndrome) is caused by haploinsufficiency of the neuronal bHLH transcription factor TCF4. *Human Molecular Genetics* 16(12): 1488–1494.

Brown, A., Bottiglieri, T., Schaefer, C., Quesenberry, C., Liu, L., Bresnahan, M., & Susser, E. (2007). Elevated prenatal homocysteine levels as a risk factor for schizophrenia. *Archives of General Psychiatry* 64(1): 31–39.

Brown, A. S. & Derkits, E. J. (2010). Prenatal infection and schizophrenia: A review of epidemiologic and translational studies. *American Journal of Psychiatry* 167(3): 261–280.

Brunetti-Pierri, N., Berg, J. S., Scaglia, F., Belmont, J., Bacino, C. A., Sahoo, T., Lalani, S. R., Graham, B., Lee, B., Shinawi, M., et al. (2008). Recurrent reciprocal 1q21.1 deletions and duplications associated with microcephaly or macrocephaly and developmental and behavioral abnormalities. *Nature Genetics* 40(12): 1466–1471.

Byrne, M., Agerbo, E., Bennedsen, B., Eaton, W. W., & Mortensen, P. B. (2007). Obstetric conditions and risk of first admission with schizophrenia: A Danish national register based study. *Schizophrenia Research* 97(1–3): 51–59.

Cannon, M., Jones, P. B., & Murray, R. M. (2002). Obstetric complications and schizophrenia: Historical and meta-analytic review. *American Journal of Psychiatry* 159(7): 1080–1092.

Cannon, T. D., Kaprio, J., Lonnqvist, J., Huttunen, M., & Koskenvuo, M. (1998). The genetic epidemiology of schizophrenia in a Finnish twin cohort: A population-based modeling study. *Archives of General Psychiatry* 55(1): 67–74.

Cardno, A. G. & Gottesman, I. (2000). Twin studies of schizophrenia: From bow-and-arrow concordances to Star Wars Mx and functional genomics. *American Journal of Medical Genetics* 97(1): 12–17.

Cardno, A. G., Marshall, E. J., Coid, B., Macdonald, A. M., Ribchester, T. R., Davies, N. J., Venturi, P., Jones, L. A., Lewis, S. W., Sham, P. C., et al. (1999). Heritability estimates for psychotic disorders: The Maudsley twin psychosis series. *Archives of General Psychiatry* 56(2): 162–168.

Cascella, N. G., Schretlen, D. J., & Sawa, A. (2009). Schizophrenia and epilepsy: Is there a shared susceptibility? *Neuroscience Research* 63(4): 227–235.

Chechik, G., Anderson, M. J., Bar-Yosef, O., Young, E. D., Tishby, N., & Nelken, I. (2006). Reduction of information redundancy in the ascending auditory pathway. *Neuron* 51(3): 359–368.

Cheverud, J. M. (2007). The relationship between development and evolution through heritable variation. *Novartis Foundation Symposium* 284: 55–65.

Christian, S. L., Brune, C. W., Sudi, J., Kumar, R. A., Liu, S., Karamohamed, S., Badner, J. A., Matsui, S., Conroy, J., McQuaid, D., et al. (2008). Novel submicroscopic chromosomal abnormalities detected in autism spectrum disorder. *Biological Psychiatry* 63(12): 1111–1117.

Cornelis, M. C., Agrawal, A., Cole, J. W., Hansel, N. N., Barnes, K. C., Beaty, T. H., Bennett, S. N., Bierut, L. J., Boerwinkle, E., Doheny, K. F., et al. (2010). The Gene, Environment Association Studies consortium (GENEVA): Maximizing the knowledge obtained from GWAS by collaboration across studies of multiple conditions. *Genetic Epidemiology* 34(4): 364–372.

Costa, E., Dong, E., Grayson, D. R., Guidotti, A., Ruzicka, W., & Veldic, M. (2007). Reviewing the role of DNA (cytosine-5) methyltransferase overexpression in the cortical GABAergic dysfunction associated with psychosis vulnerability. *Epigenetics* 2(1): 29–36.

Craddock, N. & Owen, M. J. (2007). Rethinking psychosis: The disadvantages of a dichotomous classification now outweigh the advantages. *World Psychiatry* 6(2): 84–91.

Crow, J. F. (2000). The origins, patterns and implications of human spontaneous mutation. *Nature Reviews Genetics* 1(1): 40–47.

Daly, M. J., Rioux, J. D., Schaffner, S. F., Hudson, T. J., & Lander, E. S. (2001). High-resolution haplotype structure in the human genome. *Nature Genetics* 29(2): 229–232.

Daniels, J. L., Forssen, U., Hultman, C. M., Cnattingius, S., Savitz, D. A., Feychting, M., & Sparen, P. (2008). Parental psychiatric disorders associated with autism spectrum disorders in the offspring. *Pediatrics* *121*(5):, e1357–e1362.

de Kovel, C. G., Trucks, H., Helbig, I., Mefford, H. C., Baker, C., Leu, C., Kluck, C., Muhle, H., von Spiczak, S., Ostertag, P., et al. (2009). Recurrent microdeletions at 15q11.2 and 16p13.11 predispose to idiopathic generalized epilepsies. *Brain* *133*(Pt 1): 23–32.

Dibbens, L. M., Mullen, S., Helbig, I., Mefford, H. C., Bayly, M. A., Bellows, S., Leu, C., Trucks, H., Obermeier, T., Wittig, M., et al. (2009). Familial and sporadic 15q13.3 micro-deletions in idiopathic generalized epilepsy: Precedent for disorders with complex inheritance. *Human Molecular Genetics* *18*(19): 3626–3631.

Dixon, A. L., Liang, L., Moffatt, M. F., Chen, W., Heath, S., Wong, K. C., Taylor, J., Burnett, E., Gut, I., Farrall, M., et al. (2007). A genome-wide association study of global gene expression. *Nature Genetics* *39*(10): 1202–1207.

Drachman, D. A. (2005). Do we have brain to spare? *Neurology* *64*(12): 2004–2005.

Dudbridge, F. & Gusnanto, A. (2008). Estimation of significance thresholds for genomewide association scans. *Genetic Epidemiology* *32*(3): 227–234.

Eaton, W. W., Byrne, M., Ewald, H., Mors, O., Chen, C. Y., Agerbo, E., & Mortensen, P. B. (2006). Association of schizophrenia and autoimmune diseases: Linkage of Danish national registers. *American Journal of Psychiatry* *163*(3): 521–528.

Esslinger, C., Walter, H., Kirsch, P., Erk, S., Schnell, K., Arnold, C., Haddad, L., Mier, D., Opitz von Boberfeld, C., Raab, K., et al. (2009). Neural mechanisms of a genome-wide supported psychosis variant. *Science* *324*(5927): 605.

Eyre-Walker, A. & Keightley, P. D. (1999). High genomic deleterious mutation rates in hominids. *Nature* *397*(6717): 344–347.

Fananas, L. & Bertranpetit, J. (1995). Reproductive rates in families of schizophrenic patients in a case-control study. *Acta Psychiatrica Scandinavica* *91*(3): 202–204.

Flora, A., Garcia, J. J., Thaller, C., & Zoghbi, H. Y. (2007). The E-protein Tcf4 interacts with Math1 to regulate differentiation of a specific subset of neuronal progenitors. *Proceedings of the National Academy of Sciences U.S.A.* *104*(39): 15382–15387.

Franzek, E. & Beckmann, H. (1998). Different genetic background of schizophrenia spectrum psychoses: A twin study. *American Journal of Psychiatry* *155*(1): 76–83.

Friedman, J. I., Vrijenhoek, T., Markx, S., Janssen, I. M., van der Vliet, W. A., Faas, B. H., Knoers, N. V., Cahn, W., Kahn, R. S., Edelmann, L., et al. (2008). CNTNAP2 gene dosage variation is associated with schizophrenia and epilepsy. *Molecular Psychiatry* *13*(3): 261–266.

Friedman, J. M. (1981). Genetic disease in the offspring of older fathers. *Obstetrics and Gynecology* *57*(6): 745–749.

Gabriel, S. B., Schaffner, S. F., Nguyen, H., Moore, J. M., Roy, J., Blumenstiel, B., Higgins, J., DeFelice, M., Lochner, A., Faggart, M., et al. (2002). The structure of haplotype blocks in the human genome. *Science* *296*(5576): 2225–2229.

Gejman, P. V. (2009). Combined "Freeze 1" Schizophrenia-GWAS analysis. Plenary session: The psychiatric GWAS consortium. Paper presented at the World Congress of Psychiatric Genetics, San Diego.

Gejman, P. V., Sanders, A. R., & Duan, J. (2010) The role of genetics in the etiology of schizophrenia. *Psychiatric Clinics of North America* *33*(1): 35–66.

Gerber, D. J., Hall, D., Miyakawa, T., Demars, S., Gogos, J. A., Karayiorgou, M., & Tonegawa, S. (2003). Evidence for association of schizophrenia with genetic variation in the 8p21.3 gene, PPP3CC, encoding the calcineurin gamma subunit. *Proceedings of the National Academy of Sciences U.S.A.* *100*(15): 8993–8998.

Gershon, E. S., DeLisi, L. E., Hamovit, J., Nurnberger, J. I., Jr., Maxwell, M. E., Schreiber, J., Dauphinais, D., Dingman, C. W., & Guroff, J. J. (1988). A controlled family study of chronic psychoses: Schizophrenia and schizoaffective disorder. *Archives of General Psychiatry* 45(4): 328–336.

Gershon, E. S., Hamovit, J., Guroff, J. J., Dibble, E., Leckman, J. F., Sceery, W., Targum, S. D., Nurnberger, J. I., Jr., Goldin, L. R., & Bunney, W. E., Jr. (1982). A family study of schizoaffective, bipolar I, bipolar II, unipolar, and normal control probands. *Archives of General Psychiatry* 39(10): 1157–1167.

Goes, F. S., Zandi, P. P., Miao, K., McMahon, F. J., Steele, J., Willour, V. L., Mackinnon, D. F., Mondimore, F. M., Schweizer, B., Nurnberger, J. I., Jr., et al. (2007). Mood-incongruent psychotic features in bipolar disorder: Familial aggregation and suggestive linkage to 2p11–q14 and 13q21–33. *American Journal of Psychiatry* 164(2): 236–247.

Gottesman, I. I. & Bertelsen, A. (1989). Confirming unexpressed genotypes for schizophrenia: Risks in the offspring of Fischer's Danish identical and fraternal discordant twins. *Archives of General Psychiatry* 46(10): 867–872.

Gottesman, I. I. & Gould, T. D. (2003). The endophenotype concept in psychiatry: Etymology and strategic intentions. *American Journal of Psychiatry* 160(4): 636–645.

Gottesman, I. I. & Shields, J. (1967). A polygenic theory of schizophrenia. *Proceedings of the National Academy of Sciences U.S.A.* 58(1): 199–205.

Green, E. K., Grozeva, D., Jones, I., Jones, L., Kirov, G., Caesar, S., Gordon-Smith, K., Fraser, C., Forty, L., Russell, E., et al. (2009). The bipolar disorder risk allele at CACNA1C also confers risk of recurrent major depression and of schizophrenia. *Molecular Psychiatry* 15(10): 1016–1022.

Greenwood, T. A., Braff, D. L., Light, G. A., Cadenhead, K. S., Calkins, M. E., Dobie, D. J., Freedman, R., Green, M. F., Gur, R. E., Gur, R. C., et al. (2007). Initial heritability analyses of endophenotypic measures for schizophrenia: The consortium on the genetics of schizophrenia. *Archives of General Psychiatry* 64(11): 1242–1250.

Griswold, C. K. & Whitlock, M. C. (2003). The genetics of adaptation: The roles of pleiotropy, stabilizing selection and drift in shaping the distribution of bidirectional fixed mutational effects. *Genetics* 165(4): 2181–2192.

Gulacsi, A. A. & Anderson, S. A. (2008). Beta-catenin-mediated Wnt signaling regulates neurogenesis in the ventral telencephalon. *Nature Neuroscience* 11(12): 1383–1391.

Halperin, E. & Stephan, D. A. (2009). SNP imputation in association studies. *Nature Biotechnology* 27(4): 349–351.

Hao, K., Chudin, E., McElwee, J., & Schadt, E. E. (2009). Accuracy of genome-wide imputation of untyped markers and impacts on statistical power for association studies. *BMC Genetics* 10: 27.

Harrison, P. J. & Weinberger, D. R. (2005). Schizophrenia genes, gene expression, and neuropathology: On the matter of their convergence. *Molecular Psychiatry* 10(1): 40–68.

Haukka, J., Suvisaari, J., & Lonnqvist, J. (2003). Fertility of patients with schizophrenia, their siblings, and the general population: A cohort study from 1950 to 1959 in Finland. *American Journal of Psychiatry* 160(3): 460–463.

Heckers, S. (2009). Is schizoaffective disorder a useful diagnosis? *Current Psychiatry Reports* 11(4): 332–337.

Helbig, I., Mefford, H. C., Sharp, A. J., Guipponi, M., Fichera, M., Franke, A., Muhle, H., de Kovel, C., Baker, C., von Spiczak, S., et al. (2009). 15q13.3 microdeletions increase risk of idiopathic generalized epilepsy. *Nature Genetics* 41(2): 160–162.

Herold, C., Steffens, M., Brockschmidt, F. F., Baur, M. P., & Becker, T. (2009). INTERSNP: Genome-wide interaction analysis guided by a priori information. *Bioinformatics* 25(24): 3275–3281.

Hindorff, L. A., Sethupathy, P., Junkins, H. A., Ramos, E. M., Mehta, J. P., Collins, F. S., & Manolio, T. A. (2009). Potential etiologic and functional implications of genome-wide association loci for human diseases and traits. *Proceedings of the National Academy of Sciences U.S.A. 106*(23): 9362–9367.

Hoggart, C. J., Clark, T. G., De Iorio, M., Whittaker, J. C., & Balding, D. J. (2008). Genome-wide significance for dense SNP and resequencing data. *Genetic Epidemiology 32*(2): 179–185.

Holmans, P. A., Riley, B., Pulver, A. E., Owen, M. J., Wildenauer, D. B., Gejman, P. V., Mowry, B. J., Laurent, C., Kendler, K. S., Nestadt, G., et al. (2009). Genomewide linkage scan of schizophrenia in a large multicenter pedigree sample using single nucleotide polymorphisms. *Molecular Psychiatry 14*(8): 786–795.

Huxley, J., Mayr, E., Osmond, H., & Hoffer, A. (1964). Schizophrenia as a genetic morphism. *Nature 204*: 220–221.

Hyde, T. M. & Weinberger, D. R. (1997). Seizures and schizophrenia. *Schizophrenia Bulletin 23*(4): 611–622.

Ingraham, L. J. & Kety, S. S. (2000). Adoption studies of schizophrenia. *American Journal of Medical Genetics 97*(1): 18–22.

Ioannidis, J. P. (2008). Why most discovered true associations are inflated. *Epidemiology 19*(5): 640–648.

Kallmann, F. J. (1938). *The Genetics of Schizophrenia: A Study of Heredity and Reproduction in the Families of 1,087 Schizophrenics.* New York: J. J. Augustin.

Kalscheuer, V. M., Feenstra, I., Van Ravenswaaij-Arts, C. M., Smeets, D. F., Menzel, C., Ullmann, R., Musante, L., & Ropers, H. H. (2008). Disruption of the TCF4 gene in a girl with mental retardation but without the classical Pitt-Hopkins syndrome. *American Journal of Medical Genetics A 146A*(16): 2053–2059.

Kamin, L. J. & Goldberger, A. S. (2002). Twin studies in behavioral research: A skeptical view. *Theoretical Population Biology 61*(1): 83–95.

Kasanin, J. (1933). The acute schizoaffective psychoses. *American Journal of Psychiatry 90*(1): 97–126.

Kathiresan, S., Willer, C. J., Peloso, G. M., Demissie, S., Musunuru, K., Schadt, E. E., Kaplan, L., Bennett, D., Li, Y., Tanaka, T., et al. (2009). Common variants at 30 loci contribute to polygenic dyslipidemia. *Nature Genetics 41*(1): 56–65.

Kawasaki, H. & Iwamuro, S. (2008). Potential roles of histones in host defense as antimicrobial agents. *Infectious Disorders—Drug Targets 8*(3): 195–205.

Keller, M. C. & Miller, G. (2006). Resolving the paradox of common, harmful, heritable mental disorders: Which evolutionary genetic models work best? *Behavioral and Brain Sciences 29*(4): 385–404.

Kendler, K. S. (1987). Sporadic vs familial classification given etiologic heterogeneity: I. Sensitivity, specificity, and positive and negative predictive value. *Genetic Epidemiology 4*(5): 313–330.

Kendler, K. S., McGuire, M., Gruenberg, A. M., O'Hare, A., Spellman, M., & Walsh, D. (1993). The Roscommon Family Study. I. Methods, diagnosis of probands, and risk of schizophrenia in relatives. *Archives of General Psychiatry 50*(7): 527–540.

Kendler, K. S. & Neale, M. C. (2010). Endophenotype: A conceptual analysis. *Molecular Psychiatry 15*(8): 789–797.

Kim, H. S., Cho, J. H., Park, H. W., Yoon, H., Kim, M. S., & Kim, S. C. (2002). Endotoxin-neutralizing antimicrobial proteins of the human placenta. *Journal of Immunology 168*(5): 2356–2364.

Klaning, U., Mortensen, P. B., & Kyvik, K. O. (1996). Increased occurrence of schizophrenia and other psychiatric illnesses among twins. *British Journal of Psychiatry 168*(6): 688–692.

Kleinjan, D. A. & van Heyningen, V. (2005). Long-range control of gene expression: Emerging mechanisms and disruption in disease. *American Journal of Human Genetics 76*(1): 8–32.

Konstantareas, M. M. & Hewitt, T. (2001). Autistic disorder and schizophrenia: Diagnostic overlaps. *Journal of Autism and Developmental Disorders* 31(1): 19–28.

Kraepelin, E. (1899). (English translation 1921). *Manic-Depressive Insanity and Paranoia.* Edinburgh: E. & S. Livingstone.

Kraft, P. & Hunter, D. J. (2009). Genetic risk prediction—are we there yet? *New England Journal of Medicine* 360(17): 1701–1703.

Kringlen, E. & Cramer, G. (1989). Offspring of monozygotic twins discordant for schizophrenia. *Archives of General Psychiatry* 46(10): 873–877.

Kumar, R. A., KaraMohamed, S., Sudi, J., Conrad, D. F., Brune, C., Badner, J. A., Gilliam, T. C., Nowak, N. J., Cook, E. H., Jr., Dobyns, W. B., et al. (2008). Recurrent 16p11.2 microdeletions in autism. *Human Molecular Genetics* 17(4): 628–638.

Larsson, H. J., Eaton, W. W., Madsen, K. M., Vestergaard, M., Olesen, A. V., Agerbo, E., Schendel, D., Thorsen, P., & Mortensen, P. B. (2005). Risk factors for autism: Perinatal factors, parental psychiatric history, and socioeconomic status. *American Journal of Epidemiology* 161(10): 916–928.

Lencz, T., Morgan, T. V., Athanasiou, M., Dain, B., Reed, C. R., Kane, J. M., Kucherlapati, R., & Malhotra, A. K. (2007). Converging evidence for a pseudoautosomal cytokine receptor gene locus in schizophrenia. *Molecular Psychiatry* 12(6): 572–580.

Lewis, C. M., Levinson, D. F., Wise, L. H., DeLisi, L. E., Straub, R. E., Hovatta, I., Williams, N. M., Schwab, S. G., Pulver, A. E., Faraone, S. V., et al. (2003). Genome scan meta-analysis of schizophrenia and bipolar disorder, part II: Schizophrenia. *American Journal of Human Genetics* 73(1): 34–48.

Li, M., Li, C., & Guan, W. (2008). Evaluation of coverage variation of SNP chips for genome-wide association studies. *European Journal of Human Genetics* 16(5): 635–643.

Lichtenstein, P., Bjork, C., Hultman, C. M., Scolnick, E., Sklar, P., & Sullivan, P. F. (2006). Recurrence risks for schizophrenia in a Swedish national cohort. *Psychological Medicine* 36(10): 1417–1425.

Lichtenstein, P., Yip, B. H., Bjork, C., Pawitan, Y., Cannon, T. D., Sullivan, P. F., & Hultman, C. M. (2009). Common genetic determinants of schizophrenia and bipolar disorder in Swedish families: A population-based study. *Lancet* 373(9659): 234–239.

MacCabe, J. H., Koupil, I., & Leon, D. A. (2009). Lifetime reproductive output over two generations in patients with psychosis and their unaffected siblings: The Uppsala 1915–1929 Birth Cohort Multigenerational Study. *Psychological Medicine* 39(10): 1667–1676.

Mackay, T. F. (2009). The genetic architecture of complex behaviors: Lessons from *Drosophila. Genetica* 136(2): 295–302.

Maier, W., Lichtermann, D., Franke, P., Heun, R., Falkai, P., & Rietschel, M. (2002). The dichotomy of schizophrenia and affective disorders in extended pedigrees. *Schizophrenia Research* 57(2–3): 259–266.

Maier, W., Lichtermann, D., Minges, J., Hallmayer, J., Heun, R., Benkert, O., & Levinson, D. F. (1993). Continuity and discontinuity of affective disorders and schizophrenia: Results of a controlled family study. *Archives of General Psychiatry* 50(11): 871–883.

Malaspina, D., Harlap, S., Fennig, S., Heiman, D., Nahon, D., Feldman, D., & Susser, E. (2001). Advancing paternal age and the risk of schizophrenia. *Archives of General Psychiatry* 58(4): 361–367.

Manolio, T. A., Collins, F. S., Cox, N. J., Goldstein, D. B., Hindorff, L. A., Hunter, D. J., McCarthy, M. I., Ramos, E. M., Cardon, L. R., Chakravarti, A., et al. (2009). Finding the missing heritability of complex diseases. *Nature* 461(7265): 747–753.

Mardis, E. R. (2009). New strategies and emerging technologies for massively parallel sequencing: Applications in medical research. *Genome Medicine* 1(4): 40.

Marshall, C. R., Noor, A., Vincent, J. B., Lionel, A. C., Feuk, L., Skaug, J., Shago, M., Moessner, R., Pinto, D., Ren, Y., et al. (2008). Structural variation of chromosomes in autism spectrum disorder. *American Journal of Human Genetics* 82(2): 477–488.

McCarthy, M. I., Abecasis, G. R., Cardon, L. R., Goldstein, D. B., Little, J., Ioannidis, J. P., & Hirschhorn, J. N. (2008). Genome-wide association studies for complex traits: Consensus, uncertainty and challenges. *Nature Reviews Genetics* 9(5): 356–369.

McCarthy, S. E., Makarov, V., Kirov, G., Addington, A. M., McClellan, J., Yoon, S., Perkins, D. O., Dickel, D. E., Kusenda, M., Krastoshevsky, O., et al. (2009). Microduplications of 16p11.2 are associated with schizophrenia. *Nature Genetic,* 41(11): 1223–1227.

McElroy, J. P., Nelson, M. R., Caillier, S. J., & Oksenberg, J. R. (2009). Copy number variation in African Americans. *BMC Genetics* 10: 15.

McGrath, J., Saha, S., Chant, D., & Welham, J. (2008). Schizophrenia: A concise overview of incidence, prevalence, and mortality. *Epidemiology Reviews* 30: 67–76.

Mefford, H. C., Sharp, A. J., Baker, C., Itsara, A., Jiang, Z., Buysse, K., Huang, S., Maloney, V. K., Crolla, J. A., Baralle, D., et al. (2008). Recurrent rearrangements of chromosome 1q21.1 and variable pediatric phenotypes. *New England Journal of Medicine* 359(16): 1685–1699.

Mill, J., Tang, T., Kaminsky, Z., Khare, T., Yazdanpanah, S., Bouchard, L., Jia, P., Assadzadeh, A., Flanagan, J., Schumacher, A., et al. (2008). Epigenomic profiling reveals DNA-methylation changes associated with major psychosis. *American Journal of Human Genetics* 82(3): 696–711.

Mittal, V. A., Ellman, L. M., & Cannon, T. D. (2008). Gene-environment interaction and co-variation in schizophrenia: The role of obstetric complications. *Schizophrenia Bulletin* 34(6): 1083–1094.

Moffatt, M. F., Kabesch, M., Liang, L., Dixon, A. L., Strachan, D., Heath, S., Depner, M., von Berg, A., Bufe, A., Rietschel, E., et al. (2007). Genetic variants regulating ORMDL3 expression contribute to the risk of childhood asthma. *Nature* 448(7152): 470–473.

Monsees, G. M., Tamimi, R. M., & Kraft, P. (2009). Genome-wide association scans for secondary traits using case-control samples. *Genetic Epidemiology* 33(8): 717–728.

Morris, G., Nevet, A., & Bergman, H. (2003). Anatomical funneling, sparse connectivity and redundancy reduction in the neural networks of the basal ganglia. *Journal of Physiology (Paris)* 97(4–6): 581–589.

Moskvina, V., Craddock, N., Holmans, P., Nikolov, I., Pahwa, J. S., Green, E., Owen, M. J., & O'Donovan, M. C. (2009). Gene-wide analyses of genome-wide association data sets: Evidence for multiple common risk alleles for schizophrenia and bipolar disorder and for overlap in genetic risk. *Molecular Psychiatry* 14(3): 252–260.

Mouridsen, S. E., Rich, B., Isager, T., & Nedergaard, N. J. (2008). Psychiatric disorders in individuals diagnosed with infantile autism as children: A case control study. *Journal of Psychiatric Practice* 14(1): 5–12.

Need, A. C., Ge, D., Weale, M. E., Maia, J., Feng, S., Heinzen, E. L., Shianna, K. V., Yoon, W., Kasperaviciute, D., Gennarelli, M., et al. (2009). A genome-wide investigation of SNPs and CNVs in schizophrenia. *PLoS Genetics* 5 (2): e1000373.

Ng, M. Y., Levinson, D. F., Faraone, S. V., Suarez, B. K., DeLisi, L. E., Arinami, T., Riley, B., Paunio, T., Pulver, A. E., Irmansyah, Holmans, P. A., et al. (2009). Meta-analysis of 32 genome-wide linkage studies of schizophrenia. *Molecular Psychiatry* 14(8): 774–785.

Nothnagel, M., Ellinghaus, D., Schreiber, S., Krawczak, M., & Franke, A. (2009). A comprehensive evaluation of SNP genotype imputation. *Human Genetics* 125(2): 163–171.

Nurnberger, J. I., Jr., Blehar, M. C., Kaufmann, C. A., York-Cooler, C., Simpson, S. G., Harkavy-Friedman, J., Severe, J. B., Malaspina, D., & Reich, T. (1994). Diagnostic interview for genetic studies: Rationale, unique features, and training. NIMH Genetics Initiative. *Archives of General Psychiatry* 51(11): 849–859.

O'Donovan, M. C., Craddock, N., Norton, N., Williams, H., Peirce, T., Moskvina, V., Nikolov, I., Hamshere, M., Carroll, L., Georgieva, L., et al. (2008). Identification of loci associated with schizophrenia by genome-wide association and follow-up. *Nature Genetics* 40(9): 1053–1055.

O'Rahilly, S. (2009). Human genetics illuminates the paths to metabolic disease. *Nature* 462(7271): 307–314.

Oksenberg, J. R., Baranzini, S. E., Sawcer, S., & Hauser, S. L. (2008). The genetics of multiple sclerosis: SNPs to pathways to pathogenesis. *Nature Reviews Genetics* 9(7): 516–526.

Pe'er, I., Yelensky, R., Altshuler, D., & Daly, M. J. (2008). Estimation of the multiple testing burden for genomewide association studies of nearly all common variants. *Genetic Epidemiology* 32(4): 381–385.

Pritchard, J. K. (2001). Are rare variants responsible for susceptibility to complex diseases? *American Journal of Human Genetics* 69(1): 124–137.

Purcell, S. M., Wray, N. R., Stone, J. L., Visscher, P. M., O'Donovan, M. C., Sullivan, P. F., & Sklar, P. (2009). Common polygenic variation contributes to risk of schizophrenia and bipolar disorder. *Nature* 460(7256): 748–752.

Rapoport, J., Chavez, A., Greenstein, D., Addington, A., & Gogtay, N. (2009). Autism spectrum disorders and childhood-onset schizophrenia: Clinical and biological contributions to a relation revisited. *Journal of the American Academy of Child and Adolescent Psychiatry* 48(1): 10–18.

Reich, D. E. & Lander, E. S. (2001). On the allelic spectrum of human disease. *Trends in Genetics* 17(9): 502–510.

Richter, S. H., Garner, J. P., & Wurbel, H. (2009). Environmental standardization: Cure or cause of poor reproducibility in animal experiments? *Nature Methods* 6(4): 257–261.

Risch, N. (1990). Genetic linkage and complex diseases, with special reference to psychiatric disorders. *Genetic Epidemiology* 7(1): 3–16.

Roth, T. L., Lubin, F. D., Sodhi, M., & Kleinman, J. E. (2009). Epigenetic mechanisms in schizophrenia. *Biochimica et Biophysica Acta* 1790(9): 869–877.

Rüdin, E. (1916). *Zur Vererbung und Neuenstehung der Dementia Praecox*. Berlin: Springer.

Sanders, A. R., Duan, J., Levinson, D. F., Shi, J., He, D., Hou, C., Burrell, G. J., Rice, J. P., Nertney, D. A., Olincy, A., et al. (2008). No significant association of 14 candidate genes with schizophrenia in a large European ancestry sample: Implications for psychiatric genetics. *American Journal of Psychiatry* 165(4): 497–506.

Schadt, E. E. (2009). Molecular networks as sensors and drivers of common human diseases. *Nature* 461(7261): 218–223.

Schulze, T. G., Hedeker, D., Zandi, P., Rietschel, M., & McMahon, F. J. (2006). What is familial about familial bipolar disorder? Resemblance among relatives across a broad spectrum of phenotypic characteristics. *Archives of General Psychiatry* 63(12): 1368–1376.

Sebat, J., Lakshmi, B., Malhotra, D., Troge, J., Lese-Martin, C., Walsh, T., Yamrom, B., Yoon, S., Krasnitz, A., Kendall, J., et al. (2007). Strong association of de novo copy number mutations with autism. *Science* 316(5823): 445–449.

Sharp, A. J., Mefford, H. C., Li, K., Baker, C., Skinner, C., Stevenson, R. E., Schroer, R. J., Novara, F., De Gregori, M., Ciccone, R., et al. (2008). A recurrent 15q13.3 microdeletion syndrome associated with mental retardation and seizures. *Nature Genetics* 40(3): 322–328.

Shi, J., Levinson, D. F., Duan, J., Sanders, A. R., Zheng, Y., Pe'er, I., Dudbridge, F., Holmans, P. A., Whittemore, A. S., Mowry, B. J., et al. (2009). Common variants on chromosome 6p22.1 are associated with schizophrenia. *Nature* 460(7256): 753–757.

Shi, Y. (2007). Histone lysine demethylases: Emerging roles in development, physiology and disease. *Nature Reviews Genetics 8*(11): 829–833.

Shiina, T., Inoko, H., & Kulski, J. K. (2004). An update of the HLA genomic region, locus information and disease associations: 2004. *Tissue Antigens 64*(6): 631–649.

Sipos, A., Rasmussen, F., Harrison, G., Tynelius, P., Lewis, G., Leon, D. A., & Gunnell, D. (2004). Paternal age and schizophrenia: A population based cohort study. *British Medical Journal 329*(7474): 1070.

Sklar, P., Smoller, J. W., Fan, J., Ferreira, M. A., Perlis, R. H., Chambert, K., Nimgaonkar, V. L., McQueen, M. B., Faraone, S. V., Kirby, A., et al. (2008). Whole-genome association study of bipolar disorder. *Molecular Psychiatry 13*(6): 558–569.

Spitzer, R. L., Endicott, J., & Robins, E. (1978). Research diagnostic criteria: Rationale and reliability. *Archives of General Psychiatry 35*(6): 773–782.

Sporns, O., Tononi, G., & Kotter, R. (2005). The human connectome: A structural description of the human brain. *PLoS Computational Biology 1*(4): e42.

St Clair, D., Xu, M., Wang, P., Yu, Y., Fang, Y., Zhang, F., Zheng, X., Gu, N., Feng, G., Sham, P., et al. (2005). Rates of adult schizophrenia following prenatal exposure to the Chinese famine of 1959–1961. *Journal of the American Medical Association 294*(5): 557–562.

Stahlberg, O., Soderstrom, H., Rastam, M., & Gillberg, C. (2004). Bipolar disorder, schizophrenia, and other psychotic disorders in adults with childhood onset AD/HD and/or autism spectrum disorders. *Journal of Neural Transmission 111*(7): 891–902.

Stefansson, H., Ophoff, R. A., Steinberg, S., Andreassen, O. A., Cichon, S., Rujescu, D., Werge, T., Pietilainen, O. P., Mors, O., Mortensen, P. B., et al. (2009). Common variants conferring risk of schizophrenia. *Nature 460*(7256): 744–747.

Stefansson, H., Sigurdsson, E., Steinthorsdottir, V., Bjornsdottir, S., Sigmundsson, T., Ghosh, S., Brynjolfsson, J., Gunnarsdottir, S., Ivarsson, O., Chou, T. T., et al. (2002). Neuregulin 1 and susceptibility to schizophrenia. *American Journal of Human Genetics 71*(4): 877–892.

Suarez, B. K., Duan, J., Sanders, A. R., Hinrichs, A. L., Jin, C. H., Hou, C., Buccola, N. G., Hale, N., Weilbaecher, A. N., Nertney, D. A., et al. (2006). Genomewide linkage scan of 409 European-ancestry and African American families with schizophrenia: Suggestive evidence of linkage at 8p23.3–p21.2 and 11p13.1-q14.1 in the combined sample. *American Journal of Human Genetics 78*(2): 315–333.

Sullivan, P. F., Kendler, K. S., & Neale, M. C. (2003). Schizophrenia as a complex trait: Evidence from a meta-analysis of twin studies. *Archives of General Psychiatry 60*(12): 1187–1192.

Sullivan, P. F., Lin, D., Tzeng, J. Y., van den Oord, E., Perkins, D., Stroup, T. S., Wagner, M., Lee, S., Wright, F. A., Zou, F., et al. (2008). Genomewide association for schizophrenia in the CATIE study: Results of stage 1. *Molecular Psychiatry 13*(6): 570–584.

Sun, J., Jia, P., Fanous, A. H., Webb, B. T., van den Oord, E. J., Chen, X., Bukszar, J., Kendler, K. S., & Zhao, Z. (2009). A multi-dimensional evidence-based candidate gene prioritization approach for complex diseases-schizophrenia as a case. *Bioinformatics 25*(19): 2595–2602.

Susser, E. S. & Lin, S. P. (1992). Schizophrenia after prenatal exposure to the Dutch Hunger Winter of 1944–1945. *Archives of General Psychiatry 49*(12): 983–988.

Svensson, A. C., Lichtenstein, P., Sandin, S., & Hultman, C. M. (2007). Fertility of first-degree relatives of patients with schizophrenia: A three generation perspective. *Schizophrenia Research 91*(1–3): 238–245.

Thomas, G., Jacobs, K. B., Yeager, M., Kraft, P., Wacholder, S., Orr, N., Yu, K., Chatterjee, N., Welch, R., Hutchinson, A., et al. (2008). Multiple loci identified in a genome-wide association study of prostate cancer. *Nature Genetics 40*(3): 310–315.

Torrey, E. F., Buka, S., Cannon, T. D., Goldstein, J. M., Seidman, L. J., Liu, T., Hadley, T., Rosso, I. M., Bearden, C., & Yolken, R. H. (2009). Paternal age as a risk factor for schizophrenia: How important is it? *Schizophrenia Research 114*(1–3): 1–5.

Traherne, J. A. (2008). Human MHC architecture and evolution: Implications for disease association studies. *International Journal of Immunogenetics 35*(3): 179–192.

Valles, V., van Os, J., Guillamat, R., Gutierrez, B., Campillo, M., Gento, P., & Fananas, L. (2000). Increased morbid risk for schizophrenia in families of in-patients with bipolar illness. *Schizophrenia Research 42*(2): 83–90.

van Os, J. & Kapur, S. (2009). Schizophrenia. *Lancet 374*(9690): 635–645.

Van Snellenberg, J. X. & de Candia, T. (2009). Meta-analytic evidence for familial coaggregation of schizophrenia and bipolar disorder. *Archives of General Psychiatry 66*(7): 748–755.

Veeriah, S., Taylor, B. S., Meng, S., Fang, F., Yilmaz, E., Vivanco, I., Janakiraman, M., Schultz, N., Hanrahan, A. J., Pao, W., et al. (2010). Somatic mutations of the Parkinson's disease-associated gene PARK2 in glioblastoma and other human malignancies. *Nature Genetics 42*(1): 77–82.

Viken, M. K., Blomhoff, A., Olsson, M., Akselsen, H. E., Pociot, F., Nerup, J., Kockum, I., Cambon-Thomsen, A., Thorsby, E., Undlien, D. E., et al. (2009). Reproducible association with type 1 diabetes in the extended class I region of the major histocompatibility complex. *Genes and Immunity 10*(4): 323–333.

Wang, H., Feng, R., Phillip Wang, L., Li, F., Cao, X., & Tsien, J. Z. (2008). CaMKII activation state underlies synaptic labile phase of LTP and short-term memory formation. *Current Biology 18*(20): 1546–1554.

Wassink, T. H., Piven, J., Vieland, V. J., Jenkins, L., Frantz, R., Bartlett, C. W., Goedken, R., Childress, D., Spence, M. A., Smith, M., et al. (2005). Evaluation of the chromosome 2q37.3 gene CENTG2 as an autism susceptibility gene. *American Journal of Medical Genetics Part B: Neuropsychiatric Genetics 136B*(1): 36–44.

Weedon, M. N., Lango, H., Lindgren, C. M., Wallace, C., Evans, D. M., Mangino, M., Freathy, R. M., Perry, J. R., Stevens, S., Hall, A. S., et al. (2008). Genome-wide association analysis identifies 20 loci that influence adult height. *Nature Genetics 40*(5): 575–583.

Wei, J. & Hemmings, G. P. (2000). The NOTCH4 locus is associated with susceptibility to schizophrenia. *Nature Genetics 25*(4): 376–377.

Weiss, L. A., Shen, Y., Korn, J. M., Arking, D. E., Miller, D. T., Fossdal, R., Saemundsen, E., Stefansson, H., Ferreira, M. A., Green, T., et al. (2008). Association between microdeletion and microduplication at 16p11.2 and autism. *New England Journal of Medicine 358*(7): 667–675.

Worden, F. G., Childs, B., Matthysse, S., & Gershon, E. S. (1976). Frontiers of psychiatric genetics. *Neuroscience Research Program Bulletin 14*(1): 8–86.

Wray, N. R., Goddard, M. E., & Visscher, P. M. (2007). Prediction of individual genetic risk to disease from genome-wide association studies. *Genome Research 17*(10): 1520–1528.

WTCCC. (2007). Wellcome Trust Case Control Consortium: Genome-wide association study of 14,000 cases of seven common diseases and 3,000 shared controls. *Nature 447*(7145): 661–678.

Yang, J., Visscher, P. M., & Wray, N. R. (2009). Sporadic cases are the norm for complex disease. *European Journal of Human Genetics 18*: 1039–1043.

Zeggini, E., Scott, L. J., Saxena, R., Voight, B. F., Marchini, J. L., Hu, T., de Bakker, P. I., Abecasis, G. R., Almgren, P., Andersen, G., et al. (2008). Meta-analysis of genome-wide association data and large-scale replication identifies additional susceptibility loci for type 2 diabetes. *Nature Genetics 40*(5): 638–645.

Zweier, C., de Jong, E. K., Zweier, M., Orrico, A., Ousager, L. B., Collins, A. L., Bijlsma, E. K., Oortveld, M. A., Ekici, A. B., Reis, A., et al. (2009). CNTNAP2 and NRXN1 are mutated in autosomal-recessive Pitt-Hopkins-like mental retardation and determine the level of a common synaptic protein in drosophila. *American Journal of Human Genetics* 85(5): 655–666.

CHAPTER 8

GENETIC ARCHITECTURE OF SCHIZOPHRENIA
The Contribution of Copy Number Variation

MARIA KARAYIORGOU, REBECCA J. LEVY, AND BIN XU

KEY CONCEPTS

- Rare mutations are an integral component of the genetic architecture of schizophrenia and account for a large portion of the genetic heterogeneity of the disease.
- Copy number variants (CNVs, defined as deletions or duplications larger than 1 kb) are one of the most intriguing types of variation in the human genome, the extent of which was previously unappreciated.
- Rare CNVs are important components and sources of genetic heterogeneity in the etiology of schizophrenia.
- The 22q11.2 microdeletion is the prototype rare but recurrent schizophrenia-associated CNV and one of the best known genetic risk factors for schizophrenia.
- Schizophrenia-associated rare CNVs affect a number of candidate genes involved in neural structure and function.

Schizophrenia is a devastating neuropsychiatric disorder with a lifetime prevalence of about 1% in most studied populations. It is characterized by positive psychotic symptoms such as hallucinations, delusions, and disorganized behavior; negative symptoms such as social withdrawal and apathy; and impaired cognition. Early onset, poor response to medication, frequent relapse, and chronic course impose a considerable burden on sufferers, their families, and society. Genetic epidemiology studies in schizophrenia have revealed a heritability of about 80% (Sullivan, Kendler, & Neale, 2003). However, identification of genetic risk factors for schizophrenia has been elusive despite decades of research in the etiology of the disease.

Genetic Architecture of Psychiatric Disorders

Psychiatric disorders, like other common diseases, are multifactorial in nature and have complex genetic etiologies. The genetic architecture underlying disease susceptibility is characterized by both the frequency and the penetrance of risk alleles (figure 8.1). The common disease-common allele (CDCA) hypothesis emphasizes the importance of relatively common alleles, each of small effect, acting together to increase disease risk. The common disease-rare allele (CDRA) hypothesis conversely emphasizes the impact of individually rare yet highly penetrant alleles. It is likely that both common and rare alleles contribute to the risk of psychiatric disorders, although the relative impact of each remains unknown.

Modern association studies based on the CDCA hypothesis exploit ancestral genetic variants that are now common (> 5% minor allele frequency) in the population. These studies can focus on candidate genes based on a priori functional evidence or identify candidates in an unbiased manner using genomewide association studies (GWAS) (Altshuler, Daly, & Lander, 2008). Nearly 800 candidate genes have been investigated for association with schizophrenia by more than 1,400 studies (see www.szgene.org). Although many of these are considered strong susceptibility genes, none have unequivocal statistical support (Karayiorgou

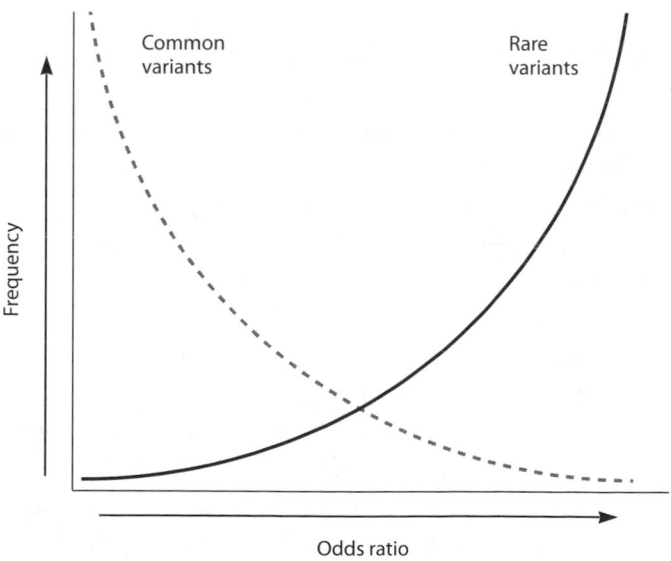

Figure 8.1. Genetic architecture of schizophrenia.
Genetic variants that are relatively common in the population (> 5%) have minimal impact on disease risk and low odds ratios (OR). In contrast, rare genetic variants (<1%) have a more substantial impact on disease risk and a high OR. (Source: Modified from Xu et al. [2009].)

& Gogos, 2006; Sanders et al., 2008; Goldstein, 2009). In addition, unbiased GWAS of psychiatric disorders have identified candidate loci for schizophrenia, as well as bipolar disorder and autism (Ferreira et al., 2008; O'Donovan et al., 2008; Wang et al., 2009). These loci await confirmation in larger-scale studies. It is interesting to note that these loci do not include any top candidate genes, such as *Neuregulin 1* or *Dysbindin*.

The CDRA hypothesis did not receive much traction until recently, primarily because of the rarity of families afflicted with psychiatric disorders in a strictly Mendelian fashion. Taking into account variable penetrance and de novo occurrences, however, one sees that rare alleles may contribute substantially to both familial and sporadic cases (Bodmer & Bonilla, 2008; ISC, 2008; Xu et al., 2008). It is not surprising that the alleles with the strongest statistical support for association with schizophrenia are rare, highly penetrant structural mutations. Identification of rare alleles in families traditionally relied on linkage studies because that approach was successful in locating rare mutations in Mendelian inherited diseases. Unfortunately, linkage studies have been less conclusive for complex conditions such as psychiatric disorders. Ironically, although the limited success of linkage studies inspired the use of GWAS for identifying common risk alleles, it was the "unexpected" use of GWAS data for copy number variation detection that, as explained in the next section, provided the strongest supporting evidence to date for the "rare variant" hypothesis.

Copy Number Variation in the Human Genome

Recently, the rapid development of new whole-genome scanning technologies has started to fill the resolution gap between the traditional cytogenetic analysis (> 2 Mb) and mutation analysis by DNA sequencing (< 1 kb). As a result, a large amount of previously undetected variation has been revealed in the human genome. One of the most intriguing types of variation, the extent of which was previously unappreciated, is copy number variation, defined as deletions or duplications larger than 1 kb.

In one of the first attempts to evaluate the prevalence of CNVs in the general population, Iafrate and colleagues used bacterial artificial chromosome probe-based array–comparative genomic hybridization (BAC-CGH) with a resolution of 1 Mb on 55 individuals, some of whom had known chromosomal abnormalities that served as an internal control of the array's sensitivity (Iafrate et al., 2004). The scan discovered 255 CNVs beyond the known abnormalities, of which about 10% had a greater than 10% prevalence. CNV location was significantly associated with segmental duplications (i.e., long segments of DNA with near-identical sequence). Independently, Sebat et al. (2004) developed another CGH system called *representational oligonucleotide microarray analysis* (ROMA) with an estimated resolution of 35 kb to investigate the extent of variation among normal individuals. In 20 normal individuals, they identified 221 CNVs in total, of which 76 were unique (Sebat et al., 2004). In line with the Iafrate et al. study, CNV locations were significantly associated with segmental duplication, suggesting a possible mechanism underlying these rearrangements. In a subsequent study of 270 controls from the HapMap sample, Redon et al. determined that CNVs cover approximately 12% of the genome in the general population (Redon et al., 2006) and encompass more nucleotide content per genome than single nucleotide polymorphisms (SNPs), highlighting their importance in contributing to total genetic variation. Overall, these and other studies unambiguously demonstrated that variation in copy number is a common source of genetic heterogeneity in the general population and that array-based CNV detection methods can be successful in discovering this type of genetic variation in the human genome.

Copy Number Variation and Schizophrenia

The 22q11.2 Microdeletion and Susceptibility to Schizophrenia

A microdeletion of 22q11.2 was the first CNV described in schizophrenia (Karayiorgou et al., 1995). Since its discovery 15 years ago, a strong and specific relationship has been established between the presence of the 22q11.2 microdeletion and psychosis in schizophrenia or schizoaffective disorder (Karayiorgou et al., 1995; Xu et al., 2008). During late adolescence and early adulthood, up to one-third of all individuals carrying this deletion develop schizophrenia or schizoaffective disorder (Pulver et al., 1994; Murphy, Jones, & Owen, 1999; Gothelf et al., 2007). A number of studies have indicated that 22q11.2 deletion syndrome (22q11DS) accounts for up to 1–2% of schizophrenia cases (Karayiorgou et al., 1995; Xu et al., 2008; ISC, 2008; Stefansson et al., 2008) and represents to date the only confirmed recurrent structural mutation responsible for introducing sporadic cases of schizophrenia into the population. This strong bidirectional association between schizophrenia and the 22q11.2 microdeletion makes this deletion one of the risk factors of greatest effect on schizophrenia, with a greater risk conferred only by being the child of two parents with schizophrenia or the monozygotic co-twin of an affected individual. Significantly, there are no major clinical differences in the core schizophrenia phenotype between individuals with schizophrenia that are 22q11.2 microdeletion carriers and those who are not (Bassett et al., 1998; Bassett et al., 2003). Moreover, many of these individuals have no obvious congenital abnormalities, and most do not have serious intellectual disabilities, making them indistinguishable from other schizophrenia patients recruited into research samples. The structural and neurocognitive anomalies that distinguish the 22q11.2 carriers who develop schizophrenia from those who do not remain unknown.

Preliminary results from a number of underpowered cross-sectional studies suggest that distinguishing features are consistent with those most consistently reported for general schizophrenia. These include larger lateral and third ventricles; generalized decreases in gray and white matter volumes, especially in frontal and temporal lobes (Chow et al., 2002; van Amelsvoort et al., 2004a); and a number of cognitive impairments that may reflect differences in the development and function of frontal brain regions (van Amelsvoort et al., 2004b; Chow et al., 2006).

Recent Copy Number Variant Discoveries in Schizophrenia

The original finding at the 22q11.2 locus raised an interesting and important question of whether the role of CNVs in the genetic makeup of complex psychiatric disorders is more widespread. Owing to rapid developments in high-density microarray technologies designed to screen for structural variants across the whole human genome and advances in statistical analysis methods, several groups in rapid succession provided evidence that rare CNVs contribute to the genetic etiology of schizophrenia and autism.

A 30 kb resolution SNP array of 359 schizophrenia and control trios (a total of 1,077 individuals) determined that de novo CNVs are significantly more common in sporadic cases than controls (10% as opposed to 1.3%) (Xu et al., 2008). Inherited rare CNVs were 1.5 times more common in sporadic cases than in controls, representing a smaller but significant increase (from 20% to 30%). Comparison of the genes affected by de novo CNVs demonstrated enrichment of neural development and RNA processing pathways. Rare inherited CNVs were also shown to be associated with familial schizophrenia. Xu et al. (2009) showed that rare inherited CNVs are almost twice as common in familial cases of schizophrenia as in sporadic cases or controls. This discovery resulted from comparing the results of a high-resolution SNP array scan on 48 schizophrenia probands plus their parents and affected relatives to those of a scan on more than 300 controls and sporadic cases, followed by validation using independent approaches. Nine of 12 families with inherited CNVs showed evidence of CNV cosegregation. The familial cases were 2.7 times more likely than controls to have genic CNVs (CNVs overlapping at least one gene, either partly or in its entirety), but there was no enrichment of de novo CNVs. These findings provided strong empirical evidence supporting the notion that multiple genetic variants, including individually rare ones that affect many different genes, contribute to the genetic risk of schizophrenia. They also highlighted some important differences in the genetic architecture of familial and nonfamilial forms of the disease: although the overall frequency of carriers of all rare structural variants is the same between the familial and sporadic cases (approximately 40%), the type of variants is markedly different. Sporadic schizophrenia is characterized by a marked enrichment of rare *new* mutations and only a modest increase in the rate of rare *inherited* CNVs, which do not appear to affect genes preferentially. By contrast, familial schizophrenia is characterized by enrichment in rare *inherited* genic CNVs (predicted to have higher penetrance), whereas *new* mutations are less prominent.

Two case-control studies that did not distinguish between familial and sporadic cases also provided evidence for a collective enrichment of rare CNVs in schizophrenia. Walsh and colleagues used ROMA on 150 individuals with schizophrenia plus controls followed by SNP-based validation and refinement (Walsh et al., 2008). They reported a significant threefold increase in rare, genic CNVs among case subjects (15% as opposed to 5%) and a fourfold increase among early-onset case subjects as opposed to controls (20% to 5%). In an independent trio sample of 83 early-onset cases, three assays for CNVs determined that rare, genic CNVs were present in 28% of cases, whereas they were present in 13% of nontransmitted parental chromosomes—a significant enrichment. The affected genes in case subjects were significantly enriched for pathways in brain development and neural function, including genes such as *ERBB4* and *Neurexin1* (*NRXN1*). Another study by the International Schizophrenia Consortium analyzed 3,391 individuals with schizophrenia and controls using SNP genotype arrays to identify CNVs greater than 100 kb (ISC, 2008). When rare (less than 1% frequency) CNVs were considered, individuals with schizophrenia had 1.15 times as many controls and 1.41 times as many genes affected by CNVs. This study confirmed that deletions in 22q11.2 were significantly associated with schizophrenia, and it identified two additional CNVs at 15q13.3 and 1q21.1 that were significantly enriched among case subjects.

Stefansson et al. (2008) provided additional evidence for a role of CNVs in schizophrenia, taking a two-step strategy. First, they identified 66 de novo CNVs in over 7,500 control European and Chinese trios and pairs (Stefansson et al., 2008). Next, they checked for associations between these 66 mutations and schizophrenia in 1,433 SGENE (Schizophrenia GENE) consortium cases and more than 33,000 controls. Three deletions at 1q21.1, 15q11.2, and 15q13.3 were nominally enriched in individuals with schizophrenia or psychosis, two of which were also reported in the ISC scan (see the previous discussion earlier in this section; ISC, 2008). On association analysis in 3,285 additional cases and 7,951 controls, all three CNVs (but not SNPs within the regions) were significantly associated with psychosis with high odds ratios. However, only 1q21.1 was significantly associated with a strict definition of schizophrenia. Several other lower-scale studies tried to assess the relevance of rare CNVs to the etiology of schizophrenia. A BAC-CGH scan of 93 Bulgarian schizophrenia trios followed by SNP array verification identified 13 rare CNVs in case subjects; these were not found in controls or the CNV database (Kirov et al., 2008). The most interesting findings were a deletion at 2p16.3 involving *Neurexin1*, carried by affected siblings and their unaffected mother; a de novo duplication at 15q13.1; and a deletion at 16p12.2 inherited from a parent who suffers from an affective disorder. Another analysis of 54 Dutch cases with a SNP array demonstrated CNVs affecting four candidate genes: *MYT1L*, *CTNND2*, *ASTN2*, and *NRXN1* (Vrijenhoek et al., 2008). On screening 752 additional cases and 706 controls for CNVs affecting these four genes, CNVs in *MYT1L*, *ASTN2*, and *NRXN1* were found only in case subjects. A study with 471 affected individuals from the United Kingdom using a SNP array and CGH validation determined that CNVs with frequency less than 1% and length greater than 1 Mb were 2.26 times more frequent in case subjects than in controls (Kirov et al., 2009). Four regions demonstrated significant association with broad schizophrenia diagnosis upon a preliminary meta-analysis of the Stefansson et al. and ISC studies: 17p12, 1q21.1, 15q11.2, and 15q13.3. Ingason et al. (2009) examined 4,345 schizophrenia patients and 35,079 controls from eight European populations for duplications and deletions at the 16p13.1 locus, using microarray data. They found a threefold excess of duplications and deletions in schizophrenia cases as opposed to controls, with duplications present in 0.30% of cases versus 0.09% of controls and deletions in 0.12% of cases and 0.04% of controls. The implicated region could be divided into three intervals defined by flanking repeats. Duplications spanning the first and second intervals showed the most significant association with schizophrenia. Notably, in a single Icelandic family, a duplication spanning these intervals was present in two cases of schizophrenia as well as in individual cases of alcoholism, attention deficit hyperactivity disorder, and dyslexia. Finally, recurrent microdeletions and microduplications of a 600 kb genomic region at an adjacent chromosomal locus (16p11.2) have been implicated in childhood-onset developmental disorders. McCarthy et al. (2009) reported an association between 16p11.2 microduplications and schizophrenia in two large cohorts. The microduplication was detected in 0.63% of cases and 0.03% of controls from the initial cohort, and in 0.34% of cases and 0.04% of controls from the replication cohort, resulting in a 14.5-fold enrichment in the combined sample.

Overall, these studies suggest that rare structural rearrangements collectively contribute to schizophrenia risk. Thus, rare CNVs represent an important source of genetic heterogeneity in the etiology of complex psychiatric diseases such as schizophrenia.

Determining the Pathogenic Nature of CNVs and Affected Genes

The identification of CNVs as an important source of variation in the human genome and the connection between rare CNVs and psychiatric disorders raises the question of how to distinguish abnormal structural mutations from neutral polymorphisms and establish a causal relationship between pathogenic CNVs and their corresponding phenotypes. Establishing causality may be easier for recurrent CNVs if a sufficient number of patients is available. In such cases, establishing a bidirectional association between CNVs and disease along the lines described here for the 22q11.2DS is important to strengthen causality and facilitate development of diagnostic assays. Specifically, in addition to enrichment among cases, unambiguous association between a CNV and schizophrenia requires demonstration of relatively high penetrance among CNV carriers (higher than the baseline rate of psychosis in mental retardation), as well as meeting full diagnostic criteria indistinguishable from those of individuals with schizophrenia that are not CNV carriers.

Establishing causality is harder for private CNVs found in only a single individual, which represent the majority of CNVs described to date in patient cohorts. In such cases, determining a possible causal connection between a specific CNV locus and a disease phenotype depends on a number of factors. For example, a rare de novo CNV is more likely to be pathogenic than a CNV inherited by an unaffected parent. For inherited CNVs, cosegregation with disease is a strong indicator of causal connection between disease and the CNV. In particular, the observation that all affected members of a family carry a rare CNV is a strong indication of pathogenicity. (It is not detrimental if unaffected members also carry it if there is incomplete penetrance.) The issue of whether a potentially pathogenic CNV segregates to all affected members within a family has not received much attention in the current literature, which is heavily based on case-control studies. This is a source of concern, as it may lead to false findings. Finally, CNVs that affect the coding region or the splicing pattern of a given gene are more likely to be pathogenic than, for example, intronic or intergenic CNVs. Overall, support for a pathogenic role can be offered by the location of a CNV in a given gene as well as by observation of recurrent incidence of independent CNVs in more than one exon of the same gene or members of the same gene family.

Help toward establishing causality may be provided by reference CNV maps across the whole genome and by online databases that are being established. The Database of Genomic Variants (DGV) (see http://projects.tcag.ca/variation) is such an accumulation of data, which as of this writing holds reports on over 8,400 CNV loci. It also provides public access to the Genome Structural Variation Consortium results from high-resolution CNV scans on 40 individuals with European or African ancestry. By offering a compendium of current findings, this database is especially valuable to determine whether newly discovered CNVs are unique to one's case population or found at relatively high frequency among controls in prior reports. However, because the CNV annotations in this database are generated by different labs, which often use different platforms and analysis algorithms, the false positive detection rate, CNV frequency, CNV size, and CNV breakpoints might vary, and all these could affect the final outcomes when used to establish a causal relation between CNVs and disease phenotypes. Another database, the Wellcome Trust Case-Control Consortium (WTCCC) (see www.wtccc.org.uk), is a collaborative effort among 50 groups in the United Kingdom, originally used to accumulate SNP genotype information across a variety of diseases for over 17,000 individuals. As this information can also be used to identify CNVs, it represents an important collection for genomic rearrangements. More recently, Conrad et al. provided a population-based CNV map by using a tiling oligonucleotide microarray of 42 million probes on 800 individuals from different ethnic groups (Conrad et al., 2010). Another recently launched international research effort, the 1000 Genomes Project, aims to establish a complete and detailed catalogue of human genetic variations, which in turn can be used for association studies relating genetic variation to disease. Once accomplished, the project will provide a map with more than 95% of the variants (e.g., SNPs, CNVs, insertions or deletions), as well as minor allele frequencies as low as 1% across the genome and 0.1–0.5% in gene regions and a high-resolution reference map for future CNV-based association studies.

Besides these reference CNV maps, several databases have also been established to collect pathogenic CNVs observed in various diseases: the Database of Chromosomal Imbalance and Phenotype in Human using Ensemble Resources (DECIPHER), the Chromosome Abnormality Database (CAD), the Mendelian Cytogenetics Network Online Database, and the European Cytogeneticists Association Register of Unbalanced Chromosome Aberrations (ECARUCA). The accumulation of recurrent CNVs in certain phenotypes will provide information on the potential connections between related diseases and might help dissect some aspects of psychiatric diseases by establishing the causal connection between intermediate phenotypes and underlying molecular mechanisms.

In addition to the challenges in establishing causality between CNVs and psychiatric diseases, accumulating evidence points toward the difficulty in pinpointing causal relationships between a specific gene or genes affected by CNVs and disease phenotypes. Even though the methods for CNV discovery are relatively well developed, a remaining problem is how to determine the exact boundaries of CNVs identified in both control populations and patient genomes. Without precise information on CNV boundaries, in many cases it might be very difficult to refine the candidate regions and determine the affected genes. High-density arrays and deep sequencing technology now provide improved resolution to fully determine the CNV boundaries in a high-throughput fashion. This technical issue notwithstanding, there are at least two ways in which the removal or duplication of genes from a region deleted or duplicated by a CNV could be acting: (1) a single dosage-sensitive gene may exert a major effect, or (2) the CNV-associated neurobehavioral phenotypes may stem from the cumulative effect of a number of gene products, acting either additively or synergistically. According to the latter model, although one or a few loci may have a greater phenotypic impact, it is the cumulative effect of the imbalance of several genes within the CNV that determines the overall phenotype. This scenario is likely to complicate gene identification efforts using traditional human genetic approaches.

Candidate Risk Genes Within Copy Number Variants

Although no large-scale systematic meta-analysis exists of the several genomewide screens to identify schizophrenia-associated CNVs, there are recurrent CNV reports as well as results from preliminary meta-analyses of a subset of the studies that have been conducted to date (Itsara et al., 2009; Kirov et al., 2009), which are summarized in table 8.1. These recurrent CNVs as well as other, rarer CNVs cover many potential candidate genes involved in neural structure and function (table 8.2).

The 22q11.2 deletion locus contains approximately 30 genes. Some potential candidates including *COMT, PRODH, ZDHH8, DGCR8,* and *TBX1* are already under investigation, and several behavioral and neuronal deficits have been associated with these genes in their respective animal models (Paterlini et al., 2005; Paylor et al., 2006; Mukai et al., 2008; Stark et al., 2008).

Another interesting candidate gene is Neurexin1 (*NRXN1*), which was identified as disrupted by CNVs at 2p16.3 in several recent genomewide array scans of schizophrenia cohorts. A targeted screen of all three Neurexin genes in 2,977 schizophrenia patients and 33,746 controls from seven European populations did not identify CNVs affecting *NRXN2* or *NRXN3* but described a significant

Table 8.1 Loci Overlapping in CNV Reports

Locus of Interest	Study	Candidate Genes
1q21.1	ISC, 2008; Stefansson et al., 2008; Kirov et al., 2009	*GJP8*
2p16.3	Kirov et al., 2008; Walsh et al., 2008; ISC, 2008; Vrijenhoek et al., 2008; Rujescu et al., 2009	*NRXN1*
15q11.2	Stefansson et al., 2008; Kirov et al., 2009	*CYFIP1*
15q13.1-q13.3	ISC, 2008; Stefansson et al., 2008; Kirov et al., 2008; Kirov et al., 2009	*CHRNA7, APBA2, NDNL2, TJP1*
17p12	Kirov et al., 2009	*PMP22*
16p11.2	Walsh et al., 2008; McCarthy et al., 2009	*MAPK3, DOC2A, SEZ6L2*
16p12.2-p12.1	Kirov et al., 2008; ISC, 2008	*EEF2K, CDR2*
16p12.4-p13.1	Kirov et al., 2009; Ingason et al., 2009	*NDE1, NXPH2, NTAN1*
22q11.2	Xu et al., 2008; ISC, 2008; Stefansson et al., 2008	*DGCR8, ZDHHC8, PRODH, COMT, TBX1*

SOURCE: Authors.

Table 8.2 Candidate Genes from CNV Reports

Study	Genes of Interest	Pathways of Interest
Walsh et al., 2008	ERBB4, NRXN1, SLC1A3, GRM7, PRKCD, SKP2, MAGI2, CAV1, PRKAG2, PTK2, DLG2, LAMA1, PTPRM	Cell adhesion, glutamate receptors, cell cycle, cell growth and extension
Kirov et al., 2008	NRXN1, APBA2, NDNL2, TJP1, EEF2K, CDR2	Cell adhesion, amyloid processing, calmodulin signaling
ISC, 2008	CHRNA7, NRXN1, CNTNAP2, NOTCH1, PAK7, GJA8	Cell adhesion, gap junctions, acetylcholine receptors
Xu et al., 2008	RAPGEF6, EphB1, DICER1	Cell signaling, Ephrin signaling, RNA processing
Stefansson et al., 2008	GJA8, CYFIP1, CHRNA7	Gap junctions, translation, acetylcholine receptors
Vrijenhoek et al., 2008	NRXN1, MYT1L, ASTN2	Cell or synaptic adhesion
Kirov et al., 2009	PMP22, NDE1, NXPH2, GJA8, CYFIP1, CHRNA7	Myelin sheath, cell adhesion
Xu et al., 2009	NRG3, RAPGEF2, PEX13, KIAA1841, AHSA2, USP34, C4orf45, PTPRN2, CSMD1, MACROD2, A26B3, LOC441956	Neural differentiation, peroxisomal targeting, ubiquitination
Ingason et al., 2009	NTAN1, NDE1	DISC1 signaling, neuronal proliferation, memory regulation

SOURCE: Authors.

association with schizophrenia and CNVs that disrupt exons of *NRXN1* (Rujescu et al., 2009). Because *NRXN1* is a cell-surface receptor involved in the formation of synaptic contacts in the central nervous system, it could have widespread effects on brain structure and connectivity (Reissner et al., 2008). It is interesting that Contactin-associated protein 2 (*CNTNAP2* or *CASPR2*) at 7q35, another member of the Neurexin family, was recently reported to be deleted in cases of schizophrenia (Friedman et al., 2008). *CNTNAP2* has also been reported as a genetic susceptibility factor in autism in CNV, linkage, and association studies (Alarcon et al., 2008; Arking et al., 2008; Bakkaloglu et al., 2008; Rossi et al., 2008). Deficits in *CNTNAP2* have also been associated with other psychiatric conditions, including Tourette's syndrome, obsessive-compulsive disorder, mental retardation (Verkerk et al., 2003), epilepsy (Strauss et al., 2006), and typical specific language impairment in children (Vernes et al., 2008). In the peripheral nervous system, CNTNAP2 regulates potassium channel clustering near nodes of Ranvier (Poliak & Peles, 2003). More recently, Abrahams et al. (2007) investigated the potential function of CNTNAP2 in the superior temporal gyrus and cerebral cortex in midgestation human fetal brains by using gene profiling and followed by selective in situ hybridization. Their results suggested that human CNTNAP2 expression was enriched in circuits involved in higher cortical functions, including language. The functional implication of CNTNAP2 in the central nervous system and recurrence of the deficits in schizophrenia, autism, and other psychiatric conditions make it a very interesting candidate.

Several genes involved in neural function were affected by CNVs in the Xu et al. studies (Xu et al., 2008; Xu et al., 2009). Notably, two members of the RAP-GEF family, *RAPGEF2* and *RAPGEF 6*, were affected by independent CNVs (Xu et al., 2008; Xu et al., 2009). This gene family is implicated in neuronal migration and arborization. Additional CNVs affected Neuregulin-3 (*NRG3*) (Xu et al., 2009) and *EphB1* (Xu et al., 2008) a receptor for ephrin, which participates in axon guidance.

Another interesting set of candidates is related to microRNA biogenesis and microRNA-mediated translation control. Besides *DGCR8* within 22q11DS, one of the top candidate genes within the 15q11.2 CNV region is *CYFIP1*, which binds the fragile X mental retardation protein FMRP1 and translation initiation factor eIF4E (Napoli et al., 2008). Both FMRP1 and eIF4E have been implicated in microRNA-mediated translational control machinery (Jin et al., 2004; Pillai et al., 2005). More interesting, DICER1, another microRNA processing enzyme, has also been shown to be affected by a de novo CNV at 14q32 (Xu et al., 2008).

Three studies reported schizophrenia-associated CNVs in 16p11.2-p13.1, which is a locus previously associated with autism, bipolar disorder, and mental retardation. Possible candidate genes in this region include *NDE1*, which binds *DISC1*, a well-known schizophrenia susceptibility gene; *NXPH2*, which binds Neurexins; *EEF2K*, a key kinase downstream of calmodulin; and *CDR2*, which is a target of autoantibodies in cerebellar diseases. A 17p12 deletion was found in four of five affected family members in the Kirov et al. study, as well as two other schizophrenia cases without neurologic symptoms (Mizuguchi et al., 2008; Kunugi et al., 2008; Kirov et al., 2009). This locus contains peripheral myelin protein 22 (*PMP22*), which causes Charcot-Marie-Tooth Syndrome, a hereditary neuropathy. Finally, 1q21.1 is a region previously reported to be deleted in cases of mental retardation and autism; one interesting candidate gene within this region is gap junction protein alpha 8/connexin50, which is associated with cataracts and corneal abnormalities.

In addition to the genes discussed here, there are several excellent candidate genes located within rarer CNVs (table 8.2) implicating a number of biological pathways, including glutamate, dopamine, and acetylcholine signaling pathways, as well as aspects of cell-cell and cell-matrix adhesion and signaling. Additionally, CNV disrupted loci may contain regulatory elements, transcription factors, or microRNAs that affect genes at a distance; thus, the known genes may not represent the full extent of the genetic information affected by these genomic rearrangements.

KEY AREAS FOR FUTURE RESEARCH

- Establish an unambiguous bidirectional association between candidate pathogenic CNVs (table 8.1) and schizophrenia according to criteria previously applied to the 22q11.2 microdeletions.
- Use larger-scale and higher-resolution scans for CNVs, with an emphasis on family-based studies.
- Identify "culprit" genes among the ones affected by CNVs.
- Identify genetic and environmental factors that determine CNV-associated disease penetrance.
- Understand the impact of pathogenic CNVs on brain structure and function through studies in patients as well as through the generation of animal models.

Selected Readings

Cirulli, E. T. & Goldstein, D. B. (2010). Uncovering the roles of rare variants in common disease through whole-genome sequencing. *Nature Reviews Genetics* 11(6): 415–425.

Goldstein, D. B. (2009). Common genetic variation and human traits. *New England Journal of Medicine* 360(17): 1696–1698.

ISC. (2008). Rare chromosomal deletions and duplications increase risk of schizophrenia. *Nature* 455(7210): 237–241.

Karayiorgou, M., Simon, T. J., & Gogos, J. A. (2010). 22q11.2 microdeletions: Linking DNA structural variation to brain dysfunction and schizophrenia. *Nature Reviews Neuroscience* 11(6): 402–416.

Redon, R., Ishikawa, S., Fitch, K. R., Feuk, L., Perry, G. H., Andrews, T. D., Fiegler, H., Shapero, M. H., Carson, A. R., Chen, W., et al. (2006). Global variation in copy number in the human genome. *Nature* 444(7118): 444–454.

Sebat, J., Lakshmi, B., Troge, J., Alexander, J., Young, J., Lundin, P., Maner, S., Massa, H., Walker, M., Chi, M., et al. (2004). Large-scale copy number polymorphism in the human genome. *Science* 305(5683): 525–528.

Xu, B., Roos, J. L., Levy, S., van Rensburg, E. J., Gogos, J. A., & Karayiorgou, M. (2008). Strong association of de novo copy number mutations with sporadic schizophrenia. *Nature Genetics* 40(7): 880–885.

References

Abrahams, B. S., Tentler, D., Perederiy, J. V., Oldham, M. C., Coppola, G., & Geschwind, D. H. (2007). Genome-wide analyses of human perisylvian cerebral cortical patterning. *Proceedings of the National Academy of Sciences U.S.A.* 104(45): 17849–17854.

Alarcon, M., Abrahams, B. S., Stone, J. L., Duvall, J. A., Perederiy, J. V., Bomar, J. M., Sebat, J., Wigler, M., Martin, C. L., Ledbetter, D. H., et al. (2008). Linkage, association, and gene-expression analyses identify CNTNAP2 as an autism-susceptibility gene. *American Journal of Human Genetics* 82(1): 150–159.

Altshuler, D., Daly, M. J., & Lander, E. S. (2008). Genetic mapping in human disease. *Science* 322(5903): 881–888.

Arking, D. E., Cutler, D. J., Brune, C. W., Teslovich, T. M., West, K., Ikeda, M., Rea, A., Guy, M., Lin, S., Cook, E. H., et al. (2008). A common genetic variant in the Neurexin superfamily member CNTNAP2 increases familial risk of autism. *American Journal of Human Genetics* 82(1): 160–164.

Bakkaloglu, B., O'Roak, B. J., Louvi, A., Gupta, A. R., Abelson, J. F., Morgan, T. M., Chawarska, K., Klin, A., Ercan-Sencicek, A. G., Stillman, A. A., et al. (2008). Molecular cytogenetic analysis and resequencing of Contactin associated protein-like 2 in autism spectrum disorders. *American Journal of Human Genetics* 82(1): 165–173.

Bassett, A. S., Chow, E. W., AbdelMalik, P., Gheorghiu, M., Husted, J., & Weksberg, R. (2003). The schizophrenia phenotype in 22q11 deletion syndrome. *American Journal of Psychiatry* 160(9): 1580–1586.

Bassett, A. S., Hodgkinson, K., Chow, E. W., Correia, S., Scutt, L. E., & Weksberg, R. (1998). 22q11 deletion syndrome in adults with schizophrenia. *American Journal of Medical Genetics* 81(4): 328–337.

Bodmer, W. & Bonilla, C. (2008). Common and rare variants in multifactorial susceptibility to common diseases. *Nature Genetics* 40(6): 695–701.

Chow, E. W., Watson, M., Young, D. A., & Bassett, A. S. (2006). Neurocognitive profile in 22q11 deletion syndrome and schizophrenia. *Schizophrenia Research* 87(1–3): 270–278.

Chow, E. W., Zipursky, R. B., Mikulis, D. J., & Bassett, A. S. (2002). Structural brain abnormalities in patients with schizophrenia and 22q11 deletion syndrome. *Biological Psychiatry* 51(3): 208–215.

Conrad, D. F., Pinto, D., Redon, R., Feuk, L., Gokcumen, O., Zhang, Y., Aerts, J., Andrews, T. D., Barnes, C., Campbell, P., et al. (2010). Origins and functional impact of copy number variation in the human genome. *Nature* 464(7289): 704–712.

Ferreira, M. A., O'Donovan, M. C., Meng, Y. A., Jones, I. R., Ruderfer, D. M., Jones, L., Fan, J., Kirov, G., Perlis, R. H., Green, E. K., et al. (2008). Collaborative genome-wide association analysis supports a role for ANK3 and CACNA1C in bipolar disorder. *Nature Genetics* 40(9): 1056–1058.

Friedman, J. I., Vrijenhoek, T., Markx, S., Janssen, I. M., van der Vliet, W. A., Faas, B. H., Knoers, N. V., Cahn, W., Kahn, R. S., Edelmann, L., et al. (2008). CNTNAP2 gene dosage variation is associated with schizophrenia and epilepsy. *Molecular Psychiatry* 13(3): 261–266.

Goldstein, D. B. (2009). Common genetic variation and human traits. *New England Journal of Medicine* 360(17): 1696–1698.

Gothelf, D., Feinstein, C., Thompson, T., Gu, E., Penniman, L., Van Stone, E., Kwon, H., Eliez, S., & Reiss, A. L. (2007). Risk factors for the emergence of psychotic disorders in adolescents with 22q11.2 deletion syndrome. *American Journal of Psychiatry* 164(4): 663–669.

Iafrate, A. J., Feuk, L., Rivera, M. N., Listewnik, M. L., Donahoe, P. K., Qi, Y., Scherer, S. W., & Lee, C. (2004). Detection of large-scale variation in the human genome. *Nature Genetics* 36(9): 949–951.

Ingason, A., Rujescu, D., Cichon, S., Sigurdsson, E., Sigmundsson, T., Pietilainen, O. P., Buizer-Voskamp, J. E., Strengman, E., Francks, C., Muglia, P., et al. (2009). Copy number variations of chromosome 16p13.1 region associated with schizophrenia. *Molecular Psychiatry* 16(1): 17–25.

ISC. (2008). Rare chromosomal deletions and duplications increase risk of schizophrenia. *Nature* 455(7210): 237–241.

Itsara, A., Cooper, G. M., Baker, C., Girirajan, S., Li, J., Absher, D., Krauss, R. M., Myers, R. M., Ridker, P. M., Chasman, D. I., et al. (2009). Population analysis of large copy number variants and hotspots of human genetic disease. *American Journal of Human Genetics* 84(2): 148–161.

Jin, P., Zarnescu, D. C., Ceman, S., Nakamoto, M., Mowrey, J., Jongens, T. A., Nelson, D. L., Moses, K., & Warren, S. T. (2004). Biochemical and genetic interaction between the fragile X mental retardation protein and the microRNA pathway. *Nature Neuroscience* 7(2): 113–117.

Karayiorgou, M. & Gogos, J.A. (2006). Schizophrenia genetics: Uncovering positional candidate genes. *European Journal of Human Genetics* 14(5): 512–519.

Karayiorgou, M., Morris, M. A., Morrow, B., Shprintzen, R. J., Goldberg, R., Borrow, J., Gos, A., Nestadt, G., Wolyniec, P. S., & Lasseter, V. K. (1995). Schizophrenia susceptibility associated with interstitial deletions of chromosome 22q11. *Proceedings of the National Academy of Sciences U.S.A.* 92(17): 7612–7616.

Kirov, G., Grozeva, D., Norton, N., Ivanov, D., Mantripragada, K. K., Holmans, P., Craddock, N., Owen, M. J., & O'Donovan, M. C. (2009). Support for the involvement of large copy number variants in the pathogenesis of schizophrenia. *Human Molecular Genetics* 18(8): 1497–1503.

Kirov, G., Gumus, D., Chen, W., Norton, N., Georgieva, L., Sari, M., O'Donovan, M. C., Erdogan, F., Owen, M. J., Ropers, H. H., et al. (2008). Comparative genome hybridization suggests a role for NRXN1 and APBA2 in schizophrenia. *Human Molecular Genetics* 17(3): 458–465.

Kunugi, H., Ozeki, Y., Mizuguchi, T., Hirabayashi, N., Ogawa, M., Ohmura, N., Moriuchie, M., Haradae, N., Matsumotob, N., & Kunugi, H. (2008). A case of schizophrenia with chromosomal microdeletion of 17p11.2 containing a myelin-related gene PMP22. *Open Psychiatry Journal* 2: 1–4.

McCarthy, S. E., Makarov, V., Kirov, G., Addington, A. M., McClellan, J., Yoon, S., Perkins, D. O., Dickel, D. E., Kusenda, M., Krastoshevsky, O., et al. (2009). Microduplications of 16p11.2 are associated with schizophrenia. *Nature Genetics* 41(11): 1223–1227.

Mizuguchi, T., Hashimoto, R., Itokawa, M., Sano, A., Shimokawa, O., Yoshimura, Y., Harada, N., Miyake, N., Nishimura, A., Saitsu, H., et al. (2008). Microarray comparative genomic hybridization analysis of 59 patients with schizophrenia. *Journal of Human Genetics* 53(10): 914–919.

Mukai, J., Dhilla, A., Drew, L. J., Stark, K. L., Cao, L., MacDermott, A. B., Karayiorgou, M., & Gogos, J. A. (2008). Palmitoylation-dependent neurodevelopmental deficits in a mouse model of 22q11 microdeletion. *Nature Neuroscience* 11(11): 1302–1310.

Murphy, K. C., Jones, L. A., & Owen, M. J. (1999). High rates of schizophrenia in adults with velo-cardio-facial syndrome. *Archives of General Psychiatry* 56(10): 940–945.

Napoli, I., Mercaldo, V., Boyl, P. P., Eleuteri, B., Zalfa, F., De Rubeis, S., Di Marino, D., Mohr, E., Massimi, M., Falconi, M., et al. (2008). The fragile X syndrome protein represses activity-dependent translation through CYFIP1, a new 4E-BP. *Cell* 134(6): 1042–1054.

O'Donovan, M. C., Craddock, N., Norton, N., Williams, H., Peirce, T., Moskvina, V., Nikolov, I., Hamshere, M., Carroll, L., Georgieva, L., et al. (2008). Identification of loci associated with schizophrenia by genome-wide association and follow-up. *Nature Genetics* 40(9): 1053–1055.

Paterlini, M., Zakharenko, S. S., Lai, W. S., Qin, J., Zhang, H., Mukai, J., Westphal, K. G., Olivier, B., Sulzer, D., Pavlidis, P., et al. (2005). Transcriptional and behavioral interaction between 22q11.2 orthologs modulates schizophrenia-related phenotypes in mice. *Nature Neuroscience* 8(11): 1586–1594.

Paylor, R., Glaser, B., Mupo, A., Ataliotis, P., Spencer, C., Sobotka, A., Sparks, C., Choi, C. H., Oghalai, J., Curran, S., et al. (2006). Tbx1 haploinsufficiency is linked to behavioral disorders in mice and humans: Implications for 22q11 deletion syndrome. *Proceedings of the National Academy of Sciences U.S.A. 103*(20): 7729–7734.

Pillai, R. S., Bhattacharyya, S. N., Artus, C. G., Zoller, T., Cougot, N., Basyuk, E., Bertrand, E., & Filipowicz, W. (2005). Inhibition of translational initiation by Let-7 MicroRNA in human cells. *Science 309*(5740): 1573–1576.

Poliak, S. & Peles, E. (2003). The local differentiation of myelinated axons at nodes of Ranvier. *Nature Reviews Neuroscience 4*(12): 968–980.

Pulver, A. E., Nestadt, G., Goldberg, R., Shprintzen, R. J., Lamacz, M., Wolyniec, P. S., Morrow, B., Karayiorgou, M., Antonarakis, S. E., Housman, D., et al. (1994). Psychotic illness in patients diagnosed with velo-cardio-facial syndrome and their relatives. *Journal of Nervous Mental Disorders 182*(8): 476–478.

Redon, R., Ishikawa, S., Fitch, K. R., Feuk, L., Perry, G. H., Andrews, T. D., Fiegler, H., Shapero, M. H., Carson, A. R., Chen, W., et al. (2006). Global variation in copy number in the human genome. *Nature 444*(7118): 444–454.

Reissner, C., Klose, M., Fairless, R., & Missler, M. (2008). Mutational analysis of the Neurexin/neuroligin complex reveals essential and regulatory components. *Proceedings of the National Academy of Sciences U.S.A. 105*(39): 15124–15129.

Rossi, E., Verri, A. P., Patricelli, M. G., Destefani, V., Ricca, I., Vetro, A. Ciccone, R., Giorda, R., Toniolo, D., Maraschio, P., et al. (2008). A 12Mb deletion at 7q33–q35 associated with autism spectrum disorders and primary amenorrhea. *European Journal of Medical Genetics 51*(6): 631–638.

Rujescu, D., Ingason, A., Cichon, S., Pietilainen, O. P., Barnes, M. R., Toulopoulou, T., Picchioni, M., Vassos, E., Ettinger, U., Bramon, E., et al. (2009). Disruption of the Neurexin 1 gene is associated with schizophrenia. *Human Molecular Genetics 18*(5): 988–996.

Sanders, A. R., Duan, J., Levinson, D. F., Shi, J., He, D., Hou, C., Burrell, G. J., Rice, J. P., Nertney, D. A., Olincy, A., et al. (2008). No significant association of 14 candidate genes with schizophrenia in a large European ancestry sample: Implications for psychiatric genetics. *American Journal of Psychiatry 165*(4): 497–506.

Sebat, J., Lakshmi, B., Troge, J., Alexander, J., Young, J., Lundin, P., Maner, S., Massa, H., Walker, M., Chi, M., et al. (2004). Large-scale copy number polymorphism in the human genome. *Science 305*(5683): 525–528.

Stark, K. L., Xu, B., Bagchi, A., Lai, W. S., Liu, H., Hsu, R., Wan, X., Pavlidis, P., Mills, A. A., Karayiorgou, M., et al. (2008). Altered brain microRNA biogenesis contributes to phenotypic deficits in a 22q11-deletion mouse model. *Nature Genetics 40*(6): 751–760.

Stefansson, H., Rujescu, D., Cichon, S., Pietilainen, O. P., Ingason, A., Steinberg, S., Fossdal, R., Sigurdsson, E., Sigmundsson, T., Buizer-Voskamp, J. E., et al. (2008). Large recurrent microdeletions associated with schizophrenia. *Nature 455*(7210): 232–236.

Strauss, K. A., Puffenberger, E. G., Huentelman, M. J., Gottlieb, S., Dobrin, S. E., Parod, J. M., Stephan, D. A., & Morton, D. H. (2006). Recessive symptomatic focal epilepsy and mutant Contactin-associated protein-like 2. *New England Journal of Medicine 354*(13): 1370–1377.

Sullivan, P. F., Kendler, K. S., & Neale, M. C. (2003). Schizophrenia as a complex trait: Evidence from a meta-analysis of twin studies. *Archives of General Psychiatry 60*(12): 1187–1192.

van Amelsvoort, T., Daly, E., Henry, J., Robertson, D., Ng, V., Owen, M., Murphy, K. C., & Murphy, D. G. (2004a). Brain anatomy in adults with velocardiofacial syndrome with and without schizophrenia: Preliminary results of a structural magnetic resonance imaging study. *Archives of General Psychiatry 61*(11); 1085–1096.

van Amelsvoort, T., Henry, J., Morris, R., Owen, M., Linszen, D., Murphy, K., & Murphy, D. (2004b). Cognitive deficits associated with schizophrenia in velo-cardio-facial syndrome. *Schizophrenia Research 70*(2–3): 223–232.

Verkerk, A. J., Mathews, C. A., Joosse, M., Eussen, B. H., Heutink, P., & Oostra, B. A. (2003). CNTNAP2 is disrupted in a family with Gilles de la Tourette syndrome and obsessive compulsive disorder. *Genomics* 82(1): 1–9.

Vernes, S. C., Newbury, D. F., Abrahams, B. S., Winchester, L., Nicod, J., Groszer, M., Alarcón, M., Oliver, P. L., Davies, K. E., Geschwind, D. H., et al. (2008). A functional genetic link between distinct developmental language disorders. *New England Journal of Medicine* 359(22): 2337–2345.

Vrijenhoek, T., Buizer-Voskamp, J. E., van der Stelt, I., Strengman, E., GROUP Consortium, Sabatti, C., Geurts van Kessel, A., Brunner, H. G., Ophoff, R. A., & Veltman, J. A. (2008). Recurrent CNVs disrupt three candidate genes in schizophrenia patients. *American Journal of Human Genetics* 83(4): 504–510.

Walsh, T., McClellan, J., McCarthy, S., Addington, A., Pierce, S., Cooper, G., Nord, A., Kusenda, M., Malhotra, D., Bhandari, A., et al. (2008). Rare structural variants disrupt multiple genes in neurodevelopmental pathways in schizophrenia. *Science* 320(5875): 539–543.

Wang, K., Zhang, H., Ma, D., Bucan, M., Glessner, J. T., Abrahams, B. S., Salyakina, D., Imielinski, M., Bradfield, J. P., Sleiman, P. M. A., et al. (2009). Common genetic variants on 5p14.1 associate with autism spectrum disorders. *Nature* 459(7246): 528–533.

Xu, B., Roos, J. L., Levy, S., van Rensburg, E. J., Gogos, J. A., & Karayiorgou, M. (2008). Strong association of de novo copy number mutations with sporadic schizophrenia. *Nature Genetics* 40(7): 880–885.

Xu, B., Woodroffe, A., Rodriguez-Murillo, L., Roos, J. L., van Rensburg, E. J., Abecasis, G. R., Gogo, J., & Karayiorgou, M. (2009). Elucidating the genetic architecture of familial schizophrenia using rare copy number variant and linkage scans. *Proceedings of the National Academy of Sciences U.S.A.* 106(39): 16746–16751.

CHAPTER 9

THE EPIGENETICS OF SCHIZOPHRENIA

IRIS CHEUNG, MIRA JAKOVCEVSKI, AND SCHAHRAM AKBARIAN

KEY CONCEPTS

- DNA methylation—the methylation of cytosine residues almost exclusively at CpG dinucleotides—and posttranslational modifications of histone tails are important epigenetic mechanisms that affect gene expression in mammals.
- Inheritance of epigenetic states across generations has been observed in different plant and animal species. Evidence for this type of epigenetic inheritance in human diseases has been described in a small number of cases.
- Changes in expression in genes involved in various neuronal functions in postmortem tissues of schizophrenic patients have been described extensively. Whether these changes are contributed by epigenetic mechanisms is a major focus of current research in schizophrenia.
- A significant contribution of epigenetic mechanisms in the pathogenesis of schizophrenia is compatible with the existing major disease models, namely the dopamine model and the diathesis stress model.
- Postmortem studies of epigenetics are complicated by both the dynamic nature of epigenetic mechanisms and influence from environmental factors.
- Recent technologic advances in mapping the epigenome will greatly facilitate research on the potential roles of epigenetic mechanisms in schizophrenia and other psychiatric disorders.

Introduction

Schizophrenia is a complex disorder defined by a concordance rate of less than 70% in monozygotic twins and non-Mendelian inheritance patterns (Kaminsky, Wang, & Petronis, 2006). Although the list of copy number variations, microdeletions, and polymorphisms associated with genetic risk for schizophrenia is steadily increasing (chapter 7, this book), identification of straightforward genetic causes is still lacking for the large majority of affected individuals (Lupski, 2008; Vrijenhoek et al., 2008; Bertolino & Blasi, 2009; Delisi, 2009; Smith, 2009). In this context, it comes as no surprise that disease models have been put forward that ascribe an important role for "epigenetic" factors to the pathophysiology of schizophrenia (Abdolmaleky, Thiagalingam, & Wilcox, 2005; Kaminsky, Wang, & Petronis, 2006). Epi- (Greek for *over* and *above*) genetics implies that changes in a phenotype or gene expression are caused by mechanisms other than alterations in genomic DNA sequence. Epigenetic marks, which on the molecular level are defined primarily by cytosine methylation of the genomic DNA and a rich cache of posttranslational modifications of histones in the core of nucleosomes, can be maintained for the remainder of the cell's life and may also last for multiple generations. Therefore, the general theme of epigenetics is of great interest to the field of schizophrenia research because (1) it could provide valid and testable alternatives to genetic heritability models and (2) exploration of chromatin structure and function in healthy and diseased brains could provide novel insights into development of the molecular pathophysiology of schizophrenia. We first discuss heritable genome modifications not associated with changes in DNA sequence and then provide an update on the growing body of clinical literature that points to changes in chromatin templates in the brains and peripheral cells of subjects with schizophrenia. The implications of both clinical and preclinical epigenetic studies for the neurobiology of the disorder are also discussed.

DNA Methylation

The methylation of cytosine residues mainly at the site of CpG dinucleotides (figure 9.1) is the epigenetic modification that directly involves genomic DNA in most eukaryotes (with notable exceptions, including yeast and *Drosophila*). CpG dinucleotides are underrepresented in the genome because of the high frequency of mutation of methylated cytosine to thymine. Nevertheless, there are regions in the genome, called *CpG islands*, in which CpG dinucleotides occur at an elevated frequency and generally are unmethylated. Variations on the theme of cytosine methylation at CpG exist in specific cell types: methylation at CpNpG (where N can be any nucleotide) can be detected in embryonic stem cells (Stine et al., 1995; Ramsahoye et al., 2000) (figure 9.1A). DNA methylation is important for genome stability, repression of parasitic DNA elements, parent-of-origin-specific gene expression, and transcriptional regulation (Suzuki & Bird, 2008). DNA methylation in proximal promoters is associated mostly with transcriptional repression. In contrast, methylation of CpGs embedded within a gene body is typical for expressed genes (Suzuki & Bird, 2008). Perhaps not surprisingly, DNA methylation and covalent histone modifications often are coregulated and functionally interconnected. For

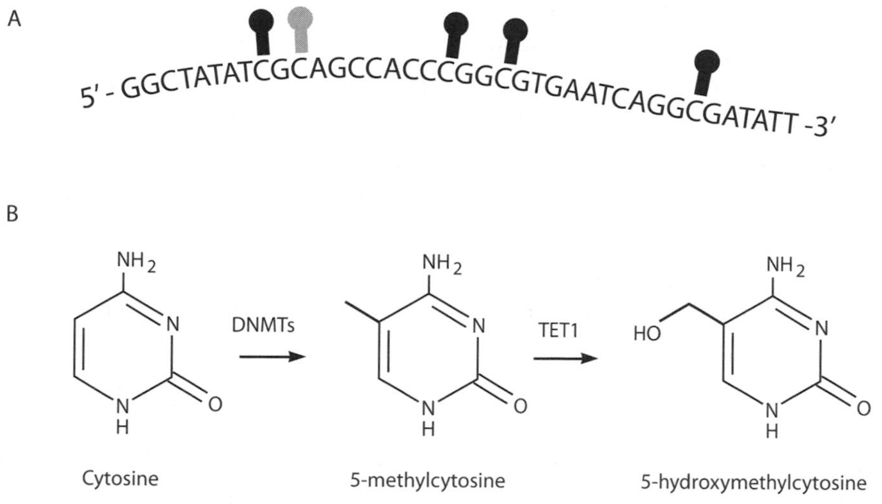

A

5' - GGCTATATCGCAGCCACCCGGCGTGAATCAGGCGATATT -3'

B

Cytosine   5-methylcytosine   5-hydroxymethylcytosine

Figure 9.1. DNA methylation.
(Source: Authors.)

example, it has been suggested that histone H3-lysine 9 (H3K9) methylation, a repressive chromatin mark, is a recruitment signal for DNA methyltransferase enzymes, which catalyze methylation of CpG dinucleotides that in turn are recognized by methyl-CpG-binding proteins associated with repressive chromatin remodeling and histone deacetylase (HDAC) activity (Fuks, 2005). Another interesting scenario involves the lysine 4 residue of histone H3. Although methylation of this particular residue is typically associated with open chromatin and active transcription, unmethylated H3K4 serves as a docking signal for DNA methyltransferases and protein complexes for chromatin remodeling involved in repression of transcription (Ciccone & Chen, 2009; Otani et al., 2009).

Recently, an unexpected layer of complexity emerged when it was discovered that a substantial portion of the methylated cytosines in Purkinje cells of the murine cerebellum exists as 5-hydroxymethylcytosine (Kriaucionis & Heintz, 2009), rather than as the typical 5-methyl-cytosine (Tahiliani et al., 2009) (figure 9.1B). Whether the two types of cytosine methylation are functionally different, and why this second type of modification is present in neurons but not in various nonneuronal cell lines, remains to be determined.

Covalent Histone Modifications

Histones and their covalent modifications play a key role in epigenetic control of gene expression and genome organization. We first provide a very brief introduction to histone modifications and chromatin function. Histones are, together with the DNA that wraps around them, the fundamental structural unit of eukaryote chromatin and thus regulate gene expression, DNA repair, and chromosome segregation, among other functions. The backbone of chromatin is provided by the core histones H2A, H2B, H3, and H4 that together form the nucleosome, a drumlike structure with 147 basepairs (bp) of genomic DNA wrapped around it (Wolffe, 1992; Hayes & Hansen, 2001) (figure 9.2). Dynamic changes in chromatin structure and accessibility of transcription factors are mediated by two molecular mechanisms: chromatin remodeling and histone tail modifications (Felsenfeld & Groudine, 2003). Chromatin remodeling is defined by the mobilization of genomic DNA wrapped around the nucleosome core particle (Peterson, 2002). Covalent modifications of specific arginine, lysine, and serine residues at the histone N-terminal tails on the nucleosome surface define a "histone code" that is differentially regulated in chromatin at sites of active gene expression (Jenuwein & Allis, 2001; Berger, 2002; Iizuka & Smith, 2003; Peterson & Laniel, 2004; Wang et al., 2004). The highly basic (positively charged) histone tails are predicted to be less structured than the histone fold regions and are believed to interact with the negatively charged DNA backbone or with other chromatin-associated proteins. In particular, the acetylation of specific lysine residues in the N-terminal tails of H3 and H4 is associated with active gene expression, whereas deacetylation of these residues results in transcriptional silencing, chromatin condensation, and hetero-

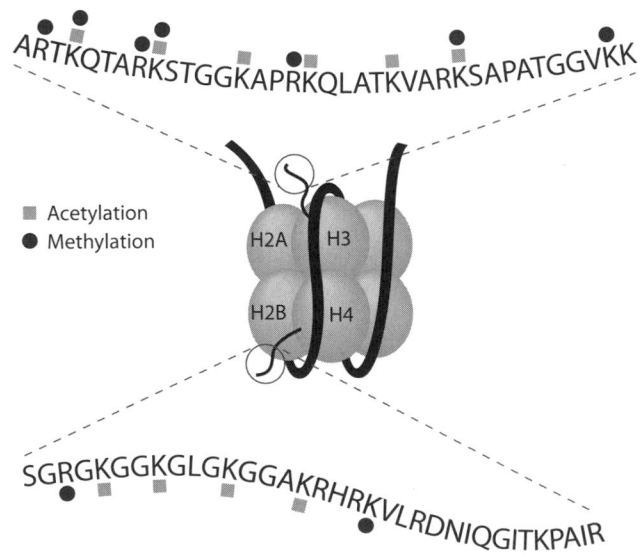

Figure 9.2. Schematic representation of the nucleosome and examples of histone modifications.
(Source: Authors.)

chromatin formation (Jenuwein & Allis, 2001; Berger, 2002; Iizuka & Smith, 2003; Peterson & Laniel, 2004; Wang et al., 2004). In addition, differential methylation, SUMOlyation and ubiquitination of specific lysine residues, and phosphorylation of specific serine and methylation of selected arginine residues of H3 and H4 are associated with transcriptional regulation in eukaryotes, including humans (Jenuwein & Allis, 2001; Berger, 2002; Fischle, Wang, & Allis, 2003; Iizuka & Smith, 2003; Peterson & Laniel, 2004; Wang et al., 2004). Among the various types of histone modifications, methylation of lysine residues appears to be one of the most highly regulated. The side chain of histone lysine residues can carry up to three methyl groups. These mono-, di-, and tri-methylated forms of specific lysine residues show cell-specific regulation during development (Biron et al., 2004) and are differentially distributed across chromatin fibers (Bernstein et al., 2005). For example, tri-methylated lysine residue 4 of histone H3 localizes to gene promoter regions, where it is associated with transcriptional activation, whereas mono-methylation of the same histone residue appears to be enriched at enhancer sequences further removed from transcription start sites (Heintzman et al., 2007). Furthermore, the mono-methylated forms of lysines 9 and 27 of histone H3, as well as lysine 20 of H4, are linked to gene activation, whereas di- or tri-methylation of the same residues are associated with repression (Barski et al., 2007).

Recent postmortem studies provide evidence that this "histone code," which differentiates chromatin at sites with active gene expression from chromatin sites with silenced gene expression (Jenuwein & Allis, 2001; Berger, 2002; Iizuka & Smith, 2003; Peterson & Laniel, 2004; Wang et al., 2004), contributes to transcriptional regulation in the human brain (Stadler et al., 2005; Huang et al., 2006; Huang et al., 2007). In addition, recent animal studies demonstrate that transcriptional regulation in a diverse set of animal models for learning- or drug-induced plasticity is accompanied by dynamic histone modification changes (Swank & Sweatt, 2001; Guan et al., 2002; Alarcon et al., 2004; Korzus, Rosenfeld, & Mayford, 2004; Li et al., 2004; Tsankova, Kumar, & Nestler, 2004; Kumar et al., 2005; Levine et al., 2005; Tsankova et al., 2006). Therefore, there is little doubt that the principles of chromatin remodeling and histone N-terminal tail modifications, which are traditionally explored in dividing cells (Jenuwein & Allis, 2001; Berger, 2002; Iizuka & Smith, 2003; Peterson & Laniel, 2004; Wang et al., 2004), also apply to the central nervous system and its postmitotic neurons (Martin & Sun, 2004; Colvis et al., 2005).

Epigenetic Heritability

Are Epigenetic Marks Passed Through the Human Germ Line?

Until recently it was believed that animals acquire epigenetic marks during development and retain some of these throughout life, except in germ cells, where the marks are erased. Erasing the imprint in the germ line ensures that the next generation has a "clean slate" with respect to epigenetic modifications, and that only truly genetic traits, encoded by actual sequence of the DNA, are inherited. For example, during spermiogenesis, the canonical histones (including their epigenetic modifications) are largely exchanged for protamines (Wykes & Krawetz, 2003), small basic proteins that form tightly packed DNA structures important for normal sperm function (Balhorn, Brewer, & Corzett, 2000). Because of this, the epigenetic contributions of sperm chromatin to embryo development have been considered extremely limited. However, it is now clear that nucleosomes are retained in 4% of the haploid genome in sperm, and these retained nucleosomes are enriched significantly at loci of developmental importance, including imprinted gene clusters, microRNA clusters, homeobox (HOX) gene clusters, and the promoters of stand-alone developmental transcription and signaling factors (Hammoud et al., 2009). Furthermore, both DNA methylation patterns and various types of histone modifications are also preserved in the portion of the genome that maintains nucleosomal organization in sperm cells {Hammoud et al., 2009). Therefore, in principle, chromatin templates, including their epigenetic markings, could be passed on to the next generation for perhaps as much as 4% of the human genome.

Epigenetic Inheritance Is Evident in Various Organisms

As already mentioned, epigenetic marks are maintained during DNA replication and hence propagated through mitotic division (Probst, Dunleavy, & Almouzni, 2009), but were thought to be erased and then reestablished between generations to ensure totipotency (Morgan et al., 2005). Although evidence for epigenetic inheritance across generations (transgenerational epigenetic inheritance) in humans has been reported only very recently (McDaniell et al., 2010), it was previously reported for a variety of organisms (Richards, 2006; Cuzin, Grandjean, & Rassoulzadegan, 2008). A classic example of such inheritance is paramutation in plants. Paramutation is a phenomenon of interallelic communication in which the presence of a specific allele (the "paramutagenic allele") modifies expression of another allele (the "paramutable allele"); this change in expression is heritable and persists even after the paramutagenic allele is removed. Although paramutation and similar phenomena have been described in several plant species, it is best studied in maize where expression of four genes ($r1$, $b1$, $p1$, and $pl1$), all of which are involved in pigmentation, is subject to regulation by paramutation (Chandler & Stam, 2004). Extensive studies in this system have provided clues that suggest the involvement of RNA in the mechanism of paramutation. In the case of $b1$, a few kilobases of tandem repeats located 100 kb away from the locus mediates paramutation at $b1$ (Stam et al., 2002). Based on the finding that both strands of the tandem repeats are transcribed, and that *mop1*—a gene initially identified as required for paramutation—is an RNA-dependent RNA polymerase, a model of RNA-mediated establishment of chromatin state was proposed (Dorweiler et al., 2000; Alleman et al., 2006).

In mice, epigenetic inheritance was first demonstrated convincingly in the dominant A^{vy} (agouti viable yellow) allele of the agouti gene (*A*) that affects coat color. A^{vy} is an insertion of a retrotransposon upstream of *A* and drives expression of the gene from its cryptic promoter. Expression of A^{vy} results in a yellow coat color, and the null allele *a* gives an agouti color. A^{vy} displays variable expressivity, leading to a spectrum of coat color in the offspring of an A^{vy}/a mother. Furthermore, the distribution of coat colors in the offspring is influenced by the phenotype of the A^{vy}/a mother: an agouti mother results in a higher frequency of agouti offspring. It is important that maternal environment was ruled out as the underlying cause, thus demonstrating epigenetic inheritance (Morgan et al., 1999). It was initially suggested that methylation status at the retrotransposon is the basis of the inheritance, but this was not supported in a subsequent study (Morgan et al., 1999; Blewitt et al., 2006). Another example of transgenerational epigenetic inheritance in mice is the *axin-fused* allele ($Axin^{Fu}$), whose expression produces a kinky tail and is influenced by the phenotype of the $Axin^{Fu}$ parent (Rakyan et al., 2003). In addition, multiple paramutation-like phenomena in the mouse have been described in which the presence of a specific allele leads to epigenetic modification of another allele, which is passed on to the next generation (Rassoulzadegan, Magliano, & Cuzin, 2002; Herman et al., 2003; Rassoulzadegan et al., 2006; Wagner et al., 2008).

Whereas these examples display transgenerational epigenetic inheritance, a different epigenetic mechanism involves heritable germ-line epimutation. *Epimutation* refers to the aberrant expression of a gene without a change in its DNA sequence. It could be a primary effect due to failure in maintaining epigenetic state, or it could be secondary to a DNA mutation, such as when the machinery for epigenetic modification itself is mutated (Lei et al., 1996; Chawla et al., 2007). Cases of epimutations producing morphologic or fruit-ripening mutants have been documented in plants (Jacobsen & Meyerowitz, 1997; Cubas, Vincent, & Coen, 1999; Manning et al., 2006). The occasional appearance of revertant tissue in a mutant plant results in fruit with an individual ripened sector (Cubas, Vincent, & Coen, 1999), or a branch with normal flower morphology accompanied by reversion of the epimutation (Manning et al., 2006) provides strong support for a causative role of the epimutation in the phenotype. In humans, epimutations affecting imprinted regions at 11p15, 14q32, or 15q11–q13 are associated with a number of disorders such as Silver-Russell syndrome, a condition defined by growth retardation and developmental delay (Buiting et al., 2003; Gicquel et al., 2005; Buiting et al., 2008). Epimutations have also been described in many types of cancers (Esteller, 2007). However, given the role of genomic instability in tumorigenesis, it is likely that at least some cases of epimutations in cancer result from DNA mutations.

Heritable germ-line epimutation, as the name suggests, is an epimutation that is inherited through the germ line. The epimutation-producing morphologic mutation in the plant *Linaria vulgaris* mentioned here is one of the few documented cases of this type of inheritance (Manning et al., 2006). There have been a number of studies reporting epimutations in the mismatch-repair genes MLH1 and MSH2 in humans, which are transmitted in specific cases of hereditary nonpolyposis colorectal cancer (Suter, Martin, & Ward, 2004; Chan et al., 2006; Hitchins and Ward, 2007; Hitchins et al., 2007). However, some of these findings have been controversial, highlighting the difficulties in establishing this type of inheritance in humans (Chong, Youngson, & Whitelaw, 2007; Hitchins & Ward, 2007).

In summary, inheritance in epigenetic states appears to be a widespread phenomenon across different organisms, even though the mechanisms behind such inheritance remain poorly explored in vertebrates, and it is likely that we have seen only the "tip of the iceberg." Some of the limitations in our knowledge result from the fact that, until recently, genomewide mapping of epigenetic marks was difficult to perform, but this is now possible with "deep" or "massively parallel" sequencing of DNA from chromatin immunoprecipitates. These techniques also paved the way for the recent discovery, mentioned already, that approximately 4% of the human genome apparently maintains nucleosomal organization and some of the epigenetic marks in germ cells (Hammoud et al., 2009). The Hammoud study and related findings from other groups (Arpanahi et al., 2009) are exciting because they identify specific sets of genes and genomic loci that are prime candidates for exploring epigenetic heritability in humans. Notably, among these are several genes regulating GABAergic signaling (Hammoud et al., 2009), which is of interest given that epigenetic marks for some of the GABA (gamma-aminobutyric acid) pathway genes are altered in the cerebral cortex of subjects with schizophrenia (see below). It is likely that, in the near future, a large number of studies will search for epigenetic heritability in schizophrenia and other brain disorders, and mechanistic insights will be driven largely by research on model organisms.

Postmortem Brain Studies of Epigenetics and Schizophrenia

Chromatin Alterations in the Brain with Schizophrenia—Evidence for a Role in Altered Gene Expression?

The molecular architecture of chromatin is of interest not only for studies of the various types of epigenetic heritability already discussed here, but also for the schizophrenia researcher who searches for molecular and cellular alterations in the diseased brain. Postmortem studies, mostly focused on the cerebral cortex and other areas of the forebrain, demonstrate alterations in gene expression, including dysregulation of transcripts involved in cellular metabolism (Middleton et al., 2002; Konradi et al., 2004; Akbarian et al., 2005), GABAergic (Akbarian & Huang, 2006; Hashimoto et al., 2008a, 2008b), glutamatergic neurotransmission (Meador-Woodruff et al., 2003; Knable et al., 2004), and myelination and other oligodendrocyte functions (Haroutunian et al., 2007; Sokolov, 2007; Karoutzou, Emerich, & Dietrich, 2008). However, very little attention has been given to the molecular mechanisms that underlie these alterations in mRNA levels, which often occur in the absence of neurodegeneration. Specifically, it is not known whether the alterations in the level of a specific mRNA are brought about by a change in transcription or mRNA turnover. Therefore, to determine whether transcription itself is altered, additional molecular assays, in combination with more traditional approaches (quantification of mRNA and protein), would be extremely useful for the postmortem field. Early studies reported various degrees of aberrant DNA CpG hypermethylation or hypomethylation in regulatory gene sequences and promoters. These include the glycoprotein *REELIN* (Abdolmaleky et al., 2005; Grayson et al., 2005); catechyl-O-methyltransferase (*COMT*, which encodes a key enzyme for catecholamine metabolism) (Abdolmaleky et al., 2006); and *SOX10*, encoding a transcription factor important for myelination and oligodendrocyte function (Iwamoto et al., 2005). It is encouraging that these disease-related methylation changes are associated with altered levels of the corresponding RNA, consistent with the repressive function of CpG methylation around transcription start sites. However, the disease-related *REELIN* and *COMT* DNA methylation changes could not be replicated in independent studies (Mill et al., 2008; Tochigi et al., 2008). Numerous factors could have contributed to these disparate findings. For example, DNA CpG methylation in a variety of tissues, including the CNS, could be sensitive to the social environment (Rampon et al., 2000; Weaver et al., 2004), ischemia (Endres et al., 2000), environmental toxins (Desaulniers et al., 2005; Bollati et al., 2007; Salnikow & Zhitkovich, 2008), nicotine (Satta et al., 2007; Satta et al., 2008), alcohol (Marutha Ravindran & Ticku, 2004), psychostimulants (Numachi et al., 2004; Numachi et al., 2007), and antipsychotic drugs (Shimabukuro et al., 2006; Cheng et al., 2008; Mill et al., 2008). It is likely that these factors also play a role in shaping DNA methylation patterns in the human brain, thereby adding significantly to sample variability in postmortem studies.

Recently, a more comprehensive DNA methylation screen of approximately 8,000 genes was conducted on the frontal cortex of schizophrenia and bipolar brains. Approximately 100 loci displayed significant methylation changes in the schizophrenia and bipolar cohorts. These loci constitute a highly heterogeneous set of genes that may regulate glutamatergic and GABAergic neurotransmission and neurodevelopment (Mill et al., 2008). That schizophrenia and bipolar disorder showed methylation changes of similar magnitude and direction at a number of loci resonates with some of the clinical, genetic, and neurochemical features common to both disorders (Craddock & Owen, 2007). Strikingly, the list of genes showing altered methylation reported by Mill et al. (2008) includes at least one locus, dysbindin, which has been associated with genetic risk for psychosis (Straub et al., 2002; Raybould et al., 2005; Pae et al., 2007). This is interesting because evidence is emerging that for a number of risk loci, epigenetic modifications in brain chromatin are influenced by local sequence polymorphisms and other genetic variations (Polesskaya, Aston, & Sokolov, 2006; Huang et al., 2007).

These studies on the frontal lobe of schizophrenic patients indicate that the total number of loci displaying DNA hyper- vs. hypomethylation was roughly equal to that of controls, making it very unlikely that schizophrenia is associated with a generalized drift toward increased (or decreased) DNA methylation in the brain. A similar conclusion was reached by an earlier study on the temporal cortex in schizophrenia that reported no significant DNA methylation changes for the 50 genes examined (Siegmund et al., 2007). Notably, in those DNA methylation studies reporting positive findings, the overall magnitude of the disease-related changes was surprisingly subtle when compared to that of controls. For example, in the Mill et al. (2008) data, disease-related DNA methylation levels in one of the most significantly changed genes *WDR18* were reported as 17% in schizophrenia patients and 25% in controls. Although it is difficult, even for single-copy genes, to extrapolate the percentages of methylated DNA extracted from a tissue homogenate to the number of cell nuclei affected, the evidence so far supports the view that many of the DNA methylation changes associated with schizophrenia are likely to involve only a subset of cells residing in the cerebral cortex.

In addition, several studies have explored changes in histone modifications in specific genes. Preference was given to the study of lysine methylation, which apparently is less affected by tissue autolysis and other postmortem confounds (Akbarian et al., 2005; Huang et al., 2006). Focusing on the distribution of trimethyl-H3K4 and -H3K27, two chromatin marks differentiating between open and repressive chromatin, a subset of subjects with schizophrenia exhibited a shift from the H3K4me3 to the H3K27me3 mark in prefrontal chromatin surrounding the transcription start site of *GAD1*, which encodes the 67 kD glutamic acid decarboxylase GABA synthesis enzyme (Huang et al., 2007). This observation is of interest because down-regulation of GAD67 RNA will affect widespread portions of the cerebral cortex, hippocampus, and other areas of the forebrain, and even the cerebellar cortex (Guidotti et al., 2000; Dracheva et al., 2004; Fatemi et al., 2005; Benes et al., 2008; Hashimoto, 2008a, 2008b). Indeed, the shift from H3K4 to H3K27 methylation in the *GAD1* gene in schizophrenia cases as opposed to the matched controls is accompanied by a deficit in GAD67 RNA (Huang et al., 2007).

Crossroad Between Genetic Studies of Schizophrenia Risk Loci and the Epigenetic Phenomena of Genomic Imprinting and Monoallelic Expression

Genomic imprinting is an epigenetic phenomenon in which certain genes are expressed in a parent-of-origin-specific manner, and typically DNA and histone lysine methylation marks at these gene loci are differentially regulated on paternal and maternal chromosomes. Imprinted genes are expressed only from the allele inherited from the mother or the father, and many, albeit not all, encode noncoding RNAs (Morison, Ramsay, & Spencer, 2005; Wood & Oakey, 2006). Fewer than 100 out of a total of 35,000 human genes show monoallelic expression due to parent-of-origin-specific regulation. An additional complexity is that for a number of imprinted genes, monoallelic expression is not consistently observed in all somatic tissues. A case in point is the 5HT2A serotonin receptor, which initially was shown to be selectively expressed from the methylated maternal chromosome in human fibroblasts (Kato et al., 1996), but a subsequent postmortem study found monoallelic expression in the brains of only a subset of individuals (Bunzel et al., 1998). In addition, single nucleotide polymorphisms within the 5HT2A gene are thought to confer genetic risk for schizophrenia (Abdolmaleky et al., 2004), possibly by contributing to differential DNA methylation and expression (Polesskaya, Aston, & Sokolov, 2006). Thus, epigenetic regulation of 5HT2A expression in the human brain apparently involves mechanisms of genomic imprinting as well as naturally occurring genetic variability in the population, and both these factors may be relevant for the neurobiology of schizophrenia.

The 5HT2A gene is not the only example of the involvement of an imprinted gene in schizophrenia. For example, *LRRTM1* (leucine-rich repeat transmembrane neuronal 1) is expressed primarily on the paternal chromosome, and certain sequence polymorphisms of the gene appear to be over-transmitted, through the paternal line, in subjects with schizophrenia and in some cases with dyslexia (Francks et al., 2007). Another example involves certain portions of chromosome 15q11–13 that contribute to Prader-Willi and Angelman syndromes, two imprinting disorders associated with defective neurodevelopment and autism (Nicholls & Knepper, 2001; Horsthemke & Wagstaff, 2008). Of note, copy number variations, microdeletions, and duplications that are located primarily somewhat more upstream on 15q12 and 15q13 confer risk for schizophrenia and related disease (Stefansson et al., 2008; Owen, Williams, & O'Donovan, 2009). It is not yet clear if the spatial proximity and partial overlap of these various risk loci for neurodevelopmental disorders in the 15q11–13 region indicate a common molecular pathology (Sharp et al., 2008).

Reproducibility of Epigenetic Alterations in Schizophrenia Postmortem Brain

Given that only a few studies have explored chromatin modifications in the schizophrenia postmortem brain thus far, it is difficult to predict whether the "epigenetic approach" will contribute to a critical advance of our knowledge about the mechanisms of the disease. Obviously, independent confirmation of reported alterations in disease tissue is required. However, recent studies suggest that DNA methylation patterns show, on a genomewide scale, considerable heterogeneity between normal individuals, with larger differences between dizygotic than between monozygotic twins (Kaminsky et al., 2009). Furthermore, the similarities in DNA methylation and histone acetylation patterns among monozygotic twin pairs tend to diminish with age (Fraga et al., 2005). Given this apparent variability in chromatin marks among individuals, which could further increase during the course of aging, it comes as no surprise that the field still awaits independent replication for the reported alterations in schizophrenia postmortem studies. For example, DNA methylation analyses for the *REELIN* promoter (encoding a glycoprotein essential for orderly brain development and neuronal connectivity) reported either no change (Mill et al., 2008) or aberrant hypermethylation at different portions of the gene in the cerebral cortex of schizophrenia patients (Abdolmaleky et al., 2005; Abdolmaleky, Thiagalingam, & Wilcox, 2005; Grayson et al., 2005). Likewise, DNA hypomethylation and increased gene expression for *COMT*, encoding a key enzyme for catecholamine metabolism, was reported in schizophrenia in one study (Abdolmaleky et al., 2006), whereas another group reported no methylation changes for the same gene (Mill et al., 2008). In addition to differences among individuals, numerous factors could have contributed to these disparate findings. It is important that, as already mentioned (see "Chromatin Alterations in the Brain with Schizophrenia—Evidence for a Role in Altered Gene Expression?"), the activity of DNA methyltransferases (the enzymes that methylate DNA) and DNA CpG methylation in a variety of tissues, including CNS, is sensitive to a variety of environmental factors. For instance, it has been documented that occupational exposure to benzene (e.g., from traffic exhaust fumes) is associated with changes in DNA methylation levels at both repetitive elements and gene-specific regions in the blood (Bollati et al., 2007). In the rat, maternal behavior has direct effects on DNA methylation and histone modification levels at the promoter of a glucocorticoid receptor gene as well as its expression in the hippocampus (Weaver et al., 2007).

Epigenetic Marks in the Brain—How Stable?

The rationale for exploring epigenetic modifications in the postmortem brain of subjects with schizophrenia is primarily driven by the question of whether changes in RNA levels are associated with alterations in DNA sequences or with histone modifications at the corresponding promoter. The underlying assumption is that changes in RNA levels observed in postmortem tissue reflect changes in steady-state RNA levels, and that any changes in DNA or histone modification will reflect a stable epigenetic alteration in the brains of subjects with schizophrenia. Whether these somewhat simplistic notions are valid is presently unknown, and little data exist about the stability or dynamic turnover of epigenetic marks in the human brain. Cell culture studies suggest that DNA methylation undergoes bidirectional changes—on the scale of minutes to hours—in response to DNA methyltransferase inhibitors (Kundakovic et al., 2007; Levenson et al., 2006) or depolarization (Martinowich et al., 2003; Nelson, Kavalali, & Monteggia, 2008). In addition, despite the fact that DNA and histone methylation were recently thought to be irreversible, molecules that mediate demethylation of CpG dinucleotides or of histone lysine residues have been identified (Klose & Zhang, 2007; Ooi & Bestor, 2008). Indeed, studies in the rodent hippocampus suggest that neuronal activity drives the expression of molecules regulating DNA methylation (Ma et al., 2009). Furthermore, learning and memory are associated with highly dynamic DNA methylation changes at *PP1*, *REELIN* and promoters regulating synaptic plasticity (Ma et al., 2009). Therefore, one could postulate that at least some of the epigenetic alterations reported in the postmortem brain of individuals with schizophrenia are not necessarily stable imprints, but instead could potentially reflect a pathophysiologic mechanism that operates on a much shorter time scale, from hours to minutes.

Implications of Epigenetics for the Neurodevelopmental Theory of Schizophrenia

The reported histone methylation changes in prefrontal *GAD1* chromatin in schizophrenia subjects (Huang et al., 2007) are also of interest for neurodevelopment. For instance, H3K4 methylation becomes progressively up-regulated in the human prefrontal cortex at a select set of GABAergic gene promoters (GAD1/GAD2/NPY/SST) during the transitions from the fetal period to childhood and then to adulthood (Huang et al., 2007). This extended course of chromatin regulation during the first two decades of life is paralleled by similar increases at the RNA level (Huang et al., 2007). These findings suggest that the prefrontal dysfunction of schizophrenia may involve chromatin remodeling and transcriptional mechanisms during development. Whether the GAD1 chromatin alterations in schizophrenia reflect disordered neurodevelopment or pathophysiology occurring later in life will be very difficult to determine in human studies but could be investigated in appropriate animal models.

From a broader perspective, evidence is emerging that epigenetic marks are highly regulated, particularly during late prenatal and early postnatal human brain development. For example, assays of DNA methylation changes at 50 gene promoters across the life span in the human temporal cortex reveal that more than half exhibit age-related methylation changes, which are particularly pronounced during the transition from the fetal period to childhood (Siegmund et al., 2007). Furthermore, maturation of the cerebellar cortex is associated with histone methylation changes in chromatin surrounding the glutamate receptor gene (Stadler et al., 2005). Future studies that map epigenetic marks on a comprehensive, genomewide scale during normal human brain development will be necessary to determine whether these developmental changes are representative for a significant portion of the genome and whether schizophrenia-related risk loci and genes show age-related changes.

Animal Models of Epigenetics and Schizophrenia

Antipsychotic Medication

As already mentioned, DNA methylation changes at selected loci have been linked to a wide range of exposures. It is interesting that studies dating back to the 1960s and 1970s observed that subjects with schizophrenia who were treated with the amino acid methionine—which is a substrate for the synthesis of the methyl-donor S-adenosylmethionine in a variety of biochemical pathways—frequently exhibited an exacerbation of their symptoms (Grayson et al., 2009). Based on preclinical studies of GABAergic gene promoters, it is possible that excessive intake of methionine may lead to aberrant DNA (and perhaps histone) methylation events at selected loci in the central nervous system, causing transcriptional dysregulation and ultimately psychosis (Grayson et al., 2009). If fine-tuning of DNA and histone methylation activities is indeed important for the neurobiology of psychosis, then one might expect that these mechanisms are affected by antipsychotic drugs. One study reported that global DNA brain methylation levels display a slight decrease in animals exposed to the antipsychotic haloperidol (Shimabukuro et al., 2006). This is consistent with the observation that methionine may exacerbate psychosis (Grayson et al., 2009). Furthermore, there is evidence from animal models—and even postmortem tissue—that expression and activity of the histone H3-lysine-4-specific methyltransferase, mixed lineage-leukemia 1 (MLL1), is up-regulated in the prefrontal cortex following exposure to the atypical antipsychotic clozapine (Huang et al., 2007; Huang & Akbarian, 2007).

There is increasing evidence that changes in the dopamine D_2-system and other receptors targeted by antipsychotics are coupled by various signaling pathways to chromatin remodeling, including DNA methylation and histone modification (Li et al., 2004; Dong et al., 2008; Costa et al., 2009). In the comprehensive study of Mill et al. (2008), DNA methylation levels in one promoter—the mitogen-activated protein kinase kinase (*MEK1*) promoter—out of approximately 8,000 showed a significant inverse association with lifetime exposure to antipsychotic medication. It is noteworthy that phosphorylation of the MEK1 protein itself is also altered in brains of animals exposed to clozapine (Browning et al., 2005), implying that antipsychotic drugs can affect MEK1 activity through multiple pathways. MEK1 and other components of the mitogen-activated kinase (MAPK) signaling pathway regulate neurodevelopment and functions of mature neurons (Rosen et al., 1994; Sweatt, 2001; Bozon et al., 2003); however, the mechanism by which they could be involved in the neurobiology of psychosis remains unclear.

Dopamine and Diathesis Stress Models

Historically, two theories dominated the modeling of certain aspects of schizophrenia in animals. These are the dopaminergic and the diathesis stress models or, when in combination, the "two-hit" model. The dopamine hypothesis is based first on the observation that amphetamine administration, which increases the levels of dopamine in meso-limbo-cortical and meso-striatal pathways, mimics the positive symptoms of schizophrenia, such as delusions and hallucinations (Laruelle et al., 1996). Second, the clinical potency of conventional antipsychotics is directly correlated with their affinity for the dopamine D_2 receptor (Laruelle et al., 1992, 1997). It is interesting that there are dynamic changes in histone acetylation and phospho-acetylation in the striatum and other brain regions of rodents and primates exposed to L-dopa, amphetamine (or other psychostimulant drugs such as cocaine), or antipsychotic drugs acting as dopamine D_2 antagonists (Shen et al., 2008; Li et al., 2004; Kumar et al., 2005; Nicholas et al., 2008). In the case of antipsychotic drugs, DNA methylation changes were also reported (Dong et al., 2008).

Although numerous mechanisms could lead to a dopamine imbalance in brains of schizophrenia patients, including but not limited to genetic variations, the diathesis stress model would be compatible with a scenario whereby yet unidentified epigenetic factors trigger the outbreak of the disease. Because brain abnormalities can be found long before the occurrence of the disease, another event (second hit) needs to fall into place to trigger the development of the disease later in life. The diathesis stress model offers a rich cache of factors that would interact in the causation of schizophrenia. For example, a genetic predisposition or environmental factor (physically or chemically disturbing the brain) could make the brain vulnerable during early prenatal or early postnatal development (first hit). Later in life, a different environmental factor triggers the acute outbreak of the disease (second hit). The environmental component of both the first or second hit might be represented by any number of adverse environmental events that cause extensive stress to the individual. In rodents, a common paradigm to investigate early environmental effects involves separating pups from the dam for a certain period each day during early development. The effects of prolonged maternal stress on histone and DNA modification patterns have been described in detail in the rat hippocampus: increased DNA methylation was observed in this brain region among rat pups that received a lower amount of maternal care (Weaver et al., 2004). It is important that maternal separation led to an exaggeration of the schizophrenia-like phenotype, including impulsivity and disinhibition, in a subset of heterozygous reeler mutant mice, which express lower levels of the developmentally regulated glycoprotein *REELIN* (Laviola et al., 2009). Notably, *REELIN* expression appears to be down-regulated in some but not all schizophrenia postmortem brain cohorts (Impagnatiello et al., 1998; Fatemi, Earle, & McMenomy, 2000; Guidotti et al., 2000; Eastwood & Harrison, 2003; Lipska et al., 2006), and this effect is associated with DNA methylation changes at the promoter (Abdolmaleky et al., 2005; Grayson et al., 2005). Therefore, it would be interesting to explore whether *REELIN* DNA methylation patterns are altered in the maternally deprived reeler animals (Laviola et al., 2009).

KEY AREAS FOR FUTURE RESEARCH

- To further research on epigenetic heritability, on a genomewide scale, explore histone modification and DNA methylation profiles in cells and tissues from subjects with schizophrenia and their family members.
- Map, for selected types of histone and DNA modifications in specific brain regions and cell types, the normal developmental trajectory and effects of aging, and include samples from schizophrenia and related diseases.
- Explore whether the two types of DNA cytosine methylation, 5-hydroxyl-methyl-cytosine and 5-methyl-cytosine, are present in human brain chromatin and altered in schizophrenia.

Selected Readings

Abdolmaleky, H. M., Thiagalingam, S., & Wilcox, M. (2005). Genetics and epigenetics in major psychiatric disorders: Dilemmas, achievements, applications, and future scope. *American Journal of Pharmacogenomics* 5(3): 149–160.

Akbarian, S. & Huang, H.S. (2006). Molecular and cellular mechanisms of altered GAD1/ GAD67 expression in schizophrenia and related disorders. *Brain Research Reviews* 52(2): 293–304.

Barski, A., Cuddapah, S., Cui, K., Roh, T. Y., Schones, D. E., Wang, Z., Wei, G., Chepelev, I., & Zhao, K. (2007). High-resolution profiling of histone methylations in the human genome. *Cell* 129(4): 823–837.

Berger, S. L. (2002). Histone modifications in transcriptional regulation. *Current Opinion in Genetics and Development* 12(2): 142–148.

Colvis, C. M., Pollock, J. D., Goodman, R. H., Impey, S., Dunn, J., Mandel, G., Champagne, F. A., Mayford, M., Korzus, E., Kumar, A., et al. (2005). Epigenetic mechanisms and gene networks in the nervous system. *Journal of Neuroscience* 25(45): 10379–10389.

Huang, H. S., Matevossian, A., Whittle, C., Kim, S. Y., Schumacher, A., Baker, S. P., & Akbarian, S. (2007). Prefrontal dysfunction in schizophrenia involves mixed-lineage leukemia 1-regulated histone methylation at GABAergic gene promoters. *Journal of Neuroscience* 27(42): 11254–11262.

Suzuki, M. M. & Bird, A. (2008). DNA methylation landscapes: Provocative insights from epigenomics. *Nature Reviews Genetics* 9(6): 465–476.

References

Abdolmaleky, H. M., Cheng, K. H., Faraone, S. V., Wilcox, M., Glatt, S. J., Gao, F., Smith, C. L., Shafa, R., Aeali, B., Carnevale, J., et al. (2006). Hypomethylation of MB-COMT promoter is a major risk factor for schizophrenia and bipolar disorder. *Human Molecular Genetics* 15(21): 3132–3145.

Abdolmaleky, H. M., Cheng, K. H., Russo, A., Smith, C. L., Faraone, S. V., Wilcox, M., Shafa, R., Glatt, S. J., Nguyen, G., Ponte, J. F., et al. (2005). Hypermethylation of the reelin (RELN) promoter in the brain of schizophrenic patients: A preliminary report. *American Journal of Medical Genetics Part B: Neuropsychiatric Genetics* 134B(1): 60–66.

Abdolmaleky, H. M., Faraone, S. V., Glatt, S. J., & Tsuang, M. T. (2004). Meta-analysis of association between the T102C polymorphism of the 5HT2a receptor gene and schizophrenia. *Schizophrenia Research* 67(1): 53–62.

Abdolmaleky, H. M., Thiagalingam, S., & Wilcox, M. (2005). Genetics and epigenetics in major psychiatric disorders: Dilemmas, achievements, applications, and future scope. *American Journal of Pharmacogenomics* 5(3): 149–160.

Akbarian, S. & Huang, H. S. (2006). Molecular and cellular mechanisms of altered GAD1/ GAD67 expression in schizophrenia and related disorders. *Brain Research Reviews* 52(2): 293–304.

Akbarian, S., Ruehl, M. G., Bliven, E., Luiz, L. A., Peranelli, A. C., Baker, S. P., Roberts, R. C., Bunney, W. E., Jr., Conley, R. C., Jones, E. G., et al. (2005). Chromatin alterations associated with down-regulated metabolic gene expression in the prefrontal cortex of subjects with schizophrenia. *Archives of General Psychiatry* 62(8): 829–840.

Alarcon, J. M., Malleret, G., Touzani, K., Vronskaya, S., Ishii, S., Kandel, E. R., & Barco, A. (2004). Chromatin acetylation, memory, and LTP are impaired in CBP+/– mice: A model for the cognitive deficit in Rubinstein-Taybi syndrome and its amelioration. *Neuron* 42(6): 947–959.

Alleman, M., Sidorenko, L., McGinnis, K., Seshadri, V., Dorweiler, J. E., White, J., Sikkink, K., & Chandler, V. L. (2006). An RNA-dependent RNA polymerase is required for paramutation in maize. *Nature* 442(7100): 295–298.

Arpanahi, A., Brinkworth, M., Iles, D., Krawetz, S. A., Paradowska, A., Platts, A. E., Saida, M., Steger, K., Tedder, P., & Miller, D. (2009). Endonuclease-sensitive regions of human spermatozoal chromatin are highly enriched in promoter and CTCF binding sequences. *Genome Research* 19(8): 1338–1349.

Balhorn, R., Brewer, L., & Corzett, M. (2000). DNA condensation by protamine and arginine-rich peptides: Analysis of toroid stability using single DNA molecules. *Molecular Reproduction and Development* 56(Suppl 2): 230–234.

Barski, A., Cuddapah, S., Cui, K., Roh, T. Y., Schones, D. E., Wang, Z., Wei, G., Chepelev, I., & Zhao, K. (2007). High-resolution profiling of histone methylations in the human genome. *Cell* 129(4): 823–837.

Benes, F. M., Lim, B., Matzilevich, D., Subburaju, S., & Walsh, J. P. (2008). Circuitry-based gene expression profiles in GABA cells of the trisynaptic pathway in schizophrenics versus bipolars. *Proceedings of the National Academy of Sciences U.S.A.* 105(52): 20935–20940.

Berger, S. L. (2002). Histone modifications in transcriptional regulation. *Current Opinion in Genetics and Development* 12(2): 142–148.

Bernstein, B. E., Kamal, M., Lindblad-Toh, K., Bekiranov, S., Bailey, D. K., Huebert, D. J., McMahon, S., Karlsson, E. K., Kulbokas, E. J., III, Gingeras, T. R., et al. (2005). Genomic maps and comparative analysis of histone modifications in human and mouse. *Cell* 120(2): 169–181.

Bertolino, A. & Blasi, G. (2009). The genetics of schizophrenia. *Neuroscience* 164(1): 288–299.

Biron, V. L., McManus, K. J., Hu, N., Hendzel, M. J., & Underhill, D. A. (2004). Distinct dynamics and distribution of histone methyl-lysine derivatives in mouse development. *Developmental Biology* 276(2): 337–351.

Blewitt, M. E., Vickaryous, N. K., Paldi, A., Koseki, H., & Whitelaw, E. (2006). Dynamic reprogramming of DNA methylation at an epigenetically sensitive allele in mice. *PLoS Genetics* 2(4): e49.

Bollati, V., Baccarelli, A., Hou, L., Bonzini, M., Fustinoni, S., Cavallo, D., Byun, H. M., Jiang, J., Marinelli, B., Pesatori, A. C., et al. (2007). Changes in DNA methylation patterns in subjects exposed to low-dose benzene. *Cancer Research* 67(3): 876–880.

Bozon, B., Kelly, A., Josselyn, S. A., Silva, A. J., Davis, S., & Laroche, S. (2003). MAPK, CREB and zif268 are all required for the consolidation of recognition memory. *Philosophical Transactions of the Royal Society B: Biological Sciences* 358(1432): 805–814.

Browning, J. L., Patel, T., Brandt, P. C., Young, K. A., Holcomb, L. A., & Hicks, P. B. (2005). Clozapine and the mitogen-activated protein kinase signal transduction pathway: Implications for antipsychotic actions. *Biological Psychiatry* 57(6): 617–623.

Buiting, K., Gross, S., Lich, C., Gillessen-Kaesbach, G., el-Maarri, O., & Horsthemke, B. (2003). Epimutations in Prader-Willi and Angelman syndromes: A molecular study of 136 patients with an imprinting defect. *American Journal of Human Genetics* 72(3): 571–577.

Buiting, K., Kanber, D., Martin-Subero, J. I., Lieb, W., Terhal, P., Albrecht, B., Purmann, S., Gross, S., Lich, C., Siebert, R., et al. (2008). Clinical features of maternal uniparental disomy 14 in patients with an epimutation and a deletion of the imprinted DLK1/GTL2 gene cluster. *Human Mutation* 29(9): 1141–1146.

Bunzel, R., Blumcke, I., Cichon, S., Normann, S., Schramm, J., Propping, P., & Nothen, M. M. (1998). Polymorphic imprinting of the serotonin-2A (5-HT2A) receptor gene in human adult brain. *Brain Research: Molecular Brain Research* 59(1): 90–92.

Chan, T. L., Yuen, S. T., Kong, C. K., Chan, Y. W., Chan, A. S., Ng, W. F., Tsui, W. Y., Lo, M. W., Tam, W. Y., Li, V. S., et al. (2006). Heritable germline epimutation of MSH2 in a family with hereditary nonpolyposis colorectal cancer. *Nature Genetics* 38(10): 1178–1183.

Chandler, V. L. & Stam, M. (2004). Chromatin conversations: Mechanisms and implications of paramutation. *Nature Reviews Genetics* 5(7): 532–544.

Chawla, R., Nicholson, S. J., Folta, K. M., & Srivastava, V. (2007). Transgene-induced silencing of Arabidopsis phytochrome A gene via exonic methylation. *Plant Journal* 52(6): 1105–1118.

Cheng, M. C., Liao, D. L., Hsiung, C. A., Chen, C. Y., Liao, Y. C., & Chen, C. H. (2008). Chronic treatment with aripiprazole induces differential gene expression in the rat frontal cortex. *International Journal of Neuropsychopharmacology* 11(2): 207–216.

Chong, S., Youngson, N. A., & Whitelaw, E. (2007). Heritable germline epimutation is not the same as transgenerational epigenetic inheritance. *Nature Genetics* 39(5): 574–575; author reply 575–576.

Ciccone, D. N. & Chen, T. (2009). Histone lysine methylation in genomic imprinting. *Epigenetics* 4(4): 216–220.

Colvis, C. M., Pollock, J. D., Goodman, R. H., Impey, S., Dunn, J., Mandel, G., Champagne, F. A., Mayford, M., Korzus, E., Kumar, A., et al. (2005). Epigenetic mechanisms and gene networks in the nervous system. *Journal of Neuroscience* 25(45): 10379–10389.

Costa, E., Chen, Y., Dong, E., Grayson, D. R., Kundakovic, M., Maloku, E., Ruzicka, W., Satta, R., Veldic, M., Zhubi, A., et al. (2009). GABAergic promoter hypermethylation as a model to study the neurochemistry of schizophrenia vulnerability. *Expert Review of Neurotherapeutics* 9(1): 87–98.

Craddock, N. & Owen, M. J. (2007). Rethinking psychosis: The disadvantages of a dichotomous classification now outweigh the advantages. *World Psychiatry* 6(2): 84–91.

Cubas, P., Vincent, C., & Coen, E. (1999). An epigenetic mutation responsible for natural variation in floral symmetry. *Nature* 401(6749): 157–161.

Cuzin, F., Grandjean, V., & Rassoulzadegan, M. (2008). Inherited variation at the epigenetic level: Paramutation from the plant to the mouse. *Current Opinion in Genetics and Development* 18(2): 193–196.

Delisi, L. E. (2009). Searching for the true genetic vulnerability for schizophrenia. *Genome Medicine* 1(1): 14.

Desaulniers, D., Xiao, G. H., Leingartner, K., Chu, I., Musicki, B., & Tsang, B. K. (2005). Comparisons of brain, uterus, and liver mRNA expression for cytochrome p450s, DNA methyltransferase-1, and catechol-o-methyltransferase in prepubertal female Sprague-Dawley rats exposed to a mixture of aryl hydrocarbon receptor agonists. *Toxicological Sciences* 86(1): 175–184.

Dong, E., Nelson, M., Grayson, D. R., Costa, E., & Guidotti, A. (2008). Clozapine and sulpiride but not haloperidol or olanzapine activate brain DNA demethylation. *Proceedings of the National Academy of Sciences U.S.A.* 105(36): 13614–13619.

Dorweiler, J. E., Carey, C. C., Kubo, K. M., Hollick, J. B., Kermicle, J. L., & Chandler, V. L. (2000). Mediator of paramutation1 is required for establishment and maintenance of paramutation at multiple maize loci. *Plant Cell* 12(11): 2101–2118.

Dracheva, S., Elhakem, S. L., McGurk, S. R., Davis, K. L., & Haroutunian, V. (2004). GAD67 and GAD65 mRNA and protein expression in cerebrocortical regions of elderly patients with schizophrenia. *Journal of Neuroscience Research* 76(4): 581–592.

Eastwood, S. L. & Harrison, P. J. (2003). Interstitial white matter neurons express less reelin and are abnormally distributed in schizophrenia: Towards an integration of molecular and morphologic aspects of the neurodevelopmental hypothesis. *Molecular Psychiatry* 8(9): 769, 821–831.

Endres, M., Meisel, A., Biniszkiewicz, D., Namura, S., Prass, K., Ruscher, K., Lipski, A., Jaenisch, R., Moskowitz, M. A., & Dirnagl, U. (2000). DNA methyltransferase contributes to delayed ischemic brain injury. *Journal of Neuroscience* 20(9): 3175–3181.

Esteller, M. (2007). Cancer epigenomics: DNA methylomes and histone-modification maps. *Nature Reviews Genetics* 8(4): 286–298.

Fatemi, S. H., Earle, J. A., & McMenomy, T. (2000). Reduction in Reelin immunoreactivity in hippocampus of subjects with schizophrenia, bipolar disorder and major depression. *Molecular Psychiatry* 5(6): 571, 654–663.

Fatemi, S. H., Stary, J. M., Earle, J. A., Araghi-Niknam, M., & Eagan, E. (2005). GABAergic dysfunction in schizophrenia and mood disorders as reflected by decreased levels of glutamic acid decarboxylase 65 and 67 kDa and Reelin proteins in cerebellum. *Schizophrenia Research* 72(2–3): 109–122.

Felsenfeld, G. & Groudine, M. (2003). Controlling the double helix. *Nature* 421(6921): 448–453.

Fischle, W., Wang, Y., & Allis, C. D. (2003). Histone and chromatin cross-talk. *Current Opinion in Cell Biology* 15(2): 172–183.

Fraga, M. F., Ballestar, E., Paz, M. F., Ropero, S., Setien, F., Ballestar, M. L., Heine-Suner, D., Cigudosa, J. C., Urioste, M., Benitez, J., et al. (2005). Epigenetic differences arise during the lifetime of monozygotic twins. *Proceedings of the National Academy of Sciences U.S.A.* 102(30): 10604–10609.

Francks, C., Maegawa, S., Lauren, J., Abrahams, B. S., Velayos-Baeza, A., Medland, S. E., Colella, S., Groszer, M., McAuley, E. Z., Caffrey, T. M., et al. (2007). LRRTM1 on chromosome 2p12 is a maternally suppressed gene that is associated paternally with handedness and schizophrenia. *Molecular Psychiatry* 12(12): 1129–1139, 1057.

Fuks, F. (2005). DNA methylation and histone modifications: Teaming up to silence genes. *Current Opinion in Genetics and Development* 15(5): 490–495.

Gicquel, C., Rossignol, S., Cabrol, S., Houang, M., Steunou, V., Barbu, V., Danton, F., Thibaud, N., Le Merrer, M., Burglen, L., et al. (2005). Epimutation of the telomeric imprinting center region on chromosome 11p15 in Silver-Russell syndrome. *Nature Genetics* 37(9): 1003–1007.

Grayson, D. R., Chen, Y., Dong, E., Kundakovic, M., & Guidotti, A. (2009). From transmethylation to cytosine methylation: Evolution of the methylation hypothesis of schizophrenia. *Epigenetics* 4(3): 144–149.

Grayson, D. R., Jia, X., Chen, Y., Sharma, R. P., Mitchell, C. P., Guidotti, A., & Costa, E. (2005). Reelin promoter hypermethylation in schizophrenia. *Proceedings of the National Academy of Sciences U.S.A.* 102(26): 9341–9346.

Guan, Z., Giustetto, M., Lomvardas, S., Kim, J. H., Miniaci, M. C., Schwartz, J. H., Thanos, D., & Kandel, E. R. (2002). Integration of long-term-memory-related synaptic plasticity involves bidirectional regulation of gene expression and chromatin structure. *Cell* 111(4): 483–493.

Guidotti, A., Auta, J., Davis, J. M., Di-Giorgi-Gerevini, V., Dwivedi, Y., Grayson, D. R., Impagnatiello, F., Pandey, G., Pesold, C., Sharma, R., et al. (2000). Decrease in reelin and glutamic acid decarboxylase67 (GAD67) expression in schizophrenia and bipolar disorder: A postmortem brain study. *Archives of General Psychiatry* 57(11): 1061–1069.

Hammoud, S. S., Nix, D. A., Zhang, H., Purwar, J., Carrell, D. T., & Cairns, B. R. (2009). Distinctive chromatin in human sperm packages genes for embryo development. *Nature* 460(7254): 473–478.

Haroutunian, V., Katsel, P., Dracheva, S., Stewart, D. G., & Davis, K. L. (2007). Variations in oligodendrocyte-related gene expression across multiple cortical regions: Implications for the pathophysiology of schizophrenia. *International Journal of Neuropsychopharmacology* 10(4): 565–573.

Hashimoto, T., Arion, D., Unger, T., Maldonado-Aviles, J. G., Morris, H. M., Volk, D. W., Mirnics, K., & Lewis, D. A. (2008a). Alterations in GABA-related transcriptome in the dorsolateral prefrontal cortex of subjects with schizophrenia. *Molecular Psychiatry 13*(2): 147–161.

Hashimoto, T., Bazmi, H. H., Mirnics, K., Wu, Q., Sampson, A. R., & Lewis, D. A. (2008b). Conserved regional patterns of GABA-related transcript expression in the neocortex of subjects with schizophrenia. *American Journal of Psychiatry 165*(4): 479–489.

Hayes, J. J. & Hansen, J. C. (2001). Nucleosomes and the chromatin fiber. *Current Opinion in Genetics and Development 11*(2): 124–129.

Heintzman, N. D., Stuart, R. K., Hon, G., Fu, Y., Ching, C. W., Hawkins, R. D., Barrera, L. O., Van Calcar, S., Qu, C., Ching, K. A., et al. (2007). Distinct and predictive chromatin signatures of transcriptional promoters and enhancers in the human genome. *Nature Genetics 39*(3): 311–318.

Herman, H., Lu, M., Anggraini, M., Sikora, A., Chang, Y., Yoon, B. J., & Soloway, P. D. (2003). Trans allele methylation and paramutation-like effects in mice. *Nature Genetics 34*(2): 199–202.

Hitchins, M. P. & Ward, R. L. (2007). Erasure of MLH1 methylation in spermatozoa—implications for epigenetic inheritance. *Nature Genetics 39*(11): 1289.

Hitchins, M. P., Wong, J. J., Suthers, G., Suter, C. M., Martin, D. I., Hawkins, N. J., & Ward, R. L. (2007). Inheritance of a cancer-associated MLH1 germ-line epimutation. *New England Journal of Medicine 356*(7): 697–705.

Horsthemke, B. & Wagstaff, J. (2008). Mechanisms of imprinting of the Prader-Willi/Angelman region. *American Journal of Medical Genetics A 146A*(16): 2041–2052.

Huang, H. S. & Akbarian, S. (2007). GAD1 mRNA expression and DNA methylation in prefrontal cortex of subjects with schizophrenia. *PLoS One 2*(8): e809.

Huang, H. S., Matevossian, A., Jiang, Y., & Akbarian, S. (2006). Chromatin immunoprecipitation in postmortem brain. *Journal of Neuroscience Methods 156*(1): 284–292.

Huang, H. S., Matevossian, A., Whittle, C., Kim, S. Y., Schumacher, A., Baker, S. P., & Akbarian, S. (2007). Prefrontal dysfunction in schizophrenia involves mixed-lineage leukemia 1-regulated histone methylation at GABAergic gene promoters. *Journal of Neuroscience 27*(42): 11254–11262.

Iizuka, M. & Smith, M. M. (2003). Functional consequences of histone modifications. *Current Opinion in Genetics and Development 13*(2): 154–160.

Impagnatiello, F., Guidotti, A. R., Pesold, C., Dwivedi, Y., Caruncho, H., Pisu, M. G., Uzunov, D. P., Smalheiser, N. R., Davis, J. M., Pandey, G. N., et al. (1998). A decrease of reelin expression as a putative vulnerability factor in schizophrenia. *Proceedings of the National Academy of Sciences U.S.A. 95*(26): 15718–15723.

Iwamoto, K., Bundo, M., Yamada, K., Takao, H., Iwayama-Shigeno, Y., Yoshikawa, T., & Kato, T. (2005). DNA methylation status of SOX10 correlates with its downregulation and oligodendrocyte dysfunction in schizophrenia. *Journal of Neuroscience 25*(22): 5376–5381.

Jacobsen, S. E. & Meyerowitz, E. M. (1997). Hypermethylated SUPERMAN epigenetic alleles in arabidopsis. *Science 277*(5329): 1100–1103.

Jenuwein, T. & Allis, C. D. (2001). Translating the histone code. *Science 293*(5532): 1074–1080.

Kaminsky, Z., Wang, S. C., & Petronis, A. (2006). Complex disease, gender and epigenetics. *Annals of Medicine 38*(8): 530–544.

Kaminsky, Z. A., Tang, T., Wang, S. C., Ptak, C., Oh, G. H., Wong, A. H., Feldcamp, L. A., Virtanen, C., Halfvarson, J., Tysk, C., et al. (2009). DNA methylation profiles in monozygotic and dizygotic twins. *Nature Genetics 41*(2): 240–245.

Karoutzou, G., Emrich, H. M., & Dietrich, D. E. (2008). The myelin-pathogenesis puzzle in schizophrenia: A literature review. *Molecular Psychiatry 13*(3): 245–260.

Kato, M. V., Shimizu, T., Nagayoshi, M., Kaneko, A., Sasaki, M. S., & Ikawa, Y. (1996). Genomic imprinting of the human serotonin-receptor (HTR2) gene involved in development of retinoblastoma. *American Journal of Human Genetics* 59(5): 1084–1090.

Klose, R. J. & Zhang, Y. (2007). Regulation of histone methylation by demethylimination and demethylation. *Nature Reviews Molecular Cell Biology* 8(4): 307–318.

Knable, M. B., Barci, B. M., Webster, M. J., Meador-Woodruff, J., & Torrey, E. F. (2004). Molecular abnormalities of the hippocampus in severe psychiatric illness: Postmortem findings from the Stanley Neuropathology Consortium. *Molecular Psychiatry* 9(6): 609–620, 544.

Konradi, C., Eaton, M., MacDonald, M. L., Walsh, J., Benes, F. M., & Heckers, S. (2004). Molecular evidence for mitochondrial dysfunction in bipolar disorder. *Archives of General Psychiatry* 61(3): 300–308.

Korzus, E., Rosenfeld, M. G., & Mayford, M. (2004). CBP histone acetyltransferase activity is a critical component of memory consolidation. *Neuron* 42(6): 961–972.

Kriaucionis, S. & Heintz, N. (2009). The nuclear DNA base 5-hydroxymethylcytosine is present in Purkinje neurons and the brain. *Science* 324(5929): 929–930.

Kumar, A., Choi, K. H., Renthal, W., Tsankova, N. M., Theobald, D. E., Truong, H. T., Russo, S. J., Laplant, Q., Sasaki, T. S., Whistler, K. N., et al. (2005). Chromatin remodeling is a key mechanism underlying cocaine-induced plasticity in striatum. *Neuron* 48(2): 303–314.

Kundakovic, M., Chen, Y., Costa, E., & Grayson, D. R. (2007). DNA methyltransferase inhibitors coordinately induce expression of the human reelin and glutamic acid decarboxylase 67 genes. *Molecular Pharmacology* 71(3): 644–653.

Laruelle, M., Abi-Dargham, A., van Dyck, C. H., Gil, R., D'Souza, C. D., Erdos, J., McCance, E., Rosenblatt, W., Fingado, C., Zoghbi, S. S., et al. (1996). Single photon emission computerized tomography imaging of amphetamine-induced dopamine release in drug-free schizophrenic subjects. *Proceedings of the National Academy of Sciences U.S.A.* 93(17): 9235–9240.

Laruelle, M., D'Souza, C. D., Baldwin, R. M., Abi-Dargham, A., Kanes, S. J., Fingado, C. L., Seibyl, J. P., Zoghbi, S. S., Bowers, M. B., Jatlow, P., et al. (1997). Imaging D2 receptor occupancy by endogenous dopamine in humans. *Neuropsychopharmacology* 17(3): 162–174.

Laruelle, M., Jaskiw, G. E., Lipska, B. K., Kolachana, B., Casanova, M. F., Kleinman, J. E., & Weinberger, D. R. (1992). D1 and D2 receptor modulation in rat striatum and nucleus accumbens after subchronic and chronic haloperidol treatment. *Brain Research* 575(1): 47–56.

Laviola, G., Ognibene, E., Romano, E., Adriani, W., & Keller, F. (2009). Gene-environment interaction during early development in the heterozygous reeler mouse: Clues for modelling of major neurobehavioral syndromes. *Neuroscience and Biobehavioral Reviews* 33(4): 560–572.

Lei, H., Oh, S. P., Okano, M., Juttermann, R., Goss, K. A., Jaenisch, R., & Li, E. (1996). De novo DNA cytosine methyltransferase activities in mouse embryonic stem cells. *Development* 122(10): 3195–3205.

Levenson, J. M., Roth, T. L., Lubin, F. D., Miller, C. A., Huang, I. C., Desai, P., Malone, L. M., & Sweatt, J. D. (2006). Evidence that DNA (cytosine-5) methyltransferase regulates synaptic plasticity in the hippocampus. *Journal of Biological Chemistry* 281(23): 15763–15773.

Levine, A. A., Guan, Z., Barco, A., Xu, S., Kandel, E. R., & Schwartz, J. H. (2005). CREB-binding protein controls response to cocaine by acetylating histones at the fosB promoter in the mouse striatum. *Proceedings of the National Academy of Sciences U.S.A.* 102(52): 19186–19191.

Li, J., Guo, Y., Schroeder, F. A., Youngs, R. M., Schmidt, T. W., Ferris, C., Konradi, C., & Akbarian, S. (2004). Dopamine D2-like antagonists induce chromatin remodeling in striatal neurons through cyclic AMP-protein kinase A and NMDA receptor signaling. *Journal of Neurochemistry* 90(5): 1117–1131.

Lipska, B. K., Peters, T., Hyde, T. M., Halim, N., Horowitz, C., Mitkus, S., Weickert, C. S., Matsumoto, M., Sawa, A., Straub, R. E., et al. (2006). Expression of DISC1 binding partners is reduced in schizophrenia and associated with DISC1 SNPs. *Human Molecular Genetics* 15(8): 1245–1258.

Lupski, J. R. (2008). Schizophrenia: Incriminating genomic evidence. *Nature* 455(7210): 178–179.

Ma, D. K., Jang, M. H., Guo, J. U., Kitabatake, Y., Chang, M. L., Pow-Anpongkul, N., Flavell, R. A., Lu, B., Ming, G. L., & Song, H. (2009). Neuronal activity-induced Gadd45b promotes epigenetic DNA demethylation and adult neurogenesis. *Science* 323(5917): 1074–1077.

Manning, K., Tor, M., Poole, M., Hong, Y., Thompson, A. J., King, G. J., Giovannoni, J. J., & Seymour, G. B. (2006). A naturally occurring epigenetic mutation in a gene encoding an SBP-box transcription factor inhibits tomato fruit ripening. *Nature Genetics* 38(8): 948–952.

Martin, K. C. & Sun, Y. E. (2004). To learn better, keep the HAT on. *Neuron* 42(6): 879–881.

Martinowich, K., Hattori, D., Wu, H., Fouse, S., He, F., Hu, Y., Fan, G., & Sun, Y. E. (2003). DNA methylation-related chromatin remodeling in activity-dependent BDNF gene regulation. *Science* 302(5646): 890–893.

Marutha Ravindran, C. R. & Ticku, M. K. (2004). Changes in methylation pattern of NMDA receptor NR2B gene in cortical neurons after chronic ethanol treatment in mice. *Brain Research: Molecular Brain Research* 121(1–2): 19–27.

McDaniell, R., Lee, B. K., Song, L., Liu, Z., Boyle, A. P., Erdos, M. R., Scott, L. J., Morken, M. A., Kucera, K. S., Battenhouse, A., et al. (2010). Heritable individual-specific and allele-specific chromatin signatures in humans. *Science* 328(5975): 235–239.

Meador-Woodruff, J. H., Clinton, S. M., Beneyto, M., & McCullumsmith, R. E. (2003). Molecular abnormalities of the glutamate synapse in the thalamus in schizophrenia. *Annals of the New York Academy of Sciences* 1003: 75–93.

Middleton, F. A., Mirnics, K., Pierri, J. N., Lewis, D. A., & Levitt, P. (2002). Gene expression profiling reveals alterations of specific metabolic pathways in schizophrenia. *Journal of Neuroscience* 22(7): 2718–2729.

Mill, J., Tang, T., Kaminsky, Z., Khare, T., Yazdanpanah, S., Bouchard, L., Jia, P., Assadzadeh, A., Flanagan, J., Schumacher, A., et al. (2008). Epigenomic profiling reveals DNA-methylation changes associated with major psychosis. *American Journal of Human Genetics* 82(3): 696–711.

Morgan, H. D., Santos, F., Green, K., Dean, W., & Reik, W. (2005). Epigenetic reprogramming in mammals. *Human Molecular Genetics* 14(Spec.1): R47–R58.

Morgan, H. D., Sutherland, H. G., Martin, D. I., & Whitelaw, E. (1999). Epigenetic inheritance at the agouti locus in the mouse. *Nature Genetics* 23(3): 314–318.

Morison, I. M., Ramsay, J. P., & Spencer, H. G. (2005). A census of mammalian imprinting. *Trends in Genetics* 21(8): 457–465.

Nelson, E. D., Kavalali, E. T., & Monteggia, L. M. (2008). Activity-dependent suppression of miniature neurotransmission through the regulation of DNA methylation. *Journal of Neuroscience* 28(2): 395–406.

Nicholas, A. P., Lubin, F. D., Hallett, P. J., Vattem, P., Ravenscroft, P., Bezard, E., Zhou, S., Fox, S. H., Brotchie, J. M., Sweatt, J. D., et al. (2008). Striatal histone modifications in models of levodopa-induced dyskinesia. *Journal of Neurochemistry* 106(1): 486–494.

Nicholls, R. D. & Knepper, J. L. (2001). Genome organization, function, and imprinting in Prader-Willi and Angelman syndromes. *Annual Review of Genomics and Human Genetics* 2: 153–175.

Numachi, Y., Shen, H., Yoshida, S., Fujiyama, K., Toda, S., Matsuoka, H., Sora, I., & Sato, M. (2007). Methamphetamine alters expression of DNA methyltransferase 1 mRNA in rat brain. *Neuroscience Letters* 414(3): 213–217.

Numachi, Y., Yoshida, S., Yamashita, M., Fujiyama, K., Naka, M., Matsuoka, H., Sato, M., & Sora, I. (2004). Psychostimulant alters expression of DNA methyltransferase mRNA in the rat brain. *Annals of the New York Academy of Sciences* 1025: 102–109.

Ooi, S. K. & Bestor, T. H. (2008). The colorful history of active DNA demethylation. *Cell* 133(7): 1145–1148.

Otani, J., Nankumo, T., Arita, K., Inamoto, S., Ariyoshi, M., & Shirakawa, M. (2009). Structural basis for recognition of H3K4 methylation status by the DNA methyltransferase 3A ATRX-DNMT3-DNMT3L domain. *EMBO Reports* 10(11): 1235–1241.

Owen, M. J., Williams, H. J., & O'Donovan, M. C. (2009). Schizophrenia genetics: Advancing on two fronts. *Current Opinion in Genetics and Development* 19(3): 266–270.

Pae, C. U., Serretti, A., Mandelli, L., Yu, H. S., Patkar, A. A., Lee, C. U., Lee, S. J., Jun, T. Y., Lee, C., Paik, I. H., et al. (2007). Effect of 5-haplotype of dysbindin gene (DTNBP1) polymorphisms for the susceptibility to bipolar 1 disorder. *American Journal of Medical Genetics Part B: Neuropsychiatric Genetics* 144(5): 701–703.

Peterson, C. L. (2002). Chromatin remodeling: Nucleosomes bulging at the seams. *Current Biology* 12(7): R245–R247.

Peterson, C. L. & Laniel, M. A. (2004). Histones and histone modifications. *Current Biology* 14(14): R546–R551.

Polesskaya, O. O., Aston, C., & Sokolov, B. P. (2006). Allele C-specific methylation of the 5-HT2A receptor gene: Evidence for correlation with its expression and expression of DNA methylase DNMT1. *Journal of Neuroscience Research* 83(3): 362–373.

Probst, A. V., Dunleavy, E., & Almouzni, G. (2009). Epigenetic inheritance during the cell cycle. *Nature Reviews Molecular Cell Biology* 10(3): 192–206.

Rakyan, V. K., Chong, S., Champ, M. E., Cuthbert, P. C., Morgan, H. D., Luu, K. V., & Whitelaw, E. (2003). Transgenerational inheritance of epigenetic states at the murine Axin(Fu) allele occurs after maternal and paternal transmission. *Proceedings of the National Academy of Sciences U.S.A.* 100(5): 2538–2543.

Rampon, C., Jiang, C. H., Dong, H., Tang, Y. P., Lockhart, D. J., Schultz, P. G., Tsien, J. Z., & Hu, Y. (2000). Effects of environmental enrichment on gene expression in the brain. *Proceedings of the National Academy of Sciences U.S.A.* 97(23): 12880–12884.

Ramsahoye, B. H., Biniszkiewicz, D., Lyko, F., Clark, V., Bird, A. P., & Jaenisch, R. (2000). Non-CpG methylation is prevalent in embryonic stem cells and may be mediated by DNA methyltransferase 3a. *Proceedings of the National Academy of Sciences U.S.A.* 97(10): 5237–5242.

Rassoulzadegan, M., Grandjean, V., Gounon, P., Vincent, S., Gillot, I., & Cuzin, F. (2006). RNA-mediated non-mendelian inheritance of an epigenetic change in the mouse. *Nature* 441(7092): 469–474.

Rassoulzadegan, M., Magliano, M., & Cuzin, F. (2002). Transvection effects involving DNA methylation during meiosis in the mouse. *EMBO Journal* 21(3): 440–450.

Raybould, R., Green, E. K., MacGregor, S., Gordon-Smith, K., Heron, J., Hyde, S., Caesar, S., Nikolov, I., Williams, N., Jones, L., et al. (2005). Bipolar disorder and polymorphisms in the dysbindin gene (DTNBP1). *Biological Psychiatry* 57(7): 696–701.

Richards, E. J. (2006). Inherited epigenetic variation—revisiting soft inheritance. *Nature Reviews Genetics* 7(5): 395–401.

Rosen, L. B., Ginty, D. D., Weber, M. J., & Greenberg, M. E. (1994). Membrane depolarization and calcium influx stimulate MEK and MAP kinase via activation of Ras. *Neuron* 12(6): 1207–1221.

Salnikow, K. & Zhitkovich, A. (2008). Genetic and epigenetic mechanisms in metal carcinogenesis and cocarcinogenesis: Nickel, arsenic, and chromium. *Chemical Research in Toxicology* 21(1): 28–44.

Satta, R., Maloku, E., Costa, E., & Guidotti, A. (2007). Stimulation of brain nicotinic acetylcholine receptors (nAChRs) decreases DNA methyltransferase 1 (DNMT1) expression in cortical and hippocampal GABAergic neurons of Swiss albino mice. *Society for Neuroscience Abstract.*

Satta, R., Maloku, E., Zhubi, A., Pibiri, F., Hajos, M., Costa, E., & Guidotti, A. (2008). Nicotine decreases DNA methyltransferase 1 expression and glutamic acid decarboxylase 67 promoter methylation in GABAergic interneurons. *Proceedings of the National Academy of Sciences U.S.A.* 105(42): 16356–16361.

Sharp, A. J., Mefford, H. C., Li, K., Baker, C., Skinner, C., Stevenson, R. E., Schroer, R. J., Novara, F., De Gregori, M., Ciccone, R., et al. (2008). A recurrent 15q13.3 microdeletion syndrome associated with mental retardation and seizures. *Nature Genetics* 40(3): 322–328.

Shen, H. Y., Kalda, A., Yu, L., Ferrara, J., Zhu, J., & Chen, J. F. (2008). Additive effects of histone deacetylase inhibitors and amphetamine on histone H4 acetylation, cAMP responsive element binding protein phosphorylation and DeltaFosB expression in the striatum and locomotor sensitization in mice. *Neuroscience* 157(3): 644–655.

Shimabukuro, M., Jinno, Y., Fuke, C., & Okazaki, Y. (2006). Haloperidol treatment induces tissue- and sex-specific changes in DNA methylation: A control study using rats. *Behavioral and Brain Functions* 2: 37.

Siegmund, K. D., Connor, C. M., Campan, M., Long, T. I., Weisenberger, D. J., Biniszkiewicz, D., Jaenisch, R., Laird, P. W., & Akbarian, S. (2007). DNA methylation in the human cerebral cortex is dynamically regulated throughout the life span and involves differentiated neurons. *PLoS One* 2(9): e895.

Smith, M. (2009). The year in human and medical genetics. Highlights of 2007–2008. *Annals of the New York Academy of Sciences* 1151: 1–21.

Sokolov, B. P. (2007). Oligodendroglial abnormalities in schizophrenia, mood disorders and substance abuse. Comorbidity, shared traits, or molecular phenocopies? *International Journal of Neuropsychopharmacology* 10(4): 547–555.

Stadler, F., Kolb, G., Rubusch, L., Baker, S. P., Jones, E. G., & Akbarian, S. (2005). Histone methylation at gene promoters is associated with developmental regulation and region-specific expression of ionotropic and metabotropic glutamate receptors in human brain. *Journal of Neurochemistry* 94(2): 324–336.

Stam, M., Belele, C., Dorweiler, J. E., & Chandler, V. L. (2002). Differential chromatin structure within a tandem array 100 kb upstream of the maize b1 locus is associated with paramutation. *Genes and Development* 16(15): 1906–1918.

Stefansson, H., Rujescu, D., Cichon, S., Pietilainen, O. P., Ingason, A., Steinberg, S., Fossdal, R., Sigurdsson, E., Sigmundsson, T., Buizer-Voskamp, J. E., et al. (2008). Large recurrent microdeletions associated with schizophrenia. *Nature* 455(7210): 232–236.

Stine, O. C., Xu, J., Koskela, R., McMahon, F. J., Gschwend, M., Friddle, C., Clark, C. D., McInnis, M. G., Simpson, S. G., & Breschel, T. S. (1995). Evidence for linkage of bipolar disorder to chromosome 18 with a parent-of-origin effect. *American Journal of Human Genetics* 57(6): 1384–1394.

Straub, R. E., Jiang, Y., MacLean, C. J., Ma, Y., Webb, B. T., Myakishev, M. V., Harris-Kerr, C., Wormley, B., Sadek, H., Kadambi, B., et al. (2002). Genetic variation in the 6p22.3 gene

DTNBP1, the human ortholog of the mouse dysbindin gene, is associated with schizophrenia. *American Journal of Human Genetics* 71(2): 337–348.

Suter, C. M., Martin, D. I., & Ward, R. L. (2004). Germline epimutation of MLH1 in individuals with multiple cancers. *Nature Genetics* 36(5): 497–501.

Suzuki, M. M. & Bird, A. (2008). DNA methylation landscapes: Provocative insights from epigenomics. *Nature Reviews Genetics* 9(6): 465–476.

Swank, M. W. & Sweatt, J. D. (2001). Increased histone acetyltransferase and lysine acetyltransferase activity and biphasic activation of the ERK/RSK cascade in insular cortex during novel taste learning. *Journal of Neuroscience* 21(10): 3383–3391.

Sweatt, J. D. (2001). The neuronal MAP kinase cascade: A biochemical signal integration system subserving synaptic plasticity and memory. *Journal of Neurochemistry* 76(1): 1–10.

Tahiliani, M., Koh, K. P., Shen, Y., Pastor, W. A., Bandukwala, H., Brudno, Y., Agarwal, S., Iyer, L. M., Liu, D. R., Aravind, L., et al. (2009). Conversion of 5-methylcytosine to 5-hydroxymethylcytosine in mammalian DNA by MLL partner TET1. *Science* 324(5929): 930–935.

Tochigi, M., Iwamoto, K., Bundo, M., Komori, A., Sasaki, T., Kato, N., & Kato, T. (2008). Methylation status of the reelin promoter region in the brain of schizophrenic patients. *Biological Psychiatry* 63(5): 530–533.

Tsankova, N. M., Berton, O., Renthal, W., Kumar, A., Neve, R. L., & Nestler, E. J. (2006). Sustained hippocampal chromatin regulation in a mouse model of depression and antidepressant action. *Nature Neuroscience* 9(4): 519–525.

Tsankova, N. M., Kumar, A., & Nestler, E. J. (2004). Histone modifications at gene promoter regions in rat hippocampus after acute and chronic electroconvulsive seizures. *Journal of Neuroscience* 24(24): 5603–5610.

Vrijenhoek, T., Buizer-Voskamp, J., van der Stelt, I., Strengman, E., Consortium, G., & Sabatti, C. (2008). Recurrent CNVs disrupt three candidate genes in schizophrenia patients. *American Journal of Human Genetics* 83(4): 504–510.

Wagner, K. D., Wagner, N., Ghanbarian, H., Grandjean, V., Gounon, P., Cuzin, F., & Rassoulzadegan, M. (2008). RNA induction and inheritance of epigenetic cardiac hypertrophy in the mouse. *Developmental Cell* 14(6): 962–969.

Wang, Y., Fischle, W., Cheung, W., Jacobs, S., Khorasanizadeh, S., & Allis, C. D. (2004). Beyond the double helix: Writing and reading the histone code. *Novartis Found Symp* 259: 3–17; discussion 17–21, 163–169.

Weaver, I. C., Cervoni, N., Champagne, F. A., D'Alessio, A. C., Sharma, S., Seckl, J. R., Dymov, S., Szyf, M., & Meaney, M. J. (2004). Epigenetic programming by maternal behavior. *Nature Neuroscience* 7(8): 847–854.

Weaver, I. C., D'Alessio, A. C., Brown, S. E., Hellstrom, I. C., Dymov, S., Sharma, S., Szyf, M., & Meaney, M. J. (2007). The transcription factor nerve growth factor-inducible protein A mediates epigenetic programming: Altering epigenetic marks by immediate-early genes. *Journal of Neuroscience* 27(7): 1756–1768.

Wolffe, A. P. (1992). New insights into chromatin function in transcriptional control. *FASEB Journal* 6(15): 3354–3361.

Wood, A. J. & Oakey, R. J. (2006). Genomic imprinting in mammals: Emerging themes and established theories. *PLoS Genetics* 2(11): e147.

Wykes, S. M. & Krawetz, S. A. (2003). The structural organization of sperm chromatin. *Journal of Biological Chemistry* 278(32): 29471–29477.

PART 2

PRECLINICAL RESEARCH ON ETIOLOGIES OF SCHIZOPHRENIA

SECTION 1
Animal Models of Environmental Factors and Schizophrenia

CHAPTER 10

ANIMAL MODELS OF THE MATERNAL INFECTION RISK FACTOR FOR SCHIZOPHRENIA

PAUL H. PATTERSON

KEY CONCEPTS

- Epidemiologic evidence highlights maternal infection as an important risk factor for schizophrenia in the offspring.
- Rodent models of viral and bacterial maternal infection yield offspring with a series of abnormal behaviors and neuropathology consistent with those found in schizophrenia. None of the behaviors or pathology is specific for schizophrenia, however.
- These models are being used to investigate the molecular and cellular pathways that mediate the effects of maternal infection on fetal brain development.
- Interventions during maternal immune activation (MIA) in utero, or even in adolescent offspring, demonstrate that the development of abnormal behavior and neuropathology can be prevented.
- Experiments with MIA in cytokine knockout and transgenic mice, as well as in candidate gene models for schizophrenia, support the gene-environment interaction paradigm of mental illness.

Birth in winter or spring months is an accepted risk factor for schizophrenia, and it is possible that the prevalence of influenza in winter months is responsible (Tochigi et al., 2004). Over 25 studies have analyzed the prevalence of schizophrenia among subjects in utero during influenza epidemics, and most have found an increased occurrence among exposed offspring. More recently, Brown and colleagues (Brown et al., 2002; Brown et al., 2004; Brown, 2006) used a prospective approach to assay prenatal serum specimens for influenza antibody in offspring drawn from a cohort of over 12,000 pregnant women, and found that influenza infection during the first trimester is associated with a sevenfold increase in the risk for schizophrenia in the offspring (Brown et al., 2004). For early to midgestation, a threefold effect was demonstrated. Because of the high prevalence of influenza infection, the authors estimated that 14–21% of schizophrenia cases would not have occurred if maternal influenza had been prevented. These findings are further supported by an association between elevated cytokines in maternal serum and schizophrenia in the offspring (Brown & Derkits, 2010). In addition, there is evidence from serologic data and obstetrics records linking maternal rubella, toxoplasma, and genital-reproductive and bacterial infections with risk for schizophrenia (reviewed by Sorensen et al., 2009; Brown & Derkits, 2010). What is most striking is that maternal rubella infection increases the risk ten- to twentyfold. Because several of these infections are nonoverlapping, an attributable risk calculation summing the influenza, toxoplasma, and genital-reproductive infection risk factors suggests that as many as 33% of schizophrenia cases would not occur if all of these maternal infections could be prevented (chapter 1, this book; Brown & Derkits, 2010).

These links are even more remarkable considering that these epidemiologic studies did not screen for susceptibility genotype. Because of the strong genetic component in schizophrenia, it is possible that maternal infection is a risk factor only in genetically susceptible individuals. Thus, the risk associated with maternal infection for individuals with the appropriate genotype may be considerably greater than those figures just cited here.

The link between maternal infection and mental illness is reinforced by findings of immune dysregulation in schizophrenia. There are many reports of abnormalities in peripheral immune cells, as well as associations between schizophrenia and autoimmunity and variants of genes for cytokines, their receptors, and the major histocompatibility complex (reviewed by Sperner-Unterweger, 2005; Muller & Schwarz, 2006; Strous & Shoenfeld, 2006; Knight et al., 2007; Potvin et al., 2008; Shi et al., 2009a; Stefansson et al., 2009). There is also evidence of abnormal expression of immune-related genes in the brains of patients with schizophrenia (Arion et al., 2007; Saetre et al., 2007). This does not appear to be classical inflammation, but rather a dysregulation. The relevance of this growing literature is, first, that the immune status of the mother and fetus is likely to be of central importance for their responses to maternal infection. Second, the diverse nature of the various types of maternal infections that increase risk for schizophrenia in the offspring indicates that the critical response mechanism is activation of the maternal immune response. This conclusion is supported by studies of animal models of maternal infection.

Questions have been raised as to whether it is possible to develop animal models that are relevant for schizophrenia, a disorder that has been termed "uniquely human." However, the goal here is not necessarily to develop an animal model of schizophrenia, but rather to determine which features of schizophrenia may be expressed in an animal model of maternal infection. Indeed, many such features can be examined in animals, including behaviors and neuropathology. Some of the behavioral tests that are relevant for schizophrenia include those for anxiety, social interaction, sensorimotor gating (prepulse inhibition, or PPI), latent inhibition, working memory, and responses to antipsychotic and psychomimetic drugs. Some of the neuropathologies that are relevant for schizophrenia include enlarged ventricles; altered dopamine neurotransmission; various changes in GABA (gamma-aminobutyric acid) neurotransmission in parvalbumin-expressing chandelier neurons in the prefrontal cortex; atrophy in the hippocampus, cerebellum, and thalamus; altered myelination; and dysregulation of immune-related molecules in the brain and periphery (Dean et al., 2009). Animal models of maternal infection that exhibit many of these features are being effectively used to explore how activation of the maternal immune system leads to changes in fetal brain development. Moreover, potential approaches to prevention and treatment of symptoms are being tested in these models. Thus, these models have both face (they reproduce features of the disease) and construct (based on environmental or genetic risk factors for the disease) validity, as well as potential therapeutic value for schizophrenia.

Mouse Model of Maternal Respiratory Infection

Given the high frequency of influenza infection in human populations, and strong evidence linking maternal influenza infection with schizophrenia, it is logical to investigate this form of respiratory infection in animals. Moreover, mice are a logical choice because of their utility in genetic studies. Exposure of pregnant C57BL/6 or BALB/C mice to a strain of human influenza virus adapted to mice results in offspring with several histologic abnormalities in the hippocampus and cortex (Fatemi et al., 1999; Fatemi et al., 2000). These include modest layer- and region-specific changes in the expression of the presynaptic marker SNAP-25, as well as in nNOS and reelin. These offspring also display a spatially restricted deficit in Purkinje cells (Shi et al., 2009b), which is commonly found in autism and also occurs in schizophrenia (Ho, Mola, & Andreasen, 2004), as well as smaller and more densely packed pyramidal cells, a finding also reminiscent of schizophrenia pathology (Fatemi et al., 2002). Changes in white matter are also reported in the cerebellum, although these alterations are inconsistent across the postnatal ages examined (Fatemi et al., 2009). In addition, neonatal mice born to infected mothers display a striking abnormality in neuronal migration to layer 2/3 in the embryonic cortex (Shi et al., 2006). This migration defect is particularly interesting because it closely resembles that observed when *DISC1* (Disrupted-in-Schizophrenia 1, a leading candidate gene for schizophrenia) is experimentally down-regulated in the mouse fetus (Kamiya et al., 2005). Immunostaining for glial fibrillary acidic protein (GFAP) reveals a striking elevation in neonatal offspring, suggesting at least a transient inflammatory state in the brain (Fatemi et al., 2004). This is potentially relevant for the signs of chronic immune dysregulation observed in schizophrenia already cited here, as well as in other animal models discussed later in this chapter. There are also several reports of changes in gene expression in the neocortex and cerebellum in postnatal offspring of infected mothers (Fatemi et al., 2008), and some of these changes have also been observed in adult subjects with schizophrenia.

Behavioral analyses demonstrate that adult mice born to infected mothers display abnormalities that are relevant to schizophrenia, including deficits in social interaction, PPI of the acoustic startle, and increased anxiety (Shi et al., 2003). It is important that the PPI deficit is ameliorated by acute administration of antipsychotic drugs (clozapine and chlorpromazine) and exacerbated by a psychomimetic drug (ketamine).

Maternal Immune Activation with Poly(I:C)

Given that influenza infection normally is restricted to the respiratory tract, it was surprising that the virus was reported to be present in the fetus following maternal infection in mice (Aronsson et al., 2002). A subsequent report was, however, unable to confirm the presence of virus in the fetus or in the newborn brain following maternal infection (Shi, Tu, & Patterson, 2005). This suggested that it is the maternal immune response that drives pathology in the fetal brain. This hypothesis receives strong support from the finding that MIA using the synthetic, double stranded RNA, poly(I:C), which acts through the toll-like receptor 3 (TLR3), is sufficient to cause all of the behavioral and histologic abnormalities seen thus far in the offspring of maternal influenza-infected mothers (Shi et al., 2003; Smith et al., 2007; Shi et al., 2009b). The poly(I:C) model of MIA has been adopted widely, and many results have been reproduced among the laboratories, including deficits in PPI, social interaction, working memory, anxiety, and latent inhibition, increased amphetamine- and MK-801-induced locomotion and altered reversal learning (Shi et al., 2003; Zuckerman et al., 2003; Zuckerman & Weiner, 2005; Meyer et al., 2006b; Ozawa et al., 2006; Meyer, Yee, & Feldon, 2007; Smith et al., 2007; Wolff & Bilkey, 2008), all of which are consistent with the schizophrenia phenotype. Reminiscent of the young-adult onset of psychosis in schizophrenia, several of the behavioral abnormalities in mice display a postpubertal onset and are corrected by acute antipsychotic drug treatment. In addition, poly(I:C) MIA offspring exhibit a postpubertal emergence of the hallmark structural abnormality in schizophrenia, ventricular enlargement (Li et al., 2009; Piontkewitz, Assaf, & Weiner, 2009).

Offspring of poly(I:C)-treated pregnant rats and mice have also been examined for neurochemical alterations. Adult offspring display increased levels of

GABAA receptor α2 immunoreactivity (Nyffeler et al., 2006) and dopamine hyperfunction (Ozawa et al., 2006) as seen in schizophrenia, as well as a delay in hippocampal myelination (Makinodan et al., 2008). Expression of NMDA receptors in the hippocampus is reduced, as are the numbers of reelin- and parvalbumin-positive cells in the prefrontal cortex (Meyer et al., 2008c). Reduced dopamine D1 and D2 receptors in the prefrontal cortex and enhanced tyrosine hydroxylyase in striatal structures have also been reported (Meyer et al., 2008b). Although some of these changes are subtle and require replication, they are clearly relevant for schizophrenia.

Very little has been published on the electrophysiologic properties of neurons and circuits in poly(I:C) offspring. Recent work on hippocampal slices indicates that CA1 pyramidal neurons in the adult offspring of poly(I:C)-treated mothers display a reduced frequency and an increased amplitude of miniature excitatory postsynaptic currents. Although no difference is observed in paired-pulse facilitation or long-term potentiation (LTP) at Schaffer collateral-CA1 synapses, temporoammonic-CA1 synapses in the poly(I:C) offspring display a significantly increased sensitivity to dopamine (Ito et al., 2010). To assess hippocampal network function in vivo, expression of the immediate early gene, *c-Fos*, was used as a surrogate measure of neuronal activity. Compared to controls, the adult offspring of poly(I:C)-treated mothers display a distinct *c-Fos* expression pattern in area CA1 following novel object exposure. Because dopamine differentially influences object and spatial information processing in the hippocampus, these findings indicate that the offspring of immune-activated mothers may have an abnormality in modality-specific information processing (Smith et al., 2008; Ito et al., 2010).

Influenza infection and poly(I:C) are known to induce cytokines, so it was natural to ask if any of the cytokines induced by poly(I:C) MIA are involved in the changes in fetal brain development that result in neuropathology and abnormal behavior. Although cytokines are just one group of molecules that are induced by MIA, they are known to regulate various aspects of normal fetal brain development (reviewed by Deverman & Patterson, 2009). Thus, cytokine changes during MIA could perturb the delicate balance required for normal development. Apart from MIA's relevance to schizophrenia, studies of the mechanism of MIA are important for understanding the many other deleterious effects that maternal infection can have on the fetus, such as those seen in periventricular leukomalacia and cerebral palsy. Two approaches have been taken in the investigation of cytokine effects: injecting or up-regulating cytokines during pregnancy in the absence of MIA, and blocking endogenous cytokines or preventing their induction during MIA. Investigation of cytokine mediation of maternal poly(I:C) effects on neuropathology and behavior in the offspring has focused on interleukin-6 (IL-6). Daily intraperitoneal injection of IL-6 in pregnant rats for three days results in profound effects on the offspring (Samuelsson et al., 2006). One hippocampal-dependent behavior—spatial memory in the water maze—was monitored in that study, and the IL-6-exposed adult offspring displayed increased escape latency and time spent near the pool wall. Thus, prolonged exposure to elevated IL-6 during fetal development causes a deficit in working memory, as is also seen in poly(I:C)-induced MIA. Remarkably, IL-6 mRNA levels in the offspring of mothers with prolonged IL-6 exposure remain elevated in the hippocampus of the offspring at four and 24 weeks of age. This is reminiscent of the permanent state of immune dysregulation in adult autistic and schizophrenia brains (Patterson, 2009). Further evidence of this parallel is the astrogliosis and elevated GFAP levels in the adult hippocampus of the IL-6-exposed offspring.

Although over-expression studies can be misleading with regard to endogenous ligand function, blocking endogenous IL-6 action during MIA supports the key role of this cytokine (Smith et al., 2007). Co-injection of a neutralizing anti-IL-6 antibody with maternal poly(I:C) blocks the effects of MIA on the behavior of the offspring (figure 10.1). Moreover, maternal injection of poly(I:C) in an IL-6 knockout mouse yields offspring with normal behavior. In addition to preventing the development of abnormal behaviors, the anti-IL-6 antibody also blocks the changes in brain gene transcription induced by maternal poly(I:C). The evidence that IL-6 is required to mediate the effects of poly(I:C) suggests that discovering where this cytokine acts could illuminate the molecular and cellular pathways that are involved in MIA-induced alterations in fetal brain development. Thus far, it is clear that poly(I:C)-induced IL-6 activates cells in both the placenta and the fetal brain (Hsiao & Patterson, 2011). Maternal injection of poly(I:C) induces downstream markers of IL-6 action (SOCS3 expression and the phosphorylation of STAT1 and STAT3) in the placenta and fetal brain. Induction of these markers requires IL-6, as shown by blocking experiments with an anti-IL-6 antibody. Immunohistochemical evidence indicates that the activation of the STAT and mitogen-activated kinase (MAPK) pathways occurs in the fetal side of the placenta. It is interesting that maternal poly(I:C) injection also induces the expression of IL-6 mRNA in both the fetal brain and the placenta, and this is also dependent on the IL-6 induced by maternal poly(I:C) (Meyer et al., 2006b; Hsiao & Patterson, 2011). This suggests a possible positive, feed-forward mechanism for chronic, subclinical inflammation in the brain. IL-6 protein as well as several chemokines are also induced in the placenta, and NFkB is activated (Koga et al., 2009). Poly(I:C) can induce cytokine and chemokine expression in a human trophoblast cell line in culture, showing that a direct effect is possible (Koga et al., 2009). Moreover, MIA activates the endogenous immune cells in the placenta, and alters placental endocrine status (Hsiao & Patterson, 2011).

The relevance of IL-6 for schizophrenia is further suggested by the fact that several extremely diverse risk factors identified by epidemiology converge to elevate maternal IL-6 (figure 10.2). In addition to IL-6, however, several other cytokines (IL-1α, IL-6, IL-10, and tumor necrosis factor α [TNF-α]) are elevated in the fetal brain by maternal poly(I:C) treatment (Meyer et al., 2006a), and cytokine

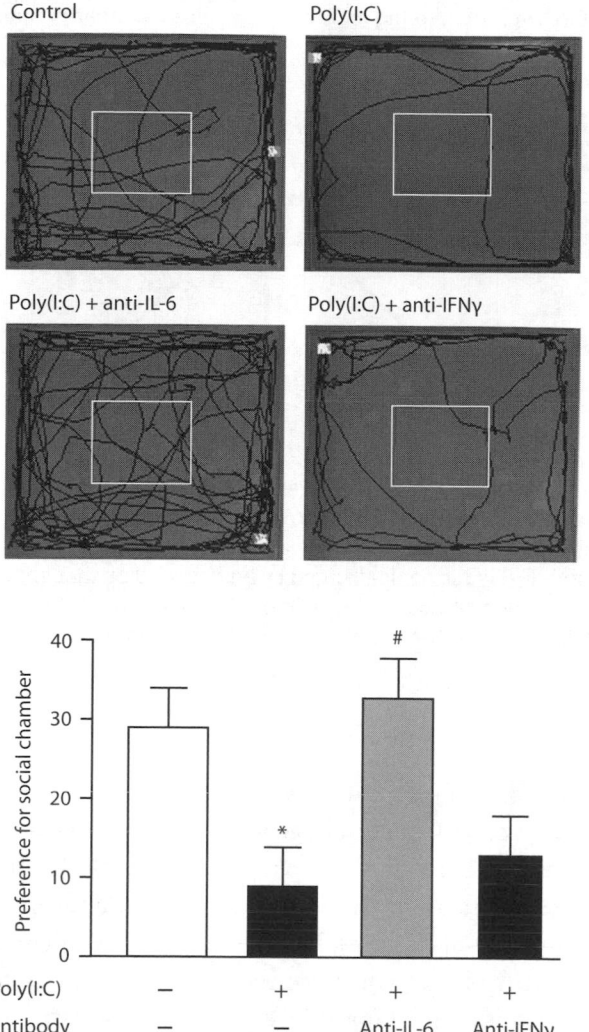

Figure 10.1. Abnormal behavior in MIA offspring is prevented by maternal treatment with anti-IL-6 antibody.

(*Top panel*) In the open field test, offspring of mice treated with poly(I:C) make fewer entries into the center than controls. Offspring of mice co-injected with anti-IL-6 and poly(I:C) enter the center as often as control mice. Offspring of mice co-injected with poly(I:C) and anti-IFNγ are not significantly different from those of controls or poly(I:C)-injected mice.

(*Bottom panel*) In the social interaction test, control mice show a strong preference for the social chamber, defined as (*percent time in social chamber*) – (*percent time in opposite chamber*), whereas the offspring of poly(I:C)-treated mice show no such preference. The deficit is corrected by maternal co-administration of IL-6 antibody along with poly(I:C).

[$F_{3,50} = 4.244$; $p < 0.01$]; *$< p < 0.05$ vs. control; #$< p < 0.05$ vs. poly(I:C). Similar results were obtained with two other behavioral assays. (Reprinted with permission from Smith et al. [2007].)

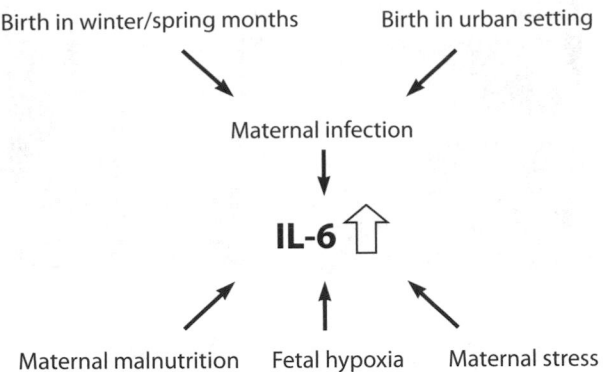

Figure 10.2. Convergence on IL-6.
Extremely divergent environmental risk factors identified by epidemiologic studies can be linked by their common ability to raise IL-6 levels in the mother. It is also suggested that birth in winter or spring months and being born in an urban environment are related to the enhanced likelihood of maternal infection in those settings. Stress increases both serum IL-6 and susceptibility to infection. IL-6 is further implicated by animal studies that show its key role in both maternal poly(I:C) and lipopolysaccharide (LPS) models, as well as the observations that this cytokine is dysregulated in the brain in both schizophrenia and autism. (Source: Author.)

expression in the neonatal offspring brain is also altered by MIA (Gilmore, Jarskog, & Vadlamudi, 2005). Conversely, genetically enforced expression of the anti-inflammatory cytokine IL-10 in macrophages attenuates the effects of poly(I:C) MIA, as measured by assays of PPI, latent inhibition, and open field anxiety in adult offspring (Meyer et al., 2008a). It is interesting that enhanced levels of IL-10 in the absence of MIA in pregnant mice leads to behavioral abnormalities in the adult offspring, illustrating the importance of the appropriate balance among cytokines that is required for normal development (Deverman & Patterson, 2009).

In addition to the brain, the peripheral immune system of poly(I:C) MIA offspring is altered, as it is in schizophrenia. For instance, compared to controls, CD4+ T cells from the spleen and mesenteric lymph nodes of adult mouse MIA offspring display significantly elevated IL-6 and IL-17 responses to in vitro stimulation (Hsiao et al., 2010; Mandal et al., 2010). Furthermore, adult MIA offspring display reduced T cell responses to antigens specific to the central nervous system, despite elevated proliferation of nonspecific T cells (Cardon et al., 2009).

The maternal poly(I:C) model is also being used for postnatal therapeutic experiments. As already mentioned, acute antipsychotic medication administration can block several of the behavioral deficits in influenza infection and poly(I:C) MIA offspring. This has been taken a step further in experiments testing such medications in immature MIA offspring, before the onset of behavioral abnormalities and ventricular enlargement (Piontkewitz, Assaf, & Weiner, 2009;

Meyer et al., 2010). Transient treatment for a week during this prodromal period during adolescence, many weeks before the onset of behavioral abnormalities and testing, is effective in preventing the emergence of abnormal behaviors as well as ventricular enlargement. This supports the notion that antipsychotic medication treatment of high-risk subjects is worthy of further investigation. It is notable, however, that clozapine treatment of offspring born to mothers injected with saline had a detrimental effect on the adolescent development of these controls, as assayed by behavioral tests (Meyer et al., 2010). Although the classic action of these antipsychotic medications involves blockade of the D2 dopamine receptor, it is worth noting in the present context that many of them can also influence cytokine expression (Pollmacher et al., 2000; Drzyzga et al., 2006).

The poly(I:C) model is also beginning to be used to explore gene-environment interactions, which is the dominant model of schizophrenia etiology. Two different mutant mouse strains of the leading schizophrenia candidate gene *DISC1* are reported to be more sensitive to poly(I:C)-induced immune activation in the mother or in the neonatal pups than wild type controls (Abazyan et al., 2010; Ibi et al., 2010). Several different behavioral assays were used. Thus, there is a gene-environment interaction worthy of further investigation. In addition, DISC1 null and heterozygote DISC1 pups born to poly(I:C)-treated heterozygote mothers display altered ultrasonic vocalizations compared to wild types (Malkova, Hsiao, & Patterson, 2010).

For expedience, all of the maternal poly(I:C) results discussed here have been summarized as if all of the laboratories are using the same protocol. In fact, some groups use mice and some rats, and some groups use intraperitoneal administration whereas others administer intravenously. Although most of the reports have yielded consistent results across laboratories, delivery site is potentially a complicating issue. It seems likely that intravenous delivery would provide access of poly(I:C) to the placenta at a higher concentration than would intraperitoneal delivery. Moreover, it is not clear whether poly(I:C) can cross the placenta. In addition, intraperitoneal delivery has the potential to more directly activate receptors in the mesenteric lymph nodes and the vagal afferents, sites important for sickness behavior and gastrointestinal responses. Various laboratories are using different salts of poly(I:C), and the manufacturers are not clear on the actual composition of the polymers they are providing. Another issue is that poly(I:C) is being injected at a variety of time points during pregnancy, and this is known to yield different results (see, for example, Meyer et al., 2006b). A final point concerns the diversity of behavioral responses observed within a treatment group, and even the diversity seen among the offspring in a single litter. This means that large numbers of animals are required for meaningful data and statistical differences between groups. But why should the behavior of individual offspring of a single mother differ significantly? One possibility is random epigenetic changes to the genome. Another explanation is related to position within the uterus, as there are known differences in placental physiology along the uterus (Ryan & Vandenbergh, 2002). Such heterogeneity of placental physiology could lead to differential responses to maternal infection and poly(I:C). Recall also that two-thirds of monozygotic human twins share the same placenta, which means that they are sharing key environmental factors that are not shared by most dizygotic twins (Patterson, 2007). This has implications for interpreting twin studies, where it is implicitly assumed that differences between monozygotic and dizygotic twins are due to genetics. All of these considerations also apply to the other animal models that will be discussed.

Another issue in all of these experiments is the potential effects of MIA on the behavior of the mother toward the pups during the early postnatal period. Cross-fostering MIA pups to surrogate control mothers does not prevent the onset of behavioral and neurochemical abnormalities in the offspring. Thus, these deficits are due in large part to the prenatal rather than postnatal effects. On the other hand, some abnormalities can be introduced in control pups raised by MIA mothers (Meyer et al., 2006b; Meyer et al., 2008b). Therefore, the behavior of the MIA mothers apparently is not completely normal. However, using the same immune-activated mother to raise her own litter is presumably more relevant to the real life situation.

Maternal Immune Activation with LPS

Another animal model of MIA is based on the maternal bacterial infection risk factor. Lipopolysaccharide (LPS), a component of bacterial cell walls that acts through TLR-4, is injected into pregnant rats, mice, rabbits, or ewes, yielding offspring with many of the same behavioral abnormalities seen in the offspring of mothers with poly(I:C)-induced MIA (reviewed by Hagberg & Mallard, 2005; Jonakait, 2007; Meyer, Yee, & Feldon, 2007; Smith & Patterson, 2008; Meyer Feldon, & Fatemi, 2009; Patterson, 2009). This is not surprising, as ligands binding TLR-4 activate many of the same signaling pathways as TLR-3 ligands. Although the specific combination of cytokines and chemokines induced by TLR-4 is slightly different from that induced by TLR-3, both poly(I:C) and LPS produce a strong, transient immune activation. Some of the behavioral abnormalities shared between the poly(I:C) and the LPS model include PPI and social interaction deficits, increased anxiety, and abnormalities in dopamine-related behaviors (Borrell et al., 2002; Fortier et al., 2004; Golan et al., 2005; Hava et al., 2006; Romero et al., 2007). Other behavioral abnormalities in the LPS model include poor performance in the beam-crossing test, deficient object recognition, and impaired water maze spatial memory (Bakos et al., 2004; Lante et al., 2007; Coyle et al., 2009). Histologic findings in the LPS model include fewer, more densely packed neurons in the hippocampus; increased microglial and GFAP staining;

altered tyrosine hydroxylase staining; decreased dopamine levels in the nucleus accumbens; decreased dendritic length; fewer oligodendrocyte precursors; and decreased myelin protein staining (Cai et al., 2000; Bell & Hallenbeck, 2002; Borrell et al., 2002; Carvey et al., 2003; Bakos et al., 2004; Ling et al., 2004; Golan et al., 2005; Elovitz, Mrinalini, & Sammel, 2006; Nitsos et al., 2006; Rousset et al., 2006; Wang et al., 2006b; Wang et al., 2007; Paintlia et al., 2008a; Paintlia et al., 2008b; Baharnoori, Brake, & Srivastava, 2009). These observations are largely consistent with schizophrenia neuropathology (Dean et al., 2009).

In one of the very few electrophysiologic studies of the offspring in the maternal LPS model, the intrinsic excitability of hippocampal CA1 pyramidal neurons was reported to be elevated and, whereas paired-pulse facilitation of the fEPSP is attenuated, long-term potentiation is normal (Lowe, Luheshi, & Williams, 2008). The authors suggest that there is a reduction in presynaptic input to CA1, with a compensatory elevation of postsynaptic glutamatergic responses. These results appear to be different from those observed in the poly(:C) model previously discussed here.

Although little attention has been paid to neurogenesis in the MIA models, maternal LPS, particularly when administered late in gestation, results in slightly fewer BrdU+ cells generated immediately after LPS (Cui et al., 2009). A larger deficit is observed in BrdU+ cells generated on postnatal day 14, and it persists for four subsequent weeks. In light of the deficit in migration to layer 2/3 observed in the poly(I:C) model, it would also be interesting to examine the migration of the newborn neurons in the LPS model.

In common with findings in the neonatal offspring of the poly(I:C) and multiple IL-6 injection models are observations of fetal and neonatal brain inflammation in maternal LPS offspring, as defined by astrogliosis (enhanced GFAP staining), altered microglial immunostaining, positron emission tomography (PET) imaging, and increased expression of proinflammatory genes such as IL-6, TNF-α, or interferon-γ (IFN- γ) (Bell & Hallenbeck, 2002; Borrell et al., 2002; Bell, Hallenbeck, & Gallo, 2004; Elovitz et al., 2006; Liverman et al., 2006; Nitsos et al., 2006; Rousset et al., 2006; Kannan et al., 2007; Paintlia et al., 2008a; Paintlia et al., 2008b; Salminen et al., 2008). Inflammatory cytokines are also induced in the placenta (Silver et al., 1997; Urakubo et al., 2001; Bell, Hallenbeck, & Gallo, 2004; Gayle et al., 2004; Ashdown et al., 2006; Elovitz & Gonzalez, 2008; Paintlia et al., 2008a; Paintlia et al., 2008b; Salminen et al., 2008). The evidence of inflammatory changes in the brains of offspring of LPS-treated mothers is consistent with the striking findings of immune dysregulation in human schizophrenia. The level and types of inflammatory markers reported for fetal brain and placenta vary, depending in part on the age, number, and site (peritoneum, cervix, uterus, or amniotic fluid) of the maternal LPS injections. An LPS protocol of maternal intraperitoneal injections every other day induces a permanent inflammatory state, as shown by elevated IL-6 and other proinflammatory cytokines in sera of adult offspring (Romero et al., 2007). Maternal LPS administration can also lead to altered responses to inflammatory challenge in adulthood (Wang et al., 2006b; Hodyl et al., 2007; Lasala & Zhou, 2007). It is interesting that the cytokine elevation in adult serum can be prevented by antipsychotic drug administration (Romero et al., 2007), as was found in the poly(I:C) model, already mentioned here. Confirming the innate inflammatory pathway in nonhuman primates, the TLR-4 antagonist TLR4A blocks the effects of intra-amniotic, LPS-induced cytokines and uterine contractions (Adams Waldorf et al., 2008).

How does maternal LPS alter fetal brain development? As with maternal poly(I:C), there is evidence of activation of inflammatory pathways in both placenta and fetal brain. The latter reaction presumably is indirect, as labeled LPS does not cross the placenta, at least when injected at E15 in the rat (Ashdown et al., 2006). A similar labeling experiment with poly(I:C) has not been reported as yet. Because cytokines can cross the placenta, at least at some stages of development, and they can be generated by the placenta, these molecules have been investigated as mediators of the effects of maternal infection on fetal brain development. Injection of anti-TNF-α antibodies or an inhibitor of TNF-α synthesis (pentoxifylline) can reduce maternal LPS-induced fetal loss and growth restriction. Conversely, injection of TNF-α alone can induce fetal loss (Silver et al., 1994; Xu et al., 2006). These effects are exacerbated significantly in IL-18 knockout mice, but not in IL-1α/α knockout mice (Wang et al., 2006a). Experiments with double knockout mice demonstrate that both TNF and IL-1 signaling are important in bacterially induced preterm labor (Hirsch, Filipovich, & Mahendroo, 2006). As in the poly(I:C) model, IL-10 is protective, mitigating white matter damage caused by maternal *E. coli* infection (Pang et al., 2005). An attractive feature of this potential therapeutic agent is that endogenous IL-10 is essential for resistance to LPS-induced preterm labor and fetal loss. Thus, administration of this cytokine enhances a natural protective mechanism by attenuating the production of proinflammatory cytokines in the uterus and placenta (Rivera et al., 1998; Terrone et al., 2001; Robertson, Skinner, & Care, 2006). Subcutaneous administration of IL-10 is nontoxic in long-term studies in mice and monkeys, although testing was not done during pregnancy (Rosenblum, Johnson, & Schmahai, 2002). It is important to note, however, that enhanced levels of IL-10 in the absence of MIA in pregnant mice leads to behavioral abnormalities in the adult offspring (Meyer et al., 2008c). Moreover, IL-10 administration can impair the response to infection (van der Poll et al., 1996). Thus, "only when the pathogenesis of obstetrical complications is more fully understood can meaningful therapeutic interventions become a realistic goal" (Elovitz, 2006). The role of IL-6 has not been investigated thoroughly in the maternal LPS model, but this cytokine is important in the neonatal brain response to intracerebral injection of LPS. An anti-IL-6 antibody attenuates ventricle dilation as well as astrocyte and microglial activation, and it improves behavioral outcome (Pang et al., 2006).

The importance of a cytokine imbalance following MIA could also be relevant postnatally. It is clear from both animal and clinical studies that acute changes in cytokines can markedly affect behavior, even to the point of inducing psychosis (reviewed by Bauer, Kerr, & Patterson, 2007). Such an imbalance could perhaps explain a series of puzzling case studies reporting the sudden onset of autistic symptoms in children and adults following encephalitis or infection with herpes simplex, varicella, or cytomegalovirus (Libbey et al., 2005). Central nervous system infections of this type are known to induce proinflammatory cytokine expression rapidly. In contrast, infections in autistic children are associated with acute amelioration of behavioral symptoms, which is also consistent with ongoing regulation of behavior by cytokines (Curran et al., 2007). Relevant to schizophrenia, there are reports (from another era) that malarial infection can ameliorate psychosis (Tempelton & Glas, 1924; Hinsie, 1929). A key point about the hypothesis of cytokines directly inducing or influencing behavior postnatally is that it raises the possibility of developing treatments based on anti-cytokine or anti-inflammatory agents. In fact, a preliminary study in 25 autistic children of the anti-inflammatory thiazolidinedione pioglitazone revealed a significant decrease in irritability, lethargy, stereotypy, and hyperactivity, with greater effects on the younger patients (Boris et al., 2007). Anti-inflammatory medication trials have also been proposed for schizophrenia (Riedel et al., 2005; Potvin et al., 2008), although the initial results have been mixed (Stolk et al., 2007). As already mentioned here, antipsychotic medications can influence cytokine expression, induce fever, and attenuate the peripheral cytokine response to poly(I:C) MIA.

Oxidative stress may also play an important role in the response to MIA, as pretreatment with the antioxidant N-acetylcysteine (NAC) prevents LPS-induced markers of stress in male fetuses and subsequent deficits in hippocampal long-term potentiation and water maze performance (Lante et al., 2007). Treatment with NAC also attenuates the induction of IL-6 in fetal blood (Beloosesky, Gayle, & Ross, 2006) as well as cytokine induction and leukocyte infiltration in the placenta (Paintlia et al., 2008a; Paintlia et al., 2008b). Various forms of prevention and treatment in the context of MIA are illustrated in figure 10.3.

Another version of the LPS model involves direct injection of LPS into the fetus, as reviewed by Wang et al. (2006b). This approach bypasses the effects of LPS on the placenta and maternal host, both of which may be critical for the development of pathology in the fetus. The same is true for models involving injection of LPS, viruses, poly(I:C), or cytokines during the early postnatal period (Pearce, 2003; Nawa & Takei, 2006; Wang et al., 2006b). Moreover, it is not clear that infection in the neonatal period increases risk for schizophrenia. The rationale for the neonatal injection models is that the very early postnatal rodent brain is thought to be at a stage of development similar to that of the human brain in the second or third trimester. However, the most recent epidemiologic data indicate

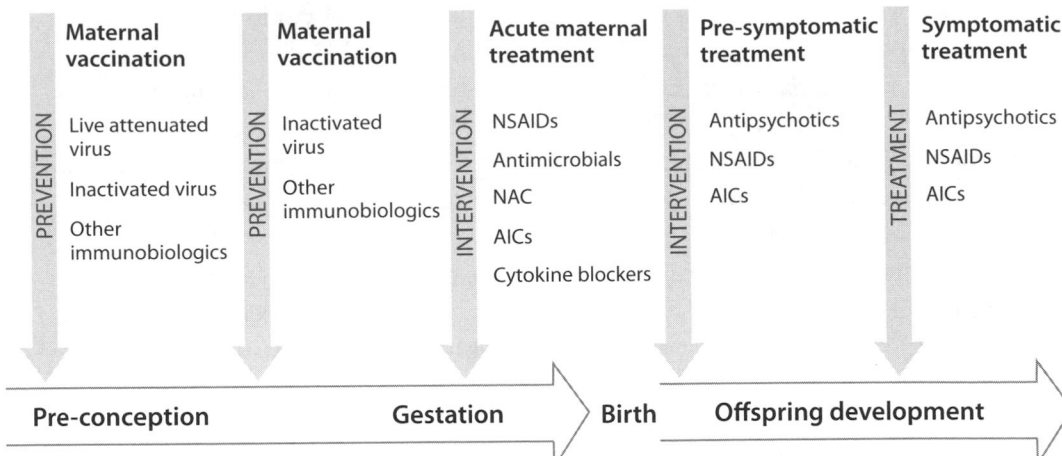

Figure 10.3. Potential prevention, intervention, and treatments for maternal infection. A timeline is depicted illustrating some of the attempts at blocking or diminishing the effects of maternal infection. Successful anti-influenza vaccination before pregnancy would be an effective and safe strategy, although it would not prevent other types of maternal infection. Vaccination during pregnancy is strongly recommended by public health authorities, although doubts have been raised about both its efficacy and its safety. Other immunobiological approaches include the use of modified bacterial toxins that are nontoxic but elicit production of antitoxins (as for diphtheria and tetanus), polysaccharides used as adjuvants (as for meningococcus), and recombinant Ig protein (as for hepatitis). Antimicrobial drugs could be used either as a preventative measure or following signs of infection. Safety for the fetus is a possible issue, however. There are a number of approaches for mitigating infection-driven inflammation, including nonsteroidal anti-inflammatory drugs (NSAIDs), N-acetyl cysteine (NAC), anti-inflammatory cytokines (AICs) (e.g., IL-10), and cytokine blockers (e.g., antibodies against IL-6, TNF blocker). All but the NSAIDS have proved effective in rodent LPS or poly(I:C) models. However, their utility under the conditions of actual maternal infection is a key issue because of the possibility of disturbing the pro- versus anti-inflammatory balance that is essential for a healthy pregnancy. A different approach that is currently being tested in the poly(:C) model involves supplementing choline in the diet of the mother—this is also being tested in human pregnancies at risk for schizophrenia outcome. Because there are clear signs of immune dysregulation in the brains and cerebral spinal fluid (CSF) of schizophrenia and autistic patients, anti-inflammatory approaches are being tested postnatally, either before or following the onset of symptoms. Antipsychotic drugs are proving effective during the prodromal period in preventing symptom onset in the poly(I:C) model, and could be acting to mitigate inflammation as well as blocking the dopamine receptors in the central nervous system. Recent experiments are also testing the utility of probiotic bacteria in preventing abnormal behaviors in the poly(I:C) model. The efficacy of these approaches following symptom onset remains to be proved. (Illustration by Elaine Hsiao.)

that the periconceptional period and the first and early second trimesters may also represent a critical window for exposure to certain maternal infections that lead to risk for schizophrenia (Brown & Derkits, 2010). Another factor to consider is the timing of immune system development. In primates, the immune system develops primarily in utero; in rats and mice, a major proportion of this development occurs during late gestation and the early postnatal period (Merlot, Couret, & Otten, 2008).

Maternal Infection with Periodontal Bacteria

Bacterial infection is associated with schizophrenia (Sorensen et al., 2009), and obstetric complications caused by such infections increase the risk for schizophrenia (Byrne et al., 2000). Intrauterine infections are associated with very low birth weight, which is correlated with neurologic disorders. Among the microorganisms isolated from the preterm placenta are gram-negative bacteria that are known to be involved in periodontal disease, *F. nucleatum*, *C. rectus*, and *P. gingivalis*. Moreover, epidemiologic evidence links periodontal disease with premature delivery (Bobetsis, Barros, & Offenbacher, 2006). In a pregnant mouse model, intravenous injection of *F. nucleatum* results in premature delivery and stillbirth (Han et al., 2004), and the infection is confined to the uterus. Fetal loss is reduced in TLR4-deficient mice and by administration of the TLR4 antagonist, TLR4A. It is interesting that TLR4A reduces fetal death and placental (decidua) necrosis without affecting bacterial colonization of the placenta, indicating the critical involvement of inflammation (Liu, Redline, & Han, 2007). Subcutaneous infection with *C. rectus* or *P. gingivalis* induces markers of inflammation in the placenta and amniotic fluid, as well as fetal growth restriction (Lin et al., 2003a; Lin et al., 2003b; Offenbacher et al., 2005; Yeo et al., 2005; Bobetsis, Barros, & Offenbacher, 2007). In an alternative mouse model using *systemic* administration of *P. gingivalis*, fetal growth restriction is observed in every litter, but not in every fetus. It is important that *P. gingivalis* DNA is found only in the placentae of affected fetuses and that those placentae show elevation of proinflammatory and reduction of anti-inflammatory cytokines (Lin et al., 2003a). These results link cytokines with fetal morbidity, and they highlight the importance of heterogeneity among placentae within the same uterus. Placental status is a key issue in interpreting genetic heritability in twin studies of schizophrenia (Patterson, 2007). An alternative model with more construct value involves *oral* infection of mice with *C. rectus*, *P. gingivalis*, or both. The mice are then mated. Examination of the placentae reveals elevated TLR4 expression in the trophoblasts, with reduced fetal weight (Arce et al., 2009).

Although there are as yet no published studies of the behavior of the offspring of mice infected with periodontal bacteria, brain neuropathology has been observed. In a preliminary report, myelin defects are seen in the corpus callosum, hippocampus, and cortex of neonatal mouse offspring of *C. rectus*-infected mothers (Offenbacher et al., 2005).

There are also a few papers on intrauterine infections with *E. coli* during late pregnancy. This results in microglial or macrophage infiltration or activation, astroglial activation, and reduced staining with myelin markers in the fetal brain.

As mentioned previously, these signs of inflammation and white matter damage are attenuated by intravenous administration of IL-10 the day after maternal infection (Pang et al., 2005). This finding is similar to the anti-inflammatory effects of IL-10 in the studies of LPS and poly(I:C) administration. Studies of gram-negative bacterial infections and TLR4 are directly relevant to the work using maternal LPS, as LPS is expressed by gram-negative bacteria and activates TLR4.

Nonhuman Primate Models

Although mouse models have the benefit of genetic manipulation, nonhuman primates display behaviors that are much more homologous to those in humans. Therefore, it would be of particular interest to evaluate behavior in nonhuman primate MIA models. However, as in schizophrenia, the key behavioral changes may have a postpubertal onset, making the experiments long-term and expensive. A preliminary MRI analysis of the effects of influenza infection in pregnant rhesus monkeys reports that the one-year-old offspring display small but significant reductions in cortical gray matter (Short et al., 2010). The largest reductions are in cingulate and parietal areas, and a slight reduction in white matter volume is seen in the parietal cortex. These offspring spend less time with their mothers than controls do, yet they emit more stress-related vocalizations. In this experiment, the early third trimester was chosen as the time of infection, which has generally not been shown to be within the window of vulnerability for the maternal infection risk factor for schizophrenia. An alternative approach is also under way, using multiple injections of poly(I:C) in rhesus monkeys during the late first trimester (Baughman et al., 2011).

Assaying for Positive Symptoms of Schizophrenia

It is important that the poly(I:C) and LPS models display many key features of schizophrenia neuropathology (particularly the enlarged ventricles seen with poly(I:C)), and that these models display a variety of behavioral abnormalities that resemble the negative symptoms of schizophrenia. However, these endophenotypes are shared with many other disorders. More specific to schizophrenia are the positive symptoms, such as hallucinations, although these can also be found in bipolar and major depressive disorders. However, this is generally considered to be a uniquely human trait or impossible to assay in animals. Nonetheless, there is a definition of hallucination that should be possible to investigate in animal models: the appearance of neuronal activity in a sensory cortex in the absence of external sensory input. This activity should also be evoked by administration of known hallucinogenic drugs and be blocked by 5-HT_{2A} receptor antagonists. Part of this paradigm has, in fact, already been achieved: injection of the hallucinogen 2,5-dimethoxy-4-iodoamphetamine (DOI) intraperitoneally in adult mice induces immediate early gene (IEG) expression in sensory cortices in the absence of external sensory stimuli (Malkova, N. & Patterson, P. H., unpublished data; also Gonzalez-Maeso et al., 2007). Such gene expression is often taken as a surrogate marker of neuronal activity. The IEG+ neurons also express 5-HT$_{2A}$ receptors (Gonzalez-Maeso et al., 2007).

Also relevant in this context is a mouse model of Wernicke-Korsakoff syndrome, which is a neuropsychiatric disorder that includes hallucinations, among a variety of other symptoms. This model is established by thiamine deprivation, as is the case in the human disorder. These mice display an elevated sensitivity to intracerebral DOI administration, as measured by increased head twitches (Nakagawasai et al., 2007). This provides an example of elevated sensitivity to a hallucinogen in a mouse model of a human disorder that involves hallucinations.

Universal Maternal Vaccination?

Given that influenza viruses mutate frequently, effective vaccination must be administered each year. Because maternal infection carries risk, it is widely recommended that women who become pregnant during or just before flu season receive the vaccine for that current year. As the animal work indicates that MIA in the absence of a pathogen is sufficient to mimic the effects of infection on the fetus, an obvious question is whether vaccination provides sufficient MIA to mimic the effects of poly(I:C) or LPS. Epidemiologic studies of human maternal vaccination do not necessarily provide a clear answer about its risk-benefit balance (Ayoub & Yazbak, 2008; Mak et al., 2008; Skowronski & De Serres, 2009); therefore, more animal work on maternal vaccination is warranted.

KEY AREAS FOR FUTURE RESEARCH

- Because mouse models with face and construct value for schizophrenia are available, and mice carrying schizophrenia candidate genes have been produced, it is now possible to test the hypothesis that a more complete schizophrenia phenotype may emerge from environmental risk factors acting on susceptibility genotypes.
- Many more aspects of schizophrenia neuropathology remain to be explored in MIA models, such as GABAergic properties of chandelier neurons and dopamine receptor occupancy.
- Multielectrode recording, functional imaging, and IEG activation studies will be important for mapping patterns of functional activity in rodent models and comparing it to functional MRI data from human patients.

- Because all available behavioral tests assay the negative and neurocognitive symptoms of schizophrenia, it will be important to develop assays for positive symptoms. Is 5-HT$_{2A}$ receptor-dependent activity in the sensory cortex in the absence of external sensory input increased in rodent models of maternal infection?
- As prenatal adjustment of the proinflammatory versus anti-inflammatory cytokine balance can prevent the effects of MIA in the offspring, and prodromal treatment with antipsychotic drugs is also effective, it seems likely that new, more efficacious drugs can be developed for presymptomatic schizophrenia.

Acknowledgments

Current work quoted from the author's laboratory is supported by grants from the National Institutes of Mental Health and General Medical Sciences, the Binational Science Foundation, the Caltech Brain Imaging Center, the Della Martin Foundation, Autism Speaks, and the Simons Foundation. Thanks to Elaine Hsiao for figure 10.3, to Patric Prado and Alan Brown for helpful comments on the manuscript, and to Laura Rodriguez for editing assistance.

Selected Readings

Brown, A. S. & Derkits, E. J. (2010). Prenatal infection and schizophrenia: A review of epidemiologic and translational studies. *American Journal of Psychiatry* 167(3): 261–280.

Meyer, U., Feldon, J., & Fatemi, S. H. (2009). In-vivo rodent models for the experimental investigation of prenatal immune activation effects in neurodevelopmental brain disorders. *Neuroscience and Biobehavioral Reviews* 33(7): 1061–1079.

Piontkewitz, Y., Assaf, Y., & Weiner, I. (2009). Clozapine administration in adolescence prevents postpubertal emergence of brain structural pathology in an animal model of schizophrenia. *Biological Psychiatry* 66(11): 1038–1046.

Robertson, S. A., Skinner, R. J., & Care, A. S. (2006). Essential role for IL-10 in resistance to lipopolysaccharide-induced preterm labor in mice. *Journal of Immunology* 177(7): 4888–4896.

Smith, S. E., Li, J., Garbett, K., Mirnics, K., & Patterson, P. H. (2007). Maternal immune activation alters fetal brain development through interleukin-6. *Journal of Neuroscience* 27(40): 10695–10702.

References

Abazyan, B., Nomura, J., Kannan, G., Ishizuka, K., Tamashiro, K. L., Nucifora, F., Pogorelov, V., Ladenheim, B., Yang, C. X., Krasnova, I. N., et al. (2010). Prenatal interaction of mutant DISC1 and immune activation produces adult psychopathology. *Biological Psychiatry* 68(12): 1172–1181.

Adams Waldorf, K. M., Persing, D., Novy, M. J., Sadowsky, D. W., & Gravett, M. G. (2008). Pretreatment with toll-like receptor 4 antagonist inhibits lipopolysaccharide-induced preterm uterine contractility, cytokines, and prostaglandins in rhesus monkeys. *Reproductive Sciences 15*(2): 121–127.

Arce, R. M., Barros, S. P., Wacker, B., Peters, B., Moss, K., & Offenbacher, S. (2009). Increased TLR4 expression in murine placentas after oral infection with periodontal pathogens. *Placenta 30*(2): 156–162.

Arion, D., Unger, T., Lewis, D. A., Levitt, P., & Mirnics, K. (2007). Molecular evidence for increased expression of genes related to immune and chaperone function in the prefrontal cortex in schizophrenia. *Biological Psychiatry 62*(7): 711–721.

Aronsson, F., Lannebo, C., Paucar, M., Brask, J., Kristensson, K., & Karlsson, H. (2002). Persistence of viral RNA in the brain of offspring to mice infected with influenza A/WSN/33 virus during pregnancy. *Journal of Neurovirology 8*(4): 353–357.

Ashdown, H., Dumont, Y., Ng, M., Poole, S., Boksa, P., & Luheshi, G. N. (2006). The role of cytokines in mediating effects of prenatal infection on the fetus: Implications for schizophrenia. *Molecular Psychiatry 11*(1): 47–55.

Ayoub, D. M. & Yazbak, F. E. (2008). A closer look at influenza vaccination during pregnancy. *Lancet Infectious Diseases 8*(11): 660–661; author reply 661–663.

Baharnoori, M., Brake, W. G., & Srivastava, L. K. (2009). Prenatal immune challenge induces developmental changes in the morphology of pyramidal neurons of the prefrontal cortex and hippocampus in rats. *Schizophrenia Research 107*(1): 99–109.

Bakos, J., Duncko, R., Makatsori, A., Pirnik, Z., Kiss, A., & Jezova, D. (2004). Prenatal immune challenge affects growth, behavior, and brain dopamine in offspring. *Annals of the New York Academy of Sciences 1018*: 281–287.

Bauer, S., Kerr, B. J., & Patterson, P. H. (2007). The neuropoietic cytokine family in development, plasticity, disease and injury. *Nature Reviews Neuroscience 8*(3): 221–232.

Baughman, M. D., Losif, A-M., Smith, S. E. P., Bregere, C., Zadran, S., Amaral, D. G., & Patterson, P. H. (2011). A Nonhuman Primate Model of Maternal Immune Activation. Washington, DC: Society for Neuroscience, in press.

Bell, M. J. & Hallenbeck, J. M. (2002). Effects of intrauterine inflammation on developing rat brain. *Journal of Neuroscience Research 70*(4): 570–579.

Bell, M. J., Hallenbeck, J. M., & Gallo, V. (2004). Determining the fetal inflammatory response in an experimental model of intrauterine inflammation in rats. *Pediatric Research 56*(4): 541–546.

Beloosesky, R., Gayle, D. A., & Ross, M. G. (2006). Maternal N-acetylcysteine suppresses fetal inflammatory cytokine responses to maternal lipopolysaccharide. *American Journal of Obstetrics and Gynecology 195*(4): 1053–1057.

Bobetsis, Y. A., Barros, S. P., Lin, D. M., Weidman, J. R., Dolinoy, D. C., Jirtle, R. L., Boggess, K. A., Beck, J. D., & Offenbacher, S. (2007). Bacterial infection promotes DNA hypermethylation. *Journal of Dental Research 86*(2): 169–174.

Bobetsis, Y. A., Barros, S. P., & Offenbacher, S. (2006). Exploring the relationship between periodontal disease and pregnancy complications. *Journal of the American Dental Association 137*(Suppl): 7S–13S.

Boris, M., Kaiser, C. C., Goldblatt, A., Elice, M. W., Edelson, S. M., Adams, J. B., & Feinstein, D. L. (2007). Effect of pioglitazone treatment on behavioral symptoms in autistic children. *Journal of Neuroinflammation 4*: 3.

Borrell, J., Vela, J. M., Arevalo-Martin, A., Molina-Holgado, E., & Guaza, C. (2002). Prenatal immune challenge disrupts sensorimotor gating in adult rats: Implications for the etiopathogenesis of schizophrenia. *Neuropsychopharmacology 26*(2): 204–215.

Brown, A. S. (2006). Prenatal infection as a risk factor for schizophrenia. *Schizophrenia Bulletin* 32(2): 200–202.

Brown, A. S., Begg, M. D., Gravenstein, S., Schaefer, C. A., Wyatt, R. J., Bresnahan, M., Babulas, V. P., & Susser, E. S. (2004). Serologic evidence of prenatal influenza in the etiology of schizophrenia. *Archives of General Psychiatry* 61(8): 774–780.

Brown, A. S. & Derkits, E. J. (2010). Prenatal infection and schizophrenia: A review of epidemiologic and translational studies. *American Journal of Psychiatry* 167(3): 261–280.

Brown, A. S., Schaefer, C. A., Wyatt, R. J., Begg, M. D., Goetz, R., Bresnahan, M. A., Harkavy-Friedman, J., Gorman, J. M., Malaspina, D., & Susser, E. S. (2002). Paternal age and risk of schizophrenia in adult offspring. *American Journal of Psychiatry* 159(9): 1528–1533.

Byrne, M., Browne, R., Mulryan, N., Scully, A., Morris, M., Kinsella, A., Takei, N., McNeil, T., Walsh, D., & O'Callaghan, E. (2000). Labour and delivery complications and schizophrenia: Case-control study using contemporaneous labour ward records. *British Journal of Psychiatry* 176: 531–536.

Cai, Z., Pan, Z. L., Pang, Y., Evans, O. B., & Rhodes, P. G. (2000). Cytokine induction in fetal rat brains and brain injury in neonatal rats after maternal lipopolysaccharide administration. *Pediatric Research* 47(1): 64–72.

Cardon, M., Ron-Harel, N., Cohen, H., Lewitus, G. M., & Schwartz, M. (2009). Dysregulation of kisspeptin and neurogenesis at adolescence link inborn immune deficits to the late onset of abnormal sensorimotor gating in congenital psychological disorders. *Molecular Psychiatry* 15(4): 415–425.

Carvey, P. M., Chang, Q., Lipton, J. W., & Ling, Z. (2003). Prenatal exposure to the bacteriotoxin lipopolysaccharide leads to long-term losses of dopamine neurons in offspring: A potential, new model of Parkinson's disease. *Frontiers in Bioscience* 8: s826–s837.

Coyle, P., Tran, N., Fung, J. N., Summers, B. L., & Rofe, A. M. (2009). Maternal dietary zinc supplementation prevents aberrant behaviour in an object recognition task in mice offspring exposed to LPS in early pregnancy. *Behavioural Brain Research* 197(1): 210–218.

Cui, K., Ashdown, H., Luheshi, G. N., & Boksa, P. (2009). Effects of prenatal immune activation on hippocampal neurogenesis in the rat. *Schizophrenia Research* 113(2–3): 288–297.

Curran, L. K., Newschaffer, C. J., Lee, L. C., Crawford, S. O., Johnston, M. V., & Zimmerman, A. W. (2007). Behaviors associated with fever in children with autism spectrum disorders. *Pediatrics* 120(6): e1386–e1392.

Dean, B., Boer, S., Gibbons, A., Money, T., & Scarr, E. (2009). Recent advances in postmortem pathology and neurochemistry in schizophrenia. *Current Opinion in Psychiatry* 22(2): 154–160.

Deverman, B. E. & Patterson, P. H. (2009). Cytokines and CNS development. *Neuron* 64(1): 61–78.

Drzyzga, L., Obuchowicz, E., Marcinowska, A., & Herman, Z. S. (2006). Cytokines in schizophrenia and the effects of antipsychotic drugs. *Brain, Behavior, and Immunology* 20(6): 532–545.

Elovitz, M. A. (2006). Anti-inflammatory interventions in pregnancy: Now and the future. *Seminars in Fetal and Neonatal Medicine* 11(5): 327–332.

Elovitz, M. A. & Gonzalez, J. (2008). Medroxyprogesterone acetate modulates the immune response in the uterus, cervix and placenta in a mouse model of preterm birth. *Journal of Maternal-Fetal and Neonatal Medicine* 21(4): 223–230.

Elovitz, M. A., Mrinalini, C., & Sammel, M. D. (2006). Elucidating the early signal transduction pathways leading to fetal brain injury in preterm birth. *Pediatric Research* 59(1): 50–55.

Fatemi, S. H., Araghi-Niknam, M., Laurence, J. A., Stary, J. M., Sidwell, R. W., & Lee, S. (2004). Glial fibrillary acidic protein and glutamic acid decarboxylase 65 and 67 kDa proteins are increased in brains of neonatal BALB/c mice following viral infection in utero. *Schizophrenia Research* 69(1): 121–123.

Fatemi, S. H., Cuadra, A. E., El-Fakahany, E. E., Sidwell, R. W., & Thuras, P. (2000). Prenatal viral infection causes alterations in nNOS expression in developing mouse brains. *Neuroreport* 11(7): 1493–1496.

Fatemi, S. H., Earle, J., Kanodia, R., Kist, D., Emamian, E. S., Patterson, P. H., Shi, L., & Sidwell, R. (2002). Prenatal viral infection leads to pyramidal cell atrophy and macrocephaly in adulthood: Implications for genesis of autism and schizophrenia. *Cellular and Molecular Neurobiology* 22(1): 25–33.

Fatemi, S. H., Emamian, E. S., Kist, D., Sidwell, R. W., Nakajima, K., Akhter, P., Shier, A., Sheikh, S., & Bailey, K. (1999). Defective corticogenesis and reduction in reelin immunoreactivity in cortex and hippocampus of prenatally infected neonatal mice. *Molecular Psychiatry* 4(2): 145–154.

Fatemi, S. H., Folsom, T. D., Reutiman, T. J., Abu-Odeh, D., Mori, S., Huang, H., & Oishi, K. (2009). Abnormal expression of myelination genes and alterations in white matter fractional anisotropy following prenatal viral influenza infection at E16 in mice. *Schizophrenia Research* 112(1–3): 46–53.

Fatemi, S. H., Folsom, T. D., Reutiman, T. J., & Sidwell, R. W. (2008). Viral regulation of aquaporin 4, connexin 43, microcephalin and nucleolin. *Schizophrenia Research* 98(1–3): 163–177.

Fortier, M. E., Joober, R., Luheshi, G. N., & Boksa, P. (2004). Maternal exposure to bacterial endotoxin during pregnancy enhances amphetamine-induced locomotion and startle responses in adult rat offspring. *Journal of Psychiatric Research* 38(3): 335–345.

Gayle, D. A., Beloosesky, R., Desai, M., Amidi, F., Nunez, S. E., & Ross, M. G. (2004). Maternal LPS induces cytokines in the amniotic fluid and corticotropin releasing hormone in the fetal rat brain. *American Journal of Physiology—Regulatory, Integrative, and Comparative Physiology* 286(6): R1024–R1029.

Gilmore, J. H., Jarskog, L. F., & Vadlamudi, S. (2005). Maternal poly I:C exposure during pregnancy regulates TNF alpha, BDNF, and NGF expression in neonatal brain and the maternal-fetal unit of the rat. *Journal of Neuroimmunology* 159(1–2): 106–112.

Golan, H. M., Lev, V., Hallak, M., Sorokin, Y., & Huleihel, M. (2005). Specific neurodevelopmental damage in mice offspring following maternal inflammation during pregnancy. *Neuropharmacology* 48(6): 903–917.

Gonzalez-Maeso, J., Weisstaub, N. V., Zhou, M., Chan, P., Ivic, L., Ang, R., Lira, A., Bradley-Moore, M., Ge, Y., Zhou, Q., et al. (2007). Hallucinogens recruit specific cortical 5-HT(2A) receptor-mediated signaling pathways to affect behavior. *Neuron* 53(3): 439–452.

Hagberg, H. & Mallard, C. (2005). Effect of inflammation on central nervous system development and vulnerability. *Current Opinion in Psychiatry* 18(2): 117–123.

Han, Y. W., Redline, R. W., Li, M., Yin, L., Hill, G. B., & McCormick, T. S. (2004). Fusobacterium nucleatum induces premature and term stillbirths in pregnant mice: Implication of oral bacteria in preterm birth. *Infection and Immunity* 72(4): 2272–2279.

Hava, G., Vered, L., Yael, M., Mordechai, H., & Mahoud, H. (2006). Alterations in behavior in adult offspring mice following maternal inflammation during pregnancy. *Developmental Psychobiology* 48(2): 162–168.

Hinsie, L. E. (1929). Malaria treatment of schizophrenia. *Psychiatric Quaterly* 2(2): 210–214.

Hirsch, E., Filipovich, Y., & Mahendroo, M. (2006). Signaling via the type I IL-1 and TNF receptors is necessary for bacterially induced preterm labor in a murine model. *American Journal of Obstetrics and Gynecology* 194(5): 1334–1340.

Ho, B. C., Mola, C., & Andreasen, N. C. (2004). Cerebellar dysfunction in neuroleptic naive schizophrenia patients: Clinical, cognitive, and neuroanatomic correlates of cerebellar neurologic signs. *Biological Psychiatry* 55(12): 1146–1153.

Hodyl, N. A., Krivanek, K. M., Lawrence, E., Clifton, V. L., & Hodgson, D. M. (2007). Prenatal exposure to a pro-inflammatory stimulus causes delays in the development of the innate immune response to LPS in the offspring. *Journal of Immunology* 190(1–2): 61–71.

Hsiao, E., Chow, J., Mazmanian, S. K., & Patterson, P. H. (2010). Modeling an autism risk factor in mice leads to permanent changes in the immune system. Paper presented at the International Meeting for Autism Research, Boston. Abstract no. 130.124.

Hsiao, E. & Patterson, P. H. (2011). Activation of the maternal immune system induces endocrine changes in the placenta via IL-6. *Brain, Behavior, and Immunity* 25: 604–615.

Ibi, D., Nagai, T., Koike, H., Kitahara, Y., Mizoguchi, H., Niwa, M., Jaaro-Peled, H., Nitta, A., Yoneda, Y., Nabeshima, T., et al. (2010). Combined effect of neonatal immune activation and mutant DISC1 on phenotypic changes in adulthood. *Behavioural Brain Research* 206(1): 32–37.

Ito, H. T., Smith, S. E. P., Hsiao, E., & Patterson, P. H. (2010). Maternal immune activation alters hippocampal information processing in adult offspring. *Brain, Behavior, & Immunity* 24: 930–941.

Jonakait, G. M. (2007). The effects of maternal inflammation on neuronal development: Possible mechanisms. *International Journal of Developmental Neuroscience* 25(7): 415–425.

Kamiya, A., Kubo, K., Tomoda, T., Takaki, M., Youn, R., Ozeki, Y., Sawamura, N., Park, U., Kudo, C., Okawa, M., et al. (2005). A schizophrenia-associated mutation of DISC1 perturbs cerebral cortex development. *Nature Cell Biology* 7(12): 1167–1178.

Kannan, S., Saadani-Makki, F., Muzik, O., Chakraborty, P., Mangner, T. J., Janisse, J., Romero, R., & Chugani, D. C. (2007). Microglial activation in perinatal rabbit brain induced by intrauterine inflammation: Detection with 11C-(R)-PK11195 and small-animal PET. *Journal of Nuclear Medicine* 48(6): 946–954.

Knight, J. G., Menkes, D. B., Highton, J., & Adams, D. D. (2007). Rationale for a trial of immunosuppressive therapy in acute schizophrenia. *Molecular Psychiatry* 12(5): 424–431.

Koga, K., Cardenas, I., Aldo, P., Abrahams, V. M., Peng, B., Fill, S., Romero, R., & Mor, G. (2009). Activation of TLR3 in the trophoblast is associated with preterm delivery. *American Journal of Reproductive Immunology* 61(3): 196–212.

Lante, F., Meunier, J., Guiramand, J., Maurice, T., Cavalier, M., de Jesus Ferreira, M. C., Aimar, R., Cohen-Solal, C., Vignes, M., & Barbanel, G. (2007). Neurodevelopmental damage after prenatal infection: Role of oxidative stress in the fetal brain. *Free Radical Biology and Medicine* 42(8): 1231–1245.

Lasala, N. & Zhou, H. (2007). Effects of maternal exposure to LPS on the inflammatory response in the offspring. *Journal of Neuroimmunology* 189(1–2): 95–101.

Li, Q., Cheung, C., Wei, R., Hui, E. S., Feldon, J., Meyer, U., Chung, S., Chua, S. E., Sham, P. C., Wu, E. X., et al. (2009). Prenatal immune challenge is an environmental risk factor for brain and behavior change relevant to schizophrenia: Evidence from MRI in a mouse model. *PLoS One* 4(7): e6354.

Libbey, J. E., Sweeten, T. L., McMahon, W. M., & Fujinami, R. S. (2005). Autistic disorder and viral infections. *Journal of Neurovirology* 11(1): 1–10.

Lin, D., Smith, M. A., Champagne, C., Elter, J., Beck, J., & Offenbacher, S. (2003a). Porphyromonas gingivalis infection during pregnancy increases maternal tumor necrosis factor alpha, suppresses maternal interleukin-10, and enhances fetal growth restriction and resorption in mice. *Infection and Immunity* 71(9): 5156–5162.

Lin, D., Smith, M. A., Elter, J., Champagne, C., Downey, C. L., Beck, J., & Offenbacher, S. (2003b). Porphyromonas gingivalis infection in pregnant mice is associated with placental dissemination, an increase in the placental Th1/Th2 cytokine ratio, and fetal growth restriction. *Infection and Immunity* 71(9): 5163–5168.

Ling, Z., Chang, Q. A., Tong, C. W., Leurgans, S. E., Lipton, J. W., & Carvey, P. M. (2004). Rotenone potentiates dopamine neuron loss in animals exposed to lipopolysaccharide prenatally. *Experimental Neurology 190*(2): 373–383.

Liu, H., Redline, R. W., & Han, Y. W. (2007). Fusobacterium nucleatum induces fetal death in mice via stimulation of TLR4-mediated placental inflammatory response. *Journal of Immunology 179*(4): 2501–2508.

Liverman, C. S., Kaftan, H. A., Cui, L., Hersperger, S. G., Taboada, E., Klein, R. M., & Berman, N. E. (2006). Altered expression of pro-inflammatory and developmental genes in the fetal brain in a mouse model of maternal infection. *Neuroscience Letters 399*(3): 220–225.

Lowe, G. C., Luheshi, G. N., & Williams, S. (2008). Maternal infection and fever during late gestation are associated with altered synaptic transmission in the hippocampus of juvenile offspring rats. *American Journal of Physiology—Regulatory, Integrative, and Comparative Physiology 295*(5): R1563–R1571.

Mak, T. K., Mangtani, P., Leese, J., Watson, J. M., & Pfeifer, D. (2008). Influenza vaccination in pregnancy: Current evidence and selected national policies. *Lancet Infectious Diseases 8*(1): 44–52.

Makinodan, M., Tatsumi, K., Manabe, T., Yamauchi, T., Makinodan, E., Matsuyoshi, H., Shimoda, S., Noriyama, Y., Kishimoto, T., & Wanaka, A. (2008). Maternal immune activation in mice delays myelination and axonal development in the hippocampus of the offspring. *Journal of Neuroscience Research 86*(10): 2190–2200.

Malkova, N., Hsiao, E. & Patterson, P. H. (2010). Maternal immune activation causes a deficit in social and communicative behavior in male mouse offspring. Program No. 561.29, Neurosci. Mtg Planner, San Diego: Soc. Neurosci., online.

Mandal, M., Marzouk, A. C., Donnelly, R., & Ponzio, N. M. (2011). Maternal immune stimulation during pregnancy affects adaptive immunity in offspring to promote development of TH17 cells. *Brain, Behavior, and Immunity*, in press.

Merlot, E., Couret, D., & Otten, W. (2008). Prenatal stress, fetal imprinting and immunity. *Brain, Behavior, and Immunity 22*(1): 42–51.

Meyer, U., Feldon, J., & Fatemi, S. H. (2009). In-vivo rodent models for the experimental investigation of prenatal immune activation effects in neurodevelopmental brain disorders. *Neuroscience & Biobehavioral Reviews 33*(7): 1061–1079.

Meyer, U., Murray, P. J., Urwyler, A., Yee, B. K., Schedlowski, M., & Feldon, J. (2008a). Adult behavioral and pharmacological dysfunctions following disruption of the fetal brain balance between pro-inflammatory and IL-10-mediated anti-inflammatory signaling. *Molecular Psychiatry 13*(2): 208–221.

Meyer, U., Nyffeler, M., Engler, A., Urwyler, A., Schedlowski, M., Knuesel, I., Yee, B. K., & Feldon, J. (2006a). The time of prenatal immune challenge determines the specificity of inflammation-mediated brain and behavioral pathology. *Journal of Neuroscience 26*(18): 4752–4762.

Meyer, U., Nyffeler, M., Schwendener, S., Knuesel, I., Yee, B. K., & Feldon, J. (2008b). Relative prenatal and postnatal maternal contributions to schizophrenia related neurochemical dysfunction after in utero immune challenge. *Neuropsychopharmacology 33*(2): 441–456.

Meyer, U., Nyffeler, M., Yee, B. K., Knuesel, I., & Feldon, J. (2008c). Adult brain and behavioral pathological markers of prenatal immune challenge during early/middle and late fetal development in mice. *Brain, Behavior, and Immunology 22*(4): 469–486.

Meyer, U., Schwendener, S., Feldon, J., & Yee, B. K. (2006b). Prenatal and postnatal maternal contributions in the infection model of schizophrenia. *Experimental Brain Research 173*(2): 243–257.

Meyer, U., Spoerri, E., Yee, B. K., Schwarz, M. J., & Feldon, J. (2010). Evaluating early preventive antipsychotic and antidepressant drug treatment in an infection-based neurodevelopmental mouse model of schizophrenia. *Schizophrenia Bulletin 36*(3): 607–623.

Meyer, U., Yee, B. K., & Feldon, J. (2007). The neurodevelopmental impact of prenatal infections at different times of pregnancy: The earlier the worse? *Neuroscientist 13*(3): 241–256.

Muller, N. & Schwarz, M. (2006). Schizophrenia as an inflammation-mediated dysbalance of glutamatergic neurotransmission. *Neurotoxicity Research 10*(2): 131–148.

Nakagawasai, O., Murata, A., Arai, Y., Ohba, A., Wakui, K., Mitazaki, S., Niijima, F., Tan-No, K., & Tadano, T. (2007). Enhanced head-twitch response to 5-HT-related agonists in thiamine-deficient mice. *Journal of Neural Transmission 114*(8): 1003–1010.

Nawa, H. & Takei, N. (2006). Recent progress in animal modeling of immune inflammatory processes in schizophrenia: Implication of specific cytokines. *Neuroscience Research 56*(1): 2–13.

Nitsos, I., Rees, S. M., Duncan, J., Kramer, B. W., Harding, R., Newnham, J. P., & Moss, T. J. (2006). Chronic exposure to intra-amniotic lipopolysaccharide affects the ovine fetal brain. *Journal of the Society for Gynecologic Investigation 13*(4): 239–247.

Nyffeler, M., Meyer, U., Yee, B. K., Feldon, J., & Knuesel, I. (2006). Maternal immune activation during pregnancy increases limbic GABAA receptor immunoreactivity in the adult offspring: Implications for schizophrenia. *Neuroscience 143*(1): 51–62.

Offenbacher, S., Riche, E. L., Barros, S. P., Bobetsis, Y. A., Lin, D., & Beck, J. D. (2005). Effects of maternal *Campylobacter rectus* infection on murine placenta, fetal and neonatal survival, and brain development. *Journal of Periodontology 76*(11 Suppl): 2133–2143.

Ozawa, K., Hashimoto, K., Kishimoto, T., Shimizu, E., Ishikura, H., & Iyo, M. (2006). Immune activation during pregnancy in mice leads to dopaminergic hyperfunction and cognitive impairment in the offspring: A neurodevelopmental animal model of schizophrenia. *Biological Psychiatry 59*(6): 546–554.

Paintlia, M. K., Paintlia, A. S., Contreras, M. A., Singh, I., & Singh, A. K. (2008a). Lipopolysaccharide-induced peroxisomal dysfunction exacerbates cerebral white matter injury: Attenuation by N-acetyl cysteine. *Experimental Neurology 210*(2): 560–576.

Paintlia, M. K., Paintlia, A. S., Singh, A. K., & Singh, I. (2008b). Attenuation of lipopolysaccharide-induced inflammatory response and phospholipids metabolism at the feto-maternal interface by N-acetyl cysteine. *Pediatric Research 64*(4): 334–339.

Pang, Y., Fan, L. W., Zheng, B., Cai, Z., & Rhodes, P. G. (2006). Role of interleukin-6 in lipopolysaccharide-induced brain injury and behavioral dysfunction in neonatal rats. *Neuroscience 141*(2): 745–755.

Pang, Y., Rodts-Palenik, S., Cai, Z., Bennett, W. A., & Rhodes, P. G. (2005). Suppression of glial activation is involved in the protection of IL-10 on maternal *E. coli* induced neonatal white matter injury. *Brain Research: Developmental Brain Research 157*(2): 141–149.

Patterson, P. H. (2007). Neuroscience: Maternal effects on schizophrenia risk. *Science 318*(5850): 576–577.

Patterson, P. H. (2009). Immune involvement in schizophrenia and autism: Etiology, pathology and animal models. *Behavioural Brain Research 204*(2): 313–321.

Pearce, B. (2003). Modeling the role of infections in the etiology of mental illness. *Clinical Neuroscience Research 3*(3): 271–282.

Piontkewitz, Y., Assaf, Y., & Weiner, I. (2009). Clozapine administration in adolescence prevents postpubertal emergence of brain structural pathology in an animal model of schizophrenia. *Biological Psychiatry 66*(11): 1038–1046.

Pollmacher, T., Haack, M., Schuld, A., Kraus, T., & Hinze-Selch, D. (2000). Effects of antipsychotic drugs on cytokine networks. *Journal of Psychiatric Research 34*(6): 369–382.

Potvin, S., Stip, E., Sepehry, A. A., Gendron, A., Bah, R., & Kouassi, E. (2008). Inflammatory cytokine alterations in schizophrenia: A systematic quantitative review. *Biological Psychiatry* 63(8): 801–808.

Riedel, M., Strassnig, M., Schwarz, M. J., & Muller, N. (2005). COX-2 inhibitors as adjunctive therapy in schizophrenia: Rationale for use and evidence to date. *CNS Drugs* 19(10): 805–819.

Rivera, D. L., Olister, S. M., Liu, X., Thompson, J. H., Zhang, X. J., Pennline, K., Azuero, R., Clark, D. A., & Miller, M. J. (1998). Interleukin-10 attenuates experimental fetal growth restriction and demise. *FASEB Journal* 12(2): 189–197.

Robertson, S. A., Skinner, R. J., & Care, A. S. (2006). Essential role for IL-10 in resistance to lipopolysaccharide-induced preterm labor in mice. *Journal of Immunology* 177(7): 4888–4896.

Romero, E., Ali, C., Molina-Holgado, E., Castellano, B., Guaza, C., & Borrell, J. (2007). Neurobehavioral and immunological consequences of prenatal immune activation in rats: Influence of antipsychotics. *Neuropsychopharmacology* 32(8): 1791–1804.

Rosenblum, I. Y., Johnson, R. C., & Schmahai, T. J. (2002). Preclinical safety evaluation of recombinant human interleukin-10. *Regulatory Toxicology and Pharmacology* 35(1): 56–71.

Rousset, C. I., Chalon, S., Cantagrel, S., Bodard, S., Andres, C., Gressens, P., & Saliba, E. (2006). Maternal exposure to LPS induces hypomyelination in the internal capsule and programmed cell death in the deep gray matter in newborn rats. *Pediatric Research* 59(3): 428–433.

Ryan, B. C. & Vandenbergh, J. G. (2002). Intrauterine position effects. *Neuroscience and Biobehavioral Reviews* 26(6): 665–678.

Saetre, P., Emilsson, L., Axelsson, E., Kreuger, J., Lindholm, E., & Jazin, E. (2007). Inflammation-related genes up-regulated in schizophrenia brains. *BMC Psychiatry* 7: 46.

Salminen, A., Paananen, R., Vuolteenaho, R., Metsola, J., Ojaniemi, M., Autio-Harmainen, H., & Hallman, M. (2008). Maternal endotoxin-induced preterm birth in mice: Fetal responses in toll-like receptors, collectins, and cytokines. *Pediatric Research* 63(3): 280–286.

Samuelsson, A. M., Jennische, E., Hansson, H. A., & Holmang, A. (2006). Prenatal exposure to interleukin-6 results in inflammatory neurodegeneration in hippocampus with NMDA/GABA(A) dysregulation and impaired spatial learning. *American Journal of Physiology—Regulatory, Integrative, and Comparative Physiology* 290(5): R1345–R1356.

Shi, J., Levinson, D. F., Duan, J., Sanders, A. R., Zheng, Y., Pe'er, I., Dudbridge, F., Holmans, P. A., Whittemore, A. S., Mowry, B. J., et al. (2009a). Common variants on chromosome 6p22.1 are associated with schizophrenia. *Nature* 460(7256): 753–757.

Shi, L., Fatemi, S. H., Sidwell, R. W., & Patterson, P. H. (2003). Maternal influenza infection causes marked behavioral and pharmacological changes in the offspring. *Journal of Neuroscience* 23(1): 297–302.

Shi, L., Malkova, N., Su, Y., Tse, D., & Patterson, P. H. (2006). Activation of the maternal immune causes altered cortical neuron positioning and a spatially restricted loss of Purkinje cells in the fetal brain. Paper presented at the Program Number 687.1. Neuroscience Meeting Planner, Atlanta, GA.

Shi, L., Smith, S. E., Malkova, N., Tse, D., Su, Y., & Patterson, P. H. (2009b). Activation of the maternal immune system alters cerebellar development in the offspring. *Brain, Behavior, and Immunology* 23(1): 116–123.

Shi, L., Tu, N., & Patterson, P. H. (2005). Maternal influenza infection is likely to alter fetal brain development indirectly: The virus is not detected in the fetus. *International Journal of Developmental Neuroscience* 23(2–3): 299–305.

Short, S. J., Lubach, G. R., Karasin, A. I., Olsen, C. W., Styner, M., Knickmeyer, R. C., Gilmore, J. H., & Coe, C. L. (2010). Maternal influenza infection during pregnancy impacts postnatal brain development in the rhesus monkey. *Biological Psychiatry* 67(10): 965–973.

Silver, R. M., Edwin, S. S., Umar, F., Dudley, D. J., Branch, D. W., & Mitchell, M. D. (1997). Bacterial lipopolysaccharide-mediated murine fetal death: The role of interleukin-1. *American Journal of Obstetrics and Gynecology* 176(3): 544–549.

Silver, R. M., Lohner, W. S., Daynes, R. A., Mitchell, M. D., & Branch, D. W. (1994). Lipopolysaccharide-induced fetal death: The role of tumor-necrosis factor alpha. *Biology of Reproduction* 50(5): 1108–1112.

Skowronski, D. M. & De Serres, G. (2009). Is routine influenza immunization warranted in early pregnancy? *Vaccine* 27(35): 4754–4770.

Smith, S. E., Li, J., Garbett, K., Mirnics, K., & Patterson, P. H. (2007). Maternal immune activation alters fetal brain development through interleukin-6. *Journal of Neuroscience* 27(40): 10695–10702.

Smith, S. E. P. & Patterson, P. H. (2008). Alteration of neurodevelopment and behavior by maternal immune activation. In A. Siegel & S. S. Zalcman (eds.), *The Neuroimmunological Basis of Behavior by Maternal Immune Activation* (pp. 111–130). Norwell, MA: Springer.

Sorensen, H. J., Mortensen, E. L., Reinisch, J. M., & Mednick, S. A. (2009). Association between prenatal exposure to bacterial infection and risk of schizophrenia. *Schizophrenia Bulletin* 35(3): 631–637.

Sperner-Unterweger, B. (2005). Immunological aetiology of major psychiatric disorders: Evidence and therapeutic implications. *Drugs* 65(11): 1493–1520.

Stefansson, H., Ophoff, R. A., Steinberg, S., Andreassen, O. A., Cichon, S., Rujescu, D., Werge, T., Pietilainen, O. P., Mors, O., Mortensen, P. B., et al. (2009). Common variants conferring risk of schizophrenia. *Nature* 460(7256): 744–747.

Stolk, P., Souverein, P. C., Leufkens, H. G., Weil, J. G., Egberts, A. C., & Heerdink, E. R. (2007). The association between exposure to COX-2 inhibitors and schizophrenia deterioration: A nested case-control study. *Pharmacopsychiatry* 40(3): 111–115.

Strous, R. D. & Shoenfeld, Y. (2006). Schizophrenia, autoimmunity and immune system dysregulation: A comprehensive model updated and revisited. *Journal of Autoimmunity* 27(2): 71–80.

Tempelton, W. L. & Glas, C. B. (1924). The effect of malarial fever upon *dementia praecox* subjects. *Journal of Mental Science* 70: 92–95.

Terrone, D. A., Rinehart, B. K., Granger, J. P., Barrilleaux, P. S., Martin, J. N., Jr., & Bennett, W. A. (2001). Interleukin-10 administration and bacterial endotoxin-induced preterm birth in a rat model. *Obstetrics and Gynecology* 98(3): 476–480.

Tochigi, M., Okazaki, Y., Kato, N., & Sasaki, T. (2004). What causes seasonality of birth in schizophrenia? *Neuroscience Research* 48(1): 1–11.

Urakubo, A., Jarskog, L. F., Lieberman, J. A., & Gilmore, J. H. (2001). Prenatal exposure to maternal infection alters cytokine expression in the placenta, amniotic fluid, and fetal brain. *Schizophrenia Research* 47(1): 27–36.

van der Poll, T., Marchant, A., Keogh, C. V., Goldman, M., & Lowry, S. F. (1996). Interleukin-10 impairs host defense in murine pneumococcal pneumonia. *Journal of Infectious Diseases* 174(5): 994–1000.

Wang, X., Hagberg, H., Mallard, C., Zhu, C., Hedtjarn, M., Tiger, C. F., Eriksson, K., Rosen, A., & Jacobsson, B. (2006a). Disruption of interleukin-18, but not interleukin-1, increases vulnerability to preterm delivery and fetal mortality after intrauterine inflammation. *American Journal of Pathology* 169(3): 967–976.

Wang, X., Hagberg, H., Zhu, C., Jacobsson, B., & Mallard, C. (2007). Effects of intrauterine inflammation on the developing mouse brain. *Brain Research 1144*: 180–185.

Wang, X., Rousset, C. I., Hagberg, H., & Mallard, C. (2006b). Lipopolysaccharide-induced inflammation and perinatal brain injury. *Seminars in Fetal and Neonatal Medicine 11*(5): 343–353.

Wolff, A. R. & Bilkey, D. K. (2008). Immune activation during mid-gestation disrupts sensorimotor gating in rat offspring. *Behavioural Brain Research 190*(1): 156–159.

Xu, D. X., Chen, Y. H., Wang, H., Zhao, L., Wang, J. P., & Wei, W. (2006). Tumor necrosis factor alpha partially contributes to lipopolysaccharide-induced intra-uterine fetal growth restriction and skeletal development retardation in mice. *Toxicology Letters 163*(1): 20–29.

Yeo, A., Smith, M. A., Lin, D., Riche, E. L., Moore, A., Elter, J., & Offenbacher, S. (2005). Campylobacter rectus mediates growth restriction in pregnant mice. *Journal of Periodontology 76*(4): 551–557.

Zuckerman, L., Rehavi, M., Nachman, R., & Weiner, I. (2003). Immune activation during pregnancy in rats leads to a postpubertal emergence of disrupted latent inhibition, dopaminergic hyperfunction, and altered limbic morphology in the offspring: A novel neurodevelopmental model of schizophrenia. *Neuropsychopharmacology 28*(10): 1778–1789.

Zuckerman, L. & Weiner, I. (2005). Maternal immune activation leads to behavioral and pharmacological changes in the adult offspring. *Journal of Psychiatric Research 39*(3): 311–323.

CHAPTER 11

DEVELOPMENTAL VITAMIN D DEFICIENCY AS A RISK FACTOR FOR SCHIZOPHRENIA

XIAOYING CUI, DARRYL W. EYLES, THOMAS H. J. BURNE, AND JOHN J. MCGRATH

KEY CONCEPTS

- Developmental vitamin D deficiency is a candidate risk factor for schizophrenia.
- Over the last decade, evidence has accumulated demonstrating that vitamin D plays a role in brain development.
- The Developmental Vitamin D (DVD) deficiency rat model demonstrates a range of altered neurobiological features, some of which are consistent with features of schizophrenia.
- The DVD deficiency model confirms the biological plausibility of this exposure for schizophrenia, but further epidemiologic research is required in order to demonstrate a link to the disease.

It is widely accepted that schizophrenia is a heterogeneous group of disorders influenced by a variety of genetic and environmental factors. Researchers have explored the association between schizophrenia and a range of candidate early life exposures that could disrupt early brain development (e.g., prenatal stress, malnutrition, infection, and obstetric complications). On the basis of the clues from epidemiology, our group proposed that low prenatal vitamin D_3 is a modifying risk factor for schizophrenia. In 1999, we developed an informative animal model—the DVD model—in which vitamin D_3 is depleted in utero. The DVD-deficient offspring reproduce several features observed in patients with schizophrenia, such as enlarged lateral ventricles and altered behavior in response to psychomimetic agents. In this chapter, we integrate findings derived from the DVD model. The first section concisely summarizes clues from the epidemiology of schizophrenia. The second section discusses the evidence regarding the biological importance of vitamin D_3 in brain development and function. The third section reviews the experimental findings in DVD rodent models, showing that maternal vitamin D_3 deficiency can lead to long-lasting neuroanatomic, neurochemical, and behavioral changes that are relevant to the disease. The final section outlines future research directions and the paradigm for testing this hypothesis in human populations.

Prenatal Low Vitamin D_3 as a Modifying Risk Factor for Schizophrenia: Clues from Epidemiology

The prenatal hypovitaminosis D_3 hypothesis was inspired by epidemiologic evidence. One of the most consistently replicated epidemiologic features of schizophrenia is the slight but significant excess of individuals with schizophrenia who were born in winter or spring months as opposed to other months of the year (Bradbury & Miller, 1985; Torrey et al., 1997; Torrey & Miller, 1997), and this feature is more prominent at high-latitude sites (Davies et al., 2003; Saha et al., 2006). Results from a large population-based Danish study showed that there was a small seasonal excess of schizophrenia births in winter and spring months (relative risk = 1.1) (Mortensen et al., 1999). Another interesting finding from this study was that the relative risk of developing schizophrenia was about 2.4-fold higher for those born in the city than for those born in the country. Other groups have also identified an excess of schizophrenia births in urban centers (Marcelis et al., 1998; Mortensen et al., 1999; Pedersen & Mortensen, 2001). Moreover, the incidence of schizophrenia is significantly higher in dark-skinned migrants to cold countries than in the native-born of those countries (Cantor-Graae, Zolkowska, & McNeil, 2005). Low prenatal vitamin D_3 "fits" these key environmental features: (1) vitamin D_3 deficiency is common during winter and at high latitude, most likely because of an decrease in sunlight duration, sunlight intensity, and outdoor activity (Holick, Matsuoka, & Wortsman, 1995); (2) city dwellers tend to have less exposure to sunlight and thus have lower 25-hydroxyvitamin D_3 (25[OH]D_3) levels (McGrath et al., 2001); and (3) hypovitaminosis D_3 is more common in dark-skinned populations (Holick, Matsuoka, & Wortsman, 1995).

In addition to these observations from ecologic epidemiology, preliminary evidence from a case-control study provides some support for the hypothesis. The 25(OH)D_3 serum levels in 26 mothers whose children developed schizophrenia were numerically (but not significantly) lower than those of 51 mothers whose children did not develop the disease (McGrath et al., 2003). In a subsample of African Americans (seven cases and 14 controls), a trend level association (p = 0.08) was found between low maternal vitamin D_3 levels and offspring who developed schizophrenia. Furthermore, vitamin D_3 supplements in the first year of life significantly reduced the risk of schizophrenia in males in a large Finnish birth cohort (McGrath et al., 2004).

Vitamin D₃ and the Brain

The Physiology of Vitamin D₃

Vitamin D_3 has long been known to control blood levels of calcium by regulating genes involved in calcium intestinal absorption, renal excretion, and movement in and out of bone (Heaney, 2007). In recent years, an ever-widening range of vitamin D_3 actions has been described, including regulation of proliferative and apoptotic activity (Reichrath et al., 2007), immunomodulation (Bouillon et al., 1995; Deluca & Cantorna, 2001), and neuroprotection (Garcion et al., 2002; Holick, 2007; McCann & Ames, 2008). In humans, vitamin D_3 is produced after ultraviolet B (UVB) light photolyzes 7-dehydrocholesterol in the skin, forming previtamin D_3 (Holick, 1988) (figure 11.1). The liver and other tissues metabolize vitamin D_3 to $25(OH)D_3$, the principal circulating form of vitamin D_3. This intermediate is then further hydroxylated by 1α-hydroxylase (1α-OHase) in the kidney to 1,25-dihydroxyvitamin D_3 $(1,25[OH]_2D_3)$, the biologically active form of the vitamin. Although some vitamin D_3 can be obtained from the diet, the majority of circulating vitamin D_3 is obtained from the action of sunlight on the skin.

1, $25(OH)_2D_3$, the active form of the vitamin D_3, can cross the blood-brain barrier (Pardridge, Sakiyama, & Coty, 1985). The concentration of $1,25(OH)_2D_3$ in normal adults has been reported as 31 pg/ml (range: 10–55) in serum and 25 pg/ml (range: 2–39) in cerebrospinal fluid (Balabanova et al., 1984). In addition, $1,25(OH)_2D_3$ can be synthesized locally in the brain. Neuronal and glial cells can absorb circulating $25(OH)D_3$ (Gascon-Barre & Huet, 1983) and produce $1,25(OH)_2D_3$ by action of 1α-OHase. 1α-OHase has been detected in the fetal (Fu et al., 1997) and the adult human brain (Eyles et al., 2005), where it is distributed in both neurons and glia in a regionally and layer-specific pattern (Eyles et al., 2005). The strongest immunohistochemical staining of 1α-OHase is in the cytoplasm of neurons in the hypothalamus and the large (presumably dopaminergic) neurons in the substantia nigra. This catalytic enzyme is also found in cerebellar Purkinje cells and neurons in the cerebral cortex (Zehnder et al., 2001). In addition, microglia in culture can metabolize $25(OH)D_3$ to produce biologically active $1,25(OH)_2D_3$ (Neveu et al., 1994).

In addition to the presence of the active vitamin D_3 and its catalyzing enzyme, the vitamin D receptor (VDR) has also been identified in the human brain (Sutherland et al., 1992; Zehnder et al., 2001; Eyles et al., 2005). The VDR is expressed in cortical and noncortical regions, including hippocampal CA1, CA2, and CA3; the caudate-putamen; the thalamus; the hypothalamus; and the cerebellum. The distribution of the VDR and the fact that it can be synthesized locally is consistent with the proposal that vitamin D operates in a fashion similar to other neurosteroids (McGrath, Feron, & Eyles, 2001).

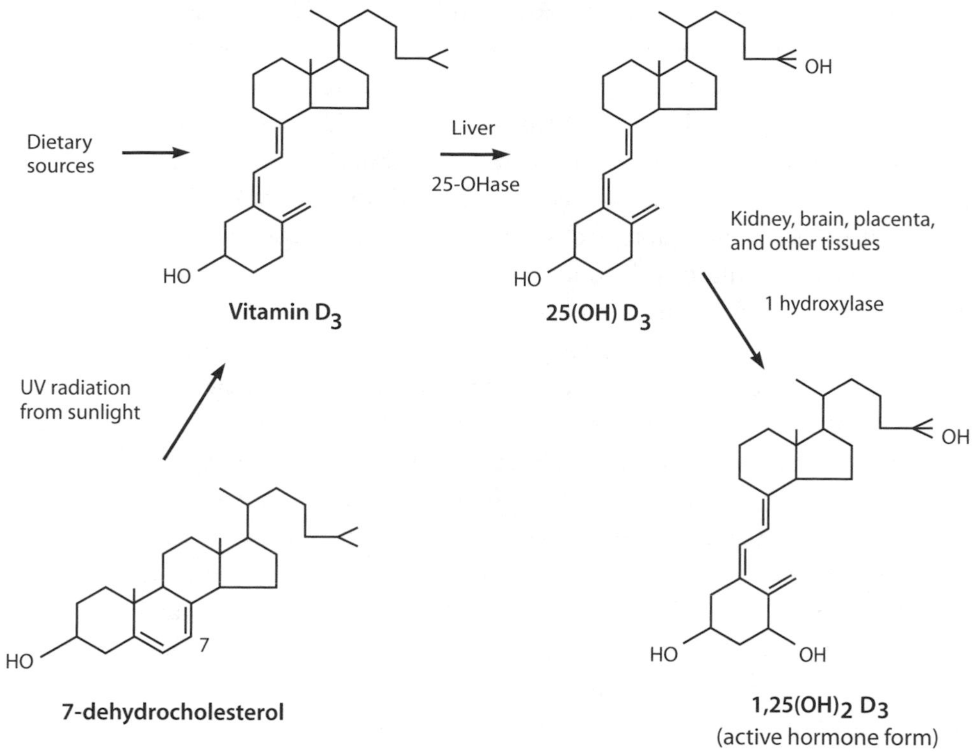

Figure 11.1. Vitamin D metabolic pathway.
In humans, although some vitamin D_3 can be obtained from the diet, the majority of circulating vitamin D_3 is obtained from the action of sunlight on the skin. Vitamin D_3 is produced after ultraviolet B (UVB) light photolyzes 7-dehydrocholesterol in the skin, forming previtamin D_3. The liver and other tissues metabolize vitamin D_3 to 25(OH)D_3, the principal circulating form of vitamin D_3. This intermediate is then further hydroxylated by 1α-hydroxylase (1α-OHase) in the kidney to 1,25-dihydroxyvitamin D_3 (1,25[OH]$_2D_3$), the biologically active form of the vitamin. (Source: Authors.)

Vitamin D_3 and Brain Development

In the rat brain, VDR expression is developmentally regulated. Its distribution is prominent within the neuroepithelium and within the differentiating fields of various areas of the brain from embryonic days 12 to 21 (Veenstra et al., 1998). Using quantitative methods, our group found that the expression of VDR mRNA and protein increased markedly between embryonic days 17 and 19, a period that correlates with the increase in apoptosis and decrease in mitosis (Burkert, McGrath, & Eyles, 2003).

The VDR is also found in the subventricular zone (SVZ), one of the major sources of neural stem cells, and this expression is particularly prominent at birth

(Cui et al., 2007). The temporal distribution pattern of VDR suggests that vitamin D_3 may influence cell differentiation in the developing brain. In addition, the influence of vitamin D has been intensively investigated in many types of cancer cells and other organs (Harrison, Wang, & Studzinski, 1999; Lin & White, 2004; Raiten & Picciano, 2004; Nagpal, Na, & Rathnachalam, 2005; Ebert et al., 2006). Our group has demonstrated that the addition of vitamin D_3 inhibits proliferation of neural progenitor cells isolated from the neonatal SVZ (Cui et al., 2007) and reduces mitotic cell number in embryonic hippocampal explants (Brown et al., 2003). In normal nervous system development, neurons are generated in numbers exceeding those found in adulthood. The surplus neurons are eliminated by programmed cell death, a process that is influenced by a range of external factors. The balance of proliferation and programmed cell death is critical for the orderly development of the brain. The effects of vitamin D_3 on neural cell number in vitro suggest a role in this critical aspect of brain development.

Taken together, several lines of evidence suggest that $1,25(OH)_2D_3$ may influence brain development and that low maternal vitamin D_3 may be an environmental risk factor for schizophrenia. A decade ago, our group developed an informative animal model—the DVD model—in which vitamin D_3 is depleted in utero. This model displays a range of subtle but informative neurochemical and behavioral features in common with the clinical phenotype of schizophrenia. In the next section, we outline the findings from this animal model with respect to brain development, brain structure, and behavior.

DVD-Deficient Rats

DVD-Deficient Rat Model

To produce the DVD-deficient model, female Sprague-Dawley rats are fed a diet that lacks vitamin D but contains normal calcium and phosphorous. The rats are housed under a 12-hour light-and-dark cycle using incandescent lighting free of UV radiation in the vitamin D_3 action spectrum (290–315 nm). After six weeks, serum vitamin D_3 depletion is confirmed before mating using a verified in-house LC/MS/MS assay ($25(OH)D_3 < 0.34$ ng/ml) (Eyles et al., 2009). The resulting dams are housed under these conditions until the birth of pups. Control animals are kept under standard lighting conditions and are supplied with standard rat chow containing vitamin D_3. All dams (both control and depleted) are kept under standard housing conditions (control rat chow and UV-emitting lighting) after giving birth. Both vitamin D_3 depleted dams and offspring remain normocalcemic. It is important to stress that the exposure to vitamin D_3 depletion is only transient. DVD-deficient offspring become vitamin D_3 replete by two weeks of age and have normal levels of vitamin D_3, calcium, and phosphorous in adulthood.

DVD Deficiency and Abnormal Brain Development in Neonates

The absence of maternal vitamin D has multiple effects on the developing brain. First, at the gross architectural level, DVD-deficient pups had cerebral hemispheres that were longer but not wider than controls. When corrected for hemispheric volume, these pups also had lateral ventricles that were larger than those of controls. In addition, after the data were normalized for whole-brain cross-sectional area, the neocortex of these pups was thinner than controls (Eyles et al., 2003).

Second, DVD deficiency increased mitosis globally across the embryonic brain. Consistent with the elevated cell division, the number of apoptotic cells was reduced in most brain regions from embryonic day 21 until birth embryonic day 23 (Ko et al., 2004). When neurosphere cultures were made from the brains of DVD-deficient neonates, neurosphere number was increased, suggesting greater rates of cell division (Cui et al., 2007). These results suggest that vitamin D exerts a pro-differentiation and proapoptotic function in the developing brain. Given that normal brain development requires precise spatial and temporal regulation of both cell proliferation and elimination, we speculate that the altered brain size and shape in DVD-deficient offspring may be the result of the disrupted normal progression of proliferation and cell death.

Low maternal vitamin D_3 also altered the gene expression profile regulating mitosis and apoptosis in the brain (Ko et al., 2004). Results from pathway-specific arrays showed that 74% of expressed apoptotic genes were down-regulated and 48% of genes related to mitosis were up-regulated in DVD-deficient pups. For example, at perinatal stages the expression of Bak, a pro-apoptotic gene, was decreased whereas cyclins A1, D1, and E, genes favoring progression of the cell cycle, were increased (Ko et al., 2004). Consistent with this pattern, both cyclin C and B, which are up-regulated by vitamin D_3 (Harrison, Wang, & Studzinski, 1999; Polly et al., 2000), were down-regulated in DVD-deficient rats. The cyclin-dependent kinase inhibitor p21cip1, which is up-regulated by vitamin D_3 in in vitro cell lines (Liu et al., 1996; Hager et al., 2001), was down-regulated in the DVD-deficient neonatal rat brain (Ko et al., 2004). In sum, at both cellular and transcriptional levels, the absence of vitamin D_3 disrupts the normal sequence of mitotic and apoptotic activity in brain development. This might explain the alterations in neonatal brain shape induced by DVD deficiency.

Apart from their role in synaptic conduction, neurotransmitters can act as trophic factors that regulate morphogenetic events such as proliferation, migration, differentiation, neurite growth, and neural circuit formation during brain development (Nguyen et al., 2001; Ruediger & Bolz, 2007). Therefore, we also examined whether neurotransmitter turnover, specifically dopamine (DA), is altered in neonatal brains. We showed that DVD deficiency induces a 45% reduction in the expression of catechol-O-methyl transferase (COMT), one of the key enzymes for

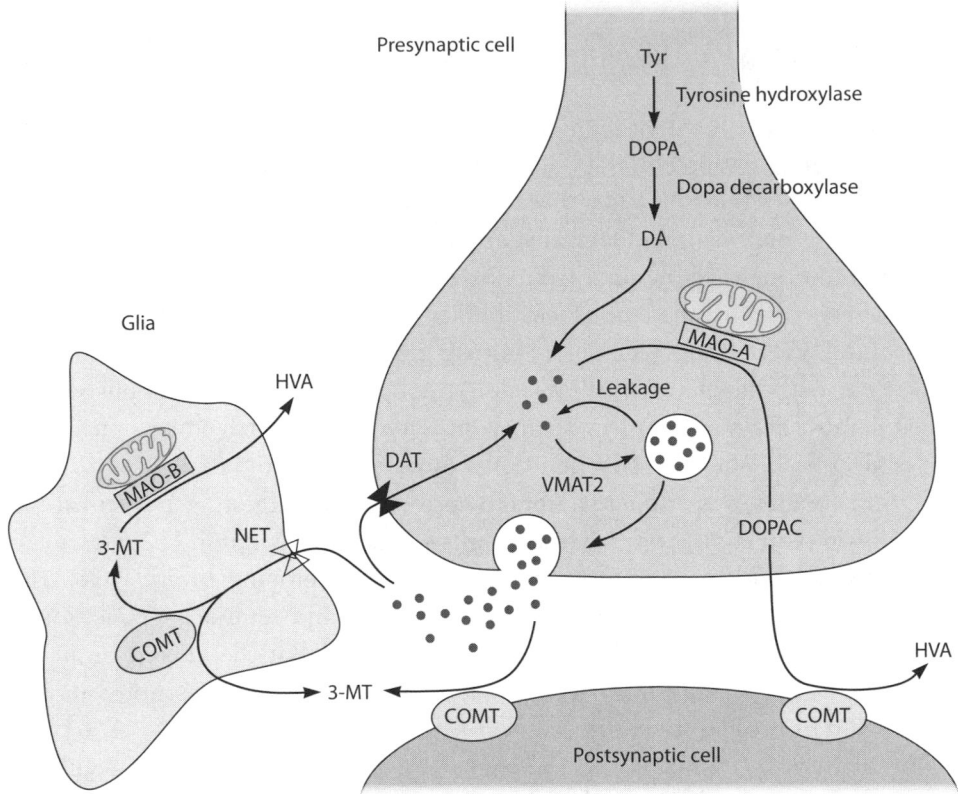

Figure 11.2. Key metabolic pathways related to dopamine neurotransmission.
The primary route of DA metabolism is through the intraneural oxidative deamination of 3,4-dihydroxyphenylacetic acid (DOPAC) by monoamine oxidase (MAO-A). DOPAC is then O-methylated extra-neuronally by catechol-O-methyl transferase (COMT), to homovanillic acid (HVA). The vesicular monoamine transporter (VMAT) avidly sequesters intracellular DA into vesicles. The vesicles are maintained within the neuron until a sufficient potential induces release at the synaptic membrane. Once released the DAT actively transports DA back into the neuron to cease signaling and allow for repacking of DA into the vesicles by VMAT. (Source: Authors.)

DA metabolism in the cortex (Kesby et al., 2009a) (figure 11.2). Although the levels of DA or DA metabolites were not altered in these brains, the ratio of the DA metabolites—3,4-dihydroxyphenylacetic acid (DOPAC) to homovanillic acid (HVA)—was significantly greater in the forebrain, reflecting decreased conversion of DOPAC to HVA by COMT. The primary route of DA metabolism is through the intraneural oxidative deamination of DA to DOPAC by monoamine oxidase. DOPAC is then O-methylated extra-neuronally by COMT to HVA. Under normal conditions within the striatum, approximately 70–80% of HVA is produced by means of this pathway (Westerink, 1985; Wood, Kim, & Marien, 1987).

In summary, our findings confirm that DVD deficiency is capable of altering aspects of brain structure, cell proliferation, apoptosis, and neurotransmission during development. In the next section, we discuss abnormalities that persist in the adult brains of DVD-deficient animals and how these might relate to the structural, neurochemical, and behavioral alterations seen in patients with schizophrenia.

DVD Deficiency and Persistent Changes in the Adult Brain

Depending on the timing of reintroduction of vitamin D_3, the DVD model also exhibits persistent changes in adult brain outcomes. Although DVD deficiency during gestation yields marginal changes in lateral ventricle volumes in adult offspring, the volume is significantly increased if the introduction of the vitamin D_3-replete diet is delayed until weaning. A proteomics study of the frontal cortex and hippocampus from these animals revealed that DVD deficiency induced a reduction in proteins directly involved with cytoskeleton maintenance such as ß tubulin and the light and medium neurofilament proteins (Almeras et al., 2007). These changes may be relevant for the structural alterations seen in the adult brains.

DVD deficiency also altered proteins involved in mitochondrial function and neurotransmission in the nucleus accumbens (Nac) (McGrath et al., 2008). Nac, one of the projection regions in the mesolimbic DA system, is of particular interest with respect to schizophrenia (Lauer, Senitz, & Beckmann, 2001). DVD deficiency was associated with alteration in 35 unique proteins. Of these, 22 were down-regulated and 13 up-regulated. Six mitochondrial proteins were down-regulated in DVD-deficient rats (NDUAA, UQCR1, ODPB, IDH3A, HKK1, VDAC2). Neurotransmssion-associated proteins were also dysregulated. Two members of the dynamin family (dynamin 1 and dynamin 1-like proteins) as well as syntaxin-binding protein, which are involved in neurotransmitter vesicle release, were significantly down-regulated in the adult DVD-deficient rats. Apart from these proteins, four calcium-binding proteins (calbindin, calbindin2, hippocalcin, and calreticulin) were significantly altered in the Nac of the adult DVD-deficient rat. Calbindin, an important component of a subset of GABAergic interneurons (those that transmit or secrete gamma-aminobutyric acid), is strongly induced by vitamin D_3 (Christakos et al., 2007), and thus it is feasible that the reduction in this protein may be a direct consequence of the early life reduction in vitamin D_3.

Vitamin D_3 depletion in utero also had significant effects on the expression of genes involved in cytoskeleton maintenance (MAP2, NF-L) and neurotransmission (GABA-Aα4) (Feron et al., 2005). In the frontal cortex and hippocampus (Eyles et al., 2007), the expression of 36 genes involved in oxidative phosphorylation, redox balance, cytoskeleton maintenance, calcium homeostasis, synaptic plasticity, neurotransmission, and chaperoning was altered. With respect to human psychiatric disorders, many of these genes have been shown to be dysregulated in schizophrenia. Most prominent among these is the dysregulation of mitochondrial proteins. In schizophrenia, adenosine triphosphate (ATP) production in the frontal and left temporal lobes is reduced (Fujimoto et al., 1992; Volz et al., 2000). It is important that a genomic-proteomic study of frontal lobes from patients with schizophrenia revealed that genes connected to mitochondria function were among the most dysregulated (Lu et al., 2000). Subjects with schizophrenia display dysregulated expression of genes involved in neurotransmission, such as synapsin-2, GAP43, Vis1, and 143G (Lu et al., 2000), as is also true of the DVD-deficient rat model. ApoE, which is low in the DVD-deficient brain, was also identified as a schizophrenia-susceptibility locus in linkage and association studies (Harrington et al., 1995).

DVD Deficiency and Behavior in the Adult Offspring

The adult offspring of DVD-deficient dams display a range of behavioral abnormalities, including hyperlocomotion, enhanced sensitivity to psychomimetic drugs, and impaired latent inhibition. Although the mechanisms mediating such behaviors are not clear, the altered behavioral phenotype demonstrates that the effects of prenatal vitamin D deficiency on brain development can persist into adulthood even after the vitamin D is reintroduced at birth.

Rats exposed to DVD deficiency had elevated levels of locomotion across a range of tests, including the hole board and elevated plus maze (Burne et al., 2004) and in the open field (Kesby et al., 2006); this has been referred to as *spontaneous hyperlocomotion*. This subtle increase in locomotion appears to be a transient response to a novel environment and is sensitive to handling procedures such as restraint (Burne et al., 2006; O'Loan et al., 2007) or restraint and injection (Kesby et al., 2006). One explanation for this phenomenon is an enhanced stress-induced activation of the hypothalamic pituitary axis in DVD-deficient rats. However, we have measured plasma corticosterone levels during and after 30 minutes of restraint stress and found no differences between control and DVD-deficient male rats (Eyles et al., 2006).

With respect to learning and memory, DVD-deficient rats have impaired latent inhibition (Becker et al., 2005). Latent inhibition is a learning phenomenon whereby irrelevant sensory information is filtered unconsciously. Latent inhibition reflects the ability to attend selectively to the important information in the environment and ignore the unimportant, a phenomenon related to both learning and attention. Attentional abnormalities are associated with schizophrenia, and acutely psychotic patients show reduced latent inhibition (Feldon, Shofel, & Weiner, 1991; Lubow & Gewirtz, 1995). Animal models with disrupted latent inhibition are thought to reflect the cognitive or attentional deficits associated with schizophrenia (Grecksch et al., 1999; Moser et al., 2000; Weiner, 2003).

In addition to the subtle and discrete behavioral alterations, DVD-deficient rats exhibit sex-specific behavioral changes in response to psychomimetic agents. DVD-deficient male rats display greater locomotor activity than do DVD-deficient female rats and control male rats in response to the noncompetitive N-methyl-D-aspartic acid receptor (NMDA-R) antagonist, MK-801, in the open field test (Kesby et al., 2006). This effect depends on the timing of the DVD deficiency, because rats experiencing the deficiency during late gestation showed this effect, whereas rats experiencing this deficiency only during early gestation did not (O'Loan et al., 2007). Both the spontaneous and the MK-801-induced hyperlocomotion were abolished by haloperidol, a DA receptor 2 (DA2) blocking agent. Psychomimetic-induced hyperlocomotion in rats has been associated with hyperactivity of mesolimbic DA neurons, a factor thought to be related to psychotic symptoms in schizophrenia (Seeman, 1987). The observation that both enhanced MK-801-induced and spontaneous locomotion in DVD-deficient animals are sensitive to the DA2 receptor blocking agent supports the suggestion that central nervous system DA signaling has been developmentally altered.

In contrast to DVD-deficient males and control females, DVD-deficient females displayed increased locomotion in response to amphetamine. Correspondingly, the density of the DA transporter (DAT) was increased by almost 40% in the caudate-putamen, and the selective affinity for DAT ligands was elevated in the Nac (Kesby et al., 2009b). Amphetamine has been used widely in animal models of schizophrenia. This drug increases striatal DA release (Bardo, Bowling, & Pierce, 1990) through multiple actions, most prominently those incorporating DAT function (Sulzer, Maidment, & Rayport, 1993; Wieczorek & Kruk, 1994; Sulzer et al., 1995; Jones, 1998). Amphetamine also induces a behavioral phenotype that can be blunted by D2 receptor blockade (O'Neill & Shaw, 1999). Hence, increased locomotor sensitivity displayed by animals in response to psychomimetic agents such as amphetamine is considered to be analogous to the enhanced subcortical dopaminergic activity observed in schizophrenia patients (Hietala et al., 1995). In schizophrenia patients, amphetamine can increase the psychotic symptoms by enhancing DA signaling. In healthy individuals, amphetamine can produce psychotic symptoms (Angrist & Vankammen, 1984). Furthermore, low doses of amphetamine that fail to induce psychotic symptoms in healthy individuals can enhance the psychotic symptoms seen in schizophrenia patients (Janowsky et al., 1973).

In conclusion, the experimental data have provided robust evidence demonstrating that DVD deficiency during gestation alters the trajectory of brain development and the structure and function of the adult brain. The DVD model appears to be an informative one for schizophrenia from several perspectives (summarized in table 11.1). With respect to brain development, DVD deficiency

Table 11.1 Summary of Key Features of the Developmental Vitamin D (DVD) Deficiency Model of Schizophrenia

Modality	DVD-Deficient Phenotype
Brain development	Enlarged lateral ventricles (Eyles et al., 2003) Increase mitosis and reduced programmed cell death (Eyles et al., 2003; Ko, McGrath, & Eyles, 2004) Increased neurosphere formation (Cui et al., 2007) Disrupted dopamine turnover (Kesby et al., 2009a)
Adult brain	Enlarged lateral ventricles (Feron et al., 2005) Mis-expression of genes and proteins involved in mitochondria function and neurotransmission (Almeras et al., 2007; McGrath et al., 2008; Kesby et al., 2009a) Increased DAT density and affinity in mesolimbic system (Kesby et al., 2009b)
Adult behavior	Hyperlocomotion (Burne et al., 2006; Kesby et al., 2006; O'Loan et al., 2007) Disrupted latent inhibition (LI) (Becker et al., 2005) Hyperlocomotion in response to MK-801(Kesby et al., 2006; O'Loan et al., 2007) Hyperlocomotion in response to amphetamine (Kesby et al., 2009b) Sensitivity to haloperidol (Kesby et al., 2006)

SOURCE: Authors.

leads to alterations in brain morphology, mitosis, programmed cell death, and expression of neurotransmitter-related genes and proteins. Most important, DVD deficiency also induces long-lasting alterations in adult brain outcomes, such as ventriculomegaly and misexpression of genes and proteins involved in mitochondrial function and neurotransmission, which have been reported to be disrupted in patients with schizophrenia. With respect to behavior, the DVD model includes the following: (1) hyperlocomotion, a predominant feature of many animal models of schizophrenia; (2) disrupted latent inhibition, an attentional deficit associated with schizophrenia; and (3) gender-specific sensitivity to psychomimetic drugs, such as MK-801 and amphetamine, as well as antipsychotics, such as haloperidol.

Future Directions and Relevance to Public Health

Although clinical research remains central to the field of psychiatry, animal models remain the only practical tool for unraveling the biological mechanisms linking early life disruptions to later neuropsychiatric disorders. The developing human brain is not open to ready observation, and experimental manipulations of normal brain development are clearly not ethical. The DVD model summarized in table 11.1 provides a tool with which to explore a candidate risk factor for schizophrenia. In addition, it has revealed previously unsuspected aspects of neurobiology.

With respect to future studies, first, the predictive validity of the DVD model for schizophrenia should be further examined. The positive symptoms of schizophrenia, such as hallucinations and delusions, are more readily recognized in patients and are generally responsive to antipsychotic medication. Reduced motivation, blunted emotions, social avoidance (negative symptoms of schizophrenia), and impaired cognitive function dramatically limit the patient's social and functional recovery and are less responsive to antipsychotics. The DVD model shows evidence for psychomotor agitation, a positive symptom of schizophrenia: the animals display increased locomotion following stimulation by psychomimetic drugs. The social and cognitive behavior of the DVD rat needs to be investigated to explore the negative and cognitive symptoms of schizophrenia. Assessment of cognitive deficits in patients with schizophrenia can include a large array of potential measures. Similarly, the assessment of attention, learning, and memory in rodent models could follow many different directions. The need to examine cognitive behaviors in animal models of schizophrenia is also timely because the pharmaceutical industry is investing strongly in the development of products that are designed primarily to ameliorate cognitive deficits rather than to reduce more traditional clinical "targets" such as hallucinations and delusions. Recently, U.S.-based researchers from the Food and Drug Administration, the National Institute of Mental Health, academia, and the pharmaceutical industry published consensus guidelines for clinical trials aimed at the treatment of cognitive symptoms of schizophrenia (Measurement and Treatment Research to Improve Cognition in Schizophrenia, or MATRICS) (Buchanan et al., 2005). The MATRICS panel has grouped the cognitive deficits associated with schizophrenia according to eight "core features" or domains (Buchanan et al., 2005). These include speed of processing, attention, vigilance, working memory, verbal learning, visual learning, reasoning and problem solving, and social cognition (Green et al., 2005). The interdisciplinary panel noted that strong animal models were currently available for working memory, attention, vigilance, and speed of processing.

Secondly, future work is required to clarify the mechanism of action linking hypovitaminosis D and the observed brain changes. In addition, it will be important to clarify how these changes are associated with altered behaviors. Finally, although the results from the DVD-deficient animal experiments indicated that brain structure and function are altered in rodents, it remains to be seen if maternal vitamin D deficiency is directly associated with schizophrenia in humans. Schizophrenia is associated with a substantial burden of disability. In the absence of major advances in the efficacy of treatments, interventions that offer the prospect of reducing the incidence of the disorder should be pursued vigorously. If future studies confirm the association between DVD deficiency and risk of schizophrenia, then it raises the tantalizing prospect of primary prevention, in a manner comparable to folate supplementation and the prevention of spina bifida.

KEY AREAS FOR FUTURE RESEARCH

- The predictive validity of the DVD model requires further exploration with psychopharmacological treatments.
- Using the domains specified by the MATRICS panel, we hope to explore further the cognitive aspects of the DVD model.
- Analytic epidemiology is required in order to explore if DVD is associated with schizophrenia.
- Explore ontological pathways linking DVD deficiency and altered brain outcomes.

Acknowledgments

We are grateful for the support of the National Health and Medical Research Council. James Kesby kindly provided figure 11.2.

Selected Readings

Eyles, D. W., Feron, F., Cui, X., Kesby, J. P., Harms, L. H., Ko, P., McGrath, J. J., & Burne, T. H. (2009). Developmental vitamin D deficiency causes abnormal brain development. *Psychoneuroendocrinology* 34 (Suppl 1): S247–S257.

Holick, M. F. (2007). Vitamin D deficiency. *North England Journal of Medicine, 357*(3): 266–281.

McCann, J. C. & Ames, B. N. (2008). Is there convincing biological or behavioral evidence linking vitamin D deficiency to brain dysfunction? *FASEB Journal* 22(4): 982–1001.

McGrath, J., Feron, F., & Eyles, D. (2001). Vitamin D: The neglected neurosteroid? *Trends in Neuroscience* 24(10): 570–572.

References

Almeras, L., Eyles, D., Benech, P., Laffite, D., Villard, C., Patatian, A., Boucraut, J., Mackay-Sim, A., McGrath, J., & Feron, F. (2007). Developmental vitamin D deficiency alters brain protein expression in the adult rat: Implications for neuropsychiatric disorders. *Proteomics* 7(5): 769–780.

Angrist, B. & Vankammen, D. P. (1984). CNS stimulants as tools in the study of schizophrenia. *Trends in Neuroscience* 7(10): 388–390.

Balabanova, S., Richter, H. P., Antoniadis, G., Homoki, J., Kremmer, N., Hanle, J., & Teller, W. M. (1984). 25-Hydroxyvitamin D, 24, 25-dihydroxyvitamin D and 1,25-dihydroxyvitamin D in human cerebrospinal fluid. *Klinische Wochenschrift* 62(22): 1086–1090.

Bardo, M. T., Bowling, S. L., & Pierce, R. C. (1990). Changes in locomotion and dopamine neurotransmission following amphetamine, haloperidol, and exposure to novel environmental stimuli. *Psychopharmacology* 101(3): 338–343.

Becker, A., Eyles, D. W., McGrath, J. J., & Grecksch, G. (2005). Transient prenatal vitamin D deficiency is associated with subtle alterations in learning and memory functions in adult rats. *Behavioural Brain Research* 161(2): 306–312.

Bouillon, R., Verstuyf, A., Branisteanu, D., Waer, M., & Mathieu, C. (1995). Immune modulation by vitamin D analogs in the prevention of autoimmune diseases. *Koninklijke Academie voor Geneeskunde van België* 57(5): 371–385; discussion 385–387.

Bradbury, T. N. & Miller, G. A. (1985). Season of birth in schizophrenia: A review of evidence, methodology, and etiology. *Psychological Bulletin* 98(3): 569–594.

Brown, J., Bianco, J. I., McGrath, J. J., & Eyles, D. W. (2003). 1,25-dihydroxyvitamin D3 induces nerve growth factor, promotes neurite outgrowth and inhibits mitosis in embryonic rat hippocampal neurons. *Neuroscience Letters* 343(2): 139–143.

Buchanan, R. W., Davis, M., Goff, D., Green, M. F., Keefe, R. S., Leon, A. C., Nuechterlein, K. H., Laughren, T., Levin, R., Stover, E., et al. (2005). A summary of the FDA-NIMH-MATRICS workshop on clinical trial design for neurocognitive drugs for schizophrenia. *Schizophrenia Bulletin* 31(1): 5–19.

Burkert, R., McGrath, J., & Eyles, D. (2003). Vitamin D receptor expression in the embryonic brain. *Neuroscience Research Communications* 33(2): 67–71.

Burne, T. H., Becker, A., Brown, J., Eyles, D. W., Mackay-Sim, A., & McGrath, J. J. (2004). Transient prenatal vitamin D deficiency is associated with hyperlocomotion in adult rats. *Behavioural Brain Research* 154(2): 549–555.

Burne, T. H., O'Loan, J., McGrath, J. J., & Eyles, D. W. (2006). Hyperlocomotion associated with transient prenatal vitamin D deficiency is ameliorated by acute restraint. *Behavioural Brain Research* 174(1): 119–124.

Cantor-Graae, E., Zolkowska, K., & McNeil, T. F. (2005). Increased risk of psychotic disorder among immigrants in Malmo: A 3-year first-contact study. *Psychological Medicine* 35(8): 1155–1163.

Christakos, S., Dhawan, P., Peng, X., Obukhov, A. G., Nowycky, M. C., Benn, B. S., Zhong, Y., Liu, Y., & Shen, Q. (2007). New insights into the function and regulation of vitamin D target proteins. *Journal of Steroid Biochemistry and Molecular Biology* 103(3–5): 405–410.

Cui, X., McGrath, J. J., Burne, T. H., Mackay-Sim, A., & Eyles, D. W. (2007). Maternal vitamin D depletion alters neurogenesis in the developing rat brain. *International Journal of Developmental Neuroscience* 25(4): 227–232.

Davies, G., Welham, J., Chant, D., Torrey, E. F., & McGrath, J. (2003). A systematic review and meta-analysis of Northern Hemisphere season of birth studies in schizophrenia. *Schizophrenia Bulletin* 29(3): 587–593.

Deluca, H. F. & Cantorna, M. T. (2001). Vitamin D: Its role and uses in immunology. *FASEB Journal* 15(14): 2579–2585.

Ebert, R., Schutze, N., Adamski, J., & Jakob, F. (2006). Vitamin D signaling is modulated on multiple levels in health and disease. *Molecular and Cellular Endocrinology* 248(1–2): 149–159.

Eyles, D., Almeras, L., Benech, P., Patatian, A., Mackay-Sim, A., McGrath, J., & Feron, F. (2007). Developmental vitamin D deficiency alters the expression of genes encoding mitochondrial, cytoskeletal and synaptic proteins in the adult rat brain. *Journal of Steroid Biochemistry and Molecular Biology* 103(3–5): 538–545.

Eyles, D., Anderson, C., Ko, P., Jones, A., Thomas, A., Burne, T., Mortensen, P. B., Norgaard-Pedersen, B., Hougaard, D. M., & McGrath, J. (2009). A sensitive LC/MS/MS assay of 25OH vitamin D3 and 25OH vitamin D2 in dried blood spots. *Clinica Chimica Acta* 403(1–2): 145–151.

Eyles, D., Brown, J., Mackay-Sim, A., McGrath, J., & Feron, F. (2003). Vitamin D3 and brain development. *Neuroscience 118*(3): 641–653.

Eyles, D. W., Rogers, F., Buller, K., McGrath, J. J., Ko, P., French, K., & Burne, T. H. (2006). Developmental vitamin D (DVD) deficiency in the rat alters adult behaviour independently of HPA function. *Psychoneuroendocrinology 31*(8): 958–964.

Eyles, D. W., Smith, S., Kinobe, R., Hewison, M., & McGrath, J. J. (2005). Distribution of the vitamin D receptor and 1 alpha-hydroxylase in human brain. *Journal of Chemical Neuroanatomy 29*(1): 21–30.

Feldon, J., Shofel, A., & Weiner, I. (1991). Latent inhibition is unaffected by direct dopamine agonists. *Pharmacology Biochemistry and Behavior 38*(2): 309–314.

Feron, F., Burne, T. H., Brown, J., Smith, E., McGrath, J. J., Mackay-Sim, A., & Eyles, D. W. (2005). Developmental vitamin D3 deficiency alters the adult rat brain. *Brain Research Bulletin 65*(2): 141–148.

Fu, G. K., Lin, D., Zhang, M. Y., Bikle, D. D., Shackleton, C. H., Miller, W. L., & Portale, A. A. (1997). Cloning of human 25-hydroxyvitamin D-1 alpha-hydroxylase and mutations causing vitamin D-dependent rickets type 1. *Molecular Endocrinology 11*(13): 1961–1970.

Fujimoto, T., Nakano, T., Takano, T., Hokazono, Y., Asakura, T., & Tsuji, T. (1992). Study of chronic schizophrenics using 31P magnetic resonance chemical shift imaging. *Acta Psychiatrica Scandinavica 86*(6): 455–462.

Garcion, E., Wion-Barbot, N., Montero-Menei, C. N., Berger, F., & Wion, D. (2002). New clues about vitamin D functions in the nervous system. *Trends in Endocrinology and Metabolism 13*(3): 100–105.

Gascon-Barre, M. & Huet, P. M. (1983). Apparent [3H]1,25-dihydroxyvitamin D3 uptake by canine and rodent brain. *American Journal of Physiology 244*(3): E266–E271.

Grecksch, G., Bernstein, H. G., Becker, A., Hollt, V., & Bogerts, B. (1999). Disruption of latent inhibition in rats with postnatal hippocampal lesions. *Neuropsychopharmacology 20*(6): 525–532.

Green, M. F., Olivier, B., Crawley, J. N., Penn, D. L., & Silverstein, S. (2005). Social cognition in schizophrenia: Recommendations from the measurement and treatment research to improve cognition in schizophrenia new approaches conference. *Schizophrenia Bulletin 31*(4): 882–887.

Hager, G., Formanek, M., Gedlicka, C., Thurnher, D., Knerer, B., & Kornfehl, J. (2001). 1,25(OH)2 vitamin D3 induces elevated expression of the cell cycle-regulating genes P21 and P27 in squamous carcinoma cell lines of the head and neck. *Acta Oto-Laryngologica 121*(1): 103–109.

Harrington, C. R., Roth, M., Xuereb, J. H., McKenna, P. J., & Wischik, C. M. (1995). Apolipoprotein E type epsilon 4 allele frequency is increased in patients with schizophrenia. *Neuroscience Letters 202*(1–2): 101–104.

Harrison, L. E., Wang, Q. M., & Studzinski, G. P. (1999). 1,25-dihydroxyvitamin D(3)-induced retardation of the G(2)/M traverse is associated with decreased levels of p34(cdc2) in HL60 cells. *Journal of Cellular Biochemistry 75*(2): 226–234.

Heaney, R. P. (2007). Vitamin D endocrine physiology. *Journal of Bone and Mineral Research 22*: V25–V27.

Hietala, J., Syvalahti, E., Vuorio, K., Rakkolainen, V., Bergman, J., Haaparanta, M., Solin, O., Kuoppamaki, M., Kirvela, O., Ruotsalainen, U., et al. (1995). Presynaptic dopamine function in striatum of neuroleptic-naive schizophrenic patients. *Lancet 346*(8983): 1130–1131.

Holick, M. F. (1988). Skin: Site of the synthesis of vitamin-D and a target tissue for the active form, 1,25-Dihydroxyvitamin-D3. *Annals of the New York Academy of Sciences 548*: 14–26.

Holick, M. F. (2007). Vitamin D deficiency. *New England Journal of Medicine* 357(3): 266–281.

Holick, M. F., Matsuoka, L. Y., & Wortsman, J. (1995). Regular use of sunscreen on vitamin D levels. *Archives of Dermatology* 131(11): 1337–1339.

Janowsky, D. S., el-Yousel, M. K., Davis, J. M., & Sekerke, H. J. (1973). Provocation of schizophrenic symptoms by intravenous administration of methylphenidate. *Archives of General Psychiatry* 28(2): 185–191.

Jones, S. R., Gainetdinov, R. R., Wightman, R. M., & Caron, M. G. (1998). Mechanisms of amphetamine action revealed in mice lacking the dopamine transporter. *Journal of Neuroscience* 18(6): 1979–1986.

Kesby, J. P., Burne, T. H., McGrath, J. J., & Eyles, D. W. (2006). Developmental vitamin D deficiency alters MK 801-induced hyperlocomotion in the adult rat: An animal model of schizophrenia. *Biological Psychiatry* 60(6): 591–596.

Kesby, J. P., Cui, X., Ko, P., McGrath, J. J., Burne, T. H., & Eyles, D. W. (2009a). Developmental vitamin D deficiency alters dopamine turnover in neonatal rat forebrain. *Neuroscience Letters* 461(2): 155–158.

Kesby, J. P., Cui, X., O'Loan, J., McGrath, J., Burne, T. H. J., & Eyles, D. W. (2009b). Developmental vitamin D deficiency alters dopamine-mediated behaviors and dopamine transporter function in adult female rats. *Psychopharmacology* 208(1): 159–168.

Ko, P., Burkert, R., McGrath, J., & Eyles, D. (2004). Maternal vitamin D3 deprivation and the regulation of apoptosis and cell cycle during rat brain development. *Brain Research: Developmental Brain Research* 153(1): 61–68.

Lauer, M., Senitz, D., & Beckmann, H. (2001). Increased volume of the nucleus accumbens in schizophrenia. *Journal of Neural Transmission* 108(6): 645–660.

Lin, R. & White, J. H. (2004). The pleiotropic actions of vitamin D. *Bioessays* 26(1): 21–28.

Liu, M., Lee, M. H., Cohen, M., Bommakanti, M., & Freedman, L. P. (1996). Transcriptional activation of the Cdk inhibitor p21 by vitamin D3 leads to the induced differentiation of the myelomonocytic cell line U937. *Genes and Development* 10(2): 142–153.

Lu, F., Selak, M., O'Connor, J., Croul, S., Lorenzana, C., Butunoi, C., & Kalman, B. (2000). Oxidative damage to mitochondrial DNA and activity of mitochondrial enzymes in chronic active lesions of multiple sclerosis. *Journal of the Neurological Sciences* 177(2): 95–103.

Lubow, R. E. & Gewirtz, J. C. (1995). Latent inhibition in humans: Data, theory, and implications for schizophrenia. *Psychological Bulletin* 117(1): 87–103.

Marcelis, M., Navarro-Mateu, F., Murray, R., Selten, J. P., & van Os, J. (1998). Urbanization and psychosis: A study of 1942–1978 birth cohorts in The Netherlands. *Psychological Medicine* 28(4): 871–879.

McCann, J. C. & Ames, B. N. (2008). Is there convincing biological or behavioral evidence linking vitamin D deficiency to brain dysfunction? *FASEB Journal* 22(4): 982–1001.

McGrath, J., Eyles, D., Mowry, B., Yolken, R., & Buka, S. (2003). Low maternal vitamin D as a risk factor for schizophrenia: A pilot study using banked sera. *Schizophrenia Research* 63(1–2): 73–78.

McGrath, J., Feron, F., & Eyles, D. (2001). Vitamin D: The neglected neurosteroid? *Trends in Neuroscience* 24(10): 570–572.

McGrath, J., Iwazaki, T., Eyles, D., Burne, T., Cui, X., Ko, P., & Matsumoto, I. (2008). Protein expression in the nucleus accumbens of rats exposed to developmental vitamin D deficiency. *PLoS One* 3(6): e2383.

McGrath, J., Saari, K., Hakko, H., Jokelainen, J., Jones, P., Järvelin, M. R., Chant, D., & Isohanni, M. (2004). Vitamin D supplementation during the first year of life and risk of schizophrenia: A Finnish birth-cohort study. *Schizophrenia Research* 67(2–3): 237–245.

McGrath, J. J., Kimlin, M. G., Saha, S., Eyles, D. W., & Parisi, A. V. (2001). Vitamin D insufficiency in south-east Queensland. *Medical Journal of Australia 174*(3): 150–151.

Mortensen, P. B., Pedersen, C. B., Westergaard, T., Wohlfahrt, J., Ewald, H., Mors, O., Andersen, P. K., & Melbye, M. (1999). Effects of family history and place and season of birth on the risk of schizophrenia. *New England Journal of Medicine 340*(8): 603–608.

Moser, P. C., Hitchcock, J. M., Lister, S., & Moran, P. M. (2000). The pharmacology of latent inhibition as an animal model of schizophrenia. *Brain Research Reviews 33*(2–3): 275–307.

Nagpal, S., Na, S., & Rathnachalam, R. (2005). Noncalcemic actions of vitamin D receptor ligands. *Endocrine Reviews 26*(5): 662–687.

Neveu, I., Naveilhan, P., Menaa, C., Wion, D., Brachet, P., & Garabedian, M. (1994). Synthesis of 1,25-dihydroxyvitamin D3 by rat brain macrophages in vitro. *Journal of Neuroscience Research 38*(2): 214–220.

Nguyen, L., Rigo, J. M., Rocher, V., Belachew, S., Malgrange, B., Rogister, B., Leprince, P., & Moonen, G. (2001). Neurotransmitters as early signals for central nervous system development. *Cell Tissue Research 305*(2): 187–202.

O'Loan, J., Eyles, D. W., Kesby, J., Ko, P., McGrath, J. J., & Burne, T. H. (2007). Vitamin D deficiency during various stages of pregnancy in the rat: Its impact on development and behaviour in adult offspring. *Psychoneuroendocrinology 32*(3): 227–234.

O'Neill, M. F. & Shaw, G. (1999). Comparison of dopamine receptor antagonists on hyperlocomotion induced by cocaine, amphetamine, MK-801 and the dopamine D-1 agonist C-APB in mice. *Psychopharmacology 145*(3): 237–250.

Pardridge, W. M., Sakiyama, R., & Coty, W. A. (1985). Restricted transport of vitamin D and A derivatives through the rat blood-brain barrier. *Journal of Neurochemistry 44*(4): 1138–1141.

Pedersen, C. B. & Mortensen, P. B. (2001). Family history, place and season of birth as risk factors for schizophrenia in Denmark: A replication and reanalysis. *British Journal of Psychiatry 179*(1): 46–52.

Polly, P., Danielsson, C., Schrader, M., & Carlberg, C. (2000). Cyclin C is a primary 1alpha,25-dihydroxyvitamin D(3) responding gene. *Journal of Cellular Biochemistry 77*(1): 75–81.

Raiten, D. J. & Picciano, M. F. (2004). Vitamin D and health in the 21st century: Bone and beyond. Executive summary. *American Journal of Clinical Nutrition 80*(6 Suppl): 1673S–1677S.

Reichrath, J., Lehmann, B., Carlberg, C., Varani, J., & Zouboulis, C. C. (2007). Vitamins as hormones. *Hormone and Metabolic Research 39*(2): 71–84.

Ruediger, T. & Bolz, J. (2007). Neurotransmitters and the development of neuronal circuits. *Advances in Experimental Medicine and Biology 621*: 104–115.

Saha, S., Chant, D. C., Welham, J. L., & McGrath, J. J. (2006). The incidence and prevalence of schizophrenia varies with latitude. *Acta Psychiatrica Scandinavica 114*(1): 36–39.

Seeman, P. (1987). Dopamine receptors and the dopamine hypothesis of schizophrenia. *Synapse 1*(2): 133–152.

Sulzer, D., Chen, T. K., Lau, Y. Y., Kristensen, H., Rayport, S., & Ewing, A. (1995). Amphetamine redistributes dopamine from synaptic vesicles to the cytosol and promotes reverse transport. *Journal of Neuroscience 15*(5): 4102–4108.

Sulzer, D., Maidment, N. T., & Rayport, S. (1993). Amphetamine and other weak bases act to promote reverse transport of dopamine in ventral midbrain neurons. *Journal of Neurochemistry 60*(2): 527–535.

Sutherland, M. K., Somerville, M. J., Yoong, L. K., Bergeron, C., Haussler, M. R., & McLachlan, D. R. (1992). Reduction of vitamin D hormone receptor mRNA levels in Alzheimer as compared to Huntington hippocampus: Correlation with calbindin-28k mRNA levels. *Brain Research: Molecular Brain Research 13*(3): 239–250.

Torrey, E., Miller, J., Rawlings, R., & Yolken, R. (1997). Seasonality of births in schizophrenia and bipolar disorder: A review of the literature. *Schizophrenia Research 28*(1): 1–38.

Torrey, E. F. & Miller, J. (1997). Season of birth and schizophrenia: Southern hemisphere data. *Australian and New Zealand Journal of Psychiatry 31*(2): 308–309.

Veenstra, T. D., Prufer, K., Koenigsberger, C., Brimijoin, S. W., Grande, J. P., & Kumar, R. (1998). 1,25-Dihydroxyvitamin D3 receptors in the central nervous system of the rat embryo. *Brain Research 804*(2): 193–205.

Volz, H. R., Riehemann, S., Maurer, I., Smesny, S., Sommer, M., Rzanny, R., Holstein, W., Czekalla, J., & Sauer, H. (2000). Reduced phosphodiesters and high-energy phosphates in the frontal lobe of schizophrenic patients: A (31)P chemical shift spectroscopic-imaging study. *Biological Psychiatry 47*(11): 954–961.

Weiner, I. (2003). The "two-headed" latent inhibition model of schizophrenia: Modeling positive and negative symptoms and their treatment. *Psychopharmacology (Berl) 169*(3–4): 257–297.

Westerink, B. H. C. (1985). Sequence and significance of dopamine metabolism in the rat brain. *Neurochemistry International 7*(2): 221–227.

Wieczorek, W. J. & Kruk, Z. L. (1994). Differential action of (+)-Amphetamine on electrically-evoked dopamine overflow in rat-brain slices containing corpus striatum and nucleus-accumbens. *British Journal of Pharmacology 111*(3): 829–836.

Wood, P. L., Kim, H. S., & Marien, M. R. (1987). Intracerebral dialysis: Direct evidence for the utility of 3-MT measurements as an index of dopamine release. *Life Sciences 41*(1): 1–5.

Zehnder, D., Bland, R., Williams, M. C., McNinch, R. W., Howie, A. J., Stewart, P. M., & Hewison, M. (2001). Extrarenal expression of 25-hydroxyvitamin d(3)-1 alpha-hydroxylase. *Journal of Clinical Endocrinology and Metabolism 86*(2): 888–894.

CHAPTER 12

ANIMAL MODELS OF PRENATAL PROTEIN MALNUTRITION RELEVANT FOR SCHIZOPHRENIA

LISA M. TARANTINO, TERESA M. REYES, AND ABRAHAM A. PALMER

KEY CONCEPTS

- Protein malnutrition during development results in behavioral, structural, and neurochemical changes in adulthood that mimic many of the characteristics of psychiatric diseases, including schizophrenia.
- Animal models have been used extensively to study the effects of protein malnutrition during development.
- Animal models have been, and will continue to be, a valuable tool for elucidating the environmental, genetic, and epigenetic consequences of protein malnutrition and its role in the development of schizophrenia and other psychiatric disorders.

Exposure to a variety of environmental challenges in utero has been shown to elevate risk for schizophrenia and other psychiatric disorders; for reviews, see Weiss & Feldon (2001) and Meyer & Feldon (2009). In particular, retrospective studies in human populations support a link between prenatal exposure to nutritional deficiency and an increased risk for development of schizophrenia (Susser & Lin, 1992; Susser et al., 1996; St Clair et al., 2005; Brown & Susser, 2008; Xu et al., 2009; see chapter 2, this book). A large natural experiment on prenatal nutrition in humans occurred at the end of World War II. A Nazi-imposed blockade that affected the six largest cities in the Netherlands resulted in a famine called the Dutch Hunger Winter. During the height of the famine, daily food rations for all residents were limited to 1,000 calories and eventually to 500 calories. Retrospective studies identified neuropsychiatric and other disorders in the offspring of women exposed to the Dutch famine during gestation. Adults conceived during the famine had an increased risk for schizophrenia (Hoek, Brown, & Susser, 1998;

Brown & Susser, 2008) and major affective disorder (Brown et al., 1995, 2000). Similar studies of offspring that were in utero during the Chinese famine of 1959–1961 confirmed an increased prevalence of schizophrenia (St Clair et al., 2005; Xu et al., 2009).

It is impossible to use human subjects to identify the causative nutrient or nutrients or to establish a mechanism for the role of prenatal nutrition in schizophrenia or other psychiatric disorders because of the obvious practical and ethical challenges. Animal models provide an alternative means to study the role of gestational environment, and particularly malnutrition, on brain development and adult behavior.

Neurodevelopmental Hypothesis of Schizophrenia

Schizophrenia is a neurodevelopmental disorder with a complex etiology resulting from both genetic and environmental factors. Evidence suggests that environmental insults acting on individuals with an existing genetic predisposition can cause developmental alterations that are present long before the onset of psychotic symptoms. Research has identified at least two windows of developmental vulnerability: the prenatal or perinatal period and early adolescence. Animal models offer the advantage of manipulating the environment at multiple points during development and measuring outcomes across the life span. Because schizophrenia symptoms normally appear in late adolescence or early adulthood, brain and behavioral abnormalities that are observed only in adult and not young animals may provide particularly attractive models for further study.

A number of early environment insults that are linked to increased risk for schizophrenia in humans have also been modeled in animals. Among the most replicated include maternal infection, maternal stress, obstetric complications, and maternal dietary malnutrition (both vitamin D and protein deprivation). These are reviewed in other chapters in this book. The present chapter provides a detailed review of early life protein malnutrition in animal models and discusses the behavioral, neurochemical, and neurophysiologic effects in relation to schizophrenia.

Animal models of nutritional deficiency have produced a number of phenotypic outcomes, including metabolic, cardiovascular, and mental disorders, among others (for a review see Armitage et al., 2004). Dietary manipulations in animals can be limited to a particular time during development, in adulthood, or across the life span. A review of all of these models would be beyond the scope of a single chapter. Instead, we limit our discussion to protein malnutrition that occurs prenatally and perinatally or postnatally. Maternal protein deprivation is defined as a dietary manipulation in females that begins before breeding and that can end at any time during pregnancy or extend through gestation and weaning into adulthood. Perinatal or postnatal protein deprivation is defined as dietary manipulations that begin during mid-gestation or immediately at birth and can last throughout weaning, into adulthood, or both. Development in rodents lags behind human development, and many relevant in utero developmental processes in humans occur in the postnatal period in rodents (Morgane et al., 1993; Clancy, Darlington, & Finlay, 2001). Therefore, studies intended to examine the entire early brain development period in humans should include protein deprivation in the early postnatal period as well as during embryogenesis in the rodent.

In animal models, protein deprivation normally is achieved by modifying the amount of casein in the diet while maintaining the caloric value by the addition of extra carbohydrates. The fraction of protein in a deficient diet ranges from 5–9%, whereas protein in normal diets ranges from 16–25%.

Protein Malnutrition and Effects on the Developing Nervous System

Most neurotransmitter systems have been implicated in schizophrenia on the basis of functional characteristics; the efficacy of receptor modulators (i.e., pharmacological manipulation with agonists and antagonists) to ameliorate, exacerbate, or mimic symptoms of the disease; or both. Evidence for a functional role of the dopaminergic, glutamatergic, serotonergic, and GABAergic systems (those that transmit or secrete gamma-aminobutyric acid) has been reviewed in detail elsewhere (Stone, Morrison, & Pilowsky, 2007; Toda & Abi-Dargham, 2007; Geyer & Vollenweider, 2008; Jones et al., 2008; Paz et al., 2008), and efforts toward understanding the effects of protein deprivation during development on each system have been assessed in animal models.

Structural Changes

Structural changes in the brain have been observed in schizophrenia, including increased ventricular volume and decreased whole brain volume (Hulshoff Pol & Kahn, 2008; Fatemi & Folsom, 2009). Although reduced brain and body weight have been reported in animals that were exposed to low protein in utero (Smart et al., 1973; Marichich, Molina, & Orsingher, 1979), gross structural abnormalities have not been observed. Rather, the deficits resulting from prenatal protein malnutrition tend to be subtle and relate to deficits within specific neurotransmitter systems, although some generalized abnormalities have been reported. For example, exposure to prenatal protein deficiency for the first two weeks of gestation in rats results in significant abnormalities in brain development in newborn pups, including delayed astrocytogenesis, abnormal neuronal differentiation (as shown by reduced microtubule-associated protein-5 [MAP-5] and increased MAP-1 expression), abnormal synaptogenesis, and decreased apoptosis (Gressens et al., 1997). It is important to note, however, that all of these deficits are normalized by adulthood (postnatal day 63). A subtle, region-specific change that has been consistently noted in response to prenatal protein malnutrition is a reduction in cell number in the hippocampus. Because the anatomy and circuitry of the hippocampus is well defined, the effect of prenatal protein malnutrition on this structure has been the focus of numerous groups. A reduced number of cells in CA1 (but no other hippocampal regions) and a reduced subiculum volume have been reported (Lister et al., 2005), whereas other groups have found changes in cell number more broadly across the dentate gyrus, CA1 and CA3, extensively detailed previously (Díaz-Cintra et al., 1991; Díaz-Cintra et al., 1994; Cintra et al., 1997a; Cintra et al., 1997b). Beyond these few notable deficits, numerous subtle changes in neurotransmitter expression and function have been identified. Yet these findings are complex and can vary in direction across different brain regions or assessment time points.

Dopamine

All currently prescribed antipsychotic medications have an affinity for dopamine (DA) D2 receptors. The long-standing DA dysfunction hypothesis of schizophrenia has been supported by the observation of increases in striatal DA D2 receptor binding and differences in DA dynamics in the brains of schizophrenic patients (Seeman et al., 1987; Joyce et al., 1988; Howes et al., 2009). An increase in D2 receptor binding in the striatum and a decrease in DA transporter binding have also been reported in rats exposed to prenatal protein deprivation (Palmer et al., 2008). Studies examining DA release and tissue concentration in the hippocampus of protein-deprived animals have been less consistent. Chen et al. (1995) reported an increased release of DA and its metabolites in hippocampal slices from prenatally protein malnourished animals, and a decrease in DA was detected in the hippocampus in prenatally malnourished animals (Kehoe et al., 2001). A decrease in basal DA was also detected (by microdialysis) in the prefrontal cortex of prenatally malnourished animals, tested as adults, as well as an absence of restraint stress-induced release of DA (Mokler et al., 2007). However, in a separate study, the expected increase in hypothalamic DA in response to isolation stress was intact in the prenatally malnourished animals tested as adults (Kehoe et al., 2001).

Serotonin (5-HT)

Serotonin dysfunction, in particular of the 5-HT2A receptor, is implicated in some symptoms of schizophrenia. This implication is based on the ability of 5-HT2A agonists, such as lysergic acid diethylamide (LSD) or psilocybin, to induce psychotic symptoms, working memory deficits, and sensorimotor gating abnormalities (Vollenweider et al., 1998; Umbricht et al., 2003). Atypical antipsychotics also have a higher affinity for 5-HT2A receptors than D2 receptors (Garzya et al., 2007).

Serotonergic changes in protein-deprived animals generally are consistent across studies. Increased 5-HT or its metabolite, 5-hydroxyindoleacetic acid (5-HIAA), or both are detected in the hippocampus (via microdialysis or in tissue) (Kehoe et al., 2001; Mokler, Galle, & Morgane, 2003; Mokler et al., 2007); throughout the brain (Resnick & Morgane, 1984); in hippocampal slices (Chen et al., 1995); and in the hypothalamus (Kehoe et al., 2001). Further, in response to stress, an increased release is detected in the hippocampus, as opposed to a decrease in control animals (Mokler et al., 2007). Animals from prenatally malnourished dams also show an altered response to dl-fenfluramine, which blocks the 5-HT transporter and stimulates 5-HT release. These offspring show a decreased behavioral response (inhibition of food intake) and reduced Fos immunoreactivity in the paraventricular nucleus of the hypothalamus in response to dl-fenfluramine (Lopes de Souza et al., 2008). Another study also detected 5-HT abnormalities within the hippocampus, including a decrease in 5-HT fiber density in the dentate gyrus and CA3; decreased 5-HT uptake in CA3 and CA1; and decreased expression of the 5-HT1A receptor in CA3 (Blatt et al., 1994). Contrary to the other reports, however, these authors did not find an increase in 5-HT within the hippocampus.

Glutamate

N-methyl-d-aspartate (NMDA) receptor blockers like phencyclidine (PCP), ketamine, and dizocipline (MK-801) produce psychotomimetic effects in healthy individuals and precipitate psychotic episodes in schizophrenia patients (Large, 2007). In addition, NMDA receptor and mGluR2/3 agonists are effective in treating schizophrenia (Javitt, 2006; Patil et al., 2007). Therefore, glutamatergic dysfunction, and particularly NMDA receptor hypofunction, is hypothesized to play a role in schizophrenia.

Abnormalities in the glutamate system have been detected in protein-deprived animals. For example, increased MK-801 binding is observed in the adult cortex, striatum, and hippocampus of rats deprived of protein prenatally, indicating decreased glutamatergic activity (Palmer et al., 2004; Palmer et al., 2008). Increased kainate receptor binding is also detected in the CA3 of animals deprived of protein prenatally. The authors speculate that this may be a compensation for reduced glutamatergic input from mossy fibers (Fiacco et al., 2003). Further, decreased sensitivity to quinolinic acid (an NMDA agonist) was detected in prenatally malnourished adult animals (Schweigert et al., 2005).

Gamma-aminobutyric Acid

GABAergic interneurons are a core component of the circuitry that controls network oscillations, information processing, and sensorimotor gating—all of which are disturbed in schizophrenia (Benes & Berretta, 2001). Therefore, alterations of the GABAergic system have been examined in protein-deprived animals as a functional model for symptoms of schizophrenia.

Defects in the GABA system have been detected in adult rodents that were protein-deprived in utero. An increase in the expression of GAD-67, a rate-limiting enzyme in GABA synthesis, is detected in the dentate gyrus of prenatally malnourished animals (Díaz-Cintra et al., 2007). Alterations in the expression of GABA-A receptors are also detected in rats that were protein-restricted prenatally, including decreased GABA-A $\gamma2L$ mRNA in the septum (Steiger et al., 2002), decreased GABA-A (alpha 1, beta 2) in the hippocampus, and an increase in alpha 3 expression in the hippocampus (Steiger et al., 2003). Higher GABA uptake by cortical and hippocampal slices is also observed in malnourished rats (Schweigert et al., 2005).

Effects of Prenatal Protein Malnutrition on Rodent Behavior

Assessing the effects of prenatal protein deprivation in animals requires the use of appropriate behavioral, neurochemical, and physiological assays that can accurately reflect human schizophrenia symptomatology. An animal model encompassing the entire spectrum of schizophrenia symptoms is impossible. Instead, the focus of animal research has been to model specific symptoms of the disease by examining endophenotypes. Human behavioral symptoms of schizophrenia can be grouped into two general categories: positive (e.g., hallucinations, delusions) and negative (e.g., social withdrawal, working memory deficits). Currently available medications for schizophrenia are more effective at treating positive rather than negative symptoms (Javitt et al., 2008). Animal models for both positive and negative symptoms exist and have been used widely in rodents (table 12.1). In addition, endophenotypes, which are traits that are enriched in affected individuals but are not symptoms of the disease, are also useful for developing animal models (Gottesman & Gould, 2003). Specific endophenotypes have been developed for schizophrenia. Models of disease symptoms and endophenotypes should provide face, predictive, and construct validity (Geyer & Markou, 1995). Many behavioral models of schizophrenia respond to human pharmacotherapies and are modulated by the same brain regions and neurotransmitter pathways (Li et al., 2009).

Table 12.1 Commonly Used Animal Models of Schizophrenia Endophenotypes and Human Correlates

	Human Correlate	Animal Model	Reference
Positive	Psychomotor agitation	Locomotor activity and response to novelty	Farrow et al., 2006; Young et al., 2007
	Disorganized behavior	Patterns of locomotor activity	Young et al., 2007
Negative	Anhedonia	Saccharine or sucrose consumption, ICSS	Berlin et al., 1998; Le Pen et al., 2002; Amitai, Semenova, & Markou, 2009
		Progressive ratio	Wiley & Compton, 2004
	Avolition (lack of motivation)	Social interaction	Sams-Dodd, 1999
	Social withdrawal	Resident intruder	Ellenbroek & Cools, 2002
		Nest building	Belforte et al., 2010
		Home cage social behavior	Torres et al., 2005
	Cognitive	Working memory (e.g., T-maze, holeboard, radial arm maze)	Damgaard et al., 2010; Arguello & Gogos, 2009; Etherton et al., 2009; Jones et al., 2008
		Visual learning (e.g., Morris water maze, novel object recognition, Barnes maze)	
		Attention (e.g., latent inhibition, sustained attention)	
		Problem solving (maze tasks)	
		Social cognition (social interaction or recognition)	
Endophenotypes	Increased sensitivity to psychostimulants (e.g., amphetamine, cocaine)	Measurement of locomotor activation following administration of psychostimulants	van den Buuse et al., 2005; Geyer & Markou, 1995
	Impaired sensorimotor gating	PPI of startle response	Turetsky et al., 2007; Powell, Zhou, & Geyer, 2009
	Impaired auditory evoked potentials	Auditory evoked potential measurement	Connolly et al., 2003
	Impaired latent inhibition	Latent inhibition	Weiner & Arad, 2009
	Impaired mismatch negativity	Mismatch negativity in anesthetized rodents	Umbricht & Krljes, 2005; Umbricht et al., 2005
Other	Alterations in neurochemistry	Neurochemistry and microdialysis measurements	Di Matteo et al., 2008; Lodge & Grace, 2008
	Sleep disturbances	EEG measurement, sleep-wake cycles	Dzirasa et al., 2006; Cohrs, 2008
	Mood (anxiety or depression)	Open field, elevated plus maze, forced swim test	Rodgers & Johnson, 1995; Cryan & Mombereau, 2004; Prut & Belzung, 2003
	Self-care	Grooming, body weight, coat condition, general health, barbering, etc.	Audet, Goulet, & Dore, 2006

Numerous studies have reported on the behavioral effects of prenatal, perinatal, or postnatal protein deprivation in adult offspring. Table 12.2 lists most of the studies that have examined the behavioral phenotype resulting from protein deprivation in utero, with a focus on animal models of behaviors that model symptoms or endophenotypes (or both) of schizophrenia.

Prepulse Inhibition

Behavioral and physiologic models of schizophrenia have focused mainly on negative symptoms and endophenotypes. Sensorimotor gating is one of the most widely studied endophenotypes. Prepulse inhibition (PPI) is a well-validated neurophysiologic test of sensorimotor gating that has almost identical human behavioral correlates and responds to atypical antipsychotics in both human (reviewed in Braff, Geyer, & Swerdlow, 2001; Swerdlow et al., 2008) and animal studies (Geyer et al., 2001; Swerdlow et al., 2008). Schizophrenia patients and asymptomatic first-degree relatives show deficits in PPI. In animal models, these deficits can be replicated by both developmental and pharmacological manipulations that affect neurotransmitter pathways and brain regions involved in the disease—most notably by DA agonists (Swerdlow et al., 1994; Geyer et al., 2001), 5-HT agonists (Dulawa et al., 2000), NMDA receptor antagonists (Geyer et al., 2001), GABA antagonists (Swerdlow et al., 1990), maternal infection and immune activation (Patterson, 2009; chapter 10, this book), maternal stress (chapter 13, this book) and neonatal ventral hippocampal lesions (Lipska et al., 1995). PPI is also disrupted in other disorders, including Alzheimer's disease (Ueki et al., 2006), bipolar disorder (Perry et al., 2001) and obsessive compulsive disorder (Shanahan et al., 2009), indicating that this behavioral deficit is not specific to schizophrenia.

Despite the widespread use of PPI as an endophenotype for schizophrenia (Swerdlow et al., 2008), only one study has been published that examined PPI following prenatal protein malnutrition. Palmer et al. (2004) reported that protein deprivation in utero is associated with lower PPI in young adult female rat offspring at postnatal day (PND) 56. However, no such deficit is observed in young adult males in this experiment. Moreover, PPI deficits are not observed in adolescent (PND 35) male or female rats exposed to maternal protein deprivation. The significant decrease in PPI in young adult female rats exposed to protein deprivation in utero is consistent with the adult onset of schizophrenia and supports the role of prenatal protein malnutrition in the development of this particular endophenotype.

Alterations in startle reactivity have been reported in patients with schizophrenia (Geyer & Braff, 1982; Braff, Grillon, & Geyer, 1992) and related disorders (Cadenhead, Geyer, & Braff, 1993), and are hypothesized to reflect a defect in central inhibitory mechanisms. Palmer et al. (2004) also observed a decrease in initial startle response in protein-deprived rats. However, a more recent study reported no

Table 12.2 Behavioral Changes in Adult Rodents After Prenatal, Perinatal, or Postnatal Exposure to Low Protein Levels

Animal Model	Strain	Diet	Low-Protein Diet Schedule	Outcome (increase [↑] or decrease [↓] as compared to normal diet)	Reference
Prenatal Malnutrition					
Rat	Sprague-Dawley	6% casein vs. 25% casein	5 weeks before mating and throughout pregnancy. Postnatal diet 25% casein.	↑ Apomorphine-induced stereotypy (females) ↑ D-amphetamine-induced locomotion (females) ↑ ^{3}H-MK-801 binding in striatum and hippocampus (females) ↑ ^{3}H-haloperidol binding in striatum (females) ↓ ^{3}H-GBR-12935 binding in striatum (females) ↑ ^{3}H-MK-801 binding in cortex (males)	Palmer et al., 2008
Rat	Wistar-Kyoto (WKY/lj-cr)	6% casein vs. 25% casein	5 weeks before mating and throughout pregnancy. Postnatal diet 25% casein.	↓ Percent prepulse inhibition (females) ↓ Acoustic startle response ↑ ^{3}H-MK-801 binding in striatum (females) ↓ Body weight (females)	Palmer et al., 2004
Rat	Sprague-Dawley	8% casein vs. 25% casein	5 weeks before mating until PND 90.	↑ Apomorphine-induced stereotypy	Leahy et al., 1978
Rat	Sprague-Dawley	8% casein vs. 25% casein	5 weeks before mating until weaning. At weaning, half of the rats from each group were switched to opposite diet.	→ Sensitivity to serotonergic agonist, DMT, in rotarod assay, DMT-induced behavior, and treadmill running behavior	Hall, Leahy, & Robertson, 1983
Rat	Sprague-Dawley	6% casein vs. 25% casein	5 weeks before mating and throughout pregnancy. Postnatal diet 25% casein.	↑ Session necessary to abolish learned alternation response in T-maze ↑ Performance in working memory task	Tonkiss & Galler, 1990
Rat	Sprague-Dawley	6% casein vs. 25% casein	5 weeks before mating and throughout pregnancy. Postnatal diet 25% casein.	↑ Responding for a food reward in a variable interval operant paradigm ↑ Responsiveness for a saccharin-solution reward	Tonkiss et al., 1990b

Species	Strain	Diet	Exposure	Findings	Reference
Rat	Sprague-Dawley	6% casein vs. 25% casein	5 weeks before mating until weaning.	↓ Transition from hyperactivity to hypoactivity in response to clonidine ↓ Wall climbing in response to clonidine	Goodlett et al., 1985
Rat	Sprague-Dawley	8% casein vs. 25% casein	5 weeks before mating until PND 112 or PND 170.	↑ Errors in delayed spatial alternation	Goodlett et al., 1986
Rat	Sprague-Dawley	6% casein vs. 25% casein	5 weeks before mating and throughout pregnancy. Postnatal diet 25% casein.	↓ Sensitivity to the amnestic effects of chlordiazepoxide in Morris Water Maze	Tonkiss et al., 2000
Rat	Sprague-Dawley	6% casein vs. 25% casein	5 weeks before mating and throughout pregnancy.	↑ Sensitization to psychomotor effects of chronic exposure to 30 mg/kg cocaine exposure ↑ Stereotypy after acute cocaine exposure (males)	Shultz, Galler, & Tonkiss, 1999
Rat	Sprague-Dawley	6% casein vs. 25% casein	5 weeks before mating to PND 55 or PND 550	↓ Time to peak activity (phase shift) in young rats ↑ Amplitude and mean value of cortical-temperature rhythm in young rats Delayed temperature acrophase (phase shift) in old rats	Castanon-Cervantes & Cintra, 2002
Rat	Sprague-Dawley	6% casein vs. 25% casein	5 weeks before mating to PND 35	↑ Wakefulness for 2 days post REM sleep deprivation ↓ Slow wave sleep for 2 days post REM sleep deprivation ↓ Amplitude of slow wave sleep Altered phase of wakefulness and REM rhythms	Cintra et al., 2002
Rat	Sprague-Dawley	6% casein vs. 25% casein	5 weeks before mating and throughout pregnancy. Postnatal diet 25% casein.	↑ REM sleep during first two hours of dark phase ↑ Wakefulness during second two hours of dark phase ↓ Slow wave sleep during second two hours of dark phase ↓ Slow wave and REM sleep following an acute restraint stress	Duran et al., 2006

(continued)

Table 12.2 (continued)

Animal Model	Strain	Diet	Low-Protein Diet Schedule	Outcome (increase [↑] or decrease [↓] as compared to normal diet)	Reference
Rat	Sprague-Dawley	6% casein vs. 25% casein	5 weeks before mating and throughout pregnancy. Postnatal diet 25% casein.	↓ Circadian activity phase	Duran et al., 2005
Rat	Sprague-Dawley	6% casein vs. 25% casein	5 weeks before mating and throughout pregnancy. Postnatal diet 25% casein.	↑ Suppression of ultrasonic vocalizations at P11 following 0.03 and 0.1 mg/kg diazepam	Tonkiss & Galler, 2007
Rat	Sprague-Dawley	6% casein vs. 25% casein	5 weeks before mating and throughout pregnancy. Postnatal diet 25% casein.	↓ Basal extracellular dopamine in the medial prefrontal cortex ↓ Release of dopamine in the prefrontal cortex following acute restraint stress	Mokler et al., 2007
Rat	Sprague-Dawley	6% casein vs. 25% casein	5 weeks before mating and throughout pregnancy. Postnatal diet 25% casein.	↑ Open arm entries in EPM ↑ Time in open arms of EPM ↓ Latency to enter open arms of EPM ↑ Head dips ↑ Rearing	Almeida, Tonkiss, & Galler, 1996b
Rat	Sprague-Dawley	6% casein vs. 25% casein	5 weeks before mating and throughout pregnancy. Postnatal diet 25% casein. Dams given injections of either saline or cocaine (30 mg/kg) 5 weeks before mating until day 18 of gestation	↑ Latency to approach nest bedding ↓ Attraction to own nest bedding	Galler, Tonkiss, & Maldonado-Irizarry, 1994; Tonkiss, Harrison, & Galler, 1996
Rat	Sprague-Dawley	6% casein vs. 25% casein	5 weeks before mating and throughout pregnancy. Postnatal diet 25% casein.	↓ Number of pins in social interaction assay ↓ Number of walkovers in social interaction assay ↓ Allogrooming (licking, nibbling of fur of other animal) ↑ Rearing	Almeida, Tonkiss, & Galler, 1996c

Species	Strain	Diet	Protocol	Outcomes	Reference
Rat	Sprague-Dawley	6% casein vs. 25% casein	5 weeks before mating and throughout pregnancy. Postnatal diet 25% casein.	↑ Percent time in open arms of ETM ↑ Rearing in ETM ↑ Head dips in ETM	Almeida, Tonkiss, & Galler, 1996a
Rat	Wistar	9% casein vs. 18% casein	Low-protein diet given at four distinct points during gestation: 0–7 days, 8–14 days, 15–22 days, and 0–22 days.	↓ Locomotor activity in males exposed to LPD during 0–7 days gestation ↓ Locomotor activity in females in all time-point groups	Bellinger, Sculley, & Langley-Evans, 2006
Rat	Sprague-Dawley	6% casein vs. 25% casein	5 weeks before mating and throughout pregnancy. Postnatal diet 25% casein.	↑ Anxiety in open field in females ↑ Immobility in forced swim test with no stressor ↓ Latency to immobility in males in forced swim test following stressor ↓ Latency to immobility in females in forced swim test following stressor	Trzctnska, Tonkiss, & Galler, 1999
Mice	MF-1	9% casein vs. 18% casein	One group of dams given diet at day of conception and throughout gestation (LPD) and another group given diet 3.5 days before breeding and then switched to 18% diet for remainder of gestation (Emb-LPD).	↑ Distance traveled, rears and jumps in open field (females only in Emb-LPD group) ↓ Seconds resting in open field (females only in Emb-LPD group)	Watkins et al., 2008a
Mice	MF-1	9% casein vs. 18% casein	Low-protein diet fed to females for 3.5 days before breeding and then returned to 18% protein diet after plug positive status determined and for remainder of gestation.	↓ Distance traveled and rears in open field in males and females ↑ Velocity in open field in males and females	Watkins et al., 2008b
Mice	Swiss	7.1% casein vs. 24.2% casein	Diet fed 6 weeks before breeding and then throughout lactation. Offspring weaned onto control diet.	↑ Reference memory errors ↑ Working memory errors ↓ Hippocampal volume	Ranade et al., 2008

(continued)

Table 12.2 (continued)

Animal Model	Strain	Diet	Low-Protein Diet Schedule	Outcome (increase [↑] or decrease [↓] as compared to normal diet)	Reference
Perinatal/Postnatal Malnutrition					
Rat	Wistar	8% casein vs. 25% casein	Pups suckled to foster mothers on experimental diet and weaned onto same diet until PND 49.	↓ Diazepam and ipsapirone dependent release in sodium chloride intake in drinking water	Almeida, de Oliveira, & Graeff, 1990
Rat	Wistar	8% casein vs. 25% casein	Pups suckled to foster mothers on experimental diet and weaned onto same diet until PND 49.	↑ Percentage of open or total arm entries ↓ Efficacy of diazepam on anxiety behaviors ↑ Efficacy of ritanserin on anxiety behaviors	Almeida, de Oliveira, & Graeff, 1991
Rat	Wistar	8% casein vs. 25% casein	Pups suckled to foster mothers on experimental diet and weaned onto experimental diet until PND 49 or PND 70.	↓ Locomotor activity at 49 but not 70 days ↓ Shock intensity threshold to display jump behavior at 49 but not 70 days ↓ Baseline and postshock inhibitory avoidance at both 49 and 70 days	Almeida et al., 1992
Rat	Wistar	8% casein vs. 25% casein	Pups suckled to foster mothers on experimental diet and weaned onto normal diet.	↑ Rearing in EPM ↑ Attempts to enter open arms in EPM	Almeida, Garcia, & de Oliveira, 1993
Rat	Wistar	6% casein vs. 16% casein	Pups suckled to foster mothers on experimental diet and weaned onto normal diet.	↓ Efficacy of diazepam on open-arm exploration in EPM ↑ Efficacy of diazepam on open-arm exploration in EPM on environmentally stimulated animals ↑ Light-dark transitions and square entries after environmental stimulation	Santucci et al., 1994
Rat	Wistar	8% casein vs. 24% casein	Diet fed from 14th day of pregnancy in dams to PND 50 in offspring.	↓ Habituation to open field ↑ Rearing in response to AMPH ↑ Locomotor response to AMPH ↑ Sensitization to locomotor effects of AMPH ↑ Dopamine and DOPAC post-AMPH ↑ Dopamine receptor binding post-AMPH	Brioni et al., 1986

Rat	Wistar	8% casein vs. 24% casein	Diet fed from 14th day of pregnancy in dams to PND 50 in offspring.	↑ Reactivity to hypothermic effects of apomorphine, naphazoline, and diazepam ↓ Reactivity to hypothermic effects of clonidine	Brioni & Orsingher, 1987
Rat	Wistar	8% casein vs. 24% casein	Diet fed from 14th day of pregnancy in dams to PND 50 in offspring.	↑ Operant behavior for sweetened milk reward under variable-rate schedule ↓ Efficiency in obtaining reward under a differential reinforcement schedule ↑ Transitions in light-dark test ↓ Efficacy of diazepam in light-dark test	Brioni & Orsingher, 1988
Rat	Wistar	8% casein vs. 24% casein	Diet fed from 14th day of pregnancy in dams to PND 50 in offspring.	↓ Anticonflict effect in response to diazepam	Brioni, Cordoba, & Orsingher, 1989
Rat	Wistar	8% casein vs. 24% casein	Diet fed from 14th day of pregnancy in dams to PND 50 in offspring.	↓ Time spent in open arms of EPM after 1.0 mg/kg diazepam ↑ Time spent in open arms of EPM after 3 and 7 days treatment with 10 mg/kg propranolol ↑ Time spent in open arms of EPM after 7 days treatment with 10 mg/kg desipramine ↑ Time spent in open arms of EPM after 7 days treatment with 10 mg/kg phenelzine	Laino, Cordoba, & Orsingher, 1993
Rat	Wistar	8% casein vs. 24% casein	Diet fed from 14th day of pregnancy in dams to PND 50 in offspring.	→ Attenuating effect of chronic desipramine treatment on apomorphine-induced hypoactivity ↓ Efficacy of desipramine treatment to reduce clonidine sedative effects ↓ Effect of chronic stress on apomorphine- and clonidine-induced hypoactivity	Keller, Molina, & Orsingher, 1990

(continued)

Table 12.2 (continued)

Animal Model	Strain	Diet	Low-Protein Diet Schedule	Outcome (increase [↑] or decrease [↓] as compared to normal diet)	Reference
Rat	Wistar	8% casein vs. 24% casein	Diet fed from 14th day of pregnancy in dams to PND 40 in offspring.	↑ Cocaine-induced locomotor activity (5 mg/kg) ↑ Sensitization of locomotor activity (5–10 mg/kg) ↑ Dopamine in nucleus accumbens core after cocaine administration in cocaine-sensitized rats	Valdomero et al., 2005
Rat	Wistar	8% casein vs. 24% casein	Diet fed from 14th day of pregnancy in dams to PND 40 in offspring.	↑ Sensitivity to cocaine-induced place preference at lower doses ↑ Cocaine place preference after preexposure to cocaine ↑ FosB expression in NA and BLA in preexposed rats	Valdomero et al., 2006
Rat	Wistar	8% casein vs. 24% casein	Diet fed from 14th day of pregnancy in dams to PND 40 in offspring.	↑ Sensitivity to morphine-induced place preference at lower doses ↑ Morphine place preference after preexposure to morphine ↑ FosB expression in NA, dorsal striatum, and BLA in preexposed rats	Valdomero et al., 2007
Rat	Wistar	8% casein vs. 24% casein	Diet fed from 14th day of pregnancy in dams to PND 40 in offspring.	↓ Ethanol preference ↓ Preference for ethanol odor	Cordoba et al., 1990
Rat	Wistar	8% casein vs. 24% casein	Diet fed from 14th day of pregnancy in dams to PND 50 in offspring.	↓ Time in open arms of elevated plus maze after acute saline, EtOH, diazepam, and pentobarbital ↑ Increased time in open arms of elevated plus maze after 1 g/kg EtOH after chronic ethanol treatment ↑ Density of GABA receptors following chronic ethanol administration	Cordoba et al., 1992

Animal	Strain	Diet	Timing	Findings	Reference
Rat	Wistar	8% casein vs. 24% casein	Diet fed from 14th day of pregnancy in dams to PND 50 in offspring.	↓ Time in open arms of EPM ↓ Tolerance to anxiolytic effects of diazepam and pentobarbital ↑ $GABA_A$ receptor affinity ↑ GABA-dependent ^{36}Cl-uptake	Borghese et al., 1998
Rat	Wistar	8% casein vs. 24% casein	Diet fed from 14th day of pregnancy in dams to PND 50 in offspring.	↓ Forepaw treading and hind limb abduction in response to 5-MeODMT and 8-OH-DPAT after chronic stress	Keller et al., 1994
Rat	Wistar	6% casein vs. 16% casein	Diet fed from PND 0 to PND 49.	↓ Inhibitory avoidance in ETM ↑ Exploration in ETM	Hernandes & Almeida, 2003
Rat	Wistar	6% casein vs. 16% casein	Diet fed from PND 0 to PND 7, PND 14, PND 21, or PND 28.	↓ Risk assessment behavior in ETM ↑ Entries into and duration of time spent in open arms of EPM ↑ Head dips in EPM ↓ Latency to enter open arm of EPM	Francolin-Silva, da Silva Hernandes, Fukuda, Valadares, & Almeida, 2006
Rat	Wistar	6% casein vs. 16% casein	Diet fed from PND 0 to PND 7, PND 14, PND 21, or PND 28.	↓ Effectiveness of diazepam ↓ Freezing time in fear-potentiated startle ↓ Reactivity to anxiolytic effects of diazepam	Francolin-Silva, Brandao, & Almeida, 2007
Rat	Wistar	6% casein vs. 16% casein	Diet fed from PND 0 to PND 49.	↑ EPM exploration but reversed by immobilization stress	Francolin-Silva & Almeida, 2004
Rat	Wistar	5% casein vs. 16% casein	Diet fed from PND 0 to PND 49.	↓ Development of social behavior ↓ Number of social contacts	Frankova, 1973

AMPH=amphetamine; BLA=basolateral amygdala; DOPAC=3,4-Dihydroxyphenylacetic acid; Emb-LPD=Embryonic Low Protein Diet; EPM=Elevated Plus Maze; ETM=Elevated T-Maze; EtOH=Ethanol; FosB=FBJ murine osteosarcoma viral oncogene homolog B; LP=Low Protein; LPD=Low Protein Diet; NA=Nucleus Accumbens; REM=rapid eye movement; PND=postnatal day.
SOURCE: Authors.

difference in startle response among protein-deprived versus control rats (Francolin-Silva, Brandao, & Almeida, 2007). There are several technical differences between this and the Palmer et al. study. Whereas Francolin-Silva limited protein malnutrition to the perinatal period, from birth up to PND 28, Palmer used a prenatal protein deprivation model that started 5 weeks before mating, lasting until PND 0. Also, the startle response amplitude measure used by Francolin-Silva, Brandao, & Almeida (2007) was averaged over 30 trials, whereas Palmer et al. (2004) observed a difference in startle response only in the initial presentations of the startle stimulus.

Cognitive Function

Cognitive deficits in schizophrenia largely drive functional outcomes for the disease and are not well managed by current antipsychotics (Fenton, Stover, & Insel, 2003). Appreciation of cognitive deficits as a core feature of the disease has generated an increased effort toward identification of appropriate animal models for screening novel pharmaceuticals for this disease domain. A National Institutes of Mental Health initiative, Measurement and Treatment Research to Improve Cognition in Schizophrenia (MATRICS), has identified seven primary cognitive domains that are affected in human schizophrenia (Green et al., 2004). A number of these cognitive features are readily measured in rodents by using basic learning and memory tasks that assess working memory, attention, visual learning, and social cognition (table 12.1). Deficits in many of these cognitive assays are observed in lesion studies of the prefrontal cortex that replicate brain structure abnormalities found in human patients and in animals genetically modified to express disease susceptibility genes, thus providing encouraging evidence for their usefulness in modeling the human disease (reviewed in Arguello & Gogos, 2009, and Kellendonk, Simpson, & Kandel, 2009). A desire to understand potential developmental causes for the cognitive deficits observed in schizophrenia patients drives research on learning and memory deficits in protein-deprived animals.

Protein deprivation during development causes lasting changes in brain regions implicated in learning and memory (Morgane et al., 1993). Perhaps one of the simplest assays of sensory and cognitive development is the homing test in which suckling animals are tested for their ability to locate the nest after displacement. Data have consistently shown that protein-malnourished animals are deficient in the ability to return to the nest (Gallo, Werboff, & Knox, 1984; Galler, Tonkiss, & Maldonado-Irizarry, 1994; Tonkiss, Harrison, & Galler, 1996).

Protein deprivation in utero or during the suckling period causes significant hippocampal alterations, including long-term potentiation deficits (Austin, Bronzino, & Morgane, 1986). The hippocampus plays a critical role in the ability to learn and remember spatial information. Tests of learning and memory indicate that prenatally malnourished rats are behaviorally inflexible (Tonkiss et al., 1993) and often show no deficits in acquisition, while being unable or unwilling to give up learned responses once acquired. For instance, prenatal protein deprivation does not affect acquisition of the alternation response in a spatial T-maze task (Goodlett et al., 1986; Tonkiss & Galler, 1990) or an operant model of the T-maze task (Tonkiss & Galler, 1990), spatial navigation in the Morris water maze (Goodlett et al., 1986; Tonkiss, Shultz, & Galler, 1994), or performance in the radial arm maze (Hall, 1983). However, rats deprived of protein in utero require more sessions to abolish learned alternation responses (Tonkiss & Galler, 1990). In conditioned taste aversion studies, prenatally malnourished rats show impaired extinction of the conditioned taste aversion response with repeated exposure (Tonkiss et al., 1993). Following continuous reinforcement in an operant task, prenatally malnourished rats exhibit impairments in acquiring a differential reinforcement of low rates of responding (DRL) task (Tonkiss et al., 1990a). These data imply that prenatal protein deprivation does not alter the ability to learn but rather makes it harder to "unlearn" once an association has been made.

There has been one report of radial arm maze performance in mice that were protein-deprived prenatally. Ranade et al. (2008) found that outbred Swiss mice make more reference memory and working memory errors—an interesting result that encourages further study of mice as animal models for the cognitive effects of prenatal protein deprivation.

Social Interaction

Impaired social interactions are a hallmark of schizophrenia, and improvement of social skills is an important element in treatment and outcomes for individuals with the disease. Two studies of social interaction behaviors in protein-malnourished rats reported a deficit in several social behaviors (Frankova, 1973; Almeida et al., 1996c). Both of these studies were performed in juvenile rats but differed in the protein deprivation protocol. Almeida and colleagues deprived prenatally until birth, whereas Frankova deprived from birth until PND 49. Contradictory results have emerged when adult offspring from dams that experienced total caloric undernutrition, as opposed to only protein malnutrition, were tested. In these studies, adult rats display increased social interaction and more aggression rather than a decrease in social interaction (Whatson, Smart, & Dobbing, 1975, 1976; Tonkiss & Smart, 1983). The extent to which age of testing, developmental period of malnutrition, or type of nutritional deficiency (overall caloric malnutrition or protein deprivation) explains these contradictory results has yet to be resolved. However, the limited results from protein-deprived juvenile rats suggest that such an experimental paradigm produces social behaviors that mimic those seen in human schizophrenia.

Sleep Abnormalities

Difficulties initiating or maintaining sleep occur in 30–80% of individuals with schizophrenia (Cohrs, 2008). Several studies have examined the result of prenatal protein deprivation on circadian and sleep behaviors. Measurement of 24-hour locomotor activity indicates that, although rats deprived of protein in utero are not impaired in spontaneous locomotor activity and show circadian rhythmicity, they do display an advanced phase shift in locomotor activity (Castanon-Cervantes & Cintra, 2002; Duran et al., 2005). Protein-deprived rats show peak activity levels before the onset of the light phase, whereas control animals show peak activity after the onset of the light phase. Duran et al. (2005) observed the phase shift in locomotor activity using standard light-dark conditions in 88-day-old rats, whereas Castanon-Cervantes and Cintra (2002) observed the phase shift in dark-dark conditions but not under a light-dark light cycle and in younger (55 days of age) but not older (550 days of age) rats. In addition, Duran and colleagues used only females, and the sex of the rats used in the Castanon-Cervantes study is not apparent from the publication.

The suprachiasmatic nucleus (SCN) of the hypothalamus is the master pacemaker for the generation and maintenance of circadian rhythms, and abnormalities in SCN development have been noted in rat pups from protein-deprived dams. Immunohistochemical examination of vasoactive intestinal peptide and arginine vasopressin neurons within the SCN revealed altered density and morphology of these two systems within this nucleus (Rojas et al., 2009).

Undernutrition-driven changes in sleep behavior are a bit more complex, but several studies indicate that the amplitude of the rhythm for both wakefulness and rapid eye movement sleep is advanced in the dark phase of the light cycle in rats that were deprived of protein in utero (Cintra et al., 2002; Duran et al., 2006) and that these changes are exacerbated by acute stress (Duran et al., 2006). A thorough review of stress and stress-related disorders and the relationship to psychiatric disorders was recently presented (Chrousos, 2009). In summary, prenatal protein malnutrition in animal models appears to alter both circadian rhythms and the sleep-wake cycle. This alteration occurs primarily at the time of light change and may provide insight into the mechanisms of sleep disturbances in schizophrenia.

Behavioral Responses to Pharmacological Challenges

Dopamine

Examination of DA-mediated behaviors in animals that were protein-deprived during development reveals lasting changes in the DA system. Most studies examining DA agonists have reported increased locomotor activity in response to amphetamine (Brioni et al., 1986; Palmer et al., 2008) and cocaine (Shultz, Galler, & Tonkiss, 1999; Valdomero et al., 2005), as well as increased stereotypy in response to apomorphine (Leahy et al., 1978; Palmer et al., 2008). Some of these differences are found in young adult female but not young adult male or adolescent rats of either sex (Palmer et al., 2008). An increase in DA release in the nucleus accumbens core following cocaine administration in cocaine-sensitized, protein-deprived rats has also been observed (Valdomero et al., 2005). These observations are consistent with the increased sensitivity to psychostimulants observed in schizophrenia (Geyer & Markou, 1995; van den Buuse et al., 2005) and indicate that prenatal protein deprivation might be a good model for DA dysfunction in human schizophrenia.

Serotonin

In behavioral studies, the 5-HT2 receptor antagonist ritanserin decreases anxiety in the open field in postnatally protein-deprived rats but had no effect on control animals (Almeida, de Oliveira, & Graeff, 1990). Postnatally deprived rats also show decreased sensitivity to the 5-HT2A receptor antagonists, 5-methoxy-dimethyltryptamine (5-MeO-DMT) and dimethyltryptamine (DMT), in rotarod and treadmill assays, and for DMT-induced behaviors (Hall, Leahy, & Robertson, 1983; Keller et al., 1994).

Gamma-aminobutyric Acid

Benzodiazepines are positive allosteric modulators of the GABA-A receptor that are commonly used as anxiolytics but also have amnesic and sedative properties. Animals that have been exposed to low protein at any time during development show a reduced sensitivity to the effects of benzodiazepines. This result has been observed repeatedly in numerous animal models of anxiety, including the elevated plus maze (Almeida, de Oliveira, & Graeff, 1991; Cordoba et al., 1992; Laino, Cordoba, & Orsingher, 1993; Santucci et al., 1994; Borghese et al., 1998; Francolin-Silva et al., 2007), light-dark (Brioni & Orsingher, 1988; Santucci et al., 1994), and fear-potentiated startle tests (Francolin-Silva & Almeida, 2004).

Rats deprived of protein prenatally also show a decreased sensitivity to the amnesic effects of chlordiazepoxide in the Morris water maze (Tonkiss et al., 2000) but show an increased behavioral sensitivity to the stimulus properties of chlordiazepoxide (Shultz, Galler, & Tonkiss, 2002), indicating that protein deprivation differentially affects other aspects of benzodiazepine action.

Drug Abuse

Drug abuse has been linked to the development of schizophrenia and, as described above, protein-deprived animals show an elevated locomotor response to psychostimulants such as cocaine, amphetamine, and apomorphine. However, there are also reports that these animals are more sensitive to the rewarding effects of cocaine (Valdomero et al., 2006) and show an increase in response for other rewarding substances, such as morphine (Valdomero et al., 2007), food (Tonkiss et al., 1990b), sweetened milk (Brioni & Orsingher, 1988), and saccharin (Tonkiss et al., 1990b), indicating that protein deprivation during development alters drug reward circuitry and may be a useful environmental manipulation for studying the role of drug reward and abuse in the development of schizophrenia.

Anxiety-Related Behaviors

Many studies have examined the role of prenatal protein malnutrition on anxiety-related behaviors. Although these behaviors are not considered to be models of schizophrenia, there is significant comorbidity between anxiety and schizophrenia that may indicate a shared liability (Buckley et al., 2009). In any case, the data on anxiety phenotypes in protein-malnourished animals provide further insight into the behavioral effects of this environmental manipulation. In general, animals exposed to protein malnutrition during early development exhibit reduced anxiety in the elevated plus maze (Almeida, de Oliveira, & Graeff, 1991; Almeida, Tonkiss, & Galler, 1996b; Francolin-Silva & Almeida, 2004), the elevated T-maze (Almeida, Tonkiss, & Galler, 1996a; Hernandes & Almeida, 2003), and the fear-potentiated startle test (Francolin-Silva, Brandao, & Almeida, 2007). An exception is the report of Borghese et al. (1998), which found a decrease in the percentage of time spent in the open arms of the elevated plus maze. However, in this experiment the animals received a daily injection of vehicle for 15 days before testing. It is possible that either the vehicle or the chronic stress of receiving daily injections had an effect on behavior in the elevated plus maze. Stress is known to interact with prenatal malnutrition to modify behavior. For instance, acute immobilization stress reverses the anxiolytic behavior observed in the elevated plus maze (Francolin-Silva & Almeida, 2004), and exposure to chronic stress reverses some of the anxiolytic and antidepressant-like effects of prenatal protein deprivation (Trzctnska, Tonkiss, & Galler, 1999).

In contrast to the assays already described here, assessment of protein-deprived animals in a different test of anxiety, the open field, has shown increased (Trzctnska, Tonkiss, & Galler, 1999; Watkins et al., 2008b), decreased (Watkins et al., 2008a), or no change in anxiety behaviors (Brioni et al., 1986). Differences among the methods used in these studies do exist and could explain the contradictory results. It is also important to note that the studies by Watkins used mice, whereas all other studies of the effects of protein malnutrition on anxiety-related behaviors have used rats. Obviously, differences in the effects of protein deprivation between mice and rats are possible, and additional studies are needed to understand the behavioral effects of low protein during development in mice.

Overall, most studies of anxiety-related behavior indicate decreased anxiety in animals that have been subjected to protein deprivation in utero, but further research is required to gain a better understanding of the mechanisms that control these behavioral responses.

The Role of Epigenetics

Epigenetic mechanisms have also been proposed as possible mediators of the effects of prenatal protein deprivation on downstream phenotypes (see chapter 9, this book). *Epigenetics* is defined as inherited phenotypic variations that are not the result of variations in the DNA sequence. This includes DNA methylation, histone modifications, and genomic imprinting, which can occur both prenatally and postnatally and can establish either transient or long-lasting changes in gene expression.

The role of diet in DNA methylation is significant. DNA methylation is catalyzed by DNA methyltransferases that transfer methyl groups from S-adenosyl-methionine (SAM) to cytosine in CpG islands. The SAM required for methylation comes, in part, from dietary methyl group intake, and the major source of methyl groups in food is methionine. If methionine is limited in the diet, the amount of SAM available is also limited and hypomethylation is found (Wainfan et al., 1989; Vachtenheim, Horakova, & Novotna, 1994). However, there also are de novo pathways (one-carbon metabolism) and other dietary sources of methyl groups, including choline, folic acid, and vitamin B12 (Niculescu & Zeisel, 2002). Limiting methionine in the diet during development is likely to result in some compensatory changes in these other pathways so that some level of methylation can occur.

Perhaps the most dramatic example of the effects of dietary methyl groups is represented by the observation that dietary supplementation of methyl groups in pregnant black pseudoagouti (A^{vy}/a) dams alters epigenetic regulation of agouti expression by increasing methylation at the long terminal repeat, resulting in increased agouti-black mottling in offspring (Wolff et al., 1998; Cooney, Dave, & Wolff, 2002). Gene-specific hypomethylation of peroxisomal proliferator-activated receptor alpha (Lillycrop et al., 2008) and the glucocorticoid receptor (Lillycrop et al., 2005) has also been observed in the offspring of rodents fed a low-protein diet, and this can be prevented with folic acid supplementation. It is interesting that methyl deficiency causing global DNA hypomethylation can occur simultaneously with gene-specific hypomethylation or hypermethylation (Singh, Murphy, & O'Reilly, 2003). A methyl-deficient diet also modifies histone methylation and increases expression of both immunoglobulin factor 2 (*Igf2*) and *H19* genes, indicating that at some loci, methyl deficiency may result in chromatin modification. It is important that hypomethylation of *Igf2* is also found in DNA samples from humans who were exposed to the Dutch famine during development (Heijmans et al., 2008).

Recent technical advances are opening up the possibility of measuring changes in methylation status on a genomewide scale (Schumacher et al., 2006). Allele-specific methylation using array-based technology allows tracking of both gene- and allele-specific changes in methylation. Paired with an experimental genetic population of animals, this technique presents a powerful tool for examining the role of prenatal nutritional environment on allele-specific methylation status and its effects on behavior.

Conclusions and Future Directions

The spectrum of data presented here reflects years of research on a variety of animal models, including work from many diverse disciplines that suggests that protein deprivation during gestation, immediately after birth, or both produces behavioral, neurochemical, and developmental changes that accurately mirror many of the symptoms of human schizophrenia.

The challenge moving forward is to integrate these environmentally induced behavioral, neurochemical, and developmental changes with the relevant genetic factors that increase susceptibility to developing schizophrenia. Numerous genes and gene expression changes have been studied in schizophrenia; for reviews, see Jones et al. (2008) and Desbonnet, Waddington, & O'Tuathaigh, (2009a, 2009b). Animal models of these can be subjected to protein deprivation to look for gene-environment interaction.

The identification of specific genetic and environmental causes of schizophrenia and other psychiatric disorders remains a challenge for the research community. Findings reviewed in this chapter highlight the importance of maternal nutrition, specifically adequate protein nutrition, within the prenatal, perinatal, and early postnatal developmental critical periods. The availability of tools for directly assessing the impact of environmental manipulations on gene structure and expression, along with a greater appreciation for the role of gene-environment interactions in complex disease, has the potential to move the field forward in the next decade.

KEY AREAS FOR FUTURE RESEARCH

- The use of protein deprivation as an environmental risk factor should be developed more systematically in mouse models, where the current genetic and genomic tools are most advanced.
- The use of mouse models would allow for a more thorough assessment of the genetic effects of prenatal protein malnutrition (i.e., strain differences, gene-environment interactions).
- As tools develop, a more systematic genomewide assessment of epigenetic changes resulting from prenatal protein deprivation should be explored.

Acknowledgments

The authors' work is supported by grants from the National Institute on Drug Abuse (DA022392 and DA023690 to L. M. Tarantino) and the National Institute of Mental Health (MH087978 and MH091372 to T. M. Reyes and MH079103 to A. A. Palmer).

Selected Readings

Meyer, U. & Feldon, J. (2009). Epidemiology-driven neurodevelopmental animal models of schizophrenia. *Progress in Neurobiology* 90(3): 285–326.

Morgane, P. J., Austin-LaFrance, R., Bronzino, J., Tonkiss, J., Diaz-Cintra, S., Cintra, L., Kemper, T., & Galler, J. R. (1993). Prenatal malnutrition and development of the brain. *Neuroscience and Biobehavioral Reviews* 17(1): 91–128.

Rutten, B. P. & Mill, J. (2009). Epigenetic mediation of environmental influences in major psychotic disorders. *Schizophrenia Bulletin* 35(6): 1045–1056.

Tonkiss, J., Galler, J., Morgane, P. J., Bronzino, J. D., & Austin-LaFrance, R. J. (1993). Prenatal protein malnutrition and postnatal brain function. *Annals of the New York Academy of Science* 678: 215–227.

van Os, J. & Rutten, B. P. (2009). Gene-environment-wide interaction studies in psychiatry. *American Journal of Psychiatry* 166(9): 964–966.

References

Almeida, S. S., de Oliveira, L. M., & Graeff, F. G. (1990). Decreased reactivity to anxiolytics caused by early protein malnutrition in rats. *Pharmacology Biochemistry and Behavior* 36(4): 997–1000.

Almeida, S. S., de Oliveira, L. M., & Graeff, F. G. (1991). Early life protein malnutrition changes exploration of the elevated plus-maze and reactivity to anxiolytics. *Psychopharmacology (Berl)* 103(4): 513–518.

Almeida, S. S., Garcia, R. A., & de Oliveira, L. M. (1993). Effects of early protein malnutrition and repeated testing upon locomotor and exploratory behaviors in the elevated plus-maze. *Physiology & Behavior* 54(2): 749–752.

Almeida, S. S., Soares, E. G., Bichuette, M. Z., Graeff, F. G., & de Oliveira, L. M. (1992). Effects of early postnatal malnutrition and chlordiazepoxide on experimental aversive situations. *Physiology & Behavior* 51(6): 1195–1199.

Almeida, S. S., Tonkiss, J., & Galler, J. R. (1996a). Prenatal protein malnutrition affects avoidance but not escape behavior in the elevated T-maze test. *Physiology and Behavior* 60(1): 191–195.

Almeida, S. S., Tonkiss, J., & Galler, J. R. (1996b). Prenatal protein malnutrition affects exploratory behavior of female rats in the elevated plus-maze test. *Physiology and Behavior* 60(2): 675–680.

Almeida, S. S., Tonkiss, J., & Galler, J. R. (1996c). Prenatal protein malnutrition affects the social interactions of juvenile rats. *Physiology and Behavior* 60(1): 197–201.

Amitai, N., Semenova, S., & Markou, A. (2009). Clozapine attenuates disruptions in response inhibition and task efficiency induced by repeated phencyclidine administration in the intracranial self-stimulation procedure. *European Journal of Pharmacology* 602(1): 78–84.

Arguello, P. A. & Gogos, J. A. (2009). Cognition in mouse models of schizophrenia susceptibility genes. *Schizophrenia Bulletin* 36(2): 289–300.

Armitage, J., Khan, I., Taylor, P., Nathanielsz, P., & Poston, L. (2004). Developmental programming of the metabolic syndrome by maternal nutritional imbalance: How strong is the evidence from experimental models in mammals? *Journal of Physiology* 561(2): 355–377.

Audet, M. C., Goulet, S., & Dore, F. Y. (2006). Repeated subchronic exposure to phencyclidine elicits excessive atypical grooming in rats. *Behavioural Brain Research* 167(1): 103–110.

Austin, K. B., Bronzino, J., & Morgane, P. J. (1986). Prenatal protein malnutrition affects synaptic potentiation in the dentate gyrus of rats in adulthood. *Brain Research* 394(2): 267–273.

Belforte, J. E., Zsiros, V., Sklar, E. R., Jiang, Z., Yu, G., Li, Y., Quinlan, E. M., & Nakazawa, K. (2010). Postnatal NMDA receptor ablation in corticolimbic interneurons confers schizophrenia-like phenotypes. *Nature Neuroscience* 13(1): 76–83.

Bellinger, L., Sculley, D. V., Langley-Evans, S. C. (2006). Exposure to undernutrition in fetal life determines fat distribution, locomotor activity and food intake in ageing rats. *International Journal of Obesity (Lond)* 30(5): 729–738.

Benes, F. M. & Berretta, S. (2001). GABAergic interneurons: Implications for understanding schizophrenia and bipolar disorder. *Neuropsychopharmacology* 25(1): 1–27.

Berlin, I., Givry-Steiner, L., Lecrubier, Y., & Puech, A. J. (1998). Measures of anhedonia and hedonic responses to sucrose in depressive and schizophrenic patients in comparison with healthy subjects. *European Psychiatry* 13(6): 303–309.

Blatt, G. J., Chen, J. C., Rosene, D. L., Volicer, L., & Galler, J. R. (1994). Prenatal protein malnutrition effects on the serotonergic system in the hippocampal formation: An immunocytochemical, ligand binding, and neurochemical study. *Brain Research Bulletin* 34(5): 507–518.

Borghese, C. M., Cordoba, N. E., Laino, C. H., Orsingher, O. A., Rubio, M. C., & Niselman, V. (1998). Lack of tolerance to the anxiolytic effect of diazepam and pentobarbital following chronic administration in perinatally undernourished rats. *Brain Research Bulletin* 46(3): 237–244.

Braff, D. L., Geyer, M. A., & Swerdlow, N. R. (2001). Human studies of prepulse inhibition of startle: Normal subjects, patient groups, and pharmacological studies. *Psychopharmacology (Berl)* 156(2–3): 234–258.

Braff, D. L., Grillon, C., & Geyer, M. A. (1992). Gating and habituation of the startle reflex in schizophrenic patients. *Archives of General Psychiatry* 49(3): 206–215.

Brioni, J. D., Cordoba, N., & Orsingher, O. A. (1989). Decreased reactivity to the anticonflict effect of diazepam in perinatally undernourished rats. *Behavioural Brain Research* 34(1–2): 159–162.

Brioni, J. D., Keller, E. A., Levin, L. E., Cordoba, N., & Orsingher, O. A. (1986). Reactivity to amphetamine in perinatally undernourished rats: Behavioral and neurochemical correlates. *Pharmacology Biochemistry and Behavior* 24(3): 449–454.

Brioni, J. D. & Orsingher, O. A. (1987). Perinatal undernutrition alters hypothermic responses to different central agonists in recovered adult rats. *Neuropharmacology* 26(7A): 771–774.

Brioni, J. D. & Orsingher, O. A. (1988). Operant behavior and reactivity to the anticonflict effect of diazepam in perinatally undernourished rats. *Physiology and Behavior* 44(2): 193–198.

Brown, A. S. & Susser, E. S. (2008). Prenatal nutritional deficiency and risk of adult schizophrenia. *Schizophrenia Bulletin* 34(6): 1054–1063.

Brown, A. S., Susser, E. S., Lin, S. P., Neugebauer, R., & Gorman, J. M. (1995). Increased risk of affective disorders in males after second trimester prenatal exposure to the Dutch hunger winter of 1944–45. *British Journal of Psychiatry* 166(5): 601–606.

Brown, A. S., van Os, J., Driessens, C., Hoek, H. W., & Susser, E. S. (2000). Further evidence of relation between prenatal famine and major affective disorder. *American Journal of Psychiatry* 157(2): 190–195.

Buckley, P. F., Miller, B. J., Lehrer, D. S., & Castle, D. J. (2009). Psychiatric comorbidities and schizophrenia. *Schizophrenia Bulletin* 35(2): 383–402.

Cadenhead, K. S., Geyer, M. A., & Braff, D. L. (1993). Impaired startle prepulse inhibition and habituation in patients with schizotypal personality disorder. *American Journal of Psychiatry* 150(12): 1862–1867.

Cannon, M., Byrne, M., Cotter, D., Sham, P., Larkin, C., & Ocallaghan, E. (1994). Further evidence for anomalies in the hand-prints of patients with schizophrenia—a study of secondary creases. *Schizophrenia Research* 13(2): 179–184.

Castanon-Cervantes, O. & Cintra, L. (2002). Circadian rhythms of occipital-cortex temperature and motor activity in young and old rats under chronic protein malnutrition. *Nutritional Neuroscience* 5(4): 279–286.

Chen, J. C., Turiak, G., Galler, J., & Volicer, L. (1995). Effect of prenatal malnutrition on release of monoamines from hippocampal slices. *Life Sciences* 57(16): 1467–1475.

Chrousos, G. P. (2009). Stress and disorders of the stress system. *Nature Reviews Endocrinology* 5(7): 374–381.

Cintra, L., Aguilar, A., Granados, L., Galván, A., Kemper, T., DeBassio, W., Galler, J., Morgane, P., Durán, P., & Díaz-Cintra, S. (1997a). Effects of prenatal protein malnutrition on hippocampal CA1 pyramidal cells in rats of four age groups. *Hippocampus* 7(22): 192–203.

Cintra, L., Duran, P., Guevara, M. A., Aguilar, A., & Castanon-Cervantes, O. (2002). Pre- and post-natal protein malnutrition alters the effect of rapid eye movements sleep-deprivation by the platform-technique upon the electrocorticogram of the circadian sleep-wake cycle and its frequency bands in the rat. *Nutritional Neuroscience* 5(2): 91–101.

Cintra, L., Granados, L., Aguilar, A., Kemper, T., DeBassio, W., Galler, J., Morgane, P., Durán, P., & Díaz-Cintra, S. (1997b). Effects of prenatal protein malnutrition on mossy fibers of the hippocampal formation in rats of four age groups. *Hippocampus* 7(2): 184–191.

Clancy, B., Darlington, R. B., & Finlay, B. L. (2001). Translating developmental time across mammalian species. *Neuroscience* 105(1): 7–17.

Cohrs, S. (2008). Sleep disturbances in patients with schizophrenia: Impact and effect of antipsychotics. *CNS Drugs* 22(11): 939–962.

Connolly, P. M., Maxwell, C. R., Kanes, S. J., Abel, T., Liang, Y., Tokarczyk, J., Bilker, W. B., Turetsky, B. I., Gur, R. E., & Siegel, S. J. (2003). Inhibition of auditory evoked potentials and prepulse inhibition of startle in DBA/2J and DBA/2Hsd inbred mouse substrains. *Brain Research* 992(1): 85–95.

Cooney, C. A., Dave, A. A., & Wolff, G. L. (2002). Maternal methyl supplements in mice affect epigenetic variation and DNA methylation of offspring. *Journal of Nutrition* 132(8 Suppl): 2393S–2400S.

Cordoba, N. E., Cuadra, G. R., Brioni, J. D., & Orsingher, O. A. (1992). Perinatal protein deprivation enhances the anticonflict effect measured after chronic ethanol administration in adult rats. *Journal of Nutrition* 122(7): 1536–1541.

Cordoba, N. E., Molina, J. C., Basso, A. M., & Orsingher, O. A. (1990). Perinatal undernutrition reduced ethanol intake preference in adult recovered rats. *Physiology & Behavior* 47(6): 1111–1116.

Cryan, J. F. & Mombereau, C. (2004). In search of a depressed mouse: Utility of models for studying depression-related behavior in genetically modified mice. *Molecular Psychiatry* 9(4): 326–357.

Damgaard, T., Larsen, D. B., Hansen, S. L., Grayson, B., Neill, J. C., & Plath, N. (2010). Positive modulation of alpha-amino-3-hydroxy-5-methyl-4-isoxazolepropionic acid (AMPA) receptors reverses sub-chronic PCP-induced deficits in the novel object recognition task in rats. *Behavioural Brain Research* 207(1): 144–150.

Desbonnet, L., Waddington, J. L., & O'Tuathaigh, C. M. (2009a). Mice mutant for genes associated with schizophrenia: Common phenotype or distinct endophenotypes? *Behavioural Brain Research* 204(2): 258–273.

Desbonnet, L., Waddington, J. L., & O'Tuathaigh, C. M. (2009b). Mutant models for genes associated with schizophrenia. *Biochemical Society Transactions* 37(Pt 1): 308–312.

Díaz-Cintra, S., Cintra, L., Galván, A., Aguilar, A., Kemper, T., & Morgane, P. (1991). Effects of prenatal protein deprivation on postnatal development of granule cells in the fascia dentata. *Journal of Comparative Neurology* 310(3): 356–364.

Díaz-Cintra, S., García-Ruiz, M., Corkidi, G., & Cintra, L. (1994). Effects of prenatal malnutrition and postnatal nutritional rehabilitation on CA3 hippocampal pyramidal cells in rats of four ages. *Brain Research* 662(1–2): 117–126.

Díaz-Cintra, S., González-Maciel, A., Morales, M. A., Aguilar, A., Cintra, L., & Prado-Alcalá, R. A. (2007). Protein malnutrition differentially alters the number of glutamic acid decarboxylase-67 interneurons in dentate gyrus and CA1-3 subfields of the dorsal hippocampus. *Experimental Neurology* 208(1): 47–53.

Di Matteo, V., Di Giovanni, G., Pierucci, M., & Esposito, E. (2008). Serotonin control of central dopaminergic function: Focus on in vivo microdialysis studies. *Progress in Brain Research* 172: 7–44.

Dulawa, S. C., Scearce-Levie, K. A., Hen, R., & Geyer, M. A. (2000). Serotonin releasers increase prepulse inhibition in serotonin 1B knockout mice. *Psychopharmacology (Berl)* 149(3): 306–312.

Duran, P., Cintra, L., Galler, J. R., & Tonkiss, J. (2005). Prenatal protein malnutrition induces a phase shift advance of the spontaneous locomotor rhythm and alters the rest/activity ratio in adult rats. *Nutritional Neuroscience* 8(3): 167–172.

Duran, P., Galler, J. R., Cintra, L., & Tonkiss, J. (2006). Prenatal malnutrition and sleep states in adult rats: Effects of restraint stress. *Physiology and Behavior* 89(2): 156–163.

Dzirasa, K., Ribeiro, S., Costa, R., Santos, L. M., Lin, S. C., Grosmark, A., Sotnikova, T. D., Gainetdinov, R. R., Caron, M. G., & Nicolelis, M. A. (2006). Dopaminergic control of sleep-wake states. *Journal of Neuroscience* 26(41): 10577–10589.

Ellenbroek, B. A. & Cools, A. R. (2002). Apomorphine susceptibility and animal models for psychopathology: Genes and environment. *Behavior Genetics* 32(5): 349–361.

Etherton, M. R., Blaiss, C. A., Powell, C. M., & Sudhof, T. C. (2009). Mouse neurexin-1 alpha deletion causes correlated electrophysiological and behavioral changes consistent with cognitive impairments. *Proceedings of the National Academy of Sciences U.S.A.* 106(42): 17998–18003.

Farrow, T. F., Hunter, M. D., Haque, R., & Spence, S. A. (2006). Modafinil and unconstrained motor activity in schizophrenia: Double-blind crossover placebo-controlled trial. *British Journal of Psychiatry* 189: 461–462.

Fatemi, S. H. & Folsom, T. D. (2009). The neurodevelopmental hypothesis of schizophrenia, revisited. *Schizophrenia Bulletin* 35(3): 528–548.

Fenton, W. S., Stover, E. L., & Insel, T. R. (2003). Breaking the log-jam in treatment development for cognition in schizophrenia: NIMH perspective. *Psychopharmacology (Berl)* 169(3–4): 365–366.

Fiacco, T. A., Rosene, D. L., Galler, J. R., & Blatt, G. J. (2003). Increased density of hippocampal kainate receptors but normal density of NMDA and AMPA receptors in a rat model of prenatal protein malnutrition. *Journal of Comparative Neurology* 456(4): 350–360.

Francolin-Silva, A. L. & Almeida, S. S. (2004). The interaction of housing condition and acute immobilization stress on the elevated plus-maze behaviors of protein-malnourished rats. *Brazilian Journal of Medical and Biological Research* 37(7): 1035–1042.

Francolin-Silva, A. L., Brandao, M. L., & Almeida, S. S. (2007). Early postnatal protein malnutrition causes resistance to the anxiolytic effects of diazepam as assessed by the fear-potentiated startle test. *Nutritional Neuroscience* 10(1–2): 23–29.

Francolin-Silva, A. L., da Silva Hernandes, A., Fukuda, M. T., Valadares, C. T., & Almeida, S. S. (2006). Anxiolytic-like effects of short-term postnatal protein malnutrition in the elevated plus-maze test. *Behavioural Brain Research* 173(2): 310–314.

Frankova, S. (1973). Effect of protein-calorie malnutrition on the development of social behavior in rats. *Developmental Psychobiology* 6(1) 33–43.

Galler, J. R., Tonkiss, J., & Maldonado-Irizarry, C. S. (1994). Prenatal protein malnutrition and home orientation in the rat. *Physiology and Behavior* 55(6): 993–996.

Gallo, P. V., Werboff, J., & Knox, K. (1984). Development of home orientation in offspring of protein-restricted cats. *Developmental Psychobiology* 17(5): 437–449.

Garzya, V., Forbes, I. T., Gribble, A. D., Hadley, M. S., Lightfoot, A. P., Payne, A. H., Smith, A. B., Douglas, S. E., Cooper, D. G., Stansfield, I. G., et al. (2007). Studies towards the identification of a new generation of atypical antipsychotic agents. *Bioorganic and Medicinal Chemistry Letters* 17(2): 400–405.

Geyer, M. A. & Braff, D. L. (1982). Habituation of the Blink reflex in normals and schizophrenic patients. *Psychophysiology* 19(1): 1–6.

Geyer, M. A., Krebs-Thomson, K., Braff, D. L., & Swerdlow, N. R. (2001). Pharmacological studies of prepulse inhibition models of sensorimotor gating deficits in schizophrenia: A decade in review. *Psychopharmacology (Berl) 156*(2–3): 117–154.

Geyer, M. A. & Markou, A. (1995). Animal models of psychiatric disorders. In F. Bloom & D. Kupfer (eds.), *Psychopharmacology: The Fourth Generation of Progress* (pp. 787–798). New York: Raven.

Geyer, M. A. & Vollenweider, F. X. (2008). Serotonin research: Contributions to understanding psychoses. *Trends in Pharmacological Sciences 29*(9): 445–453.

Goodlett, C. R., Valentino, M. L., Morgane, P. J., & Resnick, O. (1986). Spatial cue utilization in chronically malnourished rats: Task-specific learning deficits. *Developmental Psychobiology 19*(1): 1–15.

Goodlett, C. R., Valentino, M. L., Resnick, O., & Morgane, P. J. (1985). Altered development of responsiveness to clonidine in severely malnourished rats. *Pharmacology, Biochemistry, and Behavior 23*(4): 567–572.

Gottesman, I. I. & Gould, T. D. (2003). The endophenotype concept in psychiatry: Etymology and strategic intentions. *American Journal of Psychiatry 160*(4): 636–645.

Green, M. F., Nuechterlein, K. H., Gold, J. M., Barch, D. M., Cohen, J., Essock, S., Fenton, W. S., Frese, F., Goldberg, T. E., Heaton, R. K., et al. (2004). Approaching a consensus cognitive battery for clinical trials in schizophrenia: The NIMH-MATRICS conference to select cognitive domains and test criteria. *Biological Psychiatry 56*(5): 301–307.

Gressens, P., Muaku, S. M., Besse, L., Nsegbe, E., Gallego, J., Delpech, B., Gaultier, C., Evrard, P., Ketelslegers, J. M., & Maiter, D. (1997). Maternal protein restriction early in rat pregnancy alters brain development in the progeny. *Brain Research: Developmental Brain Research 103*(1): 21–35.

Hall, R. D. (1983). Is hippocampal function in the adult rat impaired by early protein or protein-calorie deficiencies? *Developmental Psychobiology 16*(5): 395–411.

Hall, R. D., Leahy, J. P., & Robertson, W. M. (1983). Hyposensitivity to serotonergic stimulation in protein malnourished rats. *Physiology and Behavior 31*(2): 187–195.

Heijmans, B. T., Tobi, E. W., Stein, A. D., Putter, H., Blauw, G. J., Susser, E. S., Slagboom, P. E., & Lumey, L. H. (2008). Persistent epigenetic differences associated with prenatal exposure to famine in humans. *Proceedings of the National Academy of Sciences U.S.A. 105*(44): 17046–17049.

Hernandes, A. S. & Almeida, S. S. (2003). Postnatal protein malnutrition affects inhibitory avoidance and risk assessment behaviors in two models of anxiety in rats. *Nutritional Neuroscience 6*(4): 213–219.

Hoek, H. W., Brown, A. S., & Susser, E. (1998). The Dutch Famine and schizophrenia spectrum disorders. *Social Psychiatry and Psychiatric Epidemiology 33*(8): 373–379.

Howes, O. D., Egerton, A., Allan, V., McGuire, P., Stokes, P., & Kapur, S. (2009). Mechanisms underlying psychosis and antipsychotic treatment response in schizophrenia: Insights from PET and SPECT imaging. *Current Pharmaceutical Design 15*(22): 2550–2559.

Hulshoff Pol, H. E. & Kahn, R. S. (2008). What happens after the first episode? A review of progressive brain changes in chronically ill patients with schizophrenia. *Schizophrenia Bulletin 34*(2): 354–366.

Javitt, D. C. (2006). Is the glycine site half saturated or half unsaturated? Effects of glutamatergic drugs in schizophrenia patients. *Current Opinion in Psychiatry 19*(2): 151–157.

Javitt, D. C., Spencer, K. M., Thaker, G. K., Winterer, G., & Hajos, M. (2008). Neurophysiological biomarkers for drug development in schizophrenia. *Nature Reviews Drug Discovery 7*(1): 68–83.

Jones, D. N. C., Gartlon, J. E., Minassian, A., Perry, W., & Geyer, M. A. (2008). Developing new drugs for schizophrenia: From animals to the clinic. In R. McArthur & F. Borsini (eds.), *Animal and Translational Models for CNS Drug Discovery* (vol. 1) (pp. 199–261). New York: Academic Press.

Joyce, J. N., Lexow, N., Bird, E., & Winokur, A. (1988). Organization of dopamine D1 and D2 receptors in human striatum: Receptor autoradiographic studies in Huntington's disease and schizophrenia. *Synapse* 2(5): 546–557.

Kehoe, P., Mallinson, K., Bronzino, J., & McCormick, C. M. (2001). Effects of prenatal protein malnutrition and neonatal stress on CNS responsiveness. *Brain Research: Developmental Brain Research* 132(1): 23–31.

Kellendonk, C., Simpson, E. H., & Kandel, E. R. (2009). Modeling cognitive endophenotypes of schizophrenia in mice. *Trends in Neuroscience* 32(6): 347–358.

Keller, E. A., Cancela, L. M., Molina, V. A., & Orsingher, O. A. (1994). Lack of adaptive changes in 5-HT sites in perinatally undernourished rats after chronic stress: Opioid influence. *Pharmacology Biochemistry and Behavior* 47(4): 789–793.

Keller, E. A., Molina, V. A., & Orsingher, O. A. (1990). Lack of neuronal adaptive changes following chronic treatments in perinatally undernourished rats. *Pharmacology, Biochemistry, and Behavior* 37(4): 675–678.

Laino, C. H., Cordoba, N. E., & Orsingher, O. A. (1993). Perinatally protein-deprived rats and reactivity to anxiolytic drugs in the plus-maze test: An animal model for screening antipanic agents? *Pharmacology Biochemistry and Behavior* 46(1): 89–94.

Large, C. H. (2007). Do NMDA receptor antagonist models of schizophrenia predict the clinical efficacy of antipsychotic drugs? *Journal of Psychopharmacology* 21(3): 283–301.

Leahy, J. P., Stern, W. C., Resnick, O., & Morgane, P. J. (1978). A neuropharmacological analysis of central nervous system catecholamine systems in development protein malnutrition. *Developmental Psychobiology* 11(4): 361–370.

Le Pen, G., Gaudet, L., Mortas, P., Mory, R., & Moreau, J. L. (2002) Deficits in reward sensitivity in a neurodevelopmental rat model of schizophrenia. *Psychopharmacology (Berl)* 161(4): 434–441.

Li, L., Du, Y., Li, N., Wu, X., & Wu, Y. (2009). Top-down modulation of prepulse inhibition of the startle reflex in humans and rats. *Neuroscience and Biobehavioral Reviews* 33(8): 1157–1167.

Lillycrop, K. A., Phillips, E. S., Jackson, A. A., Hanson, M. A., & Burdge, G. C. (2005). Dietary protein restriction of pregnant rats induces and folic acid supplementation prevents epigenetic modification of hepatic gene expression in the offspring. *Journal of Nutrition* 135(6): 1382–1386.

Lillycrop, K. A., Phillips, E. S., Torrens, C., Hanson, M. A., Jackson, A. A., & Burdge, G. C. (2008). Feeding pregnant rats a protein-restricted diet persistently alters the methylation of specific cytosines in the hepatic PPAR alpha promoter of the offspring. *British Journal of Nutrition* 100(2): 278–282.

Lipska, B. K., Swerdlow, N. R., Geyer, M. A., Jaskiw, G. E., Braff, D. L., & Weinberger, D. R. (1995). Neonatal excitotoxic hippocampal damage in rats causes post-pubertal changes in prepulse inhibition of startle and its disruption by apomorphine. *Psychopharmacology (Berl)* 122(1): 35–43.

Lister, J. P., Blatt, G. J., DeBassio, W. A., Kemper, T. L., Tonkiss, J., Galler, J. R., & Rosene, D. L. (2005). Effect of prenatal protein malnutrition on numbers of neurons in the principal cell layers of the adult rat hippocampal formation. *Hippocampus* 15(3): 393–403.

Lodge, D. J. & Grace, A. A. (2008) Hippocampal dysfunction and disruption of dopamine system regulation in an animal model of schizophrenia. *Neurotoxicity Research* 14(2–3): 97–104.

Lopes de Souza, S., Orozco-Solis, R., Grit, I., Manhães de Castro, R., & Bolaños-Jiménez, F. (2008). Perinatal protein restriction reduces the inhibitory action of serotonin on food intake. *European Journal of Neuroscience* 27(6): 1400–1408.

Marichich, E. S., Molina, V. A., & Orsingher, O. A. (1979). Persistent changes in central cate-cholaminergic system after recovery of perinatally undernourished rats. *Journal of Nutrition 109*(6): 1045–1050.

Meyer, U. & Feldon, J. (2009). Epidemiology-driven neurodevelopmental animal models of schizophrenia. *Progress in Neurobiology 90*(3): 285–326.

Mokler, D. J., Galle, J. R., & Morgane, P. J. (2003). Modulation of 5-HT release in the hip-pocampus of 30-day-old rats exposed in utero to protein malnutrition. *Brain Research: Developmental Brain Research 142*(2): 203–208.

Mokler, D. J., Torres, O. I., Galler, J. R., & Morgane, P. J. (2007). Stress-induced changes in extracellular dopamine and serotonin in the medial prefrontal cortex and dorsal hippo-campus of prenatally malnourished rats. *Brain Research 1148*: 226–233.

Morgane, P. J., Austin-LaFrance, R., Bronzino, J., Tonkiss, J., Diaz-Cintra, S., Cintra, L., Kemper, T., & Galler, J. R. (1993). Prenatal malnutrition and development of the brain. *Neuroscience and Biobehavioral Reviews 17*(1): 91–128.

Niculescu, M. D. & Zeisel, S. H. (2002). Diet, methyl donors and DNA methylation: Interac-tions between dietary folate, methionine and choline. *Journal of Nutrition 132*(8 Suppl): 2333S–2335S.

Palmer, A. A., Brown, A. S., Keegan, D., Siska, L. D., Susser, E., Rotrosen, J., & Butler, P. D. (2008). Prenatal protein deprivation alters dopamine-mediated behaviors and dopaminer-gic and glutamatergic receptor binding. *Brain Research 1237*: 62–74.

Palmer, A. A., Printz, D. J., Butler, P. D., Dulawa, S. C., & Printz, M. P. (2004). Prenatal protein deprivation in rats induces changes in prepulse inhibition and NMDA receptor binding. *Brain Research 996*(2): 193–201.

Patil, S. T., Zhang, L., Martenyi, F., Lowe, S. L., Jackson, K. A., Andreev, B. V., Avedisova, A. S., Bardenstein, L. M., Gurovich, I. Y., Morozova, M. A., et al. (2007). Activation of mGlu2/3 receptors as a new approach to treat schizophrenia: A randomized phase 2 clinical trial. *Nature Medicine 13*(9): 1102–1107.

Patterson, P. H. (2009). Immune involvement in schizophrenia and autism: Etiology, pathol-ogy and animal models. *Behavioural Brain Research 204*(2): 313–321.

Paz, R. D., Tardito, S., Atzori, M., & Tseng, K. Y. (2008). Glutamatergic dysfunction in schizo-phrenia: From basic neuroscience to clinical psychopharmacology. *European Neuropsy-chopharmacology 18*(11): 773–786.

Perry, W., Minassian, A., Feifel, D., & Braff, D. L. (2001). Sensorimotor gating deficits in bipo-lar disorder patients with acute psychotic mania. *Biological Psychiatry 50*(6): 418–424.

Powell, S. B., Zhou, X., & Geyer, M. A. (2009). Prepulse inhibition and genetic mouse models of schizophrenia. *Behavioural Brain Research 204*(2): 282–294.

Prut, L., & Belzung, C. (2003). The open field as a paradigm to measure the effects of drugs on anxiety-like behaviors: A review. *European Journal of Pharmacology 463*(1–3): 3–33.

Ranade, S. C., Rose, A., Rao, M., Gallego, J., Gressens, P., & Mani, S. (2008). Different types of nutritional deficiencies affect different domains of spatial memory function checked in a radial arm maze. *Neuroscience 152*(4): 859–866.

Resnick, O. & Morgane, P. J. (1984). Ontogeny of the levels of serotonin in various parts of the brain in severely protein malnourished rats. *Brain Research 303*(1): 163–170.

Rodgers, R. J. & Johnson, N. J. (1995). Factor analysis of spatiotemporal and ethological measures in the murine elevated plus-maze test of anxiety. *Pharmacology, Biochemistry, and Behavior 52*(2): 297–303.

Rojas, P., Montes, S., Serrano-Garcia, N., & Rojas-Castaneda, J. (2009). Effect of EGb761 supplementation on the content of copper in mouse brain in an animal model of Parkin-son's disease. *Nutrition 25*(4): 482–485.

Sams-Dodd, F. (1999). Phencyclidine in the social interaction test: An animal model of schizophrenia with face and predictive validity. *Reviews in Neurosciences* 10(1): 59–90.

Santucci, L. B., Daud, M. M., Almeida, S. S., & de Oliveira, L. M. (1994). Effects of early protein malnutrition and environmental stimulation upon the reactivity to diazepam in two animal models of anxiety. *Pharmacology Biochemistry and Behavior* 49(2): 393–398.

Schumacher, A., Kapranov, P., Kaminsky, Z., Flanagan, J., Assadzadeh, A., Yau, P., Virtanen, C., Winegarden, N., Cheng, J., Gingeras, T., et al. (2006). Microarray-based DNA methylation profiling: Technology and applications. *Nucleic Acids Research* 34(2): 528–542.

Schweigert, I. D., de Oliveira, D. L., Scheibel, F., da Costa, F., Wofchuk, S. T., Souza, D. O., & Perry, M. L. (2005). Gestational and postnatal malnutrition affects sensitivity of young rats to picrotoxin and quinolinic acid and uptake of GABA by cortical and hippocampal slices. *Brain Research: Developmental Brain Research* 154(2): 177–185.

Seeman, P., Bzowej, N. H., Guan, H. C., Bergeron, C., Reynolds, G. P., Bird, E. D., Riederer, P., Jellinger, K., & Tourtellotte, W. W. (1987). Human brain D1 and D2 dopamine receptors in schizophrenia, Alzheimer's, Parkinson's, and Huntington's diseases. *Neuropsychopharmacology* 1(1): 5–15.

Shanahan, N. A., Holick Pierz, K. A., Masten, V. L., Waeber, C., Ansorge, M., Gingrich, J. A., Geyer, M. A., Hen, R., & Dulawa, S. C. (2009). Chronic reductions in serotonin transporter function prevent 5-HT1B-induced behavioral effects in mice. *Biological Psychiatry* 65(5): 401–408.

Shultz, P. L., Galler, J. R., & Tonkiss, J. (1999). Prenatal protein restriction increases sensitization to cocaine-induced stereotypy. *Behavioural Pharmacology* 10(4): 379–387.

Shultz, P. L., Galler, J. R., & Tonkiss, J. (2002). Prenatal protein malnutrition enhances stimulus control by CDP, but not a CDP/THIP combination in rats. *Pharmacology Biochemistry and Behavior* 73(4): 759–767.

Singh, S. M., Murphy, B., & O'Reilly, R. L. (2003). Involvement of gene-diet/drug interaction in DNA methylation and its contribution to complex diseases: From cancer to schizophrenia. *Clinical Genetics* 64(6) 451–460.

Smart, J. L., Dobbing, J., Adlard, B. P., Lynch, A., & Sands, J. (1973). Vulnerability of developing brain: Relative effects of growth restriction during the fetal and suckling periods on behavior and brain composition of adult rats. *Journal of Nutrition* 103(9): 1327–1338.

St Clair, D., Xu, M., Wang, P., Yu, Y., Fang, Y., Zhang, F., Zheng, X., Gu, N., Feng, G., Sham, P., et al. (2005). Rates of adult schizophrenia following prenatal exposure to the Chinese Famine of 1959–1961. *Journal of the American Medical Association* 294: 557–562.

Steiger, J. L., Alexander, M. J., Galler, J. R., Farb, D. H., & Russek, S. J. (2003). Effects of prenatal malnutrition on GABAA receptor alpha1, alpha3 and beta2 mRNA levels. *Neuroreport* 14(13): 1731–1735.

Steiger, J. L., Galler, J. R., Farb, D. H., & Russek, S. J. (2002). Prenatal protein malnutrition reduces beta(2), beta(3) and gamma(2L) GABA(A) receptor subunit mRNAs in the adult septum. *European Journal of Pharmacology* 446(1–3): 201–202.

Stone, J. M., Morrison, P. D., & Pilowsky, L. S. (2007). Glutamate and dopamine dysregulation in schizophrenia—a synthesis and selective review. *Journal of Psychopharmacology* 21(4): 440–452.

Susser, E., Neugebauer, R., Hoek, H., Brown, A., Lin, S., Labovitz, D., & Gorman, J. (1996). Schizophrenia after prenatal famine: Further evidence. *Archives of General Psychiatry* 53: 25–31.

Susser, E. S. & Lin, S. P. (1992). Schizophrenia after prenatal exposure to the Dutch Hunger Winter of 1944–1945. *Archives of General Psychiatry* 49(12): 983–988.

Swerdlow, N. R., Braff, D. L., & Geyer, M. A. (1990). GABAergic projection from nucleus accumbens to ventral pallidum mediates dopamine-induced sensorimotor gating deficits of acoustic startle in rats. *Brain Research* 532(1–2): 146–150.

Swerdlow, N. R., Braff, D. L., Taaid, N., & Geyer, M. A. (1994). Assessing the validity of an animal model of deficient sensorimotor gating in schizophrenic patients. *Archives of General Psychiatry* 51(2): 139–154.

Swerdlow, N. R., Weber, M., Qu, Y., Light, G. A., & Braff, D. L. (2008). Realistic expectations of prepulse inhibition in translational models for schizophrenia research. *Psychopharmacology (Berl)* 199(3): 331–388.

Toda, M. & Abi-Dargham, A. (2007). Dopamine hypothesis of schizophrenia: Making sense of it all. *Current Psychiatry Reports* 9(4): 329–336.

Tonkiss, J. & Galler, J. (2007). Prenatal malnutrition alters diazepam-mediated suppression of ultrasonic vocalizations in an age dependent manner. *Behavioural Brain Research* 182(2): 337–343.

Tonkiss, J., Galler, J., Morgane, P. J., Bronzino, J. D., & Austin-LaFrance, R. J. (1993). Prenatal protein malnutrition and postnatal brain function. *Annals of the New York Academy of Sciences* 678: 215–227.

Tonkiss, J. & Galler, J. R. (1990). Prenatal protein malnutrition and working memory performance in adult rats. *Behavioural Brain Research* 40(2): 95–107.

Tonkiss, J., Galler, J. R., Formica, R. N., Shukitt-Hale, B., & Timm, R. R. (1990a). Fetal protein malnutrition impairs acquisition of a DRL task in adult rats. *Physiology and Behavior* 48(1): 73–77.

Tonkiss, J., Harrison, R. H., & Galler, J. R. (1996). Differential effects of prenatal protein malnutrition and prenatal cocaine on a test of homing behavior in rat pups. *Physiology and Behavior* 60(3): 1013–1018.

Tonkiss, J., Shukitt-Hale, B., Formica, R. N., Rocco, F. J., & Galler, J. R. (1990b). Prenatal protein malnutrition alters response to reward in adult rats. *Physiology and Behavior* 48(5): 675–680.

Tonkiss, J., Shultz, P., & Galler, J. R. (1994). An analysis of spatial navigation in prenatally protein malnourished rats. *Physiology and Behavior* 55(2): 217–224.

Tonkiss, J., Shultz, P. L., Shumsky, J. S., Fiacco, T. T., Vincitore, M., Rosene, D. L., & Galler, J. R. (2000). Chlordiazepoxide-induced spatial learning deficits: Dose-dependent differences following prenatal malnutrition. *Pharmacology Biochemistry and Behavior* 65(1): 105–116.

Tonkiss, J. & Smart, J. L. (1983). Interactive effects of genotype and early life undernutrition on the development of behavior in rats. *Developmental Psychobiology* 16(4): 287–301.

Torres, G., Meeder, B. A., Hallas, B. H., Gross, K. W., & Horowitz, J. M. (2005). Preliminary evidence for reduced social interactions in Chakragati mutants modeling certain symptoms of schizophrenia. *Brain Research* 1046(1–2): 180–186.

Trzctnska, M., Tonkiss, J., & Galler, J. R. (1999). Influence of prenatal protein malnutrition on behavioral reactivity to stress in adult rats. *Stress* 3(1): 71–83.

Turetsky, B. I., Calkins, M. E., Light, G. A., Olincy, A., Radant, A. D., & Swerdlow, N. R. (2007). Neurophysiological endophenotypes of schizophrenia: The viability of selected candidate measures. *Schizophrenia Bulletin* 33(1): 69–94.

Ueki, A., Goto, K., Sato, N., Iso, H., & Morita, Y. (2006). Prepulse inhibition of acoustic startle response in mild cognitive impairment and mild dementia of Alzheimer type. *Psychiatry and Clinical Neurosciences* 60(1): 55–62.

Umbricht, D. & Krljes, S. (2005). Mismatch negativity in schizophrenia: A meta-analysis. *Schizophrenia Research* 76(1): 1–23.

Umbricht, D., Vollenweider, F. X., Schmid, L., Grubel, C., Skrabo, A., Huber, T., & Koller, R. (2003). Effects of the 5-HT2A agonist psilocybin on mismatch negativity generation and AX-continuous performance task: Implications for the neuropharmacology of cognitive deficits in schizophrenia. *Neuropsychopharmacology* 28(1): 170–181.

Umbricht, D., Vyssotki, D., Latanov, A., Nitsch, R., & Lipp, H. P. (2005). Deviance-related electrophysiological activity in mice: Is there mismatch negativity in mice? *Clinical Neurophysiology* 116(2): 353–363.

Vachtenheim, J., Horakova, I., & Novotna, H. (1994). Hypomethylation of CCGG sites in the 3' region of H-ras protooncogene is frequent and is associated with H-ras allele loss in non-small cell lung cancer. *Cancer Research* 54(5): 1145–1148.

Valdomero, A., Bussolino, D. F., Orsingher, O. A., & Cuadra, G. R. (2006). Perinatal protein malnutrition enhances rewarding cocaine properties in adult rats. *Neuroscience* 137(1): 221–229.

Valdomero, A., Isoardi, N. A., Orsingher, O. A., & Cuadra, G. R. (2005). Pharmacological reactivity to cocaine in adult rats undernourished at perinatal age: Behavioral and neurochemical correlates. *Neuropharmacology* 48(4): 538–546.

Valdomero, A., Velazquez, E. E., de Olmos, S., de Olmos, J. S., Orsingher, O. A., & Cuadra, G. R. (2007). Increased rewarding properties of morphine in perinatally protein-malnourished rats. *Neuroscience* 150(2): 449–458.

van den Buuse, M., Garner, B., Gogos, A., & Kusljic, S. (2005). Importance of animal models in schizophrenia research. *Australian and New Zealand Journal of Psychiatry* 39(7): 550–557.

Vollenweider, F. X., Vollenweider-Scherpenhuyzen, M. F., Babler, A., Vogel, H., & Hell, D. (1998). Psilocybin induces schizophrenia-like psychosis in humans via a serotonin-2 agonist action. *Neuroreport* 9(17): 3897–3902.

Wainfan, E., Dizik, M., Stender, M., & Christman, J. K. (1989). Rapid appearance of hypomethylated DNA in livers of rats fed cancer-promoting, methyl-deficient diets. *Cancer Research* 49(15): 4094–4097.

Watkins, A. J., Ursell, E., Panton, R., Papenbrock, T., Hollis, L., Cunningham, C., Wilkins, A., Perry, V. H., Sheth, B., Kwong, W. Y., et al. (2008a). Adaptive responses by mouse early embryos to maternal diet protect fetal growth but predispose to adult onset disease. *Biological Reproduction* 78(2): 299–306.

Watkins, A. J., Wilkins, A., Cunningham, C., Perry, V. H., Seet, M. J., Osmond, C., Eckert, J. J., Torrens, C., Cagampang, F. R., Cleal, J., et al. (2008b). Low protein diet fed exclusively during mouse oocyte maturation leads to behavioural and cardiovascular abnormalities in offspring. *Journal of Physiology* 586(8): 2231–2244.

Weiner, I. & Arad, M. (2009). Using the pharmacology of latent inhibition to model domains of pathology in schizophrenia and their treatment. *Behavioural Brain Research* 204(2): 369–386.

Weiss, I. C. & Feldon, J. (2001). Environmental animal models for sensorimotor gating deficiencies in schizophrenia: A review. *Psychopharmacology (Berl)* 156(2–3): 305–326.

Whatson, T. S., Smart, J. L., & Dobbing, J. (1975). Dominance relationships among previously undernourished and well fed male rats. *Physiology and Behavior* 14(04): 425–429.

Whatson, T. S., Smart, J. L., & Dobbing, J. (1976). Undernutrition in early life: Lasting effects on activity and social behavior of male and female rats. *Developmental Psychobiology* 9(6): 529–538.

Wiley, J. L. & Compton, A. D. (2004). Progressive ratio performance following challenge with antipsychotics, amphetamine, or NMDA antagonists in adult rats treated perinatally with phencyclidine. *Psychopharmacology (Berl)* 177(1–2): 170–177.

Wolff, G. L., Kodell, R. L., Moore, S. R., & Cooney, C. A. (1998). Maternal epigenetics and methyl supplements affect agouti gene expression in Avy/a mice. *FASEB Journal 12*(11): 949–957.

Xu, M., Wen-Sheng, S., Liu, B., Feng, G., Yu, L., Yang, L., He, G., Sham, P., Susser, E., St Clair, D., et al. (2009). Prenatal malnutrition and adult schizophrenia: Further evidence from the 1959–1961 famine. *Schizophrenia Bulletin 35*(3): 568–576.

Young, J. W., Minassian, A., Paulus, M. P., Geyer, M. A., & Perry, W. (2007). A reverse-translational approach to bipolar disorder: Rodent and human studies in the Behavioral Pattern Monitor. *Neuroscience and Biobehavioral Reviews 31*(6): 882–896.

CHAPTER 13

ANIMAL MODELS OF THE MATERNAL STRESS RISK FACTOR FOR SCHIZOPHRENIA

PAUL H. PATTERSON

KEY CONCEPTS

- Epidemiologic evidence implicates maternal stress as a risk factor for schizophrenia in the offspring.
- In a variety of mammalian species, the offspring of stressed mothers display numerous altered behaviors, depending on the severity and type of the stress, its timing, and the gender of the offspring.
- Many of these behaviors are associated with disturbance of the hypothalamic-pituitary-adrenal axis and are found in human major depressive disorder and schizophrenia.
- Stress-induced elevation of maternal glucocorticoid levels is a major factor in altering fetal brain development, and the fetal brain and the placenta are targets of maternal hormone action.
- Pharmacological and environmental interventions can reverse many of the abnormalities in offspring that are exposed to maternal stress.

Concern for the health of the fetus following maternal stress has existed at least since the age of Hippocrates (Huizink et al., 2004). Highly traumatic events during pregnancy, such as death of a close relative or a severe threat to one's safety, are associated with prematurity and low birth weight in the offspring (Mulder et al., 2002; Gennaro & Hennessy, 2003; Hobel & Culhane, 2003). There is also a report of neural malformations in the offspring of mothers who experienced the death of an older child during the first trimester (Hansen, Lou, & Olsen, 2000). Regarding schizophrenia, epidemiologic studies of an ecologic nature have associated increased risk to the offspring with maternal exposure to any of a variety of stressful events (chapter 4, this book). These studies were not able to examine the risk in individual cases, however. Thus, it is important that a recent study followed the life course of subjects from gestation to adulthood and showed an increased risk for schizophrenia and psychosis in the offspring of mothers exposed to the death of a first-degree relative during the first trimester (Khashan et al., 2008). Other prospective studies reported an association of schizophrenia with unwanted pregnancy or death of the father during gestation (Huttunen & Niskanen, 1978; Myhrman et al., 1996). Maternal stress also increases the risk to the offspring of attentional deficit, hyperactivity, anxiety, and language delay (Talge, Neal, & Glover, 2007; Weinstock, 2008; Goel & Bale, 2009; Schlotz & Phillips, 2009).

It is perhaps surprising that epidemiologic studies have revealed these significant associations, as stress is a highly individual, idiosyncratic experience. What is perceived as very traumatic to one person may be a momentary setback to another. This variation is likely due to genetic background, as well as to prior life experience and available social support systems. Moreover, biomarkers of stress have not been used in these human studies, although cortisol assays have been employed in related work. It is therefore important that experiments with rodent and nonhuman primate models have provided strong support for the overall conclusions of the human studies (reviewed by Koenig, Kirkpatrick, & Lee, 2002; Kofman, 2002; Huizink et al., 2004; Bale, 2005; Viltart & Vanbesien-Mailliot, 2007; Beydoun & Saftlas, 2008; Weinstock, 2008). These animal experiments have defined various factors that can influence the outcome of maternal stress and have described structural changes in the brains of the offspring. Some of the effects of maternal stress even continue beyond the adult offspring, extending to the second generation of progeny (Drake, Walker, & Seckl, 2005). The animal studies have also revealed insights into the mechanisms mediating the effects of maternal stress on the fetus and the resulting behavioral abnormalities in the adult offspring. Most of those experiments have focused on the role of the hypothalamic-pituitary-adrenal (HPA) axis and particularly on glucocorticoids (GC) (figure 13.1).

For brevity, this review cites previous reviews instead of primary articles wherever possible.

Animal Models of Stress

Although in this field the most common terminology used is *prenatal stress*, the present review uses the term *maternal stress* because the former phrase may suggest that the stress is applied directly to the fetus, whereas the latter phrase more precisely describes the manipulation. That is, stress is applied to the mother, whose response may then affect the fetus. The types of animals used in these experiments include rats, mice, voles, guinea pigs, sheep, pigs, and nonhuman primates (rhesus monkeys, common marmosets, and African vervets). Rats have been the overwhelmingly popular choice of subject, with very few studies on mice, which is

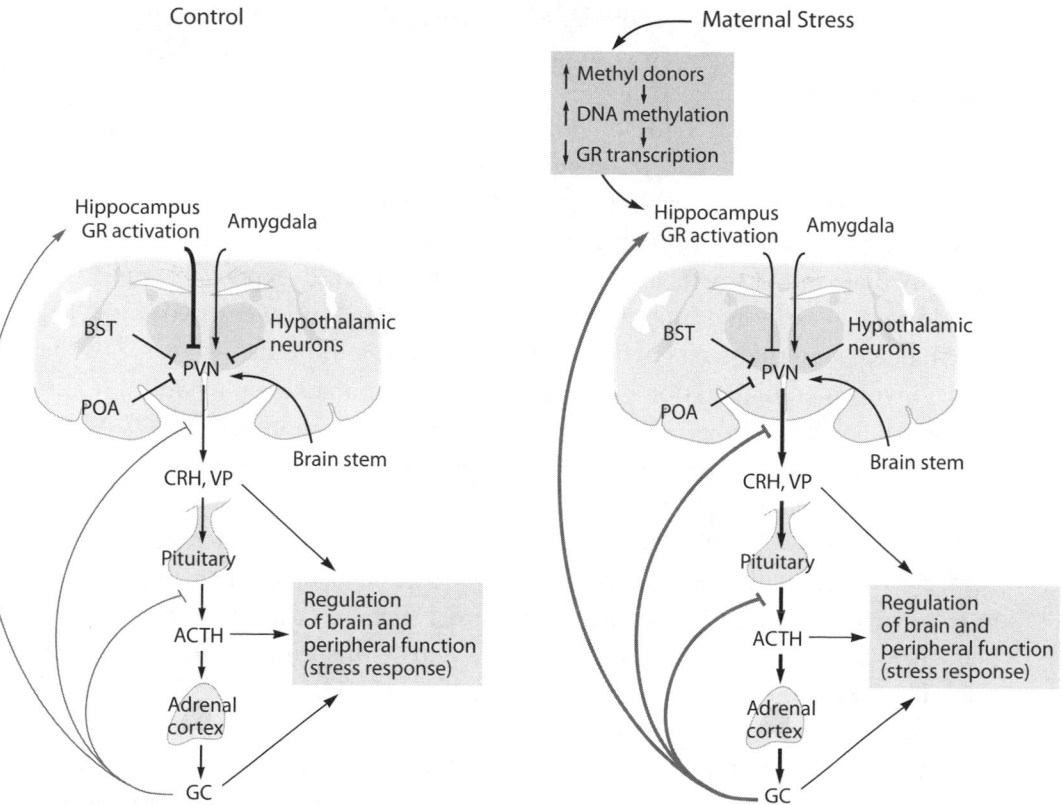

Figure 13.1. Multiple steps of the HPA axis.
A variety of types of stress activate the HPA axis. A central mediator of the stress response is the hypothalamus, where corticotropin-releasing hormone (CRH) and vasopressin are released to act on the anterior pituitary, which releases adrenocorticotropin hormone (ACTH). ACTH stimulates GC release from the adrenal cortex. This hormone mediates the adaptive stress response, but also feeds back at several levels to restore homeostasis. The hippocampus expresses both mineralocorticoid receptors (MR), which are important for controlling basal HPA axis tone and the circadian rhythm, and glucocorticoid receptors (GRs), which operate in the GC concentration range of the stress response. The paraventricular nucleus (PVN) of the hypothalamus expresses predominantly MRs. Stress down-regulates GR expression in the hippocampus and hypothalamus because of feedback by elevated GC levels. Receptor expression is regulated by GC level in a negative feedback manner. Epinephrine and norepinephrine (NE) neurons are activated by maternal stress and stimulate CRH+ neurons in the PVN. BST=bed nucleus of the stria terminalis; POA=preoptic area; VP=vasopressin. (Illustration by Elaine Hsiao.)

surprising given their utility for genetic manipulation. One form of experimental manipulation is termed *psychosocial* or *naturalistic stress*: crowding in the home cage, confrontation with an intruder in the home cage, or exposure to a novel environment or a predator. A novel form of psychological stress involves showing a pregnant rat another rat being subjected to electric shocks on the other side of a transparent wall (Abe et al., 2007). A second category of stress is termed *physical stress*: daily handling, loud noise or acoustic startle stimuli, strobe light stimulation, restraint in a ventilated plastic tube in the presence or absence of bright lights, swimming in water for 15 minutes a day, elevated or cold temperature (4° for six hrs a day), placing the cage or animal on a rotating platform, subcutaneous injection of saline, or electric foot shocks. Variable stress paradigms have also been used, such as restraint, swimming, cold exposure, fasting overnight, overcrowding social stress, lights on overnight, and cold exposure, applied in pseudorandom fashion during three periods of the day for a week (Koenig et al., 2005). Since maternal stress activates the HPA axis, a more defined form of the model involves administration of GC to the mother, mimicking the natural rise in this hormone that follows behavioral stress. This model can utilize the GC that is physiologically relevant for the species of interest, or the synthetic GC, dexamethasone (Dex), which crosses the placenta freely.

The timing of the induction of maternal stress is an important factor in the outcome for the offspring. For instance, hippocampal-dependent learning and memory in rats are influenced by the timing of the stress. Such work has also shown a dependence on the stage of the estrous cycle in female offspring and the sex of the offspring (Goel & Bale, 2009). In guinea pigs, stress applied during the period of rapid brain growth or during very late gestation produces very different effects on HPA axis activity (Kapoor & Matthews, 2008). Stress during the former period causes changes in the hippocampus, hypothalamus, anterior pituitary, and adrenal cortex. The most common treatment window in rat studies is the last week of pregnancy. However, altered behavior has also been seen in the adult offspring of dams exposed to stress as long as two weeks before conception (Shachar-Dadon, 2009). Striking results have also been obtained using variable stress during very early pregnancy in mice (E1-7) (Mueller & Bale, 2008). This is surprising given that the brain has yet not formed at this time, but it is consistent with the epidemiologic study of individual human subjects, which has implicated first-trimester exposure to maternal stress as a risk factor for schizophrenia (Khashan et al., 2008; see chapter 4, this book). This observation underscores the importance of the placenta in the response to maternal stress, and this tissue undergoes key developmental changes during this period. Another point of interest regarding the placenta is that it contains many immune cells (Koga et al., 2009), which is an important but unexplored aspect of how maternal stress evokes immune changes in the offspring. The roles of the placenta and the immune system are considered later in this review.

Effects of Maternal Stress on Offspring Behavior

The adult offspring of animals stressed during pregnancy display a variety of abnormal behaviors, including elevated levels of anxiety and responses to novelty, more learned helplessness in the forced swim test, greater vulnerability to psychostimulants, a phase advance in the circadian rhythm of locomotor activity, and an increase in paradoxical sleep (Talge, Neal, & Glover, 2007; Darnaudery & Maccari, 2008; Thomas et al., 2009). Depending on their gender, age, gestational stage, severity of the stress, and the task, adult offspring can display increased conditioned and context fear conditioning, deficits in play and other social behavior, defensive freezing, learning and memory ability, and long-term potentiation (LTP) (Griffin et al., 2003; Fumagalli et al., 2007; Mueller & Bale, 2007; Darnaudery & Maccari, 2008; Kapoor et al., 2009). Behavioral alterations have also been observed in young pups born to stressed dams (Harmon et al., 2009). Many of these changes, such as increased immobility in the forced swim test, are consistent with behaviors found in human major depressive disorder. Moreover, chronic treatment with antidepressant drugs in the adult offspring can be effective in correcting some of these behaviors in the rat maternal stress model (Morely-Fletcher et al., 2004).

As in schizophrenia, the adult offspring of pregnant rats exposed to variable stress exhibit a deficit in sensorimotor gating, as measured by the N40 auditory evoked response (Koenig et al., 2005). In contrast, in two other behavioral tests with strong relevance for schizophrenia, prepulse inhibition (PPI) and latent inhibition (LI), the results are mixed. Deficits in PPI are found in schizophrenic subjects, and in animal models with relevance to this disorder such as maternal infection, immune activation (Patterson, 2009), and neonatal ventral hippocampus lesion (Lipska & Weinberger, 2000). Moreover, both dopaminergic and glutamatergic psychomimetic drugs disrupt PPI in humans and animals. Using a variable stress paradigm with pregnant rats, Koenig et al. (2005) found a significant PPI deficit in adult male, but not female, offspring. On the other hand, Lehmann, Stohr, and Feldon (2000), using maternal restraint stress, reported increased PPI in male and female offspring, whereas Hauser, Feldon, and Pryce (2006), using the maternal Dex model, reported inconclusive PPI results. Although the different rat strains and maternal stress paradigms used in these studies undermine strict comparisons of the results, the available data do not lend strong support for a PPI deficit in the maternal stress paradigm.

Latent inhibition is another sensorimotor gating assay, but involves a neuroanatomic pathway different from that of PPI. Antipsychotic drugs can potentiate LI in schizophrenic subjects and in animals, and LI is abolished by amphetamine, which exacerbates symptoms in schizophrenia. Moreover, LI is absent in some schizophrenic subjects (Weiner, 2003). Shalev and Weiner (2001) reported that maternal restraint stress has no effect on LI in the adult offspring, whereas maternal foot shock or corticosterone administration leads to a LI deficit in the male, but not female, offspring. On the other hand, Hauser, Feldon, and Pryce (2006), using maternal Dex administration, found no evidence for LI disruption, and Bethus et al. (2005), using maternal restraint, reported an increase in LI in the offspring. If the precise method of maternal stress is critical for producing an LI deficit (Shalev & Weiner, 2001), then these studies cannot be directly compared. Moreover, different assays for LI were used. As with PPI, the available data do not provide significant support for a schizophrenia-like sensorimotor gating deficit in the maternal stress paradigm.

There is an interaction between the severity of maternal stress administered and the gender of the offspring in the outcome of behavioral changes. That is, with mild maternal stress in rats, a selective induction of anxiety in females and learning deficits in males is seen (Zagron & Weinstock, 2006). Male offspring are more likely to display deficits in learning, LTP, hippocampal neurogenesis, and dendritic spine density in the prefrontal cortex and areas CA1 and CA3 of the hippocampus (Weinstock, 2007; Martinez-Tellez et al., 2009). With stronger maternal stress, anxiogenic behavior is observed in both sexes. In fact, female offspring appear to be more prone to exhibit changes in the HPA axis and display depressive-like behavior. Differences have also been reported between the stress responses of the male and female fetal rat hypothalamus and pituitary, including hormone and neurotransmitter release (Ohkawa et al., 1991). Maternal stress in humans also causes abnormal regulation of HPA axis responses in adult female offspring. Cortisol responses are lower in maternal stress-exposed offspring than in controls following a social stress test or adrenocorticotropin hormone (ACTH) injection (Entringer et al., 2009).

Studies of maternal stress in monkeys have revealed several complexities in the analysis of offspring behavior that have not been fully appreciated in rodent work (Coe & Lubach, 2005). For instance, these "emotionally reactive" offspring tend to be lower in the group's social hierarchy as adolescents. This subordinate rank may magnify their emotionality, or may induce novel behaviors on its own. Because social rank also affects the stress response in rodents (e.g., Bartolomucci et al., 2005; Barnum, Blandino, & Deak, 2008), this could be important for a number of behavioral tests relevant for schizophrenia, such as social interaction.

Effects of Maternal Stress on Brain Development in the Offspring

A logical starting point for study of the effects of maternal stress on brain development in the offspring is the fetus. Compared with work on adult offspring, however, far less has been done on the question of how various parts of the fetal brain are altered in the early, critical stages of development. It is known that maternal stress during the last week of gestation in the rat elevates circulating GC and catecholamine levels in the fetus (Weinstock, 2007). Maternal plasma free tryptophan is also elevated, which is associated with increased fetal brain tryptophan and serotonin (5-HT) (Peters, 1990). These increases are stable until at least postnatal day 10. Time course studies estimated that the critical period for maternal stress-induced changes in brain 5-HT neurons is between E15 and birth (Peters, 1989). Cross-fostering experiments also revealed, however, that the effects of maternal stress are strongly influenced by the postnatal rearing environment (Peters, 1988). In a paradigm that tests three different levels of severity of maternal stress just before birth, increases in neuronal activity, as assessed by cFos upregulation, in the fetal paraventricular nucleus (PVN) of the hypothalamus were observed in direct relation to the amount of increase in maternal corticosterone (Fujioka et al., 2003). In the more severe stress condition, more apoptotic cells are apparent, and corticotrophin releasing hormone (CRH) is decreased, as is the total length of PVN neuronal processes. It is interesting that it was reported that short-duration, mild maternal stress has the opposite effect of strong stress: mild stress can enhance learning and LTP in adult offspring and increase neurogenesis and neuronal differentiation in the hippocampus of neonatal offspring (Fujioka et al., 2006). Another study reported that when maternal stress was applied during the last week of gestation, CRH and α-endorphin decrease in the fetal hypothalamus (Ohkawa et al., 1991). In contrast, a very short period of stress elevates CRH expression in the fetal PVN, and CRH+ neurons achieve a more mature morphology (Fujioka et al., 1999). Thus, it appears that a brief period of maternal stress may stimulate differentiation, whereas more chronic or severe stress is toxic to the fetal PVN (see figure 13.2).

It is therefore interesting that maternal stress activates epinephrine and norepinephrine (NE) neurons that stimulate CRH+ neurons in the PVN. Moreover, maternal Dex injection enhances the maturity of fetal NE neurons and their projections and induces expression of the NE transporter (Owen, Andrews, & Matthews, 2005). CRH receptors in the adult offspring cortex are elevated over those of controls, and spine frequencies and dendrite complexity in layer II/III pyramidal neurons of the anterior cingulate and orbitofrontal cortex are reduced. Serotonergic neurons also directly innervate and stimulate PVN CRH+ neurons. Maternal injection of Dex promotes 5-HT transporter development and increases hypothalamic 5-HT levels (Owen, Andrews, & Matthews, 2005). Maternal stress also induces a chronic astroglial reaction in adult offspring, which could be indicative of inflammation (Barros et al., 2006). If so, it would be a key finding. However, another study reported a reduction in hippocampal S100B, an astrocyte protein (Van den Hove et al., 2006). Synthetic GC promotes early maturation of dopamine (DA) and altered γ-aminobutyric acid (GABA) systems in the forebrain of adult rat offspring (Owen, Andrews, & Matthews, 2005). An altered inhibitory pathway is also suggested by the finding that infant and adult male offspring of stressed dams display an increased rate of kindling-induced seizures (Edwards et al., 2002). In a human study, the offspring of pregnant women treated with Dex score higher than normal on tests of emotionality, avoidance, and shyness (Trautman et al., 1996).

A typical feature of maternal stress is that the adult offspring do not regulate glucocorticoid receptor (GR) expression properly in response to increased GC.

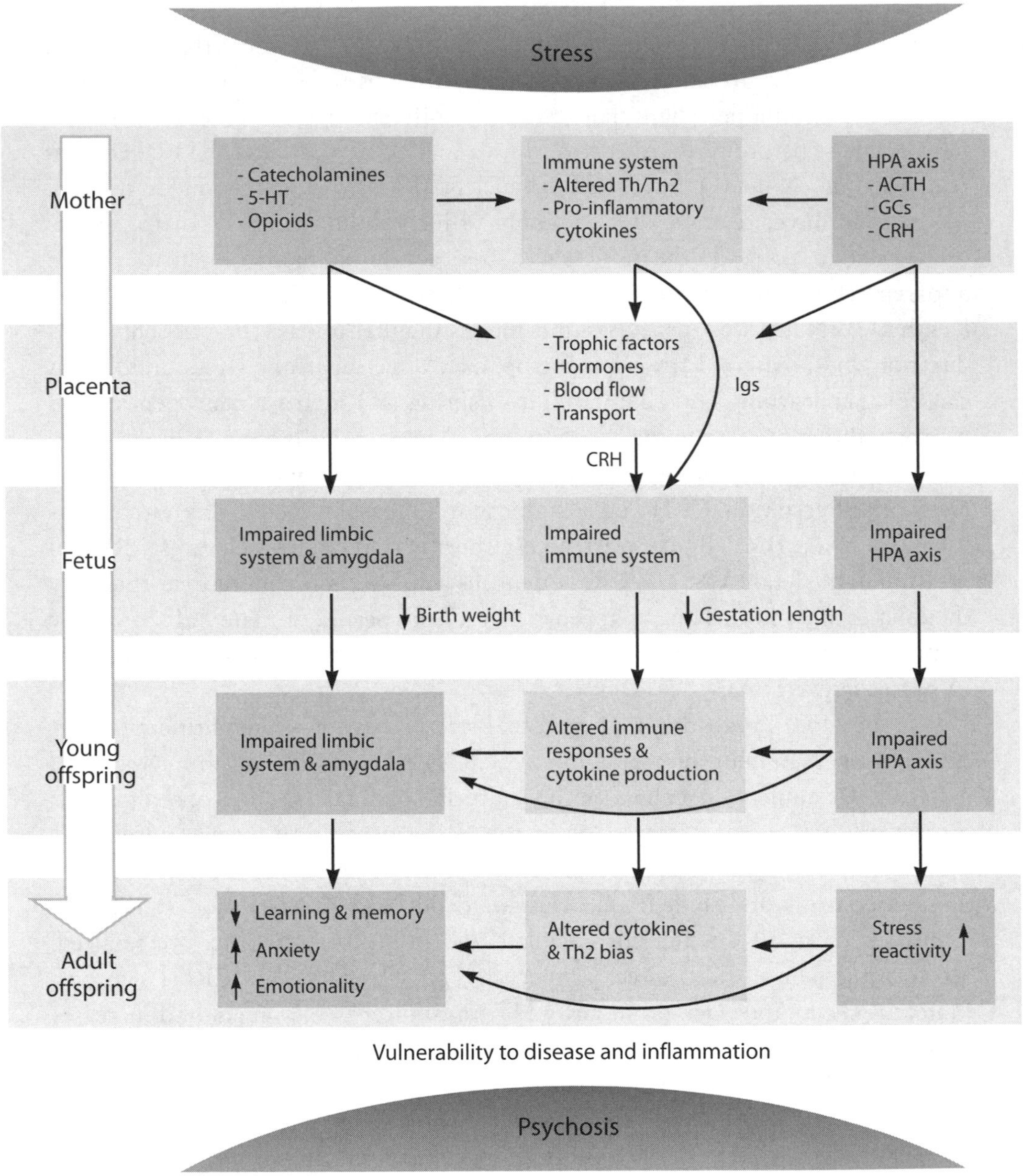

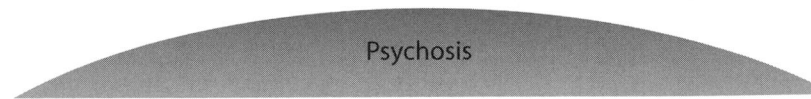

Figure 13.2. Pathways that mediate the effects of maternal stress on the offspring.
Stress impacts not only the HPA axis, but also the immune system and several neuronal
pathways. The immune system is, in turn, affected by changes in the neuronal pathways and
the HPA axis. All three systems can alter placental functions, including glucose and iron
transport, and they can likely influence fetal development directly as well. The most obvious
readouts of these changes are lower birth weight and premature birth. Changes in offspring
development can be detected at young ages, leading to altered behavior, immune balance,
and stress reactivity in adulthood. There is also increased vulnerability to inflammation and
disease, including psychosis. (Illustration by Elaine Hsiao.)

That is, there is reduced feedback in the HPA axis. Although studies of adult rat offspring have produced mixed results regarding specific changes caused by maternal stress, the data have consistently shown that induced changes in HPA axis activity are correlated with abnormalities in hippocampal negative feedback. In fact, the feedback inhibitory control is altered even in the affected fetus. In a study of fetal responses to maternal Dex injections from E17–E19, no downregulation of GRs was found in the forebrain (Slotkin et al., 2008). Another interesting observation is that late, brief maternal restraint stress decreases fetal pH, which is consistent with a hypoxic condition. In a further parallel with hypoxia, fetal plasma corticosterone and ACTH are increased (Fan et al., 2009). This provides a link to another risk factor for schizophrenia: obstetric complications in late pregnancy (see chapter 3, this book).

The amygdala perceives threats such as stressors, and through its connections with the hypothalamus it stimulates the HPA axis. The amygdala is altered in the adult offspring of stressed dams (Weinstock, 2007). The lateral nucleus is larger, with more neurons expressing nitric oxide synthase. There are also differences in the number of neurons and glia in the basolateral, central, and lateral nuclei in male offspring, and there is an increase in CRH expression in the central nucleus, as well as decreased GRs in the hippocampus (Mueller & Bale, 2008). The levels of CRH are elevated in the amygdala of the male offspring, which is relevant for their increased emotionality (Cratty et al., 1995). Cytokines of the bone morphogenetic protein (BMP) family may play a role in mediating the effects of maternal stress on the amygdala. Smad-1 transduces signaling of several BMPs, and its expression in the lateral and basolateral nuclei of the amygdala is increased in the offspring of stressed rats, whereas its response to stress in those offspring is blunted (Kaur & Salm, 2008). Further work will be necessary to assess whether BMPs are involved in the maternal stress-induced structural changes in the amygdala and the altered fear responses mediated by the amygdala.

The hippocampus displays a remarkable degree of functional and structural plasticity in response to maternal stress and GCs. There is an altered immediate early gene response to adult stress (Mairesse et al., 2007; Viltart & Vanbesien-Mailliot, 2007), which is consistent with reduced GR expression. Expression of the postsynaptic protein, homer, is altered by maternal stress (Ary et al., 2007). There is a report of reduced 5-HT transporter expression in hippocampal CA1, as well as increased levels of 5-HT receptors (Peters, 1990), both of which could underlie a greater sensitivity to citalopram, a selective 5-HT uptake inhibitor used in several assays of depressive-like behavior. A more recent study found, however, that 5-HT1A receptor levels are decreased in the region of the hippocampus involved in emotion (ventral hippocampus) but unchanged in the region involved in learning (dorsal hippocampus). Expression of 5-HT2A is not altered in either area (Van den Hove et al., 2006). Synthetic GC administration increases hypothalamic

5-HT levels and reduces 5-HT turnover in the hippocampus (Owen, Andrews, & Matthews, 2005).

Given the long-standing DA hypothesis of schizophrenia, it is important to consider the effects of maternal stress on this transmitter pathway. Positron emission tomography (PET) of young adult monkeys born to stressed mothers suggests lower DA decarboxylase and up-regulation of D2 DA receptors in the striatum. Moreover, these changes are correlated with fearful and stereotypic behaviors (Roberts et al., 2004). In contrast, down-regulation of D2 receptors is seen in the striatum of adult male mouse offspring following prolonged maternal stress. The latter study also reported increased DA turnover in striatum and lower levels of the DA transporter in both striatum and substantia-ventral tegmentum area (Son et al., 2006). In rat offspring, DA turnover is increased in female offspring, while 5-HT turnover is decreased in male offspring. In freely moving adult rat offspring of stressed dams, both basal and intraperitoneal amphetamine-induced stimulation of DA and NE output in the nucleus accumbens is higher than in controls (Silvagni et al., 2008). Increases in D2 and N-methyl-D-aspartate (NMDA) receptors in the medial and dorsal prefrontal cortices, the nucleus accumbens, and hippocampal area CA1 are found in male offspring (Henry et al., 1995; Weinstock, 2007). Moreover, phosphorylation of NMDA receptor subunits NR1 and NR2B in the prefrontal cortex in response to acute stress in adulthood is attenuated in male offspring of stressed dams (Fumagalli et al., 2009). This could be part of the molecular basis for altered feedback inhibition in the HPA stress response. It is clear that NMDA- and AMPA (2-amino-3-(5-methyl-3-oxo-1,2-oxazol-4-yl)propanoic acid)-mediated currents regulate synaptic potentiation and learning by way of GRs (e.g., Yuen et al., 2009). Regarding the relevance of D2 receptor up-regulation for schizophrenia, meta-analyses have concluded that D2 density may be only slightly elevated in the striatum of a subset of patients (Howes et al., 2009). Nonetheless, several of the observations on DA, coupled with the changes in relevant DA-mediated behaviors, can be interpreted as being consistent with a hyperdopaminergic state in schizophrenia. Ultimately, the most relevant comparisons with the human studies would be with D2 receptor occupancy and DA release in the animal striatum.

Maternal stress in rhesus monkeys decreases neurogenesis in the dentate gyrus and synapse number in the hippocampus of adult offspring, and there is a 10% decrease in hippocampal volume (Coe et al., 2003). Maternal Dex administration also reduces cell proliferation in the dentate gyrus of neonatal offspring (Tauber et al., 2006). Maternal stress in rats causes an accelerated decline in hippocampal neurogenesis with age, which is accompanied by a decrease in granule cells and is correlated with a deficit in learning in the water maze. Unlike the case with controls, there is also a failure to increase production of new neurons with training in the maze (Lemaire et al., 2000; Koehl et al., 2009). Maternal administration of Dex also reduces hippocampal size (Uno et al., 1990), and maternal stress reduces the number of granule neurons in the dentate gyrus of female rat offspring (Weinstock, 2007). In rats bred for high—but not for low—anxiety, maternal stress reduces postnatal neurogenesis in the hippocampus (Lucassen et al., 2009). Maternal stress in the rat also decreases incorporation of the cell proliferation marker, BrdU, in the fetal hippocampus and nucleus accumbens (Kawamura et al., 2006). In a human study, adult neural stem cell proliferation apparently is decreased in schizophrenia but not in depression (Reif et al., 2007).

Another putative risk factor for schizophrenia is maternal iron deficiency, which is mechanistically linked to two other such risk factors, fetal hypoxia and nutritional deprivation (Insel et al., 2008). Iron-deficient infants and children display motor and cognitive deficits in common with children who later develop schizophrenia. Moreover, iron deficiency affects aspects of the brain that are altered in schizophrenia, such as DA transmission and myelination. Thus, it is of interest that mild stress during pregnancy in monkeys results in offspring that are more vulnerable to developing iron deficiency anemia between four and eight months of age (Coe et al., 2009). Although the mechanism of this phenomenon is not yet known, it is likely that there is diminished transfer of iron from the mother to the embryo during gestation. When stressed mothers and offspring are maintained under limited iron in the diet, the one-year-olds display lower DA and higher NE levels than controls raised on the same diet.

Molecular Mediators of Maternal Stress

Much of the work on the mechanism of how maternal stress alters fetal development has been devoted to the role of the HPA axis (figure 13.1). This is largely because GC secretion is a key biological response to stress, and this hormone can exert profound effects on brain development. A particular target of GCs is the hippocampus, which expresses the highest levels of GRs in the brain. It is clear that the increase in maternal GC induced by maternal stress plays a major role in subsequent reactions to stress by the adult offspring. This was shown directly by experiments in rats in which GC levels in the dam were controlled by adrenalectomy followed by implantation of a pellet that released basal levels of GCs. Subcutaneous injection of GC was then used to increase its level to that seen in maternal stress. The adult offspring were tested for their stress response by measuring the GC response to restraint stress. The positive control yielded the expected results; raising GC levels in adrenalectomized dams up to the levels seen with maternal stress results in a normal, prolonged GC induction by stress in adult offspring as well as decreased GR levels. In contrast, the offspring of dams that were stressed, but whose GC levels were maintained at basal levels, do not display the expected, prolonged GC response to restraint stress as adults. Moreover, these offspring do not display the normal decrease in hippocampal GRs (Barbazanges et al., 1996).

Maternal adrenalectomy before stress also abolishes anxiogenic behavior and spatial memory deficits in the offspring (Zagron & Weinstock, 2006). In addition, maternal GC pellets increase GC levels, locomotor activity, and basal DA metabolism in the offspring (Fumagalli et al., 2007). In a similar manipulation, maternal ACTH administration can also mimic some of the behaviors induced by maternal stress. It will be critically important to use direct manipulations of GC levels to test if other behavioral deficits, as well as the neurochemical and neuropathologic abnormalities observed in maternal stress, are also controlled by maternal GC.

There are, however, some issues in applying this model to humans. For instance, the maternal GC response to stress decreases significantly during human pregnancy, becoming rather low by late pregnancy. Thus, at a time when there appears to be the strongest link between maternal and fetal GC levels, the maternal HPA axis is less sensitive to stress (Talge, Neal, & Glover, 2007). It is interesting that the maternal emotional state is very rapidly reflected in fetal behavior and heart rate, which is not easily explained by the slower responses of the HPA axis (Talge, Neal, & Glover, 2007). This rapid response could be mediated by the known activation of the sympathetic nervous system by stress, and unmetabolized NE can cross the placenta. Another indication for a role for catecholamines is the finding that the expected spatial learning deficits can be prevented by administration of the α-adrenergic receptor blocker, propranolol, to the pregnant rat during stress.

Cytokines may also be relevant, as physical stress such as immobilization or inescapable tail shock can increase interleukin-1 (IL-1)α in the brain, and central administration of an IL-1 receptor antagonist prevents stress-induced changes in behavior as well as altered NE, DA, and 5-HT release and plasma ACTH levels (Plata-Salaman et al., 2000). In pregnant women, stress increases plasma tumor necrosis factor (TNF)-α and IL-6, while decreasing IL-10 (Coussons-Read, Okun, & Nettles, 2007). In pregnant mice, maternal stress reduces progesterone, which influences cytokine expression in the blood and decidua (Joachim et al., 2003; Blois et al., 2004). Unfortunately, little is known about cytokine changes in the fetal brain induced by maternal stress. It is likely that such alterations occur, as they do in the related syndrome of maternal immune activation (Patterson, 2009; chapter 10, this book).

The placenta is another important candidate tissue for mediating the effects of maternal stress on the fetus. This is particularly true for the early pregnancy stress paradigm, in which stress is administered before the fetal brain has developed. The placental connection to GCs is particularly important because these hormones regulate placental size, histology, blood flow, and nutrient transporter and hormone expression (Fowden & Forhead, 2009). Moreover, a high percentage of maternal GC is inactivated by 11α-hydroxysteroid dehydrogenase type 2 (11βHSD2) in the placenta. This enzyme normally protects the fetus by breaking down the hormone, but its level is reduced by maternal stress (Darnaudery & Maccari, 2008). Thus, in many species, fetal GC concentrations parallel maternal levels during stress (Fowden & Forhead, 2009). Although maternal injection of Dex, which is not degraded by 11βHSD2, is very effective in inducing altered behavior in the offspring, late-gestation Dex treatment increases the glucose transporters (GLUTs) 1 and 3 in the placenta (Langdown & Sugden, 2001). The latter observation is inconsistent with findings that maternal stress in late gestation reduces placental 11α-HSD2 and GLUT1 expression (Mairesse et al., 2007). The GLUT1 reduction is also obtained by genetically deleting 11βHSD2 (Wyrwoll, Seckl, & Holmes, 2009). Moreover, another synthetic GC, triamcinolone, downregulates GLUT1 and 3. Inhibition of 11βHSD2 during gestation produces permanent alterations in the HPA axis and anxiety-like behavior in the offspring (Welberg, Seckl, & Holmes, 2000). In a different paradigm, a failure to increase placental 11βHSD2 after maternal stress is correlated with decreased neurogenesis in the adult offspring (Lucassen et al., 2009). Overall, these observations support the hypothesis that 11βHSD2 protects the fetus from sharp increases in maternal GC such as those that occur during maternal stress. Nonetheless, maternal stress does increase GC levels in the fetus, at least during the final week of gestation in the rat. It is also interesting that another putative risk factor for schizophrenia, maternal malnutrition (see chapter 2, this book), reduces the activity of this enzyme (Fowden & Forhead, 2009), suggesting the possibility that some of the effects of malnutrition could be mediated by maternal GCs.

In the early maternal stress model in mice, placentae of male fetuses exhibit increased levels of peroxisome proliferator-activated receptor (PPAR)α, insulin-like growth factor binding protein (IGFBP)-1, GLUT4, and hypoxia-inducible factor 3a. In contrast, female placentae display a reduced PPARα and IGFBP-1 (Mueller & Bale, 2008). PPARα expression is relevant because it regulates many cellular processes during development and is responsive to GC levels. It also regulates IGFBP-1. Given that methylation is critically important in models of postnatal stress, it is of interest that expression of DNA methyl transferase 1 (DNMT1), an enzyme involved in maintenance of methylation, is significantly lower in normal male placentae than in female placentae. Moreover, maternal stress appears to increase DNMT1 in female placentae more than in male placentae (Mueller & Bale, 2008). This suggests that the female placenta may be better able to maintain methylation under stress. In addition, hippocampal CRH and GR expression and methylation levels are altered by maternal stress in a sex-specific manner. The placenta also expresses CRH, and this is increased by GCs, unlike hypothalamic CRH expression, which is decreased by GCs (Robinson et al., 1988; King, Smith & Nicholson, 2001).

Catecholamines are important mediators of the maternal stress response, and the sympathetic nervous system plays a role in embryo implantation. Later in development, some of the maternal NE elevated by stress is not metabolized and constricts placental blood flow and glucose supply. It also activates the fetal HPA axis (Bellinger, Lubahn, & Lorton, 2008). Maternal NE is critical, as experiments with genetic deletion of DA decarboxylase suggest that NE crossing the placenta is required for survival (Thomas, Matsumoto, & Palmiter, 1995). Injection of NE into the third ventricle to stimulate the hypothalamus results in a prolonged increase in plasma GC in male but not female offspring of stressed dams. Thus, maternal stress affects activation of the HPA axis differently in male and female offspring (Reznikov, Nosenko, & Tarasenko, 1999).

Neurotrophins are secreted proteins that regulate synaptic plasticity in adulthood as well as many events during development, including neuronal survival and growth. Expression of some of them has also been found to be altered in schizophrenia. Thus, it is of interest that maternal stress results in reduced levels of brain-derived neurotrophic factor (BDNF) and basic fibroblast growth factor (FGF-2) in the prefrontal cortex of adult rat offspring. In addition, BDNF and FGF-2 expression in these offspring responds very differently to stress in adulthood than it does in controls (Fumagalli et al., 2007). Alterations in neurotrophin levels could underlie some of the neuropathology as well as changes in neurogenesis observed in the offspring of stressed dams. Evidence for a role for GCs in mediating the inhibition of cell proliferation and neurogenesis in the hippocampus caused by stress in the adult is contradictory (Mirescu & Gould, 2006).

The level of postnatal maternal care strongly affects epigenetic regulation of GR expression in the hippocampus. Methylation of DNA upstream of the GR gene is altered by maternal care, and this determines the adult response to stress (Szyf, McGowan, & Meaney, 2008). Similar experiments are starting to be done in a mouse model of maternal stress. Adult male offspring of dams exposed to stress during early pregnancy (E1-7) exhibit reduction in methylation in the CRH promoter, which is correlated with increased CRH expression in the central nucleus of the amygdala. Conversely, there is an increase in methylation of the GR promoter that correlates with a decrease in hippocampal GR expression (Mueller & Bale, 2008). These findings are also consistent with increased GC levels in these offspring.

Involvement of the Immune System

Work with nonhuman primates has revealed changes outside the nervous system that have relevance for behavior. For instance, almost all cells in the immune system have receptors for one or more of the hormones associated with the HPA axis, and mild maternal stress alters the immune system of the offspring (Coe & Lubach, 2005). In neonates, the proliferative response of mononuclear cells to antigens in vitro is deficient if the mother was stressed during late pregnancy, but it is greater than that of controls if the mother was stressed during early pregnancy. Administration of Dex during late pregnancy also decreases the response to antigens in the offspring. Maternal administration of ACTH reduces suppressor T cell activity measured in vitro in offspring that are one to two months old. These findings are consistent with the known ability of the HPA axis to modulate the immune system, and there is a moderate increase in cortisol levels in this monkey stress paradigm. On the other hand, ACTH does not cross the placenta at this stage, so action on the placenta is a possible intermediate mechanism. As already mentioned here, the placenta is a source of CRH, which can activate the fetal HPA axis to increase fetal GC levels (Challis et al., 2000). Natural killer cell activity is reduced in six-month-old offspring of stressed mothers, and at two years of age leukocytes display reduced proinflammatory responses to bacterial lipopolysaccharide in vitro. In a further indication of reduced immune status, maternal social stress lowers the level of maternal antibody in the newborn serum. This is important because the transfer of maternal IgG across the placenta during late pregnancy produces passive immunity in the infant against bacteria and viruses previously encountered by the mother. It is relevant that GCs can alter gut development, affecting the uptake of maternal immunoglobulin from the colostrum (Bellinger, Lubahn, & Lorton, 2008). Some of these changes in the immune system likely contribute to the greatly increased frequency of Shigella infections in these infants (Coe & Lubach, 2005). Altered immunity could also contribute to the observed changes in the species composition of commensal enteric bacteria in these animals. All of these phenomena are relevant for behavior because infection alters behavior, and there are striking changes in the both the immune system and the expression of immune-related molecules in the brains of schizophrenic subjects (Patterson, 2009).

In contrast to the status of the immune system in the monkey work, the picture with other mammals is mixed (Bellinger, Lubahn, & Lorton, 2008; Kohman et al., 2008; Merlot, Couret, & Otten, 2008). A study on adult offspring of stressed rats provided evidence of an enhanced immune status: increases in natural killer cells and CD8+ cells, and elevated proliferative and interferon (IFN)-γ responses to the phytohemagglutinin antigen (PHA). Surprisingly, these effects are not seen in the young offspring (Vanbesien-Mailliot et al., 2007). The latter result may explain at least some of the conflicting data from other studies on young rodents. Laviola et al. (2004) reported that juvenile offspring of stressed dams exhibit an exaggerated drop in CD4+ cells in response to the immunosuppressant cyclophosphamide. The various laboratories that conduct these studies use different intensities and timing of maternal stress. In adult rats, at least, acute stress enhances immune function whereas chronic stress suppresses it (Dhabhar & McEwen, 1997). In terms of the mechanism for how immune cells are altered by maternal stress, it is interesting that peritoneal macrophages taken from adult offspring of stressed pregnant mice display reduced phagocytosis, which can be corrected by maternal injection of the opioid antagonist naloxone (Fonseca et al., 2005).

Although there appears to be only a single human study of immune function in the offspring of stressed mothers, its findings agree with some of the animal work. In a study of healthy adult women born to mothers who experienced a major negative life event during pregnancy, cytokines from peripheral blood mononuclear cells were measured following PHA stimulation (Entringer et al., 2008). An elevation of IL-4, IL-6, and IL-10 without apparent change in IFN-γ suggests a bias toward T helper cell 2 (Th2) cytokine production. This is similar to findings with chronically depressed subjects. The women in this study, however, scored in the normal range in tests for depression and neuroticism, as well as in birth weight, postnatal care, and trauma experiences. Glucocorticoids can cause a shift from the Th1 to Th2 state, which favors humoral over cellular immunity. The Th2 bias is also similar to findings with maternal stress in mice (Pincus-Knackstedt et al., 2006), and adult offspring of stressed rats are reported to exhibit increased IL-10 and IL-6, although the results in various rat experiments are mixed, as already discussed here. If a bias toward a Th2 state is valid, there is a parallel with immune dysfunction in schizophrenia, where some reports have found evidence of such a bias in peripheral immune cells (Muller & Schwarz, 2008). Other consequences of a Th2 bias include increased susceptibility to atopic diseases such as asthma, eczema, and food allergies, as well as systemic lupus erythematosus.

Reversing the Effects of Maternal Stress

Although the effects of maternal stress can be long-lasting, postnatal manipulations such as handling, environmental enrichment, treatment with a 5-HT reuptake inhibitor, or cross-fostering to a control dam can ameliorate or reverse many of these effects (Fox, Merali, & Harrison, 2006; Laviola et al., 2008). Cross-fostering reverses maternal stress-induced abnormalities such as increased fearfulness in the defensive withdrawal test (Qian et al., 2008), deficits in spatial learning and hippocampal type 1 GRs, and the prolonged GC response to novelty (Maccari et al., 1995; Brabham et al., 2000), as well as elevated D2 receptor levels (Barros et al., 2006). In one negative finding from a study using a different rat strain and method of maternal stress, cross-fostering had no effect on the social interaction deficit in males born to stressed dams (Lee et al., 2007). In the human literature, some studies have also distinguished effects on the offspring due to prenatal versus postnatal stress in the mother (Fumagalli et al., 2007; Talge, Neal, & Glover, 2007). The rescue of behavioral deficits by cross-fostering is particularly important, as it indicates that this procedure is necessary to determine which of the many effects of that maternal stress has on the offspring are due to prenatal rather than postnatal factors. Unfortunately, this has been done in only a small fraction of experiments. On the other hand, in the natural course of events, stress on the mother during pregnancy could continue to alter her later maternal behavior. Thus, using the same stressed dam to raise her litter is more relevant to the normal situation. It is primarily in mechanistic studies that cross-fostering becomes important.

The effect of environmental enrichment is of great interest from a therapeutic point of view. Providing adolescent offspring of stressed dams a larger cage with many novel objects, places to hide, and a running wheel almost completely reverses the deficit in play behavior and hypersecretion of GC in response to acute restraint stress (Morely-Fletcher et al., 2003); depressive-like behavior in the forced swim test and morphine-induced place behavior (Yang et al., 2006); and several parameters of immune status (Laviola et al., 2004). Moreover, housing the pregnant mouse in an enriched environment also significantly attenuates the effects of maternal stress on hippocampal cell proliferation and open field behavior (Maruoka et al., 2009). An important question is whether all of these effects of environmental enrichment could be explained by exercise on the running wheel (or adoption of a healthier lifestyle), which is the case for the effect of an enriched environment on adult hippocampal neurogenesis, for instance (Pereira et al., 2007). Early postnatal manipulation of the pups can also block the adverse effects of maternal stress on the survival of newborn cells as well as the number of immature and differentiated new neurons in the hippocampus (Lemaire et al., 2006). In this case, rat pups were removed to a clean cage with a heating lamp for 15 minutes a day, from birth until weaning. Although this treatment is termed *handling*, it can also be seen as a less severe form of the maternal separation stress paradigm. Nonetheless, this handling procedure has very positive effects on neurogenesis.

While the striking success of these various postnatal manipulations in blocking (or reversing) the effects of maternal stress is encouraging from the therapeutic point of view, the results also raise several provocative questions. Does the success of the seemingly very diverse postnatal manipulations of the environment suggest that the maternal stress model lacks robustness? Does it highlight the extreme poverty of the typical home cage environment? The early postnatal environment of the typical human is vastly more enriched than the typical laboratory animal, and the experience of a woman during what we would term a stressful pregnancy would seem to be far less harsh than that used in the physical stress applied to laboratory rats. Would we then expect that laboratory animals exhibit far more severe and irreversible symptoms than those expected for humans? The problem with these questions is that it is extremely difficult to compare the human brain's response to psychologic stress, and the human symptoms of depression or schizophrenia, to those in laboratory animals, especially rodents.

Given that the maternal stress model has face validity for depression, several groups have tested antidepressant medications in this paradigm. Chronic administration of the tricyclic imipramine to adult offspring of stressed dams completely reverses their increased immobility in the forced swim test, as well as their elevated 5-HT1A mRNA expression in the frontal cortex (Morely-Fletcher et al., 2004). Postnatal administration of the selective 5-HT uptake inhibitor fluoxetine normalizes the increased GC response to restraint stress, the 5-HT turnover in the hippocampus, and the decreased dendritic spine density and synapses on CA3 pyramidal cells, and partially restores learning in the water maze test (Ishiwata, Shiga, & Okado, 2005). Tianeptine, which unlike other antidepressants, increases neuronal 5-HT uptake, reduces immobility in the forced swim test (Morely-Fletcher et al., 2003). A recent study compared several antidepressant drugs and found that imipramine, fluoxetine, tianeptine, and mirtazapine all decreased immobility time in the forced swim test, increased time in the center of the open field, and lowered stress-induced plasma GC and hippocampal GR levels (Szymanska et al., 2009). These results with drugs of various known mechanisms of action further confirm the face, construct, and predictive value of the maternal stress model for depression. One surprising result of this study is that GC and GR levels are elevated in the offspring of stressed dams, which is inconsistent with the lack of GC feedback inhibition during HPA axis hyperactivity. The finding is, however, consistent with known GC-driven hippocampal atrophy.

Neuropeptides have also been used to reverse abnormal behaviors in offspring of stressed dams. The deficits in social interaction displayed by such offspring suggest that there could be an alteration in the neuropeptide systems that regulate this behavior. Oxytocin is one such peptide that is expressed in the PVN and activates neurons in the central nucleus of the amygdala, promoting social behavior (Huber, Veinante, & Stoop, 2005; Hammock & Young, 2006). Thus, it is of interest that adult male offspring of stressed dams display a deficit in oxytocin expression and an increase in oxytocin binding in that nucleus in the amygdala. Moreover, injection of this neuropeptide into the central amygdala during a 10-minute behavioral testing period enhances social interaction in these offspring in a dose-dependent manner (Lee et al., 2007). Controls included injection of saline and vasopressin. This experiment is important for understanding the mechanism of how maternal stress alters a behavior and has clear relevance to social withdrawal in schizophrenia.

Major Depression Versus Schizophrenia

An intriguing question is whether animal models of maternal stress exhibit more features of major depression or schizophrenia. Certainly the adult offspring exhibit clear features of depression: early immobility in the forced swim test, alleviated by antidepressant drugs; enhanced emotionality; vulnerability to drugs of abuse; circadian disturbances; and an activated HPA axis. These symptoms are also shared with schizoaffective disorder, with its combination of mood disorder coupled with features of schizophrenia. There is also a significant body of evidence that schizophrenia is associated with elevated and pharmacologically induced HPA axis activity. Moreover, antipsychotic drugs reduce HPA axis activity (Walker, Mittal, & Tessner, 2007). Hippocampal volume is also reduced early in schizophrenia, which could be a sign of elevated GC toxicity. There is some evidence of reduced GR expression and increased pituitary volume as well, suggesting dysfunction in the HPA axis feedback system (Walker, Mittal, & Tessner, 2007; Takahashi et al., 2009). Although there appear to be some similarities with regard to these HPA-related phenotypes in schizophrenia and major depression, there are clearly many differences, including the presence of positive symptoms such as hallucinations and delusions, which occur only rarely in major depression. Until experimenters overcome the obstacles of assaying these symptoms in animals, however, it will be difficult to define animal models such as maternal stress more precisely using behavioral criteria. On the other hand, there are neurochemical features of the maternal stress offspring that are consistent with schizophrenia, and it may be highly informative when the most common neuromorphologic finding in schizophrenia, enlarged ventricles, is examined in this model.

KEY AREAS FOR FUTURE RESEARCH

- Future epidemiologic studies could assay for biomarkers of stress in archived maternal serum samples so as to establish objective, quantitative measures of the response to life events.
- Examining the genetic background of both the mother and offspring may also be revealing, both for subdividing the maternal population into various risk categories and for aiding in the identification of genes that confer risk to this environmental factor.
- Study of cardinal signs of schizophrenia pathology, such as ventricular enlargement and DA-related changes, should be performed in animal models of maternal stress, as well as more study of behaviors relevant for schizophrenia, such as cognitive function, PPI, LI, and amphetamine-induced activity.
- Because it is clear that maternal stress alters the immune system of the offspring, it will be informative to assay cytokines in the fetal brain and placenta in this paradigm.
- Inducing maternal stress in mice that express mutations of schizophrenia candidate genes could provide insight into gene-environment interactions.

Acknowledgments

Thanks to Elaine Hsiao for the figures, and for her and Alan Brown's helpful comments on the manuscript, and to Laura Rodriguez for editing assistance.

Selected Readings

Barbazanges, A., Piazza, P. V., Le Moal, M., & Maccari, S. (1996). Maternal glucocorticoid secretion mediates long-term effects of prenatal stress. *Journal of Neuroscience 16*(12): 3943–3949.

Khashan, A. S., Abel, K. M., McNamee, R., Pedersen, M. G., Webb, R. T., Baker, P. N., Kenny, L. C., & Mortensen, P. B. (2008). Higher risk of offspring schizophrenia following antenatal maternal exposure to severe adverse life events. *Archives of General Psychiatry 65*(2): 146–152.

Schlotz, W. & Phillips, D. I. (2009). Fetal origins of mental health: Evidence and mechanisms. *Brain, Behavior, and Immunity 23*(7): 905–916.

Weinstock, M. (2008). The long-term behavioural consequences of prenatal stress. *Neuroscience and Biobehavioral Reviews 32*(6): 1073–1086.

References

Abe, H., Hidaka, N., Kawagoe, C., Odagiri, K., Watanabe, Y., Ikeda, T., Ishizuka, Y., Hashiguchi, H., Takeda, R., Nishimori, T., et al. (2007). Prenatal psychological stress causes higher emotionality, depression-like behavior, and elevated activity in the hypothalamo-pituitary-adrenal axis. *Neuroscience Research 59*(2): 145–151.

Ary, A. W., Aguilar, V. R., Szumlinski, K. K., & Kippin, T. E. (2007). Prenatal stress alters limbo-corticostriatal Homer protein expression. *Synapse 61*(11): 938–941.

Bale, T. L. (2005). Sensitivity to stress: Dysregulation of CRF pathways and disease development. *Hormones and Behavior 48*(1): 1–10.

Barbazanges, A., Piazza, P. V., Le Moal, M., & Maccari, S. (1996). Maternal glucocorticoid secretion mediates long-term effects of prenatal stress. *Journal of Neuroscience 16*(12): 3943–3949.

Barnum, C. J., Blandino, P., Jr., & Deak, T. (2008). Social status modulates basal IL-1 concentrations in the hypothalamus of pair-housed rats and influences certain features of stress reactivity. *Brain, Behavior, and Immunity 22*(4): 517–527.

Barros, V. G., Rodriguez, P., Martijena, I. D., Perez, A., Molina, V. A., & Antonelli, M. C. (2006). Prenatal stress and early adoption effects on benzodiazepine receptors and anxiogenic behavior in the adult rat brain. *Synapse 60*(8): 609–618.

Bartolomucci, A., Palanza, P., Sacerdote, P., Panerai, A. E., Sgoifo, A., Dantzer, R., & Parmigiani, S. (2005). Social factors and individual vulnerability to chronic stress exposure. *Neuroscience and Biobehavioral Reviews 29*(1): 67–81.

Bellinger, D. L., Lubahn, C., & Lorton, D. (2008). Maternal and early life stress effects on immune function: Relevance to immunotoxicology. *Journal of Immunotoxicology 5*(4): 419–444.

Bethus, I., Lemaire, V., Lhomme, M., & Goodall, G. (2005). Does prenatal stress affect latent inhibition? It depends on the gender. *Behavioural Brain Research 158*(2): 331–338.

Beydoun, H. & Saftlas, A. F. (2008). Physical and mental health outcomes of prenatal maternal stress in human and animal studies: A review of recent evidence. *Paediatric and Perinatal Epidemiology 22*(5): 438–466.

Blois, S. M., Joachim, R., Kandil, J., Margni, R., Tometten, M., Klapp, B. F., & Arck, P. C. (2004). Depletion of CD8(+) cells abolishes the pregnancy protective effect of progesterone substitution with dydrogesterone in mice by altering the Th1/Th2 cytokine profile. *Journal of Immunology 172*(10): 5893–5899.

Brabham, T., Phelka, A., Zimmer, C., Nash, A., Lopez, J. F., & Vazquez, D. M. (2000). Effects of prenatal dexamethasone on spatial learning and response to stress is influenced by maternal factors. *American Journal of Physiology—Regulatory, Integrative and Comparative Physiology 279*(5): R1899–R1909.

Challis, J. R. G., Matthews, S. G., Gibb, W., & Lye, S. J. (2000). Endocrine and paracrine regulation of birth at term and preterm. *Endocrine Reviews 21*(5): 514–550.

Coe, C. L., Kramer, M., Czeh, B., Gould, E., Reeves, A. J., Kirschbaum, C., & Fuchs, E. (2003). Prenatal stress diminishes neurogenesis in the dentate gyrus of juvenile rhesus monkeys. *Biological Psychiatry 54*(10): 1025–1034.

Coe, C. L. & Lubach, G. R. (2005). Prenatal origins of individual variation in behavior and immunity. *Neuroscience and Biobehavioral Reviews 29*(1): 39–49.

Coe, C. L., Lubach, G. R., Bianco, L., & Beard, J. L. (2009). A history of iron deficiency anemia during infancy alters brain monoamine activity later in juvenile monkeys. *Developmental Psychobiology 51*(3): 301–309.

Coussons-Read, M. E., Okun, M. L., & Nettles, C. D. (2007). Psychosocial stress increases inflammatory markers and alters cytokine production across pregnancy. *Brain, Behavior, and Immunity 21*(3): 343–350.

Cratty, M. S., Ward, H. E., Johnson, E. A., Azzaro, A. J., & Birkle, D. L. (1995). Prenatal stress increases corticotropin-releasing factor (CRF) content and release in rat amygdala minces. *Brain Research 675*(1–2): 297–302.

Darnaudery, M. & Maccari, S. (2008). Epigenetic programming of the stress response in male and female rats by prenatal restraint stress. *Brain Research Reviews 57*(2): 571–585.

Dhabhar, F. S. & McEwen, B. S. (1997). Acute stress enhances while chronic stress suppresses cell-mediated immunity in vivo: A potential role for leukocyte trafficking. *Brain, Behavior, and Immunity 11*(4): 286–306.

Drake, A. J., Walker, B. R., & Seckl, J. R. (2005). Intergenerational consequences of fetal programming by in utero exposure to glucocorticoids in rats. *American Journal of Physiology—Regulatory, Integrative and Comparative Physiology 288*(1): R34–R38.

Edwards, H. E., Dortok, D., Tam, J., Won, D., & Burnham, W. M. (2002). Prenatal stress alters seizure thresholds and the development of kindled seizures in infant and adult rats. *Hormones and Behavior 42*(4): 437–447.

Entringer, S., Kumsta, R., Hellhammer, D. H., Wadhwa, P. D., & Wust, S. (2009). Prenatal exposure to maternal psychosocial stress and HPA axis regulation in young adults. *Hormones and Behavior 55*(2): 292–298.

Entringer, S., Kumsta, R., Nelson, E. L., Hellhammer, D. H., Wadhwa, P. D., & Wust, S. (2008). Influence of prenatal psychosocial stress on cytokine production in adult women. *Developmental Psychobiology 50*(6): 579–587.

Fan, J. M., Chen, X. Q., Jin, H., & Du, J. Z. (2009). Gestational hypoxia alone or combined with restraint sensitizes the hypothalamic-pituitary-adrenal axis and induces anxiety-like behavior in adult male rat offspring. *Neuroscience 159*(4): 1363–1373.

Fonseca, E. S., Sakai, M., Carvalho-Freitas, M. I., & Palermo Neto, J. (2005). Naloxone treatment prevents prenatal stress effects on peritoneal macrophage activity in mice offspring. *Neuroendocrinology 81*(5): 322–328.

Fowden, A. L. & Forhead, A. J., (2009). Hormones as epigenetic signals in developmental programming. *Experimental Physiology 94*(6): 607–625.

Fox, C., Merali, Z., & Harrison, C. (2006). Therapeutic and protective effect of environmental enrichment against psychogenic and neurogenic stress. *Behavioural Brain Research 175*(1): 1–8.

Fujioka, A., Fujioka, T., Ishida, Y., Maekawa, T., & Nakamura, S. (2006). Differential effects of prenatal stress on the morphological maturation of hippocampal neurons. *Neuroscience* 141(2): 907–915.

Fujioka, T., Fujioka, A., Endoh, H., Sakata, Y., Furukawa, S., & Nakamura, S. (2003). Materno-fetal coordination of stress-induced Fos expression in the hypothalamic paraventricular nucleus during pregnancy. *Neuroscience* 118(2): 409–415.

Fujioka, T., Sakata, Y., Yamaguchi, K., Shibasaki, T., Kato, H., & Nakamura, S. (1999). The effects of prenatal stress on the development of hypothalamic paraventricular neurons in fetal rats. *Neuroscience* 92(3): 1079–1088.

Fumagalli, F., Molteni, R., Racagni, G., & Riva, M. A. (2007). Stress during development: impact on neuroplasticity and relevance to psychopathology. *Progress in Neurobiology* 81(4): 197–217.

Fumagalli, F., Pasini, M., Frasca, A., Drago, F., Racagni, G., & Riva, M. A. (2009). Prenatal stress alters glutamatergic system responsiveness in adult rat prefrontal cortex. *Journal of Neurochemistry* 109(6): 1733–1744.

Gennaro, S. & Hennessy, M. D. (2003). Psychological and physiological stress: Impact on preterm birth. *Journal of Obstetric, Gynecologic, and Neonatal Nursing* 32(5): 668–675.

Goel, N. & Bale, T. L. (2009). Examining the intersection of sex and stress in modelling neuropsychiatric disorders. *Journal of Neuroendocrinology* 21(4): 415–420.

Griffin, W. C., Skinner, H. D., Salm, A. K., & Birkle, D. L. (2003). Mild prenatal stress in rats is associated with enhanced conditioned fear. *Physiology and Behavior* 79(2): 209–215.

Hammock, E. A. & Young, L. J. (2006). Oxytocin, vasopressin and pair bonding: Implications for autism. *Philosophical Transactions of the Royal Society B: Biological Sciences* 361(1476): 2187–2198.

Hansen, D., Lou, H.C., & Olsen, J. (2000). Serious life events and congenital malformations: A national study with complete follow-up. *Lancet* 356(9233): 875–880.

Harmon, K. M., Greenwald, M. L., McFarland, A., Beckwith, T., & Cromwell, H. C. (2009). The effects of prenatal stress on motivation in the rat pup. *Stress (Amsterdam, Netherlands)* 12(3): 250–258.

Hauser, J., Feldon, J., & Pryce, C. R. (2006). Prenatal dexamethasone exposure, postnatal development, and adulthood prepulse inhibition and latent inhibition in Wistar rats. *Behavioural Brain Research* 175(1): 51–61.

Henry, C., Guegant, G., Cador, M., Arnauld, E., Arsaut, J., Le Moal, M., & Demotes-Mainard, J. (1995). Prenatal stress in rats facilitates amphetamine-induced sensitization and induces long-lasting changes in dopamine receptors in the nucleus accumbens. *Brain Research* 685(1–2): 179–186.

Hobel, C. & Culhane, J. (2003). Role of psychosocial and nutritional stress on poor pregnancy outcome. *Journal of Nutrition* 133(5 Suppl 2): 1709S–1717S.

Howes, O. D., Egerton, A., Allan, V., McGuire, P., Stokes, P., & Kapur, S. (2009). Mechanisms underlying psychosis and antipsychotic treatment response in schizophrenia: Insights from PET and SPECT imaging. *Current Pharmaceutical Design* 15(22): 2550–2559.

Huber, D., Veinante, P., & Stoop, R. (2005). Vasopressin and oxytocin excite distinct neuronal populations in the central amygdala. *Science* 308(5719): 245–248.

Huizink, A. C., Mulder, E. J., Robles de Medina, P. G., Visser, G. H., & Buitelaar, J. K. (2004). Is pregnancy anxiety a distinctive syndrome? *Early Human Development* 79(2): 81–91.

Huttunen, M. O. & Niskanen, P. (1978). Prenatal loss of father and psychiatric disorders. *Archives of General Psychiatry* 35(4): 429–431.

Insel, B. J., Schaefer, C. A., McKeague, I. W., Susser, E. S., & Brown, A. S. (2008). Maternal iron deficiency and the risk of schizophrenia in offspring. *Archives of General Psychiatry* 65(10): 1136–1144.

Ishiwata, H., Shiga, T., & Okado, N. (2005). Selective serotonin reuptake inhibitor treatment of early postnatal mice reverses their prenatal stress-induced brain dysfunction. *Neuroscience 133*(4): 893–901.

Joachim, R., Zenclussen, A. C., Polgar, B., Douglas, A. J., Fest, S., Knackstedt, M., Klapp, B. F., & Arck, P. C. (2003). The progesterone derivative dydrogesterone abrogates murine stress-triggered abortion by inducing a Th2 biased local immune response. *Steroids 68*(10–13): 931–940.

Kapoor, A., Kostaki, A., Janus, C., & Matthews, S. G. (2009). The effects of prenatal stress on learning in adult offspring is dependent on the timing of the stressor. *Behavioural Brain Research 197*(1): 144–149.

Kapoor, A. & Matthews, S. G. (2008). Prenatal stress modifies behavior and hypothalamic-pituitary-adrenal function in female guinea pig offspring: Effects of timing of prenatal stress and stage of reproductive cycle. *Endocrinology 149*(12): 6406–6415.

Kaur, G. & Salm, A. K. (2008). Blunted amygdalar anti-inflammatory cytokine effector response to postnatal stress in prenatally stressed rats. *Brain Research 1196*: 1–12.

Kawamura, T., Chen, J., Takahashi, T., Ichitani, Y., & Nakahara, D. (2006). Prenatal stress suppresses cell proliferation in the early developing brain. *Neuroreport 17*(14): 1515–1518.

Khashan, A. S., Abel, K. M., McNamee, R., Pedersen, M. G., Webb, R. T., Baker, P. N., Kenny, L. C., & Mortensen, P. B. (2008). Higher risk of offspring schizophrenia following antenatal maternal exposure to severe adverse life events. *Archives of General Psychiatry 65*(2): 146–152.

King, B. R., Smith, R., & Nicholson, R. C. (2001). The regulation of human corticotrophin-releasing hormone gene expression in the placenta. *Peptides 22*(11): 1941–1947.

Koehl, M., Lemaire, V., Le Moal, M., & Abrous, D. N. (2009). Age-dependent effect of prenatal stress on hippocampal cell proliferation in female rats. *European Journal of Neuroscience 29*(3): 635–640.

Koenig, J. I., Elmer, G. I., Shepard, P. D., Lee, P. R., Mayo, C., Joy, B., Hercher, E., & Brady, D. L. (2005). Prenatal exposure to a repeated variable stress paradigm elicits behavioral and neuroendocrinological changes in the adult offspring: Potential relevance to schizophrenia. *Behavioural Brain Research 156*(2): 251–261.

Koenig, J. I., Kirkpatrick, B., & Lee, P. (2002). Glucocorticoid hormones and early brain development in schizophrenia. *Neuropsychopharmacology 27*(2): 309–318.

Kofman, O. (2002). The role of prenatal stress in the etiology of developmental behavioural disorders. *Neuroscience and Biobehavioral Reviews 26*(4): 457–470.

Koga, K., Cardenas, I., Aldo, P., Abrahams, V. M., Peng, B., Fill, S., Romero, R., & Mor, G. (2009). Activation of TLR3 in the trophoblast is associated with preterm delivery. *American Journal of Reproductive Immunology 61*(3): 196–212.

Kohman, R. A., Tarr, A. J., Day, C. E., McLinden, K. A., & Boehm, G. W. (2008). Influence of prenatal stress on behavioral, endocrine, and cytokine responses to adulthood bacterial endotoxin exposure. *Behavioural Brain Research 193*(2): 257–268.

Langdown, M. L. & Sugden, M. C. (2001). Enhanced placental GLUT1 and GLUT3 expression in dexamethasone-induced fetal growth retardation. *Molecular and Cellular Endocrinology 185*(1–2): 109–117.

Laviola, G., Hannan, A. J., Macri, S., Solinas, M., & Jaber, M. (2008). Effects of enriched environment on animal models of neurodegenerative diseases and psychiatric disorders. *Neurobiology of Disease 31*(2): 159–168.

Laviola, G., Rea, M., Morley-Fletcher, S., Di Carlo, S., Bacosi, A., De Simone, R., Bertini. M., & Pacifici, R. (2004). Beneficial effects of enriched environment on adolescent rats from stressed pregnancies. *European Journal of Neuroscience 20*(6): 1655–1664.

Lee, P. R., Brady, D. L., Shapiro, R. A., Dorsa, D. M., & Koenig, J. I. (2007). Prenatal stress generates deficits in rat social behavior: Reversal by oxytocin. *Brain Research 1156*: 152–167.

Lehmann, J., Stohr, T., & Feldon, J. (2000). Long-term effects of prenatal stress experiences and postnatal maternal separation on emotionality and attentional processes. *Behavioural Brain Research 107*(1–2): 133–144.

Lemaire, V., Koehl, M., Le Moal, M., & Abrous, D. N. (2000). Prenatal stress produces learning deficits associated with an inhibition of neurogenesis in the hippocampus. *Proceedings of the National Academy of Sciences U.S.A. 97*(20): 11032–11037.

Lemaire, V., Lamarque, S., Le Moal, M., Piazza, P. V., & Abrous, D. N. (2006). Postnatal stimulation of the pups counteracts prenatal stress-induced deficits in hippocampal neurogenesis. *Biological Psychiatry 59*(9): 786–792.

Lipska, B. K. & Weinberger, D. R. (2000). To model a psychiatric disorder in animals: Schizophrenia as a reality test. *Neuropsychopharmacology 23*(3): 223–239.

Lucassen, P. J., Bosch, O. J., Jousma, E., Kromer, S. A., Andrew, R., Seckl, J. R., & Neumann, I. D. (2009). Prenatal stress reduces postnatal neurogenesis in rats selectively bred for high, but not low, anxiety: Possible key role of placental 11beta-hydroxysteroid dehydrogenase type 2. *European Journal of Neuroscience 29*(1): 97–103.

Maccari, S., Piazza, P. V., Kabbaj, M., Barbazanges, A., Simon, H., & Le Moal, M. (1995). Adoption reverses the long-term impairment in glucocorticoid feedback induced by prenatal stress. *Journal of Neuroscience 15*(1 Pt 1): 110–116.

Mairesse, J., Viltart, O., Salome, N., Giuliani, A., Catalani, A., Casolini, P., Morley-Fletcher, S., Nicoletti, F., & Maccari, S. (2007). Prenatal stress alters the negative correlation between neuronal activation in limbic regions and behavioral responses in rats exposed to high and low anxiogenic environments. *Psychoneuroendocrinology 32*(7): 765–776.

Martinez-Tellez, R. I., Hernandez-Torres, E., Gamboa, C., & Flores, G. (2009). Prenatal stress alters spine density and dendritic length of nucleus accumbens and hippocampus neurons in rat offspring. *Synapse 63*(9): 794–804.

Maruoka, T., Kodomari, I., Yamauchi, R., Wada, E., & Wada, K. (2009). Maternal enrichment affects prenatal hippocampal proliferation and open-field behaviors in female offspring mice. *Neuroscience Letters 454*(1): 28–32.

Merlot, E., Couret, D., & Otten, W. (2008). Prenatal stress, fetal imprinting and immunity. *Brain, Behavior, and Immunity 22*(1): 42–51.

Mirescu, C. & Gould, E. (2006). Stress and adult neurogenesis. *Hippocampus 16*(3): 233–238.

Morley-Fletcher, S., Darnaudery, M., Koehl, M., Casolini, P., Van Reeth, O., & Maccari, S. (2003). Prenatal stress in rats predicts immobility behavior in the forced swim test: Effects of a chronic treatment with tianeptine. *Brain Research 989*(2): 246–251.

Morley-Fletcher, S., Darnaudery, M., Mocaer, E., Froger, N., Lanfumey, L., Laviola, G., Casolini, P., Zuena, A. R., Marzano, L., Hamon, M., et al. (2004). Chronic treatment with imipramine reverses immobility behaviour, hippocampal corticosteroid receptors and cortical 5-HT(1A) receptor mRNA in prenatally stressed rats. *Neuropharmacology 47*(6): 841–847.

Mueller, B. R. & Bale, T. L. (2007). Early prenatal stress impact on coping strategies and learning performance is sex dependent. *Physiology and Behavior 91*(1): 55–65.

Mueller, B. R. & Bale, T. L. (2008). Sex-specific programming of offspring emotionality after stress early in pregnancy. *Journal of Neuroscience 28*(36): 9055–9065.

Mulder, E. J., Robles de Medina, P. G., Huizink, A. C., Van den Bergh, B. R., Buitelaar, J. K., & Visser, G. H. (2002). Prenatal maternal stress: Effects on pregnancy and the (unborn) child. *Early Human Development 70*(1–2): 3–14.

Muller, N. & Schwarz, M. J. (2008). A psychoneuroimmunological perspective to Emil Krae-pelins dichotomy: Schizophrenia and major depression as inflammatory CNS disorders. *European Archives of Psychiatry and Clinical Neuroscience 258* (Suppl 2): 97–106.

Myhrman, A., Rantakallio, P., Isohanni, M., Jones, P., & Partanen, U. (1996). Unwantedness of a pregnancy and schizophrenia in the child. *British Journal of Psychiatry 169*(5): 637–640.

Ohkawa, T., Rohde, W., Takeshita, S., Dorner, G., Arai, K., & Okinaga, S. (1991). Effect of an acute maternal stress on the fetal hypothalamo-pituitary-adrenal system in late gestational life of the rat. *Experimental and Clinical Endocrinology 98*(2): 123–129.

Owen, D., Andrews, M. H., & Matthews, S. G. (2005). Maternal adversity, glucocorticoids and programming of neuroendocrine function and behaviour. *Neuroscience and Biobe-havioral Reviews 29*(2): 209–226.

Patterson, P. H. (2009), Immune involvement in schizophrenia and autism: Etiology, pathology and animal models. *Behavioural Brain Research 204*(2): 313–321.

Pereira, A. C., Huddleston, D. E., Brickman, A. M., Sosunov, A. A., Hen, R., McKhann, G. M., Sloan, R., Gage, F. H., Brown, T. R., & Small, S. A. (2007). An in vivo correlate of exercise-induced neurogenesis in the adult dentate gyrus. *Proceedings of the National Academy of Sciences U.S.A. 104*(13): 5638–5643.

Peters, D. A. (1988). Both prenatal and postnatal factors contribute to the effects of maternal stress on offspring behavior and central 5-hydroxytryptamine receptors in the rat. *Pharmacology Biochemistry and Behavior 30*(3): 669–673.

Peters, D. A. (1989). Effects of maternal stress during different gestational periods on the se-rotonergic system in adult rat offspring. *Pharmacology Biochemistry and Behavior 31*(4): 839–843.

Peters, D. A. (1990). Maternal stress increases fetal brain and neonatal cerebral cortex 5-hydroxytryptamine synthesis in rats: A possible mechanism by which stress influences brain development. *Pharmacology Biochemistry and Behavior 35*(4): 943–947.

Pincus-Knackstedt, M. K., Joachim, R. A., Blois, S. M., Douglas, A. J., Orsal, A. S., Klapp, B. F., Wahn, U., Hamelmann, E., & Arck, P. C. (2006). Prenatal stress enhances susceptibility of murine adult offspring toward airway inflammation. *Journal of Immunology 177*(12): 8484–8492.

Plata-Salamán, C. R., Ilyin, S. E., Turrin, N. P., Gayle, D., Flynn, M. C., Bedard, T., Merali, Z., & Anisman, H. (2000). Neither acute nor chronic exposure to a naturalistic (predator) stressor influences the interleukin-1beta system, tumors necrosis factor-alpha, transforming growth factor-1beta, and neuropeptide mRNAs in specific brain regions. *Brain Research Bulletin 51*(2): 187–193.

Qian, J., Zhou, D., Pan, F., Liu, C. X., & Wang, Y. W. (2008). Effect of environmental enrichment on fearful behavior and gastrin-releasing peptide receptor expression in the amygdala of prenatal stressed rats. *Journal of Neuroscience Research 86*(13): 3011–3017.

Reif, A., Schmitt, A., Fritzen, S., & Lesch, K. P. (2007). Neurogenesis and schizophrenia: Dividing neurons in a divided mind? *European Archives of Psychiatry and Clinical Neuroscience 257*(5): 290–299.

Reznikov, A. G., Nosenko, N. D., & Tarasenko, L. V. (1999). Prenatal stress and glucocorticoid effects on the developing gender-related brain. *Journal of Steroid Biochemistry and Molecular Biology 69*(1–6): 109–115.

Roberts, A. D., Moore, C. F., DeJesus, O. T., Barnhart, T. E., Larson, J. A., Mukherjee, J., Nick-les, R. J., Schueller, M. J., Shelton, S. E., & Schneider, M. L. (2004). Prenatal stress, moderate fetal alcohol, and dopamine system function in rhesus monkeys. *Neurotoxicology and Teratology 26*(2): 169–178.

Robinson, B. G., Emanuel, R. L., Frim, D. M., & Majzoub, J. A. (1988). Glucocorticoid stimulates expression of corticotropin-releasing hormone gene in human placenta. *Proceedings of the National Academy of Sciences U.S.A.* 85(14): 5244–5248.

Schlotz, W. & Phillips, D. I. (2009). Fetal origins of mental health: Evidence and mechanisms. *Brain, Behavior, and Immunity* 23(7): 905–916.

Shachar-Dadon, A. (2009). Adversity before conception will affect adult progeny in rats. *Developmental Psychology* 1: 9–16.

Shalev, U. & Weiner, I. (2001). Gender-dependent differences in latent inhibition following prenatal stress and corticosterone administration. *Behavioural Brain Research* 126(1–2): 57–63.

Silvagni, A., Barros, V. G., Mura, C., Antonelli, M. C., & Carboni, E. (2008). Prenatal restraint stress differentially modifies basal and stimulated dopamine and noradrenaline release in the nucleus accumbens shell: An "in vivo" microdialysis study in adolescent and young adult rats. *European Journal of Neuroscience* 28(4): 744–758.

Slotkin, T. A., Seidler, F. J., Wood, C. R., & Lau, C. (2008). Development of glucocorticoid receptor regulation in the rat forebrain: Implications for adverse effects of glucocorticoids in preterm infants. *Brain Research Bulletin* 76(5): 531–535.

Son, G. H., Geum, D., Chung, S., Kim, E. J., Jo, J. H., Kim, C. M., Lee, K. H., Kim, H., Choi, S., Kim, H. T., et al. (2006). Maternal stress produces learning deficits associated with impairment of NMDA receptor-mediated synaptic plasticity. *Journal of Neuroscience* 26(12): 3309–3318.

Szyf, M., McGowan, P., & Meaney, M. J. (2008). The social environment and the epigenome. *Environmental and Molecular Mutagenesis* 49(1): 46–60.

Szymanska, M., Budziszewska, B., Jaworska-Feil, L., Basta-Kaim, A., Kubera, M., Leskiewicz, M., Regulska, M., & Lason, W. (2009). The effect of antidepressant drugs on the HPA axis activity, glucocorticoid receptor level and FKBP51 concentration in prenatally stressed rats. *Psychoneuroendocrinology* 34(6): 822–832.

Takahashi, T., Malhi, G. S., Wood, S. J., Walterfang, M., Yucel, M., Lorenzetti, V., Soulsby, B., Suzuki, M., Velakoulis, D., & Pantelis, C. (2009). Increased pituitary volume in patients with established bipolar affective disorder. *Progress in Neuro-Psychopharmacology and Biological Psychiatry* 33(7): 1245–1249.

Talge, N. M., Neal, C., & Glover, V. (2007). Antenatal maternal stress and long-term effects on child neurodevelopment: How and why? *Journal of Child Psychology and Psychiatry* 48(3–4): 245–261.

Tauber, S. C., Schlumbohm, C., Schilg, L., Fuchs, E., Nau, R., & Gerber, J. (2006). Intrauterine exposure to dexamethasone impairs proliferation but not neuronal differentiation in the dentate gyrus of newborn common marmoset monkeys. *Brain Pathology* 16(3): 209–217.

Thomas, M. B., Hu, M., Lee, T. M., Bhatnagar, S., & Becker, J. B. (2009) Sex-specific susceptibility to cocaine in rats with a history of prenatal stress. *Physiology and Behavior* 997(2): 270–277.

Thomas, S. A., Matsumoto, A. M., & Palmiter, R. D. (1995). Noradrenaline is essential for mouse fetal development. *Nature* 374(6523): 643–646.

Trautman, P. D., Meyer-Bahlburg, H. F., Postelnek, J., & New, M. I. (1996). Mothers' reactions to prenatal diagnostic procedures and dexamethasone treatment of congenital adrenal hyperplasia. *Journal of Psychosomatic Obstetrics and Gynecology* 17(3): 175–181.

Uno, H., Lohmiller, L., Thieme, C., Kemnitz, J. W., Engle, M. J., Roecker, E. B., & Farrell, P. M. (1990). Brain damage induced by prenatal exposure to dexamethasone in fetal rhesus macaques. I. Hippocampus. *Brain Research: Developmental Brain Research* 53(2): 157–167.

Van den Hove, D. L., Steinbusch, H. W., Scheepens, A., Van de Berg, W. D., Kooiman, L. A., Boosten, B. J., Prickaerts, J., & Blanco, C. E. (2006). Prenatal stress and neonatal rat brain development. *Neuroscience 137*(1): 145–155.

Vanbesien-Mailliot, C. C. A., Wolowczuk, I., Mairesse, J., Viltart, O., Delacre, M., Khalife, J., Chartier-Harlin, M. C., & Maccari, S. (2007) Prenatal stress has pro-inflammatory consequences on the immune system in adult rats. *Psychoneuroendocrinology 32*(2): 114–124.

Viltart, O. & Vanbesien-Mailliot, C. C. (2007). Impact of prenatal stress on neuroendocrine programming. *Scientific World Journal 7*: 1493–1537.

Walker, E., Mittal, V., & Tessner, K. (2008). Stress and the hypothalamic pituitary adrenal axis in the developmental course of schizophrenia. *Annual Review of Clinical Psychology 4*: 189–216.

Weiner, I. (2003). The "two-headed" latent inhibition model of schizophrenia: Modeling positive and negative symptoms and their treatment. *Psychopharmacology (Berl) 169*(3–4): 257–297.

Weinstock, M. (2007). Gender differences in the effects of prenatal stress on brain development and behaviour. *Neurochemical Research 32*(10): 1730–1740.

Weinstock, M. (2008). The long-term behavioural consequences of prenatal stress. *Neuroscience and Biobehavioral Reviews 32*(6): 1073–1086.

Welberg, L. A., Seckl, J. R., & Holmes, M. C. (2000). Inhibition of 11beta-hydroxysteroid dehydrogenase, the foeto-placental barrier to maternal glucocorticoids, permanently programs amygdala GR mRNA expression and anxiety-like behaviour in the offspring. *European Journal of Neuroscience 12*(3): 1047–1054.

Wyrwoll, C. S., Seckl, J. R., & Holmes, M. C. (2009). Altered placental function of 11beta-hydroxysteroid dehydrogenase 2 knockout mice. *Endocrinology 150*(3): 1287–1293.

Yang, J., Li, W., Liu, X., Li, Z., Li, H., Yang, G., Xu, L., & Li, L. (2006). Enriched environment treatment counteracts enhanced addictive and depressive-like behavior induced by prenatal chronic stress. *Brain Research 1125*(1): 132–137.

Yuen, E. Y., Liu, W. H., Karatsoreos, I. N., Feng, J., McEwen, B. S., & Yan, Z. (2009). Acute stress enhances glutaminergic transmission in prefrontal cortex and facilitates working memory. *Proceeedings of the National Academy of Sciences of the United States of America 106*: 14075–14079.

Zagron, G. & Weinstock, M. (2006). Maternal adrenal hormone secretion mediates behavioural alterations induced by prenatal stress in male and female rats. *Behavioural Brain Research 175*(2): 323–328.

SECTION 2
Animal Models of Genetic Factors and Schizophrenia

CHAPTER 14

DISC1

A New Paradigm for Schizophrenia and Biological Psychiatry

DAVID PORTEOUS

KEY CONCEPTS

- The Disrupted-in-Schizophrenia gene (*DISC1*) is a causal genetic risk factor for schizophrenia and related psychiatric disorders.
- The DISC1 protein plays a key role in neurodevelopment and neurosignaling.
- The DISC1 pathway is a potential target for novel, knowledge-based interventions.

St Clair and colleagues (1990) first reported a Scottish family with a high loading of psychiatric illness that cosegregated with a balanced translocation between chromosomes 1 and 11 (Log of the Odds [LOD] = 3.4). In a major follow-up of family members and newly located relatives, Blackwood and colleagues (2001) reported on 87 family members, 37 of whom carried the translocation. Of 29 individuals carrying the translocation and for whom a psychiatric assessment was possible, seven had a diagnosis of schizophrenia, one had a diagnosis of bipolar disorder, and 10 had recurrent major depressive disorder. Thus, 18 of 29 (70%) translocation carriers had a diagnosis of major mental illness, whereas none of 38 nontranslocation carriers had such a diagnosis. This provides compelling statistical evidence for a causal link between the t(1;11) and the psychiatric liability in this unique family. Indeed, the updated LOD score of 3.6 for schizophrenia alone and of 7.1 for the broad diagnosis of major mental illness remains to this day one of the single most striking linkage findings in the psychiatric field. It is important to note that the psychiatric presentations were typical, with no other distinguishing clinical features. Moreover, Blackwood et al. (2001) also reported that the latency and amplitude of the event-related potential (ERP) P300, a measure of the speed and efficiency of information processing, was indistinguishable between unaffected and affected translocation carriers and that as a group the translocation carriers showed the characteristically abnormal ERP P300 that is associated with schizophrenia and bipolar disorder. The pattern of inheritance in the Scottish t(1;11) family was thus consistent with a simple dominant mode of inheritance of a broad spectrum of major psychiatric illness, with incomplete penetrance, and with altered ERP P300 as a correlated phenotype. Secondary and independently segregating genetic risk factors, variable environmental exposures, stochastic events, or all three may influence the presence or absence of clinical signs and the specific psychiatric diagnosis at the age of ascertainment, but it is clear that the t(1;11) accounts for essentially all of the transmitted genetic risk in this family.

At the time, this finding was viewed skeptically by many as it challenged two fervently held precepts: on the clinical side, the etiologic distinction between schizophrenia, bipolar disorder, and major depressive disorder, and on the genetic side, the notion that these psychiatric conditions were "always" complex, non-Mendelian disorders. In the intervening period, the validity of the Kraepelinian dichotomy between schizophrenia and bipolar disorder has been vigorously debated, with genetic findings becoming more prominent (Craddock & Owen, 2005; Craddock, O'Donovan, & Owen, 2006). The evidence for a major influence of genetic factors in risk of schizophrenia and bipolar disorder is beyond dispute (reviewed in Harrison & Weinberger, 2005, and Ross et al., 2006), but in truth, families that "breed true" for only schizophrenia or bipolar disorder are the rare exception rather than the rule (Blackwood et al., 1996). Monozygotic twin studies have shown that the concordance rates for schizophrenia are about 50% and for bipolar disorder higher still, but what is not so widely recognized is that the incidence of bipolar disorder in the monozygotic co-twin of a proband with schizophrenia, and vice versa, is much higher (10–15%) than expected by chance (1% population average), providing additional evidence for shared genetic risk between bipolar disorder and schizophrenia (Cardno et al., 2002). Putting the matter beyond dispute, the recent major epidemiologic study of the Swedish incidence of schizophrenia and bipolar disorder estimates the genetic risk is shared between these illnesses about half the time (Lichtenstein et al., 2009). Thus, the evidence for a simple, shared genetic liability for a broad spectrum of mental illness that includes recurrent major depressive disorder in the Scottish t(1;11) family should be seen as entirely consistent with this revisionist view of diagnostic criteria and their validity (Craddock et al., 2006).

Positional Cloning of *DISC1*

Molecular cytogenetics is a powerful and underutilized tool for gene searches in psychiatric disease (McIntyre et al., 2003; Pickard et al., 2005b). In the postgenome era, mapping a chromosome translocation is facile. Metaphase chromosomes from patient blood samples are probed by fluorescently labeled in situ hybridization using genomic clones of known map location. Once narrowed down to a few kilobases of DNA, polymerase chain reaction (PCR) mapping and sequencing of the breakpoint can quickly follow. But in the pregenome era, all of the mapping reagents, including human-mouse somatic cell hybrids and dedicated clone libraries, had to be built from scratch; mapping was both technically difficult and slow (Fletcher et al., 1993; Evans et al., 1995). Consequently, it was a full decade after reporting the t(1;11) translocation family that the breakpoint was finally cloned and analyzed (Millar et al., 2000). Sequencing of the translocation breakpoint revealed not one but two affected genes, both novel. The first coded for a protein, which took the name Disrupted-in-Schizophrenia 1, or *DISC1*; the second was an RNA-only gene, named *DISC2*.

DISC2 is a very large, spliced RNA-only gene that runs antiparallel to *DISC1* on chromosome 1 (Millar et al., 2000). In common with other RNA-only genes, it is poorly conserved across species (Taylor et al., 2003) and its function still remains uncertain, but by analogy with other examples, it may regulate *DISC1* expression. On first discovery, the function of DISC1 was also far from clear as it showed no obvious similarity to other known genes or proteins (Millar et al., 2000). De novo biochemical and expression studies have since established that DISC1 is a multifunctional, developmentally regulated scaffold protein (see Chubb et al., 2008, and references therein for a comprehensive review).

The scaffold function of DISC1 helps resolve the genetics paradox. Many of the proteins known to interact with DISC1 have a role in neurodevelopment; neurosignaling; and cytoskeletal, centrosomal, or synaptic function, or all three (Camargo et al., 2007). Thus, these interactors have the potential to simultaneously affect a wide range of plausible risk processes in schizophrenia susceptibility (reviewed in Carter, 2006; Mackie, Millar, & Porteous, 2007; Chubb et al., 2008; Jaaro-Peled et al., 2009). Indeed, several of the DISC1 interactors, such as NDE1, PDE4B, PDE4D (reviewed in Chubb et al., 2008), and PCM1 (Gurling et al., 2006; Kamiya et al., 2008), turn out to be codependent or independent genetic risk factors for schizophrenia. Furthermore, as first pointed out by Carter (2006) and discussed in detail by Jaaro-Peled et al. (2009), there is growing evidence for convergence between the biological pathways influenced by DISC1 and NRG1, another prominent candidate risk gene for schizophrenia (Harrison & Weinberger, 2005).

DISC1: A Causal Genetic Risk Factor for Schizophrenia and Related Psychiatric Disorders

As the likely biological function of DISC1 was being elucidated, so the genetics community started to report evidence in support of a genetic role for *DISC1* in the general population. Again, statistical support came not just from studies of schizophrenia, but also from studies of bipolar disorder and unipolar disorder (reviewed in Chubb et al., 2008). Indeed, the spectrum of disorders in which *DISC1* appeared to play a role extended to include schizoaffective disorder (Hamshere et al., 2005), autism spectrum disorder (Kilpinin et al., 2008), and possibly Alzheimer's disease (Beecham et al., 2009). There is also evidence from brain imaging studies that common genetic variants of *DISC1* explain variation in hippocampal and cortical function (Callicott et al., 2005; Di Giorgio et al., 2008; Prata et al., 2008; Szeszko et al., 2008).

But as for all putative risk factors in major mental illness, the picture is still complex. *DISC1* is a large gene, extending over some 450 kb of genomic DNA, which is poorly tagged by second-generation Affymetrics and Illumina genomewide association study (GWAS) chips. Despite this, the DISC1 locus does generate a modest association signal in GWAS (Sullivan et al., 2008). Further to this point, Hennah et al. (2009) recently reported a detailed association study of the DISC locus in four European cohorts and reported association for bipolar disorder in the Finnish cohort at rs1538979 (OR = 2.73, CI 1.42–5.27) and at rs821577 in the London cohort (OR = 1.64, CI 1.2–2.19). Dividing the cohorts into subgroups based on these two single nucleotide polymorphisms (SNPs) revealed a third significant SNP association at rs821633, which modified risk according to the presence or absence of the other two SNPs. Because none of these three SNPs are on the Illumina550 chip and only rs821577 is present on the Affy500 chip, this finding would be missed using these platforms, and likewise these specific SNPs were not tested in a locus-specific association study. This rather novel concept of intergenic allelic interplay has its antecedent in an earlier study by Hennah et al. (2007), which identified a *DISC1* risk haplotype by genomewide linkage analysis and repeated the analysis based on its presence or absence, thus identifying a second *DISC1*-dependent locus as *NDE1*, a known DISC1 interactor.

NDE1 and NDEL1 are two highly related neurodevelopmental proteins that dimerize and heteromultimerize when binding to DISC1 (Hayashi et al., 2005; Leliveld et al., 2008; Bradshaw et al., 2009). Burdick et al. (2008) reported evidence for a genetic and biological interaction between the common *DISC1* missense mutation S704C and differential binding of NDE1 and NDEL1. Moreover, the common *DISC1* missense variants L607F and S704C may modify DISC1 function in schizophrenia, bipolar disorder, and indeed normal individuals (Thomson et al., 2005; Leliveld et al., 2008, 2009; Eastwood, Hodgkinson, & Harrison, 2009).

Song et al. (2008) reported the results of genomic resequencing of *DISC1* coding sequence and splice junctions in 288 schizophrenia samples and identified eight new, ultrarare variants that were not seen in controls. They estimated that 2% of all schizophrenia subjects had *DISC1* missense mutations. Large-scale resequencing studies are under way in our laboratory and others that will no doubt discover additional, rare missense mutations. Resequencing of the SNP and haplotype regions of reported association may refine the source of the statistical signals, the underlying casual variants, and the mechanism or mechanisms by which they exert their effects. It is, however, now beyond debate that there are several *DISC1* variants, both coding and noncoding, that do influence brain function and personality within the psychopathic and normal range.

Repeating the *DISC1* Cytogenetic Paradigm

It is worth noting that *DISC1* is not the only gene for schizophrenia to be identified through molecular cytogenetics (reviewed in MacIntyre et al., 2003; Pickard et al., 2005b). The Edinburgh laboratory alone has reported on the positional cloning and substantiation of not just *DISC1*, but also *PDE4B* (Millar et al., 2005), *GRIK4* (Pickard et al., 2006), *NPAS3* (Pickard et al., 2009), and *ABCA13* (Knight et al., 2009) association with schizophrenia. Thus, molecular cytogenetics has made a significant contribution to candidate gene discovery in psychiatry, arguably matching, if not exceeding, that of GWAS (Porteous, 2008; Mitchell & Porteous, 2009; Purcell et al., 2009). Critically, these atypical genetic presentations allow gene-specific hypotheses of biological plausibility to be proposed and tested (Porteous, 2008).

GRIK4, a kainate-type ionotropic glutamate receptor on chromosome 11q23.3, was identified as being disrupted as part of a complex chromosomal aneuploidy in a patient with chronic schizophrenia that was comorbid with learning disability and mild mental retardation. Of the several genes influenced by the complex chromosome rearrangement in this subject, GRIK4 was considered the best candidate because of the glutamate hypothesis in schizophrenia. This hypothesis arose from the observation that PCP and ketamine, antagonists of ionotropic glutamate receptors, can induce psychosis (Goff & Wine, 1997; Javitt, 2004). Pickard et al. (2006) strengthened the case for GRIK4 by providing supportive genetic evidence from the general population, in the form of a risk haplotype for schizophrenia (p=0.0005, OR=1.45) and a protective haplotype against bipolar disorder (p=0.0002; OR=0.62). In follow-up studies, the bipolar disorder protective haplotype finding was replicated in a second case-association study, shown also to affect GRIK4 brain transcript abundance (Pickard et al., 2008) and to modulate hippocampal function in a functional MRI (fMRI) facial affect-processing task (Whalley et al., 2009).

NPAS3 is an attractive biological candidate for involvement in schizophrenia because it is a neuronal transcription factor that plays a key role in adult hippocampal neurogenesis (Pieper et al., 2005), and mouse mutants in NPAS3 display behavioral proxies for schizophrenia, including altered startle response, diminished social recognition, and hyperactivity (Erbel-Sieler et al., 2004). NPAS3 maps to chromosome 14 and was found disrupted by a balanced t(9,14)(q34.2;q13) translocation in a mother and daughter with schizophrenia and learning disability and mild mental retardation (Pickard et al., 2009). Association with schizophrenia and bipolar disorder was also demonstrated: the picture was complex, with four distinct regions of risk and protection identified. When considered jointly, these identified regions allowed a calculation of the net genetic load and the likelihood of schizophrenia or bipolar disorder developing (Pickard et al., 2009). The result was a distribution of likelihoods from protective (OR = 0.78) to risk (OR = 1.17).

ABCA13 is a member of the ATP-binding cassette (ABC) superfamily of transmembrane transporters. This large, 62-exon gene was found disrupted by a t(7;8) (p12.3;p23) translocation in a single male patient with chronic schizophrenia (Knight et al., 2009). Sequencing key functional domains in a discovery set of 100 schizophrenia cases identified 10 missense mutations in ABCA13, several of which were shown to segregate in families with psychiatric illness across a wide spectrum, from schizophrenia through bipolar disorder to major and minor depression (combined Z score of 4.18, LOD score of 4.38 for all of these disorders). Some mutations were seen exclusively in cases and across a spectrum of diagnoses; others were seen occasionally in controls, but were enriched in cases; and several were predicted by homology and structural modeling to be of functional significance (Knight et al., 2009).

As we will now discuss, the phosphodiesterase PDE4B is very much part of the DISC1 story, being a direct interactor and key mediator of cAMP signaling (Millar et al., 2005).

DISC1 Plays a Key Role in Neurodevelopment and Neurosignaling

The real catalysts for taking DISC1 seriously as a telling light upon the etiology of psychotic and mood disorders came from two highly complementary research directions in 2005, which were highlighted as "scientific breakthroughs" that year by *Science*. The first introduced a critical new genetic player and direct protein interactor with DISC1. A fragment of the phosphodiesterase gene type 4B, PDE4B, was one in a very long list of putative protein interactors identified by Camargo et al. (2007) in their comprehensive yeast-2-hybrid screen. In parallel, our laboratory identified a single case of a subject with schizophrenia who had a cousin with psychotic disorder in whom the *PDE4B* gene was disrupted by a cytogenetic breakpoint (Millar et al., 2005), genetic evidence that was subsequently substantiated by association analysis (Pickard et al., 2007; Numata et al., 2008; Tomppo et al., 2009). It is important that Millar et al. (2005) showed that DISC1 interacted dynamically with PDE4B to modulate cAMP in a protein kinase A (PKA)- and phosphorylation-dependent fashion. Phosphodiesterases, of which there are over 20 different forms, are the sole means of catabolizing cAMP, a key signaling molecule in the brain. The PDE4 isoforms (A, B, C, and D) are linked to memory formation and mood disorder, respectively, through cognate fly mutants and from gene knockout studies of the B and D isoforms in the mouse. Moreover, PDE4 is the target for rolipram, a well-known antidepressant and mood stabilizer (reviewed by Mackie, Millar, & Porteous, 2007). Subsequent peptide mapping studies identified both consensus and PDE4 isoform-specific binding domains on DISC1 (Murdoch et al., 2007), which is discussed further later in the chapter.

At the same time, Akira Sawa's laboratory at Johns Hopkins University was undertaking a novel approach to *Disc1* gene modulation in the mouse by electroporation of gene constructs in utero and studying the effects on early postnatal brain development (Kamiya et al., 2005). They showed that short hairpin loop RNA oligonucleotides could transiently repress expression of endogenous mouse *Disc1*. Down-regulation of *Disc1* resulted in a striking phenotype of reduced migration out of the subventricular zone to the cortical plate. This was accompanied by altered cell polarity and reduced arborization of processes. They reported a similar phenotype when truncated human *DISC1* cDNA was over-expressed. This study demonstrated for the first time in vivo a direct role for DISC1 in early brain development, consistent with the neurodevelopmental hypothesis of schizophrenia (Weinberger, 1987; Jones & Murray, 1991).

Shortly thereafter, a series of transgenic and mutant mouse models of DISC1 were reported, each of which gave rise to subtle neurodevelopmental and behavioral phenotypes (individual and social) that modeled important aspects of the human conditions, including deficits in prepulse inhibition, latent inhibition, and working memory (reviewed in Chubb et al., 2008). Intriguingly, two independent ENU mutagen-induced, missense mouse models of *Disc1*, Q31L and L100P, were shown to exhibit rather different behaviors in standardized tests, suggesting a depression-like and schizophrenia-like phenotype respectively (Clapcote et al., 2007). These mutation-specific behaviors responded differentially to typical and atypical antipsychotics and to antidepressants (Clapcote et al., 2007). The Q31L and L100P mutations map to two distinct DISC1-PDE4B-selective binding domains (Murdoch et al., 2007), which may provide a mechanistic explanation for their differential behaviors and responses to antipsychotic and antidepressant treatment.

The DISC1 Pathway: A Potential Target for Novel, Knowledge-Based Interventions

Taking the next big step beyond Kamiya et al. (2005), Duan et al. (2007) used an elegant, retrovirally mediated, single-cell RNA interference strategy to selectively suppress mouse *Disc1* expression in vivo in differentiating hippocampal neuronal precursor cells. They made the striking observation that if *Disc1* was selectively suppressed in neuronal precursor cells, the result was over-migration, aberrant integration, and misfiring of differentiated neurons. In a follow-up study,

Kim et al. (2009) demonstrated that the critical function of DISC1 in postnatal hippocampal neurogenesis is mediated in large part by interaction with KIA1212, also known as *Girdin* (Girders of actin filaments). Parallel work by Enomoto et al. (2009) suggested much the same. Kim et al. (2009) further demonstrated that this interaction with Girdin suppresses signaling by the serine-threonine-specific kinase AKT and, remarkably, that the gross effects of *Disc1* suppression could be largely rescued by rapamycin, which inhibits the mammalian target or rapamycin (mTOR), an effector pathway activated by AKT signaling. There are important points of difference between these two studies (reviewed by Porteous & Millar, 2009) that hinge around how DISC1 and Girdin bind and the manner and extent to which this mediates an effect on AKT signaling, but this potential link between DISC1 and AKT1—and thus a second major brain signaling pathway—is tantalizing. Indeed, Enomoto and colleagues (2005) had previously reported that AKT1, a key serine-threonine-specific kinase with multiple signaling properties, regulates actin organization and cell motility by way of Girdin, which directly binds actin at the leading edge of migrating cells. The genetic evidence for AKT being a risk factor for schizophrenia is modest by comparison to that for DISC1, but there is a growing body of evidence from human and mouse studies that the AKT pathway may indeed be important (reviewed by Arguello & Gogos, 2008). Genetic variants in AKT1 have been reported to be associated with schizophrenia. AKT1 activity and AKT-dependent phosphorylation of glycogen synthase kinase 3 beta (GSK3β) is decreased in postmortem schizophrenic brains. *Akt1* knockout mice show impaired prepulse inhibition of the startle response, a corollary of the altered salience typical of schizophrenia. Both typical and atypical antipsychotics enhance AKT signaling by activating AKT or by increasing phosphorylation of GSK3β.

The Wnt pathway and α-catenin neurosignaling are also firmly in the frame of DISC1 influence as a result of the work of Mao et al. (2009), who had identified GSK3β as a novel DISC1 interactor. GSK3β is inhibited by both AKT signaling and by DISC1, and GSK3β is a known target for lithium chloride, still widely used to treat bipolar disorder. Mao et al. (2009) further reported that administration of the GSK3β-specific inhibitor SB216763 could rescue the behavioral effects of lentivirus-induced *Disc1* suppression in the adult dentate gyrus.

The effects of rolipram and other psychiatric drugs on *Disc1* missense mouse mutants (Clapcote et al., 2007), of rapamycin on *Disc1* suppression (Kim et al., 2009), and of SB216763 (and lithium chloride) on GSK3β (Mao et al., 2009) are positive portents of future therapeutic strategies, but it remains critical to determine exactly which aspects of the DISC1 pathway must be corrected and when during brain development, as well as how behavioral responses in mouse models translate to symptom control in human subjects. Furthermore, none of these medications is without side effects. The real challenge will be to use this new knowledge to devise more selective and specific treatments that achieve a level of compliance and clinical effectiveness that has so far eluded the field of psychiatric medicine (Insel, 2009). What should not be underestimated, however, is the considerable value this recent research adds to future DISC1 pathway research, and to biological psychiatry in general, as a consequence of landing on signaling pathways that are the subject of intense interest, substantial research, and development investment by both academia and industry in relation to cancer and cardiovascular and inflammatory diseases.

A full understanding of the structure-function relationships of DISC1 complexes and their interactors, and of the impact of genetic variation, awaits more detailed biophysical characterization. We know that DISC1 is composed of a highly disordered N-terminal head domain and a C-terminal tail with multiple coiled-coil domains, and we also know that almost the entire length of DISC1 interacts with one protein or another (reviewed in Chubb et al., 2008). The binding domains for PDE4, GSK3β, and Girdin at least partially overlap with one another. Both DISC1 and Girdin dimerize and both bind NDEL1, which in turn binds NDE1 and thus LIS1, yet another key protein in brain development (Porteous & Millar, 2009). In the postmortem brain, a significant fraction of DISC1 forms higher-order aggregates in chronic psychiatric case subjects, but not in normal controls (Leliveld et al., 2008). Moreover, DISC1 aggregation appears to abrogate the binding of NDE1 (Leliveld et al., 2008) and is sensitive to polymorphic variation at the Ser704Cys position (Leliveld et al., 2009). This is the same polymorphism previously related by structural and functional MRI to altered brain function (Callicott et al., 2005; Szeszko et al., 2008; Di Giorgio et al., 2008; Prata et al., 2008) and also to altered brain expression of DISC1 partners (Lipska et al., 2006).

When considering which proteins DISC1 interacts with, and where and when in the developing and adult brain they are expressed, it is important to take account of the growing evidence for multiple transcripts and protein isoforms of DISC1 and their developmental regulation (reviewed in Chubb et al., 2008). This has taken on further significance in light of recent evidence for as many as 50 different isoforms and for a dramatic difference in their prenatal and postnatal brain expression profiles (Nakata et al., 2009).

Although it is the classical reductionist approach, studying DISC1-protein interactions in pairwise fashion is bound to oversimplify the biology and potentially mislead research. Defining the DISC1 proteome by cell type and lineage during prenatal and postnatal development and in the adult brain may be necessary for a full understanding of the multiplicity of DISC1 functions and how these relate to the full spectrum of DISC1-related psychopathology and its variation within the normal range of personality and cognition.

The estimate of 2% of schizophrenic individuals having a DISC1 missense mutation (Song et al., 2008) does not take into account the evidence from genetic association studies that point to the additional effects of common, noncoding variants of *DISC1*, *PDE4B*, *PDE4D*, *NDE1* (reviewed in Chubb et al., 2008), and *PCM1* (Gurling et al., 2006; Kamiya et al., 2008). We have recently shown that a group of six common variants within or immediately flanking the *DISC1* gene alter expression levels of DISC1 itself by up to 20% (Hennah & Porteous, 2009). Through the scaffold function of DISC1, these modest reductions of *DISC1* expression may exert subtle but pervasive effects on neurodevelopment and neurophysiology. We also showed that common variants in *DISC1*, *PDE4B*, *PDE4D*, and *NDE1* are transcriptional modulators of cAMP signaling, cytoskeletal, synaptogenic, neurodevelopmental, and sensory perception proteins (Hennah & Porteous, 2009). Furthermore, when we examined the Ingenuity Pathway Analysis database (www.ingenuity.com) for genes that were current targets of psychiatric drug development targets, seven of these 139 (5% of total, p=0.007) were regulated by *DISC1* pathway genetic variants (Hennah & Porteous, 2009). Thus, the dual impact of rare, highly penetrant and of common, low-penetrant gene variants within the *DISC1* pathway may contribute to a sizable fraction of the genetic variance in schizophrenia and related major mental disorders.

The example of *DISC1* and other candidate genes identified by molecular cytogenetic methods points to a high level of locus and allelic heterogeneity in schizophrenia and challenges the still prevailing (but conspicuously waning) dogma that schizophrenia is a "common, complex disorder" that must be due to "common, ancient (single nucleotide) polymorphisms" (McClellan, Susser, & King, 2007; Porteous, 2008; Goldstein, 2009; Mitchell & Porteous, 2009). Multiple studies have very recently reported higher than expected levels of copy number variations in schizophrenia (Stefansson et al., 2008; Walsh et al., 2008; Xu et al., 2008; McCarthy et al., 2009; see chapter 8, this book). Just as was required for DISC1, these findings demand genetic validation and testing for biological plausibility. Added to the examples from molecular cytogenetics (McIntyre et al., 2003; Pickard et al., 2005a), however, their discovery strengthens the argument for a "multiple, rare mutation" model of causality (McClellan, Susser, & King, 2007; Porteous, 2008; Goldstein, 2009; Mitchell & Porteous, 2009) and against the "polygene" model of common, ancient SNP variants, which may be only a modest contributor to the sum of genetic variance (Purcell et al., 2009). As genetic evidence challenges and transcends classical DSM (*Diagnostic and Statistical Manual of Mental Disorders*) diagnostic criteria, so we may see a shift toward gene-centric diagnoses and treatments for "DISCopathies" and other "GENEopathies." This will certainly raise challenges to the "one size fits all" philosophy that has dominated the approach in industry and not succeeded over the last 60 years to produce a single, novel antipsychotic drug that was not a D2 antagonist similar to those previously in use (Insel, 2009). Led by the example of *DISC1*, the evidence base is steadily growing for genetic mechanisms and a number of pathways of causality in major mental illness. As a consequence, new opportunities are emerging for evidence-based drug development targeting particular steps in these pathways. We recently described DISC1 as the "orchestrator of a suite of protein-protein interactions harmonized in time and space" (Porteous & Millar, 2009). We suggested that the conventional models of signal transduction and metabolic flux—depicted as linear pathways, feedback loops, and "upstream-downstream" molecules—fail to convey the highly structured and compartmentalized nature of cells. This new concept (Porteous & Millar, 2009) is of "the DISC1 complex as the pathway": whether in the nucleus, or at the growth cone, the centrosome, the mitochondria, or the presynaptic and postsynaptic density, each pathway is defined by locally determined isoforms, interactions, cAMP concentrations, and phosphorylation states. It is around this concept that we would seek and expect to devise evidence-based molecular therapies that are effective, safe, and relevant to a sizable fraction of those suffering from psychotic or mood disorders, or both.

KEY AREAS FOR FUTURE RESEARCH

- Identify the full spectrum of genetic risk variants in *DISC1* and its core interacting partners.
- Biophysically characterize the DISC1 complex and the functional impact of genetic risk variants.
- Produce and characterize molecular, cellular, and animal models of *DISC1* pathway variants, including mouse, rat, zebrafish, and patient-derived induced pluripotent stem cells.
- Develop novel, knowledge-based biotherapeutics based on the aforementiond.

Acknowledgments

I thank the MRC, Wellcome Trust, and NARSAD for grant aided support and my colleagues in the Medical Genetics Section for all their contributions to the science discussed here. Any opinions expressed are my own.

Selected Readings

Chubb, J. E., Bradshaw, N. J., Soares, D. C., Porteous, D. J., & Millar, J. K. (2008). The DISC locus in psychiatric illness. *Molecular Psychiatry 13*(1): 36–64.

Harrison, P. J. & Weinberger, D. R. (2005). Schizophrenia genes, gene expression, and neuropathology: On the matter of their convergence. *Molecular Psychiatry 10*(1): 40–68.

Mackie, S., Millar, J. K., & Porteous, D. J. (2007). Role of DISC1 in neural development and schizophrenia. *Current Opinion in Neurobiology 17*(1): 95–102.

Porteous, D. (2008). Genetic causality in schizophrenia and bipolar disorder: Out with the old and in with the new. *Current Opinion in Genetics and Development 18*(3): 229–234.

Porteous, D. & Millar, K. (2009). How DISC1 regulates postnatal brain development: Girdin gets in on the AKT. *Neuron 63*(6): 711–713.

Ross, C. A., Margolis, R. L., Reading, S. A., Pletnikov, M., & Coyle, J. T. (2006). Neurobiology of schizophrenia. *Neuron 52*(1): 139–153.

References

Arguello, P. A. & Gogos, J. A. (2008). A signaling pathway AKTing up in schizophrenia. *Journal of Clinical Investigation 118*(6): 2018–2021.

Beecham, G. W., Martin, E. R., Li, Y. J., Slifer, M. A., Gilbert, J. R., Haines, J. L., & Pericak-Vance, M. A. (2009). Genome-wide association study implicates a chromosome 12 risk locus for late-onset Alzheimer disease. *American Journal of Human Genetics 84*(1): 35–43.

Blackwood, D. H., Fordyce, A., Walker, M. T., St Clair, D. M., Porteous, D. J., & Muir, W. J. (2001). Schizophrenia and affective disorders—cosegregation with a translocation at chromosome 1q42 that directly disrupts brain-expressed genes: Clinical and P300 findings in a family. *American Journal of Human Genetics 69*(2): 428–433.

Blackwood, D. H., He, L., Morris, S. W., McLean, A., Whitton, C., Thomson, M., Walker, M. T., Woodburn, K., Sharp, C. M., Wright, A. F., et al. (1996). A locus for bipolar affective disorder on chromosome 4p. *Nature Genetics 12*(4): 427–430.

Bradshaw, N. J., Christie, S., Soares, D. C., Carlyle, B. C., Porteous, D. J., & Millar, J. K. (2009). NDE1 and NDEL1: Multimerisation, alternate splicing and DISC1 interaction. *Neuroscience Letters 449*(3): 228–233.

Burdick, K. E., Kamiya, A., Hodgkinson, C. A., Lencz, T., DeRosse, P., Ishizuka, K., Elashvili, S., Arai, H., Goldman, D., Sawa, A., et al. (2008). Elucidating the relationship between DISC1, NDEL1 and NDE1 and the risk for schizophrenia: Evidence of epistasis and competitive binding. *Human Molecular Genetics 17*(16): 2462–2473.

Callicott, J. H., Straub, R. E., Pezawas, L., Egan, M. F., Mattay, V. S., Hariri, A. R., Verchinski, B. A., Meyer-Lindenberg, A., Balkissoon, R., Kolachana, B., et al. (2005). Variation in DISC1 affects hippocampal structure and function and increases risk for schizophrenia. *Proceedings of the National Academy of Sciences U.S.A. 102*(24): 8627–8632.

Camargo, L. M., Collura, V., Rain, J. C., Mizuguchi, K., Hermjakob, H., Kerrien, S., Bonnert, T. P., Whiting, P. J., & Brandon, N. J. (2007). Disrupted in schizophrenia 1 interactome: Evidence for the close connectivity of risk genes and a potential synaptic basis for schizophrenia. *Molecular Psychiatry 12*(1): 74–86.

Cardno, A. G., Rijsdijk, F. V., Sham, P. C., Murray, R. M., & McGuffin, P. (2002). A twin study of genetic relationships between psychotic symptoms. *American Journal of Psychiatry 159*(4): 539–545.

Carter, C. J. (2006). Schizophrenia susceptibility genes converge on interlinked pathways related to glutamatergic transmission and long-term potentiation, oxidative stress and oligodendrocyte viability. *Schizophrenia Research 86*(1–3): 1–4.

Chubb, J. E., Bradshaw, N. J., Soares, D. C., Porteous, D. J., & Millar, J. K. (2008). The DISC locus in psychiatric illness. *Molecular Psychiatry 13*(1): 36–64.

Clapcote, S. J., Lipina, T. V., Millar, J. K., Mackie, S., Christie, S., Ogawa, F., Lerch, J. P., Trimble, K., Uchiyama, M., Sakuraba, Y., et al. (2007). Behavioral phenotypes of Disc1 missense mutations in mice. *Neuron 54*(3): 387–402.

Craddock, N., O'Donovan, M. C., & Owen, M. J. (2006). Genes for schizophrenia and bipolar disorder? Implications for psychiatric nosology. *Schizophrenia Bulletin 32*(1): 9–16.

Craddock, N. & Owen, M. J. (2005). The beginning of the end for the Kraepelinian dichotomy. *British Journal of Psychiatry 186*: 364–366.

Di Giorgio, A., Blasi, G., Sambataro, F., Rampino, A., Papazacharias, A., Gambi, F., Romano, R., Caforio, G., Rizzo, M., Latorre, V., et al. (2008). Association of the SerCys DISC1 polymorphism with human hippocampal formation gray matter and function during memory encoding. *European Journal of Neuroscience 28*(10): 2129–2136.

Duan, X., Chang, J. H., Ge, S., Faulkner, R. L., Kim, J. Y., Kitabatake, Y., Liu, X.-B., Yang, C.-H., Jordan, J. D., Ma, D. K., et al. (2007). Disrupted-in-schizophrenia 1 regulates integration of newly generated neurons in the adult brain. *Cell 130*(6): 1146–1158.

Eastwood, S. L., Hodgkinson, C. A., & Harrison, P. J. (2009). DISC-1 Leu607Phe alleles differentially affect centrosomal PCM1 localization and neurotransmitter release. *Molecular Psychiatry 14*(6): 556–557.

Enomoto, A., Asai, N., Namba, T., Wang, Y., Kato, T., Tanaka, M., Tatsumi, H., Taya, S., Tsuboi, D., Kuroda, K., et al. (2009). Roles of disrupted-in-schizophrenia 1-interacting protein girdin in postnatal development of the dentate gyrus. *Neuron: 63*(6): 774–787.

Enomoto, A., Murakami, H., Asai, N., Morone, N., Watanabe, T., Kawai, K., Murakumo, Y., Usukura, J., Kaibuchi, K., & Takahashi, M. (2005). Akt/PKB regulates actin organization and cell motility via Girdin/APE. *Developmental Cell 9*(3): 389–402.

Erbel-Sieler, C., Dudley, C., Zhou, Y., Wu, X., Estill, S. J., Han, T., Diaz-Arrastia, R., Brunskill, E. W., Potter, S. S., & McKnight, S. L. (2004). Behavioral and regulatory abnormalities in mice deficient in the NPAS1 and NPAS3 transcription factors. *Proceedings of the National Academy of Sciences U.S.A. 101*(37): 13648–13653.

Evans, K. L., Brown, J., Shibasaki, Y., Devon, R. S., He, L., Arveiler, B., Christie, S., Maule, J. C., Baillie, D., Slorach, E. M., et al. (1995). A contiguous clone map over 3 Mb on the long arm of chromosome 11 across a balanced translocation associated with schizophrenia. *Genomics 28*(3): 420–428.

Fletcher, J. M., Evans, K., Baillie, D., Byrd, P., Hanratty, D., Leach, S., Julier, C., Gosden, J. R., Muir, W., Porteous, D. J., et al. (1993). Schizophrenia-associated chromosome 11q21 translocation: Identification of flanking markers and development of chromosome 11q fragment hybrids as cloning and mapping resources. *American Journal of Human Genetics 52*(3): 478–490.

Goff, D. C. & Wine, L. (1997). Glutamate in schizophrenia: Clinical and research implications. *Schizophrenia Research 27*(2–3): 157–168.

Goldstein, D. B. (2009). Common genetic variation and human traits. *New England Journal of Medicine 360*(17): 1696–1698.

Gurling, H. M. D., Critchley, H., Datta, S. R., McQuillin, A., Blaveri, E., Thirumalai, S., Pimm, J., Krasucki, R., Kalsi, G., Quested, D., et al. (2006). Genetic association and brain morphology studies and the chromosome 8p22 pericentriolar material 1 (PCM1) gene in susceptibility to schizophrenia. *Archives of General Psychiatry 63*(8): 844–854.

Hamshere, M. L., Bennett, P., Williams, N., Segurado, R., Cardno, A., Norton, N., Lambert, D., Williams, H., Kirov, G., Corvin, A., et al. (2005). Genomewide linkage scan in schizoaffective disorder: Significant evidence for linkage at 1q42 close to DISC1, and suggestive evidence at 22q11 and 19p13. *Archives of General Psychiatry 62*(10): 1081–1088.

Harrison, P. J. & Weinberger, D. R. (2005). Schizophrenia genes, gene expression, and neuropathology: On the matter of their convergence. *Molecular Psychiatry 10*(1): 40–68.

Hayashi, M. A. F., Portaro, F. C. V., Bastos, M. F., Guerreiro, J. R., Oliveira, V., Gorrão, S. S., Tambourgi, D. V., Sant'Anna, O. A., Whiting, P. J., Camargo, L. M., et al. (2005). Inhibition of NUDEL (nuclear distribution element-like)-oligopeptidase activity by disrupted-in-schizophrenia 1. *Proceedings of the National Academy of Sciences U.S.A. 102*(10): 3828–3833.

Hennah, W. & Porteous, D. (2009). The DISC1 pathway modulates expression of neurodevelopmental, synaptogenic and sensory perception genes. *PLoS One 4*(3): e4906.

Hennah, W., Thomson, P., McQuillin, A., Bass, N., Loukola, A., Anjorin, A., Blackwood, D., Curtis, D., Deary, I. J., Harris, S. E., et al. (2009). DISC1 association, heterogeneity and interplay in schizophrenia and bipolar disorder. *Molecular Psychiatry* 14(9): 865–873.

Hennah, W., Tomppo, L., Hiekkalinna, T., Palo, O. M., Kilpinen, H., Ekelund, J., Tuulio-Henriksson, A., Silander, K., Partonen, T., Paunio, T., et al. (2007). Families with the risk allele of DISC1 reveal a link between schizophrenia and another component of the same molecular pathway, NDE1. *Human Molecular Genetics* 16(5): 453–462.

Insel, T. R. (2009). Translating scientific opportunity into public health impact: A strategic plan for research on mental illness. *Archives of General Psychiatry* 66(2): 128–133.

Jaaro-Peled, H., Hayashi-Takagi, A., Seshadri, S., Kamiya, A., Brandon, N. J., & Sawa, A. (2009). Neurodevelopmental mechanisms of schizophrenia: Understanding disturbed postnatal brain maturation through neuregulin-1-ErbB4 and DISC1. *Trends in Neurosciences* 32(9): 485–495.

Javitt, D. C. (2004). Glutamate as a therapeutic target in psychiatric disorders. *Molecular Psychiatry* 9(11): 984–997, 979.

Jones, P. & Murray, R. M. (1991). The genetics of schizophrenia is the genetics of neurodevelopment. *British Journal of Psychiatry* 158: 615–623.

Kamiya, A., Kubo, K., Tomoda, T., Takaki, M., Youn, R., Ozeki, Y., Sawamura, N., Park, U., Kudo, C., Okawa, M., et al. (2005). A schizophrenia-associated mutation of DISC1 perturbs cerebral cortex development. *Nature Cell Biology* 7(12): 1167–1178.

Kamiya, A., Tan, P. L., Kubo, K., Engelhard, C., Ishizuka, K., Kubo, A., Tsukita, S., Pulver, A. E., Nakajima, K., Cascella, N. G., et al. (2008). Recruitment of PCM1 to the centrosome by the cooperative action of DISC1 and BBS4: A candidate for psychiatric illnesses. *Archives of General Psychiatry* 65(9): 996–1006.

Kilpinen, H., Ylisaukko-Oja, T., Hennah, W., Palo, O. M., Varilo, T., Vanhala, R., Nieminen-von Wendt, T., von Wendt, L., Paunio, T., & Peltonen, L. (2008). Association of DISC1 with autism and Asperger syndrome. *Molecular Psychiatry* 13(2): 187–196.

Kim, J. Y., Duan, X., Liu, C. Y., Jang, M. H., Guo, J. U., Pow-anpongkul, N., Kang, E., Song, H., & Ming, G. L. (2009). DISC1 regulates new neuron development in the adult brain via modulation of AKT-mTOR signaling through KIAA1212. *Neuron* 63(6): 761–773.

Knight, H. M., Pickard, B. S., Maclean, A., Malloy, M. P., Soares, D. C., McRae, A. F., Condie, A., White, A., Hawkins, W., McGhee, K., et al. (2009). A cytogenetic abnormality and rare coding variants identify ABCA13 as a candidate gene in schizophrenia, bipolar disorder, and depression. *American Journal of Human Genetics* 85(6): 833–846.

Lichtenstein, P., Yip, B. H., Bjork, C., Pawitan, Y., Cannon, T. D., Sullivan, P. F., & Hultman, C. M. (2009). Common genetic determinants of schizophrenia and bipolar disorder in Swedish families: A population-based study. *Lancet* 373(9659): 234–239.

Leliveld, S. R., Bader, V., Hendriks, P., Prikulis, I., Sajnani, G., Requena, J. R., & Korth, C. (2008). Insolubility of disrupted-in-schizophrenia 1 disrupts oligomer-dependent interactions with nuclear distribution element 1 and is associated with sporadic mental disease. *Journal of Neuroscience* 28(15): 3839–3845.

Leliveld, S. R., Hendriks, P., Michel, M., Sajnani, G., Bader, V., Trossbach, S., Prikulis, I., Hartmann, R., Jonas, E., Willbold, D., et al. (2009). Oligomer assembly of the C-terminal DISC1 domain (640–854) is controlled by self-association motifs and disease-associated polymorphism S704C. *Biochemistry* 48(32): 7746–7755.

Lipska, B. K., Peters, T., Hyde, T. M., Halim, N., Horowitz, C., Mitkus, S., Weickert, C. S., Matsumoto, M., Sawa, A., Straub, R. E., et al. (2006). Expression of DISC1 binding partners is reduced in schizophrenia and associated with DISC1 SNPs. *Human Molecular Genetics* 15(8): 1245–1258.

Mao, Y., Ge, X., Frank, C. L., Madison, J. M., Koehler, A. N., Doud, M. K., Tassa, C., Berry, E. M., Soda, T., Singh, K. K., et al. (2009). Disrupted in schizophrenia 1 regulates neuronal progenitor proliferation via modulation of GSK3beta/beta-catenin signaling. *Cell 136*(6): 1017–1031.

MacIntyre, D. J., Blackwood, D. H., Porteous, D. J., Pickard, B. S., & Muir, W. J. (2003). Chromosomal abnormalities and mental illness. *Molecular Psychiatry 8*(3): 275–287.

Mackie, S., Millar, J. K., & Porteous, D. J. (2007). Role of DISC1 in neural development and schizophrenia. *Current Opinion in Neurobiology 17*(1): 95–102.

McCarthy, S. E., Makarov, V., Kirov, G., Addington, A. M., McClellan, J., Yoon, S., Perkins, D. O., Dickel, D. E., Kusenda, M., Krastoshevsky, O., et al. (2009). Microduplications of 16p11.2 are associated with schizophrenia. *Nature Genetics 41*(11): 1223–1227.

McClellan, J. M., Susser, E., & King, M. C. (2007). Schizophrenia: A common disease caused by multiple rare alleles. *British Journal of Psychiatry 190*: 194–199.

Millar, J. K., Pickard, B. S., Mackie, S., James, R., Christie, S., Buchanan, S. R., Malloy, M. P., Chubb, J. E., Huston, E., Baillie, G. S., et al. (2005). DISC1 and PDE4B are interacting genetic factors in schizophrenia that regulate cAMP signaling. *Science 310*(5751): 1187–1191.

Millar, J. K., Wilson-Annan, J. C., Anderson, S., Christie, S., Taylor, M. S., Semple, C. A. M., Devon, R. S., Clair, D. M. S., Muir, W. J., Blackwood, D. H. R., et al. (2000). Disruption of two novel genes by a translocation co-segregating with schizophrenia. *Human Molecular Genetics 9*(9): 1415–1423.

Mitchell, K. J. & Porteous, D. J. (2009). GWAS for psychiatric disease: Is the framework built on a solid foundation? *Molecular Psychiatry 14*(8): 740–741.

Murdoch, H., Mackie, S., Collins, D. M., Hill, E. V., Bolger, G. B., Klussmann, E., Porteous, D. J., Millar, J. K., & Houslay, M. D. (2007). Isoform-selective susceptibility of DISC1/phosphodiesterase-4 complexes to dissociation by elevated intracellular cAMP levels. *Journal of Neuroscience 27*(35): 9513–9524.

Nakata, K., Lipska, B. K., Hyde, T. M., Ye, T., Newburn, E. N., Morita, Y., Vakkalanka, R., Barenboim, M., Sei, Y., Weinberger, D. R., et al. (2009). DISC1 splice variants are upregulated in schizophrenia and associated with risk polymorphisms. *Proceedings of the National Academy of Sciences U.S.A. 106*(37): 15873–15878.

Numata, S., Ueno, S., Iga, J., Song, H., Nakataki, M., Tayoshi, S., Sumitani, S., Tomotake, M., Itakura, M., Sano, A., et al. (2008). Positive association of the PDE4B (phosphodiesterase 4B) gene with schizophrenia in the Japanese population. *Journal of Psychiatric Research 43*(1): 7–12.

Pickard, B. S., Christoforou, A., Thomson, P. A., Fawkes, A., Evans, K. L., Morris, S. W., Porteous, D. J., Blackwood, D. H., & Muir, W. J. (2009). Interacting haplotypes at the NPAS3 locus alter risk of schizophrenia and bipolar disorder. *Molecular Psychiatry 14*(9): 874–884.

Pickard, B. S., Knight, H. M., Hamilton, R. S., Soares, D. C., Walker, R., Boyd, J. K. F., Machell, J., Maclean, A., McGhee, K. A., Condie, A., et al. (2008). A common variant in the 3'UTR of the GRIK4 glutamate receptor gene affects transcript abundance and protects against bipolar disorder. *Proceedings of the National Academy of Sciences U.S.A. 105*(39): 14940–14945.

Pickard, B. S., Malloy, M. P., Christoforou, A., Thomson, P. A., Evans, K. L., Morris, S. W., Hampson, M., Porteous, D. J., Blackwood, D. H., & Muir, W. J. (2006). Cytogenetic and genetic evidence supports a role for the kainate-type glutamate receptor gene, GRIK4, in schizophrenia and bipolar disorder. *Molecular Psychiatry 11*(9): 847–857.

Pickard, B. S., Malloy, M. P., Porteous, D. J., Blackwood, D. H., & Muir, W. J. (2005a). Disruption of a brain transcription factor, NPAS3, is associated with schizophrenia and learning disability. *American Journal of Medical Genetics Part B: Neuropsychiatric Genetics* *136B*(1): 26–32.

Pickard, B. S., Millar, J. K., Porteous, D. J., Muir, W. J., & Blackwood, D. H. (2005b). Cytogenetics and gene discovery in psychiatric disorders. *Pharmacogenomics Journal* *5*(2): 81–88.

Pickard, B. S., Thomson, P. A., Christoforou, A., Evans, K. L., Morris, S. W., Porteous, D. J., Blackwood, D. H., & Muir, W. J. (2007). The PDE4B gene confers sex-specific protection against schizophrenia. *Psychiatric Genetics* *17*(3): 129–133.

Pieper, A. A., Wu, X., Han, T. W., Estill, S. J., Dang, Q., Wu, L. C., Reece-Fincanon, S., Dudley, C. A., Richardson, J. A., Brat, D. J., et al. (2005). The neuronal PAS domain protein 3 transcription factor controls FGF-mediated adult hippocampal neurogenesis in mice. *Proceedings of the National Academy of Sciences U.S.A.* *102*(39): 14052–14057.

Porteous, D. (2008). Genetic causality in schizophrenia and bipolar disorder: Out with the old and in with the new. *Current Opinion in Genetics and Development* *18*(3): 229–234.

Porteous, D. & Millar, K. (2009). How DISC1 regulates postnatal brain development: Girdin gets in on the AKT. *Neuron* *63*(6): 711–713.

Prata, D. P., Mechelli, A., Fu, C. H. Y., Picchioni, M., Kane, F., Kalidindi, S., McDonald, C., Kravariti, E., Toulopoulou, T., Miorelli, A., et al. (2008). Effect of disrupted-in-schizophrenia-1 on pre-frontal cortical function. *Molecular Psychiatry* *13*(10): 915–917, 909.

Purcell, S. M., Wray, N. R., Stone, J. L., Visscher, P. M., O'Donovan, M. C., Sullivan, P. F., & Sklar, P. (2009). Common polygenic variation contributes to risk of schizophrenia and bipolar disorder. *Nature* *460*(7256): 748–752.

Ross, C. A., Margolis, R. L., Reading, S. A., Pletnikov, M., & Coyle, J. T. (2006). Neurobiology of schizophrenia. *Neuron* *52*(1): 139–153.

Song, W., Li, W., Feng, J., Heston, L. L., Scaringe, W. A., & Sommer, S. S. (2008). Identification of high risk DISC1 structural variants with a 2% attributable risk for schizophrenia. *Biochemical and Biophysical Research Communications* *367*(3): 700–706.

Stefansson, H., Rujescu, D., Cichon, S., Pietilainen, O. P. H., Ingason, A., Steinberg, S., Fossdal, R., Sigurdsson, E., Sigmundsson, T., Buizer-Voskamp, J. E., et al. (2008). Large recurrent microdeletions associated with schizophrenia. *Nature* *455*(7210): 232–236.

St Clair, D., Blackwood, D., Muir, W., Walker, M., Carothers, A., Spowart, G., Gosden, C., & Evans, H. J. (1990). Association within a family of a balanced autosomal translocation with major mental illness. *Lancet* *336*(8706): 13–16.

Sullivan, P. F., Lin, D., Tzeng, J. Y., van den Oord, E., Perkins, D., Stroup, T. S., Wagner, M., Lee, S., Wright, F. A., Zou, F., et al. (2008). Genomewide association for schizophrenia in the CATIE study: Results of stage 1. *Molecular Psychiatry* *13*(6): 570–584.

Szeszko, P. R., Hodgkinson, C. A., Robinson, D. G., DeRosse, P., Bilder, R. M., Lencz, T., Burdick, K. E., Napolitano, B., Betensky, J. D., Kane, J. M., et al. (2008). DISC1 is associated with prefrontal cortical gray matter and positive symptoms in schizophrenia. *Biological Psychology* *79*(1): 103–110.

Taylor, M. S., Devon, R. S., Millar, J. K., & Porteous, D. J. (2003). Evolutionary constraints on the disrupted in schizophrenia locus. *Genomics* *81*(1): 67–77.

Thomson, P. A., Harris, S. E., Starr, J. M., Whalley, L. J., Porteous, D. J., & Deary, I. J. (2005). Association between genotype at an exonic SNP in DISC1 and normal cognitive aging. *Neuroscience Letters* *389*(1): 41–45.

Tomppo, L., Hennah, W., Lahermo, P., Loukola, A., Tuulio-Henriksson, A., Suvisaari, J., Partonen, T., Ekelund, J., Lönnqvist, J., & Peltonen, L. (2009). Association between genes of disrupted in schizophrenia 1 (DISC1) interactors and schizophrenia supports the role of the DISC1 pathway in the etiology of major mental illnesses. *Biological Psychiatry* *65*(12): 1055–1062.

Walsh, T., McClellan, J. M., McCarthy, S. E., Addington, A. M., Pierce, S. B., Cooper, G. M., Nord, A. S., Kusenda, M., Malhotra, D., Bhandari, A., et al. (2008). Rare structural variants disrupt multiple genes in neurodevelopmental pathways in schizophrenia. *Science* 320(5875): 539–543.

Weinberger, D. R. (1987). Implications of normal brain development for the pathogenesis of schizophrenia. *Archives of General Psychiatry* 44(7): 660–669.

Whalley, H. C., Pickard, B. S., McIntosh, A. M., Zuliani, R., Johnstone, E. C., Blackwood, D. H. R., Lawrie, S. M., Muir, W. J., & Hall, J. (2009). A GRIK4 variant conferring protection against bipolar disorder modulates hippocampal function. *Molecular Psychiatry* 14(5): 467–468.

Xu, B., Roos, J. L., Levy, S., van Rensburg, E. J., Gogos, J. A., & Karayiorgou, M. (2008). Strong association of de novo copy number mutations with sporadic schizophrenia. *Nature Genetics* 40(7): 880–885.

CHAPTER 15

MUTANT MODELS OF *Nrg1* AND *ErbB4*
Abnormalities of Brain Structures, Functions, and Behaviors Relevant to Schizophrenia

YACHI CHEN, LORNA W. ROLE, AND DAVID A. TALMAGE

KEY CONCEPTS

- Multiple studies provide evidence that *NRG1* and *ERBB4* are candidate susceptibility genes for schizophrenia.
- Mice with genetic disruption in *Nrg1* or *ErbB4* display enlarged lateral ventricles and reduced spine density on hippocampal subicular dendrites, which are characteristics of schizophrenia neuropathology.
- *Nrg1* and *ErbB4* mutant mice also display hyperlocomotor activity, impaired sensorimotor gating, abnormal social interactions, and diminished performance in learning and memory tasks. These abnormalities are consistent with alterations in cortico–limbic functions that often are severely compromised in patients with schizophrenia.

Structure and Function of Neuregulin 1

The neuregulin proteins (NRGs) represent a large family of growth factors encoded by four individual genes (*NRG1-4*). Of these four genes, *NRG1* is the best characterized. *NRG1* is located on the short arm of chromosome 8, where Stefansson et al. (2002) identified *NRG1* as a putative schizophrenia susceptibility gene. In the central nervous system (CNS), NRG1 plays critical roles in neuronal migration, synapse formation, and plasticity; the last of these is based on NRG1 regulation of neurotransmitter receptor expression and function (Falls, 2003; Corfas et al., 2004; Harrison & Law, 2006; Mei & Xiong, 2008). Alterations in regulation of one or more of these key processes by NRG1 are thought to contribute to the pathophysiology of schizophrenia.

The NRG1 proteins are classified into six subtypes (Types I–VI) based on type-specific sequences and the structural domains located in the NH$_2$-terminal region (figure 15.1A) (Falls, 2003; Mei & Xiong, 2008). Within the NH$_2$-terminal region, the immunoglobulin (Ig)-like domain is present in Types I, II, IV, and V, whereas a hydrophobic cysteine-rich domain (CRD) is present only in Type III. Alternative splicing in the juxtamembrane stalk region and the intracellular domain (ICD) generates additional variants of each major subtype. Differential levels and patterns of the expression of the three major types, I–III, occur in various tissues including the brain (Meyer & Birchmeier, 1995). In addition, mice with targeted mutations disrupting certain classes of NRG1 isoforms have distinct defects in neural development (Falls, 2003). Together, these results demonstrate isoform-specific expression and function of NRG1.

Proteolytic Processing of NRG1

A majority of NRG1 isoforms are produced as single-pass transmembrane pro-proteins. However, Type III NRG1 pro-proteins span the membrane twice be-cause of the presence of the hydrophobic CRD. Proteolytic processing in the ex-tracellular, juxtamembrane region of NRG1 releases the ecotodomain containing the epidermal growth factor (EGF)-like domain, which participates in paracrine signaling by activating ERBB kinases (figure 15.1B) (Falls, 2003; Mei & Xiong, 2008). For Type III NRG1 isoforms, the cleaved ecto-domain containing the EGF-like domain remains tethered to the membrane by the CRD and is believed to signal through ERBB receptor kinases in a contact-dependent, juxtacrine man-ner (Wolpowitz et al., 2000; Leimeroth et al., 2002; Falls, 2003). Type III NRG1 undergoes a second, intramembranous, γ-secretase-dependent cleavage to release ICD from the membrane (Bao et al., 2003). The released ICD translocates to the nucleus and regulates gene expression (Bao et al., 2003, 2004). Thus, Type III NRG1 can signal by means of the activation of ERBB kinases and by means of the ICD.

NRG1 Signaling Through ERBB Receptor Tyrosine Kinases

NRG1 serves as one of the ligands of ERBB receptor tyrosine kinases. EGFR/ERBB1, ERBB2, ERBB3, and ERBB4 are members of the ERBB kinase family. Binding of NRG1 to homo- or hetero-dimerized ERBB receptors by way of the EGF-like domain leads to stimulation of the kinase activity of ERBB, activation of intracellular signaling networks, and induction of cellular responses. Among the ERBB family members, EGFR and ERBB2 do not bind NRG1 but do have

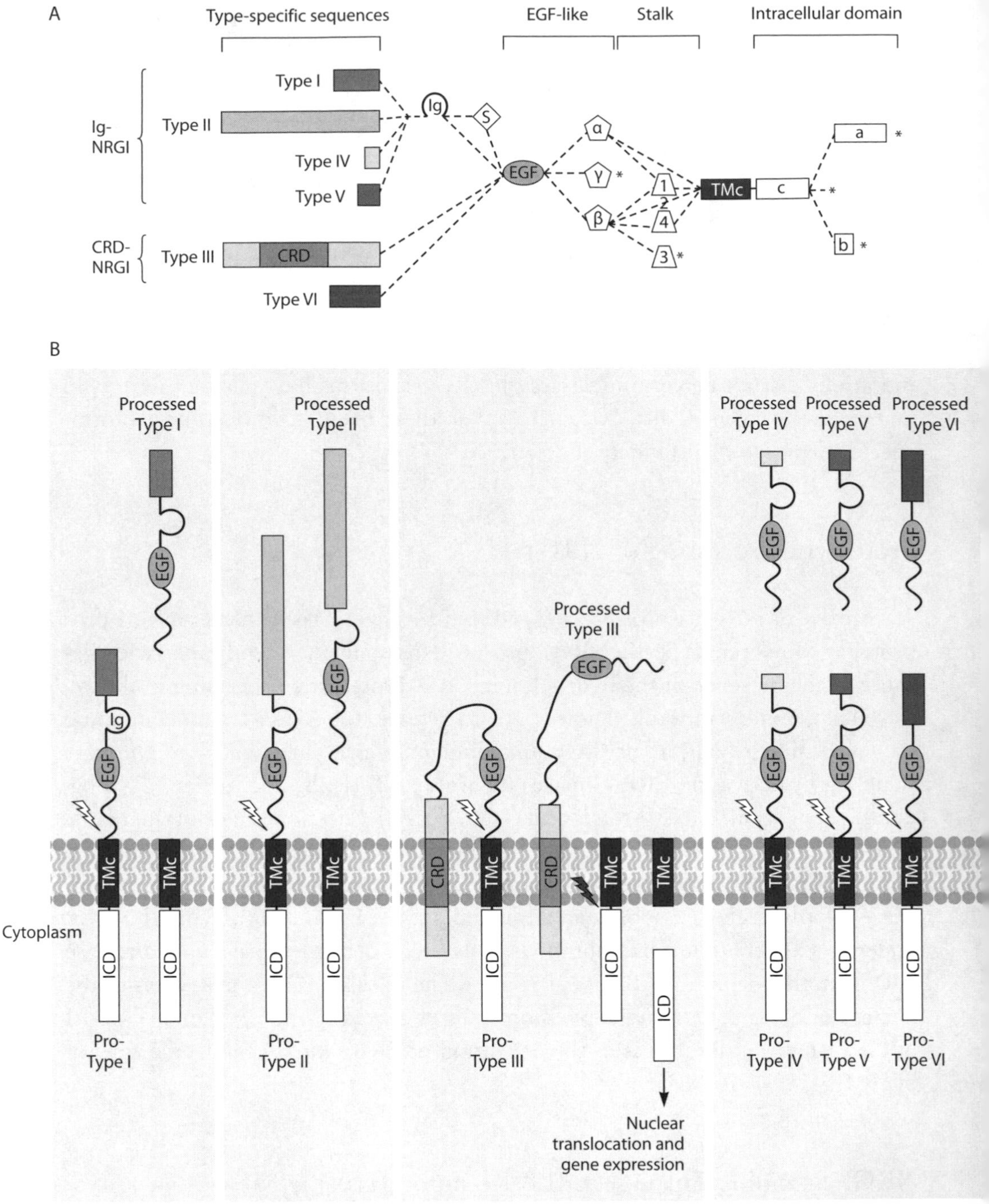

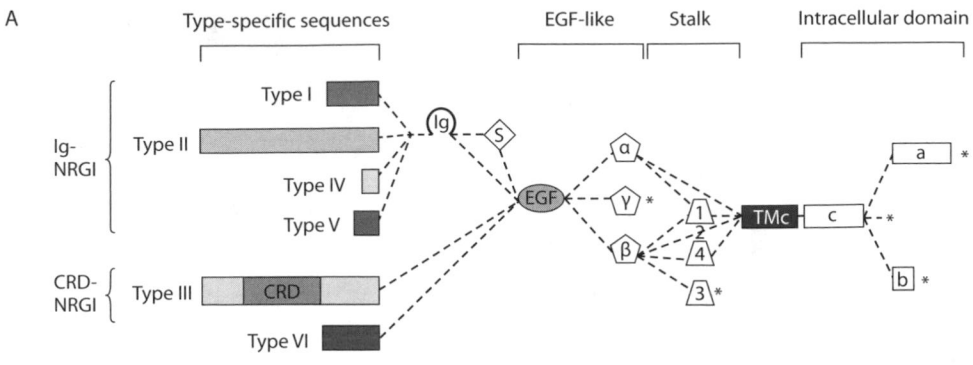

Figure 15.1. Illustration of different types of NRG1 and their proteolytic processing events. (A) The NRG1 proteins are classified into six major types based on distinct NH_2-terminal type-specific sequences that arise from the unique usage of multiple promoters. Types I, II, IV, and V NRG1 are sometimes referred to as Ig-NRG1 because of the presence of an immunoglobulin (Ig)-like domain, which is connected to the epidermal growth factor (EGF)-like domain by a spacer region (S) in certain isoforms. Type III NRG1 has a cysteine-rich domain (CRD) and is therefore sometimes referred to as CRD-NRG1. Because the CRD is hydrophobic, it acts as the second transmembrane anchor in addition to the first transmembrane

functional kinase domains. In contrast, ERBB3 binds to NRG1 but has an impaired kinase function. Most importantly, ERBB4 interacts with NRG1 and has a functional kinase domain. Since EGFR and ERBB2 do not bind NRG1, the catalytically active ERBB dimers that are most capable of transducing NRG1 signals are ERBB2–ERBB3, ERBB2–ERBB4, ERBB3–ERBB4, and ERBB4–ERBB4.

NRG1 and Neurotransmission

In view of the diverse set of cognitive functions and behaviors that are thought to be compromised in schizophrenia, it is not surprising that many neurotransmitter systems and neuromodulatory circuits have been implicated in its etiology. As such, it is important to consider how the dysregulation of NRG1/ERBB signaling might disrupt neurotransmitter systems affected in schizophrenia.

The schizophrenia literature has focused on alterations in four major transmitter systems and circuits as key players in the etiology and symptomatology of schizophrenia. The first consists of the meso-limbic and meso-cortical dopamine signaling systems that have been implicated because of the profound response of patients to pharmacotherapeutics that target the dopamine system. The second candidate dysregulated system involves cortical inhibitory interneurons that utilize gamma-aminobutyric acid for neurotransmission (i.e., GABAergic interneurons).

domain (TMc) at the COOH-terminus. The NH_2-terminal regions of Types III and VI NRG1 are connected directly to the EGF-like domain. The EGF-like domain present in all six types of NRG1 proteins interacts with the ERBB receptor tyrosine kinases. Alternative splicing of sequences within the stalk region and the intracellular domain at the COOH-terminus yields different isoforms of each type of NRG1. The asterisk marks the stop codon.

(B) A majority of NRG1 isoforms are synthesized as single-pass transmembrane pro-proteins, with the NH_2-terminal region containing the EGF-like domain located on the extracellular side. However, Type III NRG1 spans the membrane twice and the NH_2-terminal and COOH-terminal regions are both located on the cytoplasmic side. Proteolytic processing (represented by the light-shaded lightning arrow) of NRG1 pro-proteins by tumor necrosis factor-α converting enzyme (TACE), β-site of amyloid precursor protein cleaving enzyme (BACE), or meltrin β releases the ecto-domain containing the EGF-like domain, which binds to and activates ERBB receptor tyrosine kinase. In the case of Type III NRG1, the cleaved ecto-domain is tethered to the membrane by the CRD and activates ERBB kinase in a contact-dependent manner. Moreover, Type III NRG1 undergoes a second intramembranous cleavage that is, at least in part, γ-secretase-dependent (indicated by the dark-shaded lightning arrow), and this results in the release of NRG1 intracellular domain (ICD) from the membrane (Bao et al., 2003). The released ICD translocates to the nucleus, where it regulates gene expression (Bao et al., 2003, 2004). Thus, Type III NRG1 can signal bidirectionally, through the activation of ERBB kinases and through the ICD. Although the processing of Types IV, V, and VI isoforms of NRG1 pro-proteins is less clear, it most likely resembles that of Types I and II. (Source: Authors, based on Falls [2003]; Mei & Xiong [2008].)

The third neurotransmitter system implicated in schizophrenia is based on recent literature focusing on an important role for alterations in cortico-limbic glutamatergic synaptic transmission in schizophrenia pathology, with particular emphasis on N-methyl-D-aspartate (NMDA) receptor pathways. Finally, we discuss alterations in cholinergic signaling, which have long been noted as being associated with the pathophysiology of schizophrenia, and also the strong comorbidity of schizophrenia with nicotine abuse.

NRG1 and Dopaminergic Transmission

The literature on the neurobiology of schizophrenia strongly implicates alterations in dopamine signaling at the core of the disease. The important role of imbalances in dopamine signaling is supported by (1) findings of hyperdopaminergic signaling (increased D2 receptor activation) in subcortical areas and (2) findings consistent with hypodopaminergic signaling in cortical regions. The former is thought to underlie the "positive" symptoms of schizophrenia, whereas the latter may be responsible for the impairments in cognitive functions and behavior (Guillin, Abi-Dargham, & Laruelle, 2007). Attempts to dissect how the imbalance in dopamine signaling could lead to the manifestations of positive and negative symptoms have been avidly pursued in animal models. In fact, the selective manipulation of schizophrenia susceptibility genes reveals an important role for NRG1/ERBB signaling components in dopamine transmission. Several studies implicate NRG1/ERBB signaling in the development of central dopaminergic neurons (Steiner et al., 1999). Infusion of exogenous NRG1 (beta peptide) induces substantial increases in striatal dopamine release (Yurek et al., 2004). Perhaps most intriguing are recent probes into the effects of NRG1/ERBB signaling in the regulation of long-term potentiation (LTP) in the hippocampus—an established model for dissecting the synaptic underpinnings of memory. Addition of soluble NRG1 regulates LTP by increasing dopamine release, leading to activation of dopamine D4 receptors (Kwon et al., 2008). The shift in dopamine signaling, in turn, regulates glutamatergic transmission, leading to an inhibition or reversal of glutamatergic LTP in the hippocampus (Neddens et al., 2009). Another study manipulated NRG1/ERBB signaling by expressing a dominant negative ERBB4 receptor and found altered dopaminergic tone, as evidenced by increased levels of dopamine receptors (D1R, D2R) and DAT transporter (Roy et al., 2007).

NRG1 and GABAergic Synapses

Postmortem analyses of brains from schizophrenia patients have demonstrated reduction in the synapses between GABAergic, fast-spiking chandelier interneurons and layer 3 pyramidal neurons (Lewis, 2000; Volk & Lewis, 2002; Hashimoto et al., 2003, 2007; Lewis, Volk, & Hashimoto, 2004; Lewis, Hashimoto, & Volk, 2005). Chandelier interneurons are believed to impose synchrony on excitatory output from the cortex, and deficits in chandelier neuronal function are likely to contribute to impairments in higher-level cortical processing or the integration of thalamo-cortical signaling, or both.

Several studies have implicated NRG1 signaling in the development, maintenance, or plasticity of GABAergic cortical interneurons. During early embryonic development, the tangential migration of interneurons into the neocortex requires NRG1/ERBB4 signaling (Flames et al., 2004; Flames & Marin, 2005; Lopez-Bendito et al., 2006). Adult mice that are heterozygous for disruption of Type III *Nrg1* have a decreased number of GABAergic interneurons that stain strongly for parvalbumin (PV) within the prelimbic and infralimbic cortex (Johnson, 2007). In vitro, NRG1 signaling regulates the expression of GABA-A receptors (Rieff et al., 1999; Okada & Corfas, 2004). Cortical GABAergic axon terminals contain ERBB4, and activation of presynaptic ERBB4 modulates the probability of GABA release (Mei & Xiong, 2008; Woo et al., 2007). In addition, in PV-*ErbB4*$^{-/-}$ mice a selective loss of ERBB4 in PV-positive interneurons prevents NRG1 from stimulating GABA release (Wen et al., 2010). Thus, NRG1/ERBB4 signaling modulates the strength of GABAergic transmission. Given that alterations in GABA signaling appear to depend on the type, timing, and method of NRG1 manipulation, animal models present an important opportunity to sort out the differential role of NRG1/ERBB signaling during development and in adulthood.

NRG1 and Glutamatergic Plasticity

Functional imaging, pharmacological, and postmortem studies all point to aberrant cortical glutamatergic transmission in schizophrenia (Harrison et al., 2003; Laruelle et al., 2003; Coyle, 2004; Coyle & Tsai, 2004; Harrison & Weinberger, 2005). NRG1/ERBB signaling plays an important role in the development and plasticity of thalamo-cortical and cortico-cortical glutamatergic circuits. First, NRG1/ERBB signaling appears to be a key player in the radial migration of differentiating excitatory pyramidal neurons (Anton et al., 1997) as well as in the targeting of glutamatergic thalamo-cortical projections (Lopez-Bendito et al., 2006). In the adult, NRG1/ERBB signaling modulates activity-dependent synaptic plasticity by regulating NMDA and AMPA receptor phosphorylation and trafficking (Ozaki et al., 1997; Stefansson et al., 2002; Gu et al., 2005; Kwon et al., 2005; Hahn et al., 2006; Bjarnadottir et al., 2007; Li et al., 2007). Although the results are complex and to some extent contradictory, these studies point to the need for a fine balance of NRG1/ERBB signaling in which both deficient and excessive signaling interfere with synaptic plasticity (Gu et al., 2005; Kwon et al., 2005;

Hahn et al., 2006; Bjarnadottir et al., 2007; Li et al., 2007; Role & Talmage, 2007). Such findings also underscore the important role of studies in animal models where different aspects of the signaling can be selectively disrupted or up-regulated and where the precise nature of the change or changes in glutamatergic synapses can be assessed directly.

NRG1 and Cholinergic Modulation of Circuits

The *CHRNA7* gene, which encodes the $\alpha 7$ subunit of the nicotinic acetylcholine receptors, $\alpha 7^*$nAChRs, has been linked to schizophrenia and, in particular, to endophenotypes associated with sensory gating deficits (Martin et al., 2007). Recent genomewide association studies (GWAS) that identified DNA copy number variations associated with schizophrenia converged on multiple regions of 15 q, with the common domain being the upstream regulatory domain of the *CHRNA7* gene (International Schizophrenia Consortium, 2008). Postmortem studies have also demonstrated region-specific reductions in $\alpha 7^*$nAChRs in patients with schizophrenia and further showed that these reductions were associated with risk single nucleotide polymorphisms (SNPs) in *NRG1* (Leonard et al., 2002; Gault et al., 2003; Mathew et al., 2007; Stephens et al., 2009). Animal studies demonstrate that NRG1 signaling regulates the expression and presynaptic targeting of $\alpha 7^*$nAChRs (Yang et al., 1998; Liu et al., 2001; Kawai, Zago, & Berg, 2002; Hancock et al., 2008; Talmage, 2008; Zhong et al., 2008). In view of the strong comorbidity of smoking and schizophrenia, a systematic investigation into the mechanisms by which NRG1 signaling alters cholinergic and cholinoceptive systems is important. In particular, studies linking alterations in NRG1/ERBB signaling components and the functional profile of cholinergic receptor expression in circuits affected in schizophrenia should be pursued.

NRG1 and ERBB4 as Schizophrenia Susceptibility Genes

In 2002, a group from deCode reported an association between schizophrenia and a cluster of sequence polymorphisms near the 5-prime end of *NRG1* (Stefansson et al., 2002). This so-called Icelandic risk haplotype (Ice$_{HAP}$) was estimated to confer a population-attributable risk of 16%. *NRG1* has been evaluated specifically as a schizophrenia susceptibility gene in more than 30 subsequent studies, about 60% of which showed positive association either with the Ice$_{HAP}$ or other polymorphisms spanning essentially the entire locus. In at least two instances, risk-conferring interactions between *NRG1* and *ERBB4* sequence polymorphism were reported (Norton et al., 2006; Shiota et al., 2008). Altered hippocampal or prefrontal cortical expression of *NRG1* isoforms and *ERBB4* isoforms, or both, is associated with specific risk alleles in postmortem brains (Law et al., 2006, 2007; Nicodemus et al., 2009). The observed changes are predicted to alter signaling in the NRG1/ERBB4 system. The increase in Type I and IV NRG1 expression would increase paracrine signaling, whereas the decrease in Type III NRG1 expression would decrease juxtacrine NRG1 signaling (figure 15.1). Increased expression of the JMa/CYT-1 isoform of ERBB4 would selectively increase signaling via phosphatidylinositol 3-kinase (PI3K) (figure 15.2).

Further evidence in support of a role for altered NRG1 function in the etiology of schizophrenia comes from a series of studies demonstrating the link between specific *NRG1* risk alleles and particular schizophrenia-associated endophenotypes, including enlarged lateral ventricles (Mata et al., 2009), altered hippocampal activity measured with functional magnetic resonance imaging (fMRI) (Kircher et al., 2009b), verbal fluency (Kircher et al., 2009a), P300 event-related potential (ERP) (Bramon et al., 2008), various psychosocial measures (e.g., Keri et al., 2009), and expression of *CHRNA7* (Mathew et al., 2007). Whether, and how, changes in the levels and type of NRG1/ERBB4 signaling contribute to these phenotypes is not clear, but these findings raise an important set of questions that can be addressed in mouse genetic models. Progress along these avenues is discussed in detail below.

Mutant Mouse Models

Whereas ERBB2 and ERBB3 require heterodimerization for kinase activation, ERBB4 can undergo homodimerization to transduce NRG1 signals, indicating that neuronal expression of ERBB4, in particular, may be of functional significance. There is evidence that genetic interaction between variants of *NRG1* and *ERBB4* loci increases susceptibility to schizophrenia (Norton et al., 2006; Shiota et al., 2008). Furthermore, *ERBB2* and *ERBB3* are not known schizophrenia susceptibility genes (Kanazawa et al., 2007; Watanabe et al., 2007), and mice heterozygous for targeted disruption of *ErbB2* or *ErbB3* do not show behaviors reminiscent of schizophrenia (Gerlai, Pisacane, & Erickson, 2000). Hence, we will focus on NRG1 and ERBB4 functional alterations associated with schizophrenia by reviewing studies of the currently available mutant mouse models of *Nrg1* and *ErbB4*.

Many mouse lines carrying mutations in the *Nrg1* or *ErbB4* gene have been generated. Homozygous deletions of *Nrg1* or *ErbB4* lead to embryonic or perinatal lethality because of heart malformations, thus limiting their usefulness to studies of early brain development. However, heterozygous mutant mice with targeted disruption of *Nrg1* or *ErbB4* are viable and fertile, and these animals have been used for investigating the effects of reduced NRG1 or ERBB4 expression in adult brains. Additionally, several mouse lines carrying conditional muta-

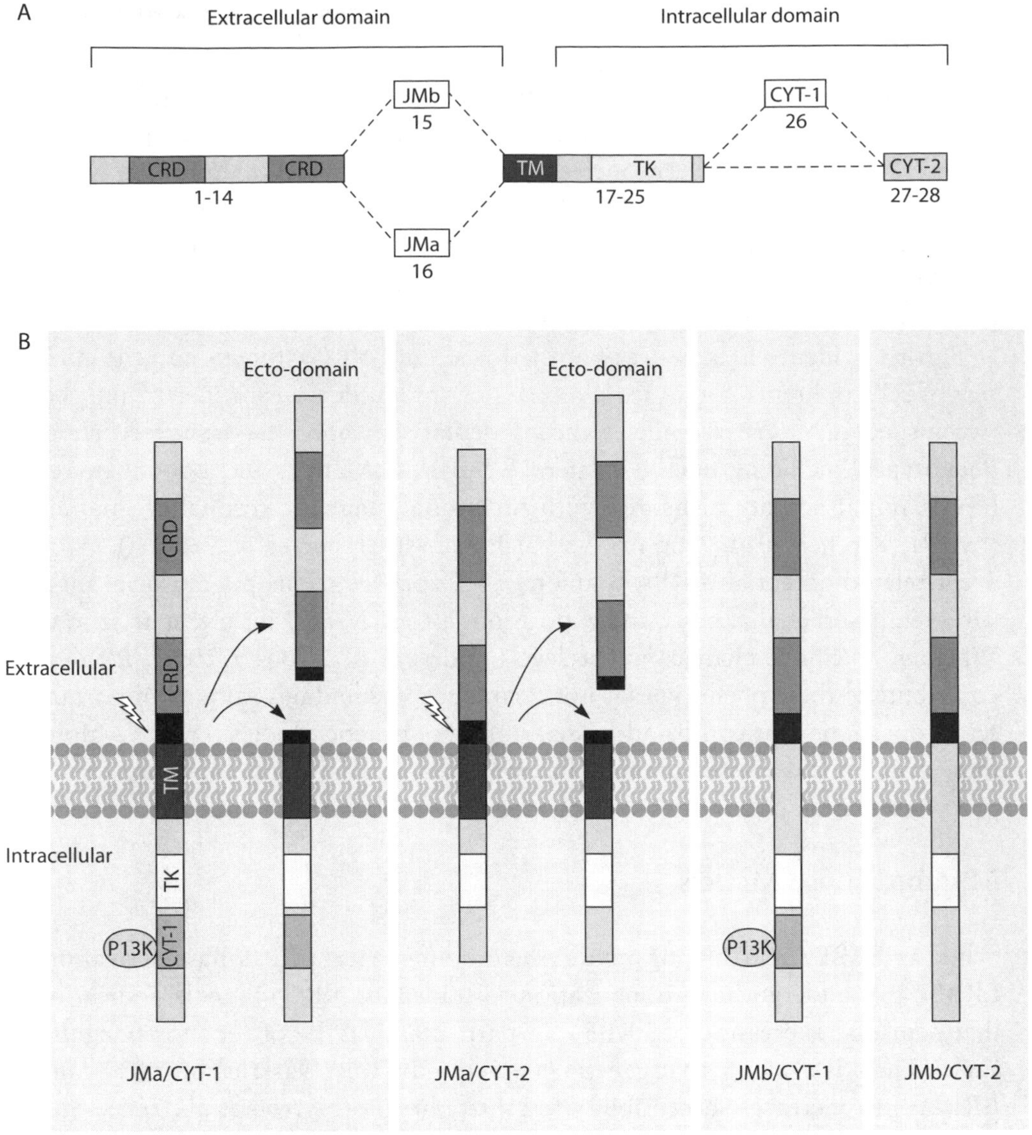

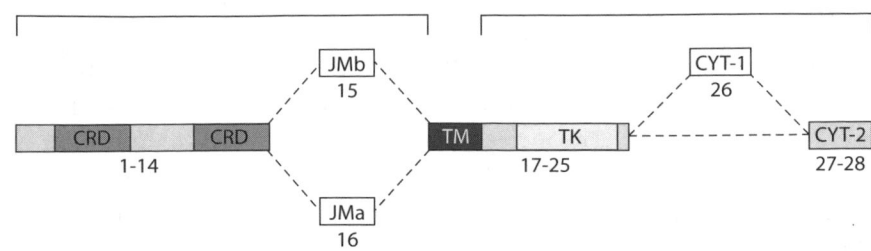

Figure 15.2. Structural organization and processing of four ERBB4 splice variants.
(A) Differential usage of exon 15 and 16 encoding the extracellular juxtamembrane sequences results in the generation of the juxtamembrane-b (JMb) or juxtamembrane-a (JMa) isoforms, respectively. The JMa and JMb isoforms can be further differentiated on the basis of the presence (cytoplasmic-1, CYT-1) or absence (cytoplasmic-2, CYT-2) of exon 26-encoded sequences within the cytoplasmic region. Therefore, four *ERBB4* isoforms are JMa/CYT-1, JMa/CYT-2, JMb/CYT-1, and JMb/CYT-2. Corresponding exon numbers are shown at the bottom of the domain structures. CRD = cysteine-rich domain; TK = tyrosine kinase domain; TM = transmembrane domain.
(B) The ERBB4 isoforms interact with NRG1 through their ecto-domains. Following ligand-binding, the JMa isoform but not the JMb isoform is proteolytically processed (represented by the lightning arrow) by TACE to produce two fragments: a soluble ecto-domain that is subsequently shed, and a second fragment that contains the intracellular cytoplasmic domain. Within the intracellular domain, only the CYT-1 isoform contains the interaction motif that recruits the p85 subunit of phosphatidylinositol 3-kniase (PI3K), which subsequently activates Akt kinase. (Source: Authors, based on Falls [2003]; Mei & Xiong [2008].)

tions of *ErbB4* or a dominant negative allele of *ErbB4* are available for functional characterization of NRG1/ERBB signaling. Table 15.1 lists heterozygous *Nrg1* mutant mouse models that eliminate all or specific isoforms of *Nrg1* as well as a transgenic mouse line over-expressing Type I *Nrg1*. Table 15.2 lists *ErbB4* mutant mice that have been analyzed. A variety of structural and functional studies as well as behavioral assays have been performed on *Nrg1* and *ErbB4* mutant mice to probe the function of CNS circuits underlying schizophrenia-associated endophenotypes.

Anatomic or Structural Defects and Alterations in Synaptic Functions in *Nrg1* and *ErbB4* Mutant Mice

Enlargement of Lateral Ventricles

The lateral ventricles represent a brain region that circulates the cerebrospinal fluid and helps protect against physical trauma. A review of structural MRI data of schizophrenia patients has revealed enlargement of the lateral ventricles in approximately 80% of the studies (McCarley et al., 1999). Ventriculomegaly is therefore the most robust MRI finding in schizophrenia. Recently, a variant of *NRG1* was associated with increased lateral ventricle volume in patients with first-episode schizophrenia (Mata et al., 2009). It is interesting that Type III-*Nrg1*$^{+/-}$ mutant mice also exhibit age-dependent, enlarged lateral ventricles (Chen et al., 2008).

Selective Loss of Parvalbumin-Positive GABAergic Interneurons in the Prefrontal Cortex

Abnormal neural synchrony due to deficits in the GABAergic neurotransmission has been implicated in schizophrenia. Consistent with this is a selective reduction of immunoreactivity in a specific subtype of inhibitory GABAergic interneuron—PV-positive interneurons—in the prefrontal cortex of patients with schizoprenia (Beasley & Reynolds, 1997; Hashimoto et al., 2003; Lewis, Hashimoto, & Volk, 2005). Similarly, there is a striking decrease in the PV-positive, but not the calbindin-positive, population of GABAergic interneurons in the infralimbic and prelimbic areas of the prefrontal cortex of adult Type III-*Nrg1*$^{+/-}$ mutant mice (Johnson, 2007). This cell- and region-specific effect of reduced levels of Type III NRG1 was further demonstrated by a lack of changes in the PV-positive GABAergic interneuron population in the dorso-peduncular prefrontal area (Johnson, 2007). In addition, young (postnatal day 20) *ErbB4*$^{-/-}$ HER4^{heart} mutant mice (table 15.2) show a decrease in the number of GABAergic interneurons at

Table 15.1 Summary of *Nrg1* Mouse Lines

EGF-*Nrg1*$^{+/-}$ mice
- Developed by Erickson et al., 1997
- Disruption of the exon encoding the N-terminal half of the EGF-like-domain; all NRG1 isoforms do not bind and activate ERBB receptors
- Reference for behavioral studies: Gerlai, Pisacane, & Erickson, 2000 (maintained in a C57BL/6 X 129/SVEV background)

EGF-*Nrg1*$^{+/-}$ mice
- Developed by Meyer & Birchmeier, 1995
- Targeted disruption of exons 7, 8, and 9, which encode the C-terminus of the EGF-like domain of all NRG1 isoforms; all NRG1 isoforms do not bind and activate ERBB receptors
- References for behavioral studies: Duffy et al., 2008 (maintained in a C57BL/6 background); Moy et al., 2009 (maintained in a B6D2F1/CrlBR background); Ehrlichman et al., 2009 (maintained in a C57BL/6 X 129/SVEV background)

Ig-*Nrg1*$^{+/-}$ mice
- Developed by Kramer et al., 1996
- Targeted mutation of exon 3 that inactivates all Ig-NRG1 isoforms
- Reference for behavioral studies: Rimer et al., 2005 (maintained in a C57BL/6 background)

TM-*Nrg1*$^{+/-}$ mice
- Developed by Liu et al., 1998
- Targeted deletion of exon 11 encoding the transmembrane domain
- References for behavioral studies: Stefansson et al., 2002 (maintained in a C57BL/6 X 129/SVEV hybrid background); Liu et al., 1998; O'Tuathaigh et al., 2006; Boucher et al., 2007; Karl et al., 2007; O'Tuathaigh et al., 2007; O'Tuathaigh et al., 2008; van den Buuse et al., 2009 (maintained in a C57BL/6 background)

Type III (or CRD)-*Nrg1*$^{+/-}$ mice
- Developed by (Wolpowitz et al., 2000)
- Type III NRG1 is inactivated due to disruption of exon 7 encoding the CRD; Ig-NRG1 expression is normal
- Reference for behavioral studies: Chen et al., 2008 (maintained in a C57BL/6 X 129/SVEV hybrid background)

*Nrg1*α$^{-/-}$ mice
- Developed by Li et al., 2002
- Targeted mutation of exon 7 that inactivates all NRG1 isoforms with an α-type EGF-like domain; the expression of isoforms with β-type EGF-like domain is normal
- Behavioral phenotypes have not been determined.

Nrg1$^{Type\ I\text{-}tg}$ mice
- Developed by Michailov et al., 2004
- Transgenic mice over-express the β1a isoform of Type I *Nrg1* from the murine Thy1.2 promoter, which is active in postnatal motor neurons and DRG neurons, and show altered central myelination.
- Reference for behavioral studies: Deakin et al., 2009 (maintained in a C57BL/6 background)

SOURCE: Authors.

Table 15.2 Summary of *ErbB4* Mouse Lines

ErbB4⁺/⁻ mice

- Targeted disruption of exon 2 generated by Gassmann et al., 1995.
- Reference for behavioral studies: Stefansson et al., 2002 (maintained in a C57BL/6 background).

*ErbB4*ᶠˡᵒˣ/⁻ **Nes-Cre mice**

- The *ErbB4*ᶠˡᵒˣ/⁻ Nes-Cre mutant mice (Golub, Germann, & Lloyd, 2004; Thuret et al., 2004) were generated by crossing "floxed" *ErbB4* mice containing two *lox*P sites in introns 1 and 2 of the *ErbB4* locus (Long et al., 2003) with *Nes-Cre* mice expressing Cre recombinase from the rat promoter of the neural marker protein nestin (Tronche et al., 1999). ERBB4 protein was not detected in the brain of the *ErbB4*ᶠˡᵒˣ/⁻ Nes-Cre mice (Thuret et al., 2004).
- References for behavioral studies: Golub, Germann, & Lloyd, 2004 (maintained in a C57BL/6J background); Thuret et al., 2004 (the strain background was not specified).

*ErbB4*ᶠˡᵒˣ/⁻ **hGFAP-Cre mice**

- The *ErbB4*ᶠˡᵒˣ/⁻ hGFAP-Cre mutant mice (Anton et al., 2004) were generated by crossing "floxed" *ErbB4* mice containing two *lox*P sites in introns 1 and 2 of the *ErbB4* locus (Long et al., 2003) with hGFAP-Cre mice expressing Cre recombinase from the human promoter of the astrocytic marker protein GFAP (glial fibrillary acidic protein) (Zhuo et al., 2001).
- Reference for behavioral studies: Moy et al., 2009 (maintained in a C57BL/6J X 129S1/SvImJ hybrid background).

DN-*ErbB4* mice

- The DN-*ErbB4* mutant mice (Chen et al., 2006) express a dominant negative *ErbB4* (DN-*ErbB4*) from the promoter of CNP (2',3'-cyclic nucleotide 3'-phosphodiesterase), an enzyme found in oligodendrocytes and myelinating Schwann cells. Expression of DN-*ErbB4* inhibits ERBB2, ERBB3, and ERBB4 signaling and function in cells including oligodendrocytes and myelinating Schwann cells (Chen et al., 2006; Roy et al., 2007).
- Reference for behavioral studies: Roy et al., 2007 (FVB/N background).

ErbB2/B4-CNSko **mice**

- The *ErbB2/B4-CNSko* mutant mice were generated by crossing a mouse line homozygous for loxP-flanked *ErbB2* and *ErbB4* alleles (Leu et al., 2003; Long et al., 2003) with hGFAP-Cre mice expressing Cre recombinase from the human GFAP promoter (Zhuo et al., 2001).
- Reference for behavioral studies: Barros et al., 2009 (the strain background was not specified).

ErbB4⁻/⁻ ᴴᴱᴿ⁴ ʰᵉᵃʳᵗ **mice**

- The *ErbB4*⁻/⁻ HER4 *(or ErbB4)*ʰᵉᵃʳᵗ mutant mice (Flames et al., 2004) were generated by crossing *ErbB4*⁺/⁻ mice (Gassmann et al., 1995) with transgenic mice expressing *ErbB4* (or *HER4*) under the control of the cardiac-specific, alpha-myosin heavy chain promoter (Tidcombe et al., 2003).
- Behavioral phenotypes have not been determined.

PV-*ErbB4*⁻/⁻ mice

- The PV-*ErbB4*⁻/⁻ mutant mice (Wen et al., 2010) were generated by crossing *ErbB4*ˡᵒˣᴾ/ˡᵒˣᴾ mice containing two *lox*P sequences flanking exon 2 of the *ErbB4* locus (Garcia-Rivello et al., 2005) with PV-Cre mice expressing Cre recombinase from the endogenous *Pvalb*, parvalbumin, locus (Hippenmeyer et al., 2005).
- Reference for behavioral studies: Wen et al., 2010 (the strain background was not specified).

SOURCE: Authors.

midcortical and caudal cortical levels and in the hippocampus (Flames et al., 2004). It remains to be seen whether there will be a reduction in the number of PV-positive GABAergic interneurons in the schizophrenia-linked prefrontal cortical region in $ErbB4^{-/-}$ $HER4^{heart}$ mutant animals after the inhibitory circuitry has fully developed in adulthood.

Decreased Spine Density of Pyramidal Neurons in the Subiculum of the Ventral Hippocampus

Dendritic spines are the major sites of postsynaptic contact of excitatory synapses in the cortex. Moreover, spines are believed to be the anatomic structures involved in learning and memory (Bourne & Harris, 2007). Postmortem studies of schizophrenia have revealed decreased density of dendritic spines in the subicular region of the ventral hippocampus as well as in the prefrontal cortex, suggesting impaired synaptic function in these regions (Garey et al., 1998; Glantz & Lewis, 2000; Rosoklija et al., 2000). A similar reduction in the spine density of apical dendrites of pyramidal neurons in the subiculum of the ventral hippocampus has been shown in Type III-$Nrg1^{+/-}$ mutant mice (Chen et al., 2008). In addition, there is a decrease in the spine density of pyramidal neurons in the CA1 and prefrontal cortical regions in $ErbB2/B4$-$CNSko$ mutant mice (Barros et al., 2009). Clozapine, the atypical antipsychotic drug used to treat schizophrenia patients (Krakowski et al., 2006), increases spine density of hippocampal neurons in both wild-type mice and $ErbB2/B4$-$CNSko$ mutants, thereby normalizing the spine defects in the mutant mice (Barros et al., 2009). Finally, addition of recombinant NRG1 to cultured hippocampal neurons from wild-type mice leads to an increase in spine density (Barros et al., 2009). Together, these studies demonstrate a crucial role of NRG1/ERBB signaling in spine development, and they implicate altered NRG1/ERBB function in the abnormal neuroconnectivity that may underlie schizophrenia.

Functional Alterations in the Hippocampal and Prefrontal Cortical Regions

The anatomic and structural alterations observed in schizophrenia likely translate into functional and behavioral alterations. fMRI mapping of neuronal activity has been used to study functional changes associated with schizophrenia and revealed alterations in the hippocampal CA1 subfield, orbitofrontal cortex, and dorsolateral prefrontal cortex of schizophrenia patients (Schobel et al., 2009), as well as regional deficits in activation of the hippocampus, anterior cingulate, and precuneus during working memory tasks in individuals carrying *NRG1* risk alleles (Kircher et al., 2009a, 2009b). Similarly, abnormalities in the hippocampus and prefrontal cortex have also been reported in fMRI studies of Type III-*Nrg1*$^{+/-}$ mutant mice (Chen et al., 2008).

NRG1 and Myelination

Postmortem microarray studies by Hakak et al. (2001) revealed decreased expression of the NRG1 receptor, ERBB3, as well as other genes predominantly expressed in mature oligodendrocytes in tissue from patients with schizophrenia. These findings raised the possibility that reductions in the number or function of oligodendrocytes might contribute to the disease. Studies in *Nrg1* mutant mice and in the in vitro culture systems have demonstrated that NRG1 signaling is essential for proper myelination of peripheral nerves by Schwann cells (Michailov et al., 2004; Taveggia et al., 2005; Nave & Salzer, 2006). However, a role for NRG1 signaling in CNS myelination by oligodendrocytes is less clear. Minor and track-specific deficits have been seen in Type III-*Nrg1*$^{+/-}$ mutant mice, and inhibition of ERBB signaling in oligodendrocytes by the expression of a dominant negative *ErbB4* transgene reduces the CNS myelination (Roy et al., 2007; Taveggia et al., 2008). In contrast, when Brinkmann et al. (2008) totally eliminated ERBB or NRG1 expression in the CNS using conditional gene deletion, they failed to see any effect on CNS myelination. In sum, these studies make it unlikely that NRG1 is a major regulator of CNS myelination and leave open the question of the role of disrupted oligodendroctye function in the etiology of schizophrenia.

Behavioral Abnormalities of *Nrg1* and *ErbB4* Mutant Mice

Behavioral Studies of Hypomorphic Nrg1 Mutant Animals

HYPERLOCOMOTOR ACTIVITY. Hyperactivity and stereotypic behaviors are often measured in animal models of schizophrenia-associated phenotypes. Studies on a variety of *Nrg1* mutant animals revealed hyperlocomotor activity. TM-*Nrg1*$^{+/-}$ and EGF-*Nrg1*$^{+/-}$ mutant mice display increased locomotion in a novel open-field environment (Gerlai, Pisacane, & Erickson, 2000; Stefansson et al., 2002; O'Tuathaigh et al., 2006, 2007; Boucher et al., 2007; Karl et al., 2007; Duffy et al., 2008; van den Buuse et al., 2009). Moreover, as opposed to the results in wild-type animals, hyperlocomotor activity observed in TM-*Nrg1*$^{+/-}$ mutant mice is not affected by the psychotropic drug amphetamine (van den Buuse et al.,

2009). In line with a hyperactive phenotype, TM-$Nrg1^{+/-}$ and EGF-$Nrg1^{+/-}$ mutant mice show an increased number of arm-compartment entries in various behavioral paradigms (Boucher et al., 2007; O'Tuathaigh et al., 2007; Duffy et al., 2008; Ehrlichman et al., 2009; Moy et al., 2009) and EGF-$Nrg1^{+/-}$ mutant animals demonstrate better motor performance (i.e., balance and coordination) on the accelerating rotarod than their wild-type counterparts in the rotarod paradigm (Gerlai, Pisacane, & Erickson, 2000). Clozapine normalizes hyperlocomotor activity in TM-$Nrg1^{+/-}$ mutant mice (Stefansson et al., 2002), providing indirect evidence that the hyperactivity observed in $Nrg1^{+/-}$ mutant mice is related to altered dopaminergic signaling.

Studies of Ig-$Nrg1^{+/-}$ mutant animals, however, did not reveal increased locomotor activity in the open field test or running-wheel activity assay (Rimer et al., 2005). Type III $Nrg1^{+/-}$ mutant mice also show normal locomotor activity in the open field or home cage environment (Chen et al., 2008; Luca, E., Role, L. W., & Talmage, D. A., unpublished results). In addition, both TM-$Nrg1^{+/-}$ and Type III-$Nrg1^{+/-}$ mutant mice show normal hyperlocomotor responses (i.e., equivalent to wild-type littermate controls) to amphetamine challenge (van den Buuse et al., 2009; Chen, Y. J., Talmage, D. A. & Role, L. W., unpublished results). It is likely that the discrepancy between the locomotor results from mutants heterozygous for TM domain-, EGF domain-, Ig domain-, or Type III-specific $Nrg1$ mutations reflects disruption of a greater number of $Nrg1$ isoforms by the TM and EGF domain deletions.

It is interesting that EGF-$Nrg1^{+/-}$ mutant animals, which are hyperactive in an open field environment, show normal locomotor activity in a home cage environment (Gerlai, Pisacane, & Erickson, 2000; Duffy et al., 2008; Ehrlichman et al., 2009). This raises the possibility that the hyperlocomotion phenotype reflects altered responses to stressful situations such as exposure to a novel open field.

ABNORMAL EXPLORATORY BEHAVIOR AND IMPAIRED HABITUATION. Impaired processing of novel environmental stimuli and disruption of habituation are considered relevant to the cognitive dysfunction observed in schizophrenia (Grossberg, 2000). It is interesting that male TM-$Nrg1^{+/-}$ mutant mice exhibit gender-specific abnormalities in certain aspects of their exploratory behaviors, such as higher levels of sifting (i.e., sifting movements of the front paws through cage bedding material) and reduced grooming in an open field-type environment (O'Tuathaigh et al., 2006). During the subsequent habituation phase of exploration, male TM-$Nrg1^{+/-}$ mutants show increased grooming (O'Tuathaigh et al., 2006). Moreover, adult (four to seven months of age) TM-$Nrg1^{+/-}$ mutant animals show an age-specific increase in the frequency of exploration-related behaviors, such as head dipping and vertical activity in an open field activity test, a light-dark emergence test, and a hole board task (Boucher et al., 2007; Karl et al., 2007). In sum, this increase in the frequency of exploratory behaviors is in line with the hyperlocomotor activity phenotype of TM-*Nrg1*$^{+/-}$ mutant mice.

IMPAIRED SOCIAL INTERACTION. Impaired social interaction is a key feature of the symptoms of schizophrenia (Freedman, 2003). Increased aggression is observed in some schizophrenia patients (Krakowski et al., 2006). Several studies on *Nrg1*-deficient mouse models have revealed alterations in social approach and increased aggression. TM-*Nrg1*$^{+/-}$ and EGF-*Nrg1*$^{+/-}$ mutant mice exhibit a selective disruption in their behavioral response to social novelty by showing no preference to the novel conspecific in a resident-intruder paradigm (O'Tuathaigh et al., 2007, 2008; Ehrlichman et al., 2009; Moy et al., 2009). TM-*Nrg1*$^{+/-}$ mutant animals also display more nonsocial, aggressive exploratory behaviors toward the conspecific (O'Tuathaigh et al., 2007, 2008).

PREPULSE INHIBITION, LATENT INHIBITION, AND MISMATCH NEGATIVITY DEFICITS. Prepulse inhibition (PPI) and latent inhibition (LI) paradigms are used for assaying information processing deficits related to cognitive dysfunction in schizophrenia. PPI is a behavioral paradigm in which there is a decrease in the magnitude of startle response to an intense stimulus when preceded by a weaker prestimulus. PPI is commonly used as a measure of sensory-motor gating, which is a preattentional mechanism critical to selective processing of external stimuli (Swerdlow, Braff, & Geyer, 2000). Patients with schizophrenia show deficits in PPI (Powell & Geyer, 2002; Weike et al., 2000). Analyses of Type III-*Nrg1*$^{+/-}$ and TM-*Nrg1*$^{+/-}$ mutant mice reveal PPI deficits (Stefansson et al., 2002; Chen et al., 2008). Moreover, chronic nicotine administration in Type III-*Nrg1*$^{+/-}$ mutant animals ameliorates PPI deficits (Chen et al., 2008), a result reminiscent of the nicotine effect on the functional impairments of schizophrenia (George et al., 2006; Kumari & Postma, 2005; Postma et al., 2006). Although one report of PPI in TM-*Nrg1*$^{+/-}$ mutant animals showed a deficit (Stefansson et al., 2002), two other studies demonstrated normal PPI (Boucher et al., 2007; van den Buuse et al., 2009). The observed difference in PPI phenotype could be due to variations in the genetic background of the mouse lines. Studies of EGF-*Nrg1*$^{+/-}$ mutants also did not reveal a baseline PPI deficit (Duffy et al., 2008; Ehrlichman et al., 2009). However, EGF-*Nrg1*$^{+/-}$ mutant mice exhibit a PPI deficit following the administration of the NMDA receptor antagonist, MK801 (Duffy et al., 2008). Treatment of TM-*Nrg1*$^{+/-}$ mutant animals with the 5-HT$_{1A}$ receptor agonist, 8-OH-DPAT, similarly resulted in the disruption of PPI, along with a marked reduction of startle amplitude (van den Buuse et al., 2009). Together, these results imply that NRG1 has a role in sensorimotor gating involving glutamatergic, cholinergic, and serotonergic neurotransmission, which have been shown to contribute to the etiology and pathophysiology of schizophrenia.

LI measures an animal's ability to ignore irrelevant stimuli. In one form of the LI test, prior exposure to a tone makes the tone less likely to reduce ambulatory activity in a test chamber. The reduction in LI observed in schizophrenia is thought to reflect a selective attention deficit (Lubow, 2005). Ig-*Nrg1*$^{+/-}$ mutant animals display more greatly impaired LI than littermate controls by showing a greater decrease in ambulatory distance traveled in response to the acoustic conditioned stimulus (Rimer et al., 2005).

Mismatch negativity (MMN) is a behavioral paradigm that assesses the mismatch response in electroencephalography (EEG) to an odd stimulus within a sequence of otherwise regular stimuli. Auditory MMN can occur in response to deviance in sound pitch, intensity, or duration and has been shown to be impaired in patients with schizophrenia (Shelley et al., 1991). Auditory MMN is disrupted in EGF-*Nrg1*$^{+/-}$ mutant mice, indicating abnormal auditory sensory processing in these mutants (Ehrlichman et al., 2009).

DEFICITS IN LEARNING AND WORKING MEMORY. Patients with schizophrenia show a broad range of cognitive dysfunction, including deficits in learning and working memory (Nuechterlein et al., 2004). To assess short-term or working memory, Type III-*Nrg1*$^{+/-}$ mutant mice were tested in delayed, alternating choice T-maze tasks. In these tasks, using alternating trials, animals learn to find the arm that is baited. Type III-*Nrg1*$^{+/-}$ mutant mice had been shown to perform this task with less accuracy than control animals, thereby demonstrating cognitive dysfunction (Chen et al., 2008).

The Barnes maze task is another behavioral paradigm for assessing working memory in which performance is dependent on the memory of the location of an escape hole. During initial learning sessions of this test, male TM-*Nrg1*$^{+/-}$ mutant mice spend more time finding and entering the escape hole, and then commit a greater number of errors, indicating impaired spatial learning or memory (O'Tuathaigh et al., 2007).

Contextual fear conditioning involves placing an animal in a novel test environment to deliver an aversive stimulus such as a foot shock during the training session and then returning it to the home cage. During the testing period, on returning to the same test environment, the animal shows a freezing response to fear if it had learned to associate the test environment with the aversive stimulus. When tested in the contextual fear paradigm, EGF-*Nrg1*$^{+/-}$ mutant mice display less freezing than the controls, indicating impaired memory function (Ehrlichman et al., 2009).

In sum, *Nrg1* mutant mice exhibit performance abnormalities on tasks designed to probe phenotypes observed in patients with schizophrenia. Although some behaviors are altered in a majority of *Nrg1* mutants studied, others are only found in animals with disruption of certain *Nrg1* isoforms. In general, *Nrg1* mutant animals display hyperactivity in a novel open field, have abnormal exploratory behavior and impaired habituation, show altered information processing and sensorimotor gating, and have impaired social interactions and disrupted working memory.

Behavioral Studies of Transgenic Mice Over-Expressing Type I NRG1

Results from postmortem studies revealing elevated levels of Type I *NRG1* transcripts in the hippocampus and prefrontal cortex of patients with schizophrenia (Hashimoto et al., 2004; Law et al., 2006) have stimulated the generation of transgenic mice over-expressing Type I *Nrg1* (i.e., *Nrg1*[Type I-tg]). The *Nrg1*[Type I-tg] animals show robust over-expression of Type I NRG1 in the brain, particularly in the hippocampus and cortex, but not in the striatum or cerebellum (Deakin et al., 2009). These animals were also studied in behavioral assays similar to paradigms used for *Nrg1* hypomorphs. Female *Nrg1*[Type I-tg] mice are slightly less active and show mild increases in some anxiety measures (Deakin et al., 2009). *Nrg1*[Type I-tg] mice have a movement-related tremor (Michailov et al., 2004; Brinkmann et al., 2008; Deakin et al., 2009) and show poor performance on the accelerating rotarod (Deakin et al., 2009). In addition, these animals exhibit PPI deficits indicative of sensorimotor gating deficits, but with an increased baseline acoustic startle response (Deakin et al., 2009). Thus, behavioral changes observed in *Nrg1*[Type I-tg] mice are not entirely reciprocal with those detected in *Nrg1* hypomorphs. Nonetheless, these results strongly support the idea that an optimal level of NRG1/ERBB signaling is essential for normal behavior and synaptic plasticity (Role & Talmage, 2007).

Behavioral Studies of ErbB4 Mutant Animals

In comparison to analyses on *Nrg1* mutant animals, there are relatively fewer studies on the schizophrenia-related behavioral phenotypes of *ErbB4* mutant mice.

LOCOMOTOR ACTIVITY AND MOTOR PERFORMANCE. Both *ErbB4*[+/−] mutant mice and conditional mutants of *ErbB4* have been analyzed for the locomotor phenotype. When evaluated in an open field test, *ErbB4*[+/−] mutant animals exhibit a hyperlocomotor phenotype that is less robust than that observed in TM-*Nrg1*[+/−] mutant mice (Stefansson et al., 2002). Mice with a conditional deletion of *ErbB4* in astrocytes (i.e., *ErbB4*[flox/−] hGFAP-Cre mutant mice) as well as mice with a selective loss of *ErbB4* in PV-positive interneurons (i.e. PV-*ErbB4*[−/−] mutant mice) also show enhanced locomotor activity (Moy et al., 2009; Wen et al.,

2010). However, double mutant mice with conditional deletions of *ErbB2* and *ErbB4* alleles in astrocytes (i.e., *ErbB2/B4-CNSko* mutant mice) display normal locomotor behavior (Barros et al., 2009). Although mice with a nervous-system-specific conditional mutation of *ErbB4* (i.e, *ErbB4*^{flox/–} Nes-Cre mutant mice) show hyperactivity in the open field before weaning (postnatal day 21), these animals become hypoactive at an older age (postnatal day 66) (Golub, Germann, & Lloyd, 2004). DN-*ErbB4* mutant mice also display hypoactivity when exploring an open field (Roy et al., 2007). It is not clear why locomotor activity phenotypes are not consistent in mice with disrupted ERBB4 signaling, but the age of animals tested is an important variable. In the open field test, the locomotor activity of three- to four-month-old wild-type male mice is almost twice as high as that of four- to six-month-old wild-type male animals (Karl et al., 2007). In studies demonstrating a normal or hypoactive phenotype, some or all test animals in cohorts were less than four months of age (Golub, Germann, & Lloyd, 2004; Roy et al., 2007; Barros et al., 2009). Therefore, it is likely that the inclusion of younger animals with higher locomotor activity may raise the baseline activity levels used for comparison.

The accelerating rotarod paradigm measures motor performance (i.e., balance and coordination). EGF-*Nrg1*^{+/–} mutant animals show enhanced performance on the rotarod (Gerlai et al., 2000), whereas *Erbb4*^{flox/–} hGFAP-Cre and *Erbb4*^{flox/–} Nes-Cre mutant mice display normal performance in this test (Thuret et al., 2004; Moy et al., 2009) indicating normal sensorimotor coordination.

ABNORMAL SOCIAL INTERACTIONS. A variety of *ErbB4* mutant mice have been analyzed in social interaction assays similar to those used for *Nrg1*^{+/–} mutants. Whereas TM-*Nrg1*^{+/–} and EGF-*Nrg1*^{+/–} mice exhibit a selective disruption in their response to social novelty by showing no preference for the novel stranger (O'Tuathaigh et al., 2007, 2008), *ErbB4*^{flox/–} hGFAP-Cre mice show normal responses in the resident-intruder paradigm (Moy et al., 2009). The *ErbB2/B4-CNSko* mice, however, display increased aggression—including biting, kicking, and wrestling—toward novel conspecifics similar to the reported behavior of TM-*Nrg1*^{+/–} mutant animals in a resident-intruder paradigm (O'Tuathaigh et al., 2007, 2008; Barros et al., 2009). The aggressive behavior of *ErbB2/B4-CNSko* mutant mice is normalized by clozapine treatment (Barros et al., 2009). It is interesting that DN-*ErbB4* mutant mice exhibit social dysfunction by showing increased latency in investigating a novel intruder and significantly less dominance-related mounting behavior (Roy et al., 2007). The observed social dysfunctions in DN-*ErbB4* mutants are reminiscent of the negative symptoms of social withdrawal seen in patients with chronic schizophrenia (Blanchard & Cohen, 2006).

PREPULSE INHIBITION DEFICITS. PV-*ErbB4*^{–/–} mutant mice and male *ErbB2/B4-CNSko* mice show schizophrenia-like PPI deficits that have been previously found in Type III-*Nrg1*$^{+/-}$ and TM-*Nrg1*$^{+/-}$ mutant animals (Stefansson et al., 2002; Chen et al., 2008; Barros et al., 2009; Wen et al., 2010). The hyperactive *ErbB4*$^{+/-}$ mutant animals also display minor PPI deficits (Stefansson et al., 2002). The PPI deficits of male *ErbB2/B4-CNSko* mice are alleviated by clozapine treatment (Barros et al., 2009). In addition, the disrupted PPI in PV-*ErbB4*$^{-/-}$ mice is ameliorated by diazepam, a GABA enhancer, further indicating that alterations in ERBB4 regulation of GABAergic neurotransmission may underlie schizophrenia-associated PPI deficits (Wen et al., 2010).

DEFICITS IN LEARNING AND MEMORY. Both TM-*Nrg1*$^{+/-}$ and Type III-*Nrg1*$^{+/-}$ mutant mice exhibit impaired short-term or working memory (O'Tuathaigh et al., 2007; Chen et al., 2008). Male *ErbB4*$^{flox/-}$ mice show similar deficits in learning and memory in the Morris water navigation task. In this paradigm, the animal is released into a pool of water and learns to escape from it by using visual cues placed around the pool to locate a platform that is submerged in the water. The measure of learning is the latency in finding the hidden platform. Male *ErbB4*$^{flox/-}$ mutant animals display longer latencies; this indicates poor spatial learning and memory performance (Golub, Germann, & Lloyd, 2004). PV-*ErbB4*$^{-/-}$ mutant mice also were evaluated for deficits in working memory based on their performance in the automated radial eight-arm maze task. During the training phase, food-restricted mice were trained to retrieve food pellets from the end of each arm. Mice were allowed to freely access eight arms baited with food pellets during the test phase and were analyzed for the number of wrong entries (i.e., repeated entries to an already visited arm or omission of an arm) and the number of correct entries within the first entries. Compared to controls, PV-*ErbB4*$^{-/-}$ mutant mice show increased wrong entries and decreased correct entries, thereby demonstrating impaired working memory (Wen et al., 2010).

Collectively, studies of behavioral phenotypes of *ErbB4* mutant mice have revealed altered locomotor activity, abnormal social interactions, sensorimotor gating deficits, and impaired working memory. The abnormal phenotypes present in *ErbB4* mutants are shared by various *Nrg1* mutants, and these results reinforce the idea that NRG1/ERBB4 interactions play a prominent role in the development or function, or both, of neural circuits underlying behaviors altered in schizophrenia. The conditional *ErbB4* mutant mouse lines with genetic disruptions of *ErbB4* in neurons, oligodendrocytes, astrocytes, or PV-positive interneurons will undoubtedly prove very useful in studying schizophrenia-associated alterations that may potentially be caused by disrupted functions of specific cell populations.

Conclusion

In summary, the anatomic, structural, and functional alterations found in *Nrg1* and *ErbB4* mutant mice most likely contribute to schizophrenia-related behavioral abnormalities in these animals. Thus, genetic susceptibility involving NRG1/ERBB signaling contributes to an array of circuit and behavioral changes that are strikingly reminiscent of schizophrenia phenotypes. Together with results from linkage analyses and association studies, these findings provide strong evidence for altered NRG1 and ERBB function in schizophrenia. Furthermore, transgenic mice that model alterations in schizophrenia at the levels of anatomy, structure, synaptic function, and behavior should aid significantly the understanding of the etiology and pathophysiology of this disabling disease, thereby enhancing the development of novel treatment therapeutics.

KEY AREAS FOR FUTURE RESEARCH

- Many schizophrenia-associated *NRG1* SNPs have been identified in the noncoding or coding regions of the *NRG1* locus. How these *NRG1* mutations affect susceptibility to schizophrenia remains to be elucidated. Studies are needed to further our understanding of the mechanisms by which these SNPs contribute to the changes in brain function that lead to schizophrenia.
- An in-depth understanding of the cellular and molecular mechanisms underlying the etiologically heterogeneous disorder called schizophrenia is essential for the identification of potential molecular targets in novel therapy development.
- Because the etiology of schizophrenia involves a combination of multiple susceptibility genes and environmental factors, studies of gene-gene or gene-environment interactions should provide fundamental insights into pathophysiologic mechanisms underlying this complex disease.
- Currently available medications for schizophrenia have limited efficacy and severe side effects. Therefore, novel therapeutic strategies are needed in the clinical management of schizophrenia. Mouse models exhibiting phenotypic changes relevant to schizophrenia are of high utility in the screening of new potential compounds.

Selected Readings

Bao, J., Wolpowitz, D., Role, L. W., & Talmage, D. A. (2003). Back signaling by the Nrg-1 intracellular domain. *Journal of Cell Biology* 161(6): 1133–1141.

Chen, Y.-J. J., Johnson, M. A., Lieberman, M. D., Goodchild, R. E., Schobel, S., Lewandowski, N., Rosoklija, G., Liu, R.-C., Gingrich, J. A., Small, S., et al. (2008). Type III neuregulin-1 is required for normal sensorimotor gating, memory-related behaviors, and corticostriatal circuit components. *Journal of Neuroscience 28*(27): 6872–6883.

Falls, D. L. (2003). Neuregulins: Functions, forms, and signaling strategies. *Experimental Cell Research 284*(1): 14–30.

Mei, L. & Xiong, W. C. (2008). Neuregulin 1 in neural development, synaptic plasticity and schizophrenia. *Nature Reviews Neuroscience 9*(6): 437–452.

Role, L. W. & Talmage, D. A. (2007). Neurobiology: New order for thought disorders. *Nature 448*(7151) : 263–265.

Stefansson, H., Sigurdsson, E., Steinthorsdottir, V., Bjornsdottir, S., Sigmundsson, T., Ghosh, S., Brynjolfsson, J., Gunnarsdottir, S., Ivarsson, O., Chou, T. T., et al. (2002). Neuregulin 1 and susceptibility to schizophrenia. *American Journal of Human Genetics 71*(4): 877–892.

References

Anton, E. S., Ghashghaei, H. T., Weber, J. L., McCann, C., Fischer, T. M., Cheung, I. D., Gassmann, M., Messing, A., Klein, R., Schwab, M. H., et al. (2004). Receptor tyrosine kinase ErbB4 modulates neuroblast migration and placement in the adult forebrain. *Nature Neuroscience 7*(12): 1319–1328.

Anton, E. S., Marchionni, M. A., Lee, K. F., & Rakic, P. (1997). Role of GGF/neuregulin signaling in interactions between migrating neurons and radial glia in the developing cerebral cortex. *Development 124*(18): 3501–3510.

Bao, J., Lin, H., Ouyang, Y., Lei, D., Osman, A., Kim, T. W., Mei, L., Dai, P., Ohlemiller, K. K., & Ambron, R. T. (2004). Activity-dependent transcription regulation of PSD-95 by neuregulin-1 and Eos. *Nature Neuroscience 7*(11): 1250–1258.

Bao, J., Wolpowitz, D., Role, L. W., & Talmage, D. A. (2003). Back signaling by the Nrg-1 intracellular domain. *Journal of Cell Biology 161*(6): 1133–1141.

Barros, C. S., Calabrese, B., Chamero, P., Roberts, A. J., Korzus, E., Lloyd, K., Stowers, L., Mayford, M., Halpain, S., & Muller, U. (2009). Impaired maturation of dendritic spines without disorganization of cortical cell layers in mice lacking NRG1/ErbB signaling in the central nervous system. *Proceedings of the National Academy of Sciences U.S.A. 106*(11): 4507–4512.

Beasley, C. L. & Reynolds, G. P. (1997). Parvalbumin-immunoreactive neurons are reduced in the prefrontal cortex of schizophrenics. *Schizophrenia Research 24*(3): 349–355.

Bjarnadottir, M., Misner, D. L., Haverfield-Gross, S., Bruun, S., Helgason, V. G., Stefansson, H., Sigmundsson, A., Firth, D. R., Nielsen, B., Steffansdottir, R., et al. (2007). Neuregulin1 (NRG1) signaling through Fyn modulates NMDA receptor phosphorylation: Differential synaptic function in NRG1+/– knock-outs compared with wild-type mice. *Journal of Neuroscience 27*(17): 4519–4529.

Blanchard, J. J. & Cohen, A. S. (2006). The structure of negative symptoms within schizophrenia: Implications for assessment. *Schizophrenia Bulletin 32*(2): 238–245.

Boucher, A. A., Arnold, J. C., Duffy, L., Schofield, P. R., Micheau, J., & Karl, T. (2007). Heterozygous neuregulin 1 mice are more sensitive to the behavioural effects of Delta(9)-tetrahydrocannabinol. *Psychopharmacology (Berl) 192*(3): 325–336.

Bourne, J. & Harris, K. M. (2007). Do thin spines learn to be mushroom spines that remember? *Current Opinion in Neurobiology 17*(3): 381–386.

Bramon, E., Dempster, E., Frangou, S., Shaikh, M., Walshe, M., Filbey, F. M., McDonald, C., Sham, P., Collier, D. A., & Murray, R. (2008). Neuregulin-1 and the P300 waveform—a preliminary association study using a psychosis endophenotype. *Schizophrenia Research 103*(1–3): 178–185.

Brinkmann, B. G., Agarwal, A., Sereda, M. W., Garratt, A. N., Muller, T., Wende, H., Stassart, R. M., Nawaz, S., Humml, C., Velanac, V., et al. (2008). Neuregulin-1/ErbB signaling serves distinct functions in myelination of the peripheral and central nervous system. *Neuron* 59(4): 581–595.

Chen, S., Velardez, M. O., Warot, X., Yu, Z. X., Miller, S. J., Cros, D., & Corfas, G. (2006). Neuregulin 1-erbB signaling is necessary for normal myelination and sensory function. *Journal of Neuroscience* 26(12): 3079–3086.

Chen, Y. J., Johnson, M. A., Lieberman, M. D., Goodchild, R. E., Schobel, S., Lewandowski, N., Rosoklija, G., Liu, R. C., Gingrich, J. A., Small, S., et al. (2008). Type III neuregulin-1 is required for normal sensorimotor gating, memory-related behaviors, and corticostriatal circuit components. *Journal of Neuroscience* 28(27): 6872–6883.

Corfas, G., Roy, K., & Buxbaum, J. D. (2004). Neuregulin 1-erbB signaling and the molecular/cellular basis of schizophrenia. *Nature Neuroscience* 7(6): 575–580.

Coyle, J. T. (2004). The GABA-glutamate connection in schizophrenia: Which is the proximate cause? *Biochemical Pharmacology* 68(8): 1507–1514.

Coyle, J. T. & Tsai, G. (2004). NMDA receptor function, neuroplasticity, and the pathophysiology of schizophrenia. *International Review of Neurobiology* 59: 491–515.

Deakin, I. H., Law, A. J., Oliver, P. L., Schwab, M. H., Nave, K. A., Harrison, P. J., & Bannerman, D. M. (2009). Behavioural characterization of neuregulin 1 type I overexpressing transgenic mice. *Neuroreport* 20(17): 1523–1528.

Duffy, L., Cappas, E., Scimone, A., Schofield, P. R., & Karl, T. (2008). Behavioral profile of a heterozygous mutant mouse model for EGF-like domain neuregulin 1. *Behavioral Neuroscience* 122(4): 748–759.

Ehrlichman, R. S., Luminais, S. N., White, S. L., Rudnick, N. D., Ma, N., Dow, H. C., Kreibich, A. S., Abel, T., Brodkin, E. S., Hahn, C. G., et al. (2009). Neuregulin 1 transgenic mice display reduced mismatch negativity, contextual fear conditioning and social interactions. *Brain Research* 1294: 116–127.

Erickson, S. L., O'Shea, K. S., Ghaboosi, N., Loverro, L., Frantz, G., Bauer, M., Lu, L. H., & Moore, M. W. (1997). ErbB3 is required for normal cerebellar and cardiac development: A comparison with ErbB2-and heregulin-deficient mice. *Development* 124(24): 4999–5011.

Falls, D. L. (2003). Neuregulins: Functions, forms, and signaling strategies. *Experimental Cell Research* 284(1): 14–30.

Flames, N., Long, J. E., Garratt, A. N., Fischer, T. M., Gassmann, M., Birchmeier, C., Lai, C., Rubenstein, J. L., & Marin, O. (2004). Short- and long-range attraction of cortical GABAergic interneurons by neuregulin-1. *Neuron* 44(2): 251–261.

Flames, N. & Marin, O. (2005). Developmental mechanisms underlying the generation of cortical interneuron diversity. *Neuron* 46(3): 377–381.

Freedman, R. (2003). Schizophrenia. *New England Journal of Medicine* 349(18): 1738–1749.

Garcia-Rivello, H., Taranda, J., Said, M., Cabeza-Meckert, P., Vila-Petroff, M., Scaglione, J., Ghio, S., Chen, J., Lai, C., Laguens, R. P., et al. (2005). Dilated cardiomyopathy in Erb-b4-deficient ventricular muscle. *American Journal of Physiology, Heart and Circulatory Physiology* 289(3): H1153–H1160.

Garey, L. J., Ong, W. Y., Patel, T. S., Kanani, M., Davis, A., Mortimer, A. M., Barnes, T. R., & Hirsch, S. R. (1998). Reduced dendritic spine density on cerebral cortical pyramidal neurons in schizophrenia. *Journal of Neurology, Neurosurgery, and Psychiatry* 65(4): 446–453.

Gassmann, M., Casagranda, F., Orioli, D., Simon, H., Lai, C., Klein, R., & Lemke, G. (1995). Aberrant neural and cardiac development in mice lacking the ErbB4 neuregulin receptor. *Nature* 378(6555): 390–394.

Gault, J., Hopkins, J., Berger, R., Drebing, C., Logel, J., Walton, C., Short, M., Vianzon, R., Olincy, A., Ross, R. G., et al. (2003). Comparison of polymorphisms in the alpha7 nicotinic receptor gene and its partial duplication in schizophrenic and control subjects. *American Journal of Medical Genetics Part B: Neuropsychiatric Genetics 123*(1): 39–49.

George, T. P., Termine, A., Sacco, K. A., Allen, T. M., Reutenauer, E., Vessicchio, J. C., & Duncan, E. J. (2006). A preliminary study of the effects of cigarette smoking on prepulse inhibition in schizophrenia: Involvement of nicotinic receptor mechanisms. *Schizophrenia Research 87*(1–3): 307–315.

Gerlai, R., Pisacane, P., & Erickson, S. (2000). Heregulin, but not ErbB2 or ErbB3, heterozygous mutant mice exhibit hyperactivity in multiple behavioral tasks. *Behavioural Brain Research 109*(2): 219–227.

Glantz, L. A. & Lewis, D. A. (2000). Decreased dendritic spine density on prefrontal cortical pyramidal neurons in schizophrenia. *Archives of General Psychiatry 57*(1): 65–73.

Golub, M. S., Germann, S. L., & Lloyd, K. C. (2004). Behavioral characteristics of a nervous system-specific erbB4 knock-out mouse. *Behavioural Brain Research 153*(1): 159–170.

Grossberg, S. (2000). The imbalanced brain: From normal behavior to schizophrenia. *Biological Psychiatry 48*(2): 81–98.

Gu, Z., Jiang, Q., Fu, A. K., Ip, N. Y., & Yan, Z. (2005). Regulation of NMDA receptors by neuregulin signaling in prefrontal cortex. *Journal of Neuroscience 25*(20): 4974–4984.

Guillin, O., Abi-Dargham, A., & Laruelle, M. (2007). Neurobiology of dopamine in schizophrenia. *International Review of Neurobiology 78*: 1–39.

Hahn, C. G., Wang, H. Y., Cho, D. S., Talbot, K., Gur, R. E., Berrettini, W. H., Bakshi, K., Kamins, J., Borgmann-Winter, K. E., Siegel, S. J., et al. (2006). Altered neuregulin 1-erbB4 signaling contributes to NMDA receptor hypofunction in schizophrenia. *Nature Medicine 12*(7): 824–828.

Hakak, Y., Walker, J., Li, C., Wong, W., Davis, K., Buxbaum, J., Haroutunian, V., & Fienberg, A. (2001). Genome-wide expression analysis reveals dysregulation of myelination-related genes in chronic schizophrenia. *Proceedings of the National Academy of Sciences U.S.A. 98*(8): 4746–4751.

Hancock, M. L., Canetta, S. E., Role, L. W., & Talmage, D. A. (2008). Presynaptic type III neuregulin1-ErbB signaling targets (alpha)7 nicotinic acetylcholine receptors to axons. *Journal of Cell Biology 181*(3): 511–521.

Harrison, P. J. & Law, A. J. (2006). Neuregulin 1 and schizophrenia: Genetics, gene expression, and neurobiology. *Biological Psychiatry 60*(2): 132–140.

Harrison, P. J., Law, A. J., & Eastwood, S. L. (2003). Glutamate receptors and transporters in the hippocampus in schizophrenia. *Annals of the New York Academy of Sciences 1003*: 94–101.

Harrison, P. J. & Weinberger, D. R. (2005). Schizophrenia genes, gene expression, and neuropathology: On the matter of their convergence. *Molecular Psychiatry 10*(1): 40–68.

Hashimoto, R., Straub, R. E., Weickert, C. S., Hyde, T. M., Kleinman, J. E., & Weinberger, D. R. (2004). Expression analysis of neuregulin-1 in the dorsolateral prefrontal cortex in schizophrenia. *Molecular Psychiatry 9*(3): 299–307.

Hashimoto, T., Arion, D., Unger, T., Maldonado-Aviles, J. G., Morris, H. M., Volk, D. W., Mirnics, K., & Lewis, D. A. (2007). Alterations in GABA-related transcriptome in the dorsolateral prefrontal cortex of subjects with schizophrenia. *Molecular Psychiatry 13*(2): 147–161.

Hashimoto, T., Volk, D. W., Eggan, S. M., Mirnics, K., Pierri, J. N., Sun, Z., Sampson, A. R., & Lewis, D. A. (2003). Gene expression deficits in a subclass of GABA neurons in the prefrontal cortex of subjects with schizophrenia. *Journal of Neuroscience 23*(15): 6315–6326.

Hippenmeyer, S., Vrieseling, E., Sigrist, M., Portmann, T., Laengle, C., Ladle, D. R., & Arber, S. (2005). A developmental switch in the response of DRG neurons to ETS transcription factor signaling. *PLoS Biology* 3(5): e159.

International Schizophrenia Consortium. (2008). Rare chromosomal deletions and duplications increase risk of schizophrenia. *Nature* 455(7210): 237–241.

Johnson, M. (2007). The role of Type III Neuregulin 1 in birth and migration of neurons in the embryonic and adult forebrain interneurons. Ph.D. dissertation, Columbia University, New York.

Kanazawa, T., Glatt, S. J., Tsutsumi, A., Kikuyama, H., Koh, J., Yoneda, H., & Tsuang, M. T. (2007). Schizophrenia is not associated with the functional candidate gene ERBB3: Results from a case-control study. *American Journal of Medical Genetics Part B: Neuropsychiatric Genetics* 144B(1) : 113–116.

Karl, T., Duffy, L., Scimone, A., Harvey, R. P., & Schofield, P. R. (2007). Altered motor activity, exploration and anxiety in heterozygous neuregulin 1 mutant mice: Implications for understanding schizophrenia. *Genes, Brain and Behavior* 6(7): 677–687.

Kawai, H., Zago, W., & Berg, D. K. (2002). Nicotinic alpha 7 receptor clusters on hippocampal GABAergic neurons: Regulation by synaptic activity and neurotrophins. *Journal of Neuroscience* 22(18): 7903–7912.

Keri, S., Kiss, I., Seres, I., & Kelemen, O. (2009). A polymorphism of the neuregulin 1 gene (SNP8NRG243177/rs6994992) affects reactivity to expressed emotion in schizophrenia. *American Journal of Medical Genetics Part B: Neuropsychiatric Genetics* 150B(3): 418–420.

Kircher, T., Krug, A., Markov, V., Whitney, C., Krach, S., Zerres, K., Eggermann, T., Stocker, T., Shah, N. J., Treutlein, J., et al. (2009a). Genetic variation in the schizophrenia-risk gene neuregulin 1 correlates with brain activation and impaired speech production in a verbal fluency task in healthy individuals. *Human Brain Mapping* 30(10): 3406–3416.

Kircher, T., Thienel, R., Wagner, M., Reske, M., Habel, U., Kellermann, T., Frommann, I., Schwab, S., Wolwer, W., von Wilmsdorf, M., et al. (2009b). Neuregulin 1 ICE-single nucleotide polymorphism in first episode schizophrenia correlates with cerebral activation in fronto-temporal areas. *European Archives of Psychiatry and Clinical Neuroscience* 259(2): 72–79.

Krakowski, M. I., Czobor, P., Citrome, L., Bark, N., & Cooper, T. B. (2006). Atypical antipsychotic agents in the treatment of violent patients with schizophrenia and schizoaffective disorder. *Archives of General Psychiatry* 63(6): 622–629.

Kramer, R., Bucay, N., Kane, D. J., Martin, L. E., Tarpley, J. E., & Theill, L. E. (1996). Neuregulins with an Ig-like domain are essential for mouse myocardial and neuronal development. *Proceedings of the National Academy of Sciences U.S.A.* 93(10): 4833–4838.

Kumari, V. & Postma, P. (2005). Nicotine use in schizophrenia: The self medication hypotheses. *Neuroscience and Biobehavioral Reviews* 29(6): 1021–1034.

Kwon, O. B., Longart, M., Vullhorst, D., Hoffman, D. A., & Buonanno, A. (2005). Neuregulin-1 reverses long-term potentiation at CA1 hippocampal synapses. *Journal of Neuroscience* 25(41): 9378–9383.

Kwon, O. B., Paredes, D., Gonzalez, C. M., Neddens, J., Hernandez, L., Vullhorst, D., & Buonanno, A. (2008). Neuregulin-1 regulates LTP at CA1 hippocampal synapses through activation of dopamine D4 receptors. *Proceedings of the National Academy of Sciences U.S.A.* 105(40): 15587–15592.

Laruelle, M., Kegeles, L. S., & Abi-Dargham, A. (2003). Glutamate, dopamine, and schizophrenia: From pathophysiology to treatment. *Annals of the New York Academy of Sciences* 1003: 138–158.

Law, A. J., Kleinman, J. E., Weinberger, D. R., & Weickert, C. S. (2007). Disease-associated intronic variants in the ErbB4 gene are related to altered ErbB4 splice-variant expression in the brain in schizophrenia. *Human Molecular Genetics 16*(2): 129–141.

Law, A. J., Lipska, B. K., Weickert, C. S., Hyde, T. M., Straub, R. E., Hashimoto, R., Harrison, P. J., Kleinman, J. E., & Weinberger, D. R. (2006). Neuregulin 1 transcripts are differentially expressed in schizophrenia and regulated by 5' SNPs associated with the disease. *Proceedings of the National Academy of Sciences U.S.A. 103*(17): 6747–6752.

Leimeroth, R., Lobsiger, C., Lussi, A., Taylor, V., Suter, U., & Sommer, L. (2002). Membrane-bound neuregulin1 type III actively promotes Schwann cell differentiation of multipotent Progenitor cells. *Developmental Biology 246*(2): 245–258.

Leonard, S., Gault, J., Hopkins, J., Logel, J., Vianzon, R., Short, M., Drebing, C., Berger, R., Venn, D., Sirota, P., et al. (2002). Association of promoter variants in the alpha7 nicotinic acetylcholine receptor subunit gene with an inhibitory deficit found in schizophrenia. *Archives of General Psychiatry 59*(12): 1085–1096.

Leu, M., Bellmunt, E., Schwander, M., Farinas, I., Brenner, H. R., & Muller, U. (2003). Erbb2 regulates neuromuscular synapse formation and is essential for muscle spindle development. *Development 130*(11): 2291–2301.

Lewis, D. A. (2000). GABAergic local circuit neurons and prefrontal cortical dysfunction in schizophrenia. *Brain Research, Brain Research Reviews 31*(2–3): 270–276.

Lewis, D. A., Hashimoto, T., & Volk, D. W. (2005). Cortical inhibitory neurons and schizophrenia. *Nature Reviews Neuroscience 6*(4): 312–324.

Lewis, D. A., Volk, D. W., & Hashimoto, T. (2004). Selective alterations in prefrontal cortical GABA neurotransmission in schizophrenia: A novel target for the treatment of working memory dysfunction. *Psychopharmacology (Berl) 174*(1): 143–150.

Li, B., Woo, R. S., Mei, L., & Malinow, R. (2007). The neuregulin-1 receptor erbB4 controls glutamatergic synapse maturation and plasticity. *Neuron 54*(4): 583–597.

Li, L., Cleary, S., Mandarano, M. A., Long, W., Birchmeier, C., & Jones, F. E. (2002). The breast proto-oncogene, HRGalpha regulates epithelial proliferation and lobuloalveolar development in the mouse mammary gland. *Oncogene 21*(32): 4900–4907.

Liu, X., Hwang, H., Cao, L., Buckland, M., Cunningham, A., Chen, J., Chien, K. R., Graham, R. M., & Zhou, M. (1998). Domain-specific gene disruption reveals critical regulation of neuregulin signaling by its cytoplasmic tail. *Proceedings of the National Academy of Sciences U.S.A. 95*(22): 13024–13029.

Liu, Y., Ford, B., Mann, M. A., & Fischbach, G. D. (2001). Neuregulins increase alpha7 nicotinic acetylcholine receptors and enhance excitatory synaptic transmission in GABAergic interneurons of the hippocampus. *Journal of Neuroscience 21*(15): 5660–5669.

Long, W., Wagner, K. U., Lloyd, K. C., Binart, N., Shillingford, J. M., Hennighausen, L., & Jones, F. E. (2003). Impaired differentiation and lactational failure of Erbb4-deficient mammary glands identify ERBB4 as an obligate mediator of STAT5. *Development 130*(21): 5257–5268.

Lopez-Bendito, G., Cautinat, A., Sanchez, J. A., Bielle, F., Flames, N., Garratt, A. N., Talmage, D. A., Role, L. W., Charnay, P., Marin, O., et al. (2006). Tangential neuronal migration controls axon guidance: A role for neuregulin-1 in thalamocortical axon navigation. *Cell 125*(1): 127–142.

Lubow, R. E. (2005). Construct validity of the animal latent inhibition model of selective attention deficits in schizophrenia. *Schizophrenia Bulletin 31*(1): 139–153.

Martin, L. F., Leonard, S., Hall, M. H., Tregellas, J. R., Freedman, R., & Olincy, A. (2007). Sensory gating and alpha-7 nicotinic receptor gene allelic variants in schizoaffective disorder, bipolar type. *American Journal of Medical Genetics Part B: Neuropsychiatric Genetics 144B*(5): 611–614.

Mata, I., Perez-Iglesias, R., Roiz-Santianez, R., Tordesillas-Gutierrez, D., Gonzalez-Mandly, A., Vazquez-Barquero, J. L., & Crespo-Facorro, B. (2009). A neuregulin 1 variant is associated with increased lateral ventricle volume in patients with first-episode schizophrenia. *Biological Psychiatry* 65(6): 535–540.

Mathew, S. V., Law, A. J., Lipska, B. K., Davila-Garcia, M. I., Zamora, E. D., Mitkus, S. N., Vakkalanka, R., Straub, R. E., Weinberger, D. R., Kleinman, J. E., et al. (2007). Alpha7 nicotinic acetylcholine receptor mRNA expression and binding in postmortem human brain are associated with genetic variation in neuregulin 1. *Human Molecular Genetics* 16(23): 2921–2932.

McCarley, R. W., Wible, C. G., Frumin, M., Hirayasu, Y., Levitt, J. J., Fischer, I. A., & Shenton, M. E. (1999). MRI anatomy of schizophrenia. *Biological Psychiatry* 45(9): 1099–1119.

Mei, L. & Xiong, W. C. (2008). Neuregulin 1 in neural development, synaptic plasticity and schizophrenia. *Nature Reviews Neuroscience,* 9(6): 437–452.

Meyer, D. & Birchmeier, C. (1995). Multiple essential functions of neuregulin in development. *Nature* 378(6555): 386–390.

Michailov, G. V., Sereda, M. W., Brinkmann, B. G., Fischer, T. M., Haug, B., Birchmeier, C., Role, L., Lai, C., Schwab, M. H., & Nave, K. A. (2004). Axonal neuregulin-1 regulates myelin sheath thickness. *Science* 304(5671): 700–703.

Moy, S. S., Ghashghaei, H. T., Nonneman, R. J., Weimer, J. M., Yokota, Y., Lee, D., Lai, C., Threadgill, D., & Anton, E. S. (2009). Deficient NRG1-ERBB signaling alters social approach: Relevance to genetic models of schizophrenia. *Journal of Neurodevelopmental Disorders* 1(4): 302–312.

Nave, K. A. & Salzer, J. L. (2006). Axonal regulation of myelination by neuregulin 1. *Current Opinion in Neurobiology* 16(5): 492–500.

Neddens, J., Vullhorst, D., Paredes, D., & Buonanno, A. (2009). Neuregulin links dopaminergic and glutamatergic neurotransmission to control hippocampal synaptic plasticity. *Communicative and Integrative Biology* 2(3): 261–264.

Nicodemus, K. K., Law, A. J., Luna, A., Vakkalanka, R., Straub, R. E., Kleinman, J. E., & Weinberger, D. R. (2009). A 5' promoter region SNP in NRG1 is associated with schizophrenia risk and type III isoform expression. *Molecular Psychiatry* 14(8): 741–743.

Norton, N., Moskvina, V., Morris, D. W., Bray, N. J., Zammit, S., Williams, N. M., Williams, H. J., Preece, A. C., Dwyer, S., & Wilkinson, J. C. (2006). Evidence that interaction between neuregulin 1 and its receptor erbB4 increases susceptibility to schizophrenia. *American Journal of Medical Genetics Part B: Neuropsychiatric Genetics* 141B(1): 96–101.

Nuechterlein, K. H., Barch, D. M., Gold, J. M., Goldberg, T. E., Green, M. F., & Heaton, R. K. (2004). Identification of separable cognitive factors in schizophrenia. *Schizophrenia Research* 72(1): 29–39.

Okada, M. & Corfas, G. (2004). Neuregulin1 downregulates postsynaptic GABAA receptors at the hippocampal inhibitory synapse. *Hippocampus* 14(3): 337–344.

O'Tuathaigh, C. M., Babovic, D., O'Meara, G., Clifford, J. J., Croke, D. T., & Waddington, J. L. (2007). Susceptibility genes for schizophrenia: Characterisation of mutant mouse models at the level of phenotypic behaviour. *Neuroscience and Biobehavioral Reviews* 31(1): 60–78.

O'Tuathaigh, C. M., Babovic, D., O'Sullivan, G. J., Clifford, J. J., Tighe, O., Croke, D. T., Harvey, R., & Waddington, J. L. (2007). Phenotypic characterization of spatial cognition and social behavior in mice with "knockout" of the schizophrenia risk gene neuregulin 1. *Neuroscience* 147(1): 18–27.

O'Tuathaigh, C. M., O'Connor, A. M., O'Sullivan, G. J., Lai, D., Harvey, R., Croke, D. T., & Waddington, J. L. (2008). Disruption to social dyadic interactions but not emotional/

anxiety-related behaviour in mice with heterozygous "knockout" of the schizophrenia risk gene neuregulin-1. *Progress in Neuropsychopharmacology & Biological Psychiatry* 32(2): 462–466.

O'Tuathaigh, C. M., O'Sullivan, G. J., Kinsella, A., Harvey, R. P., Tighe, O., Croke, D. T., & Waddington, J. L. (2006). Sexually dimorphic changes in the exploratory and habituation profiles of heterozygous neuregulin-1 knockout mice. *Neuroreport* 17(1): 79–83.

Ozaki, M., Sasner, M., Yano, R., Lu, H. S., & Buonanno, A. (1997). Neuregulin-beta induces expression of an NMDA-receptor subunit. *Nature* 390(6661): 691–694.

Postma, P., Gray, J. A., Sharma, T., Geyer, M., Mehrotra, R., Das, M., Zachariah, E., Hines, M., Williams, S. C., and Kumari, V. (2006). A behavioural and functional neuroimaging investigation into the effects of nicotine on sensorimotor gating in healthy subjects and persons with schizophrenia. *Psychopharmacology (Berl)* 184(3–4): 589–599.

Powell, S. B. & Geyer, M. A. (2002). Developmental markers of psychiatric disorders as identified by sensorimotor gating. *Neurotoxicity Research* 4(5–6): 489–502.

Rieff, H. I., Raetzman, L. T., Sapp, D. W., Yeh, H. H., Siegel, R. E., & Corfas, G. (1999). Neuregulin induces GABA(A) receptor subunit expression and neurite outgrowth in cerebellar granule cells. *Journal of Neuroscience* 19(24): 10757–10766.

Rimer, M., Barrett, D. W., Maldonado, M. A., Vock, V. M., & Gonzalez-Lima, F. (2005). Neuregulin-1 immunoglobulin-like domain mutant mice: Clozapine sensitivity and impaired latent inhibition. *Neuroreport* 16(3): 271–275.

Role, L. W. & Talmage, D. A. (2007). Neurobiology: New order for thought disorders. *Nature* 448(7151): 263–265.

Rosoklija, G., Toomayan, G., Ellis, S. P., Keilp, J., Mann, J. J., Latov, N., Hays, A. P., & Dwork, A. J. (2000). Structural abnormalities of subicular dendrites in subjects with schizophrenia and mood disorders: Preliminary findings. *Archives of General Psychiatry* 57(4): 349–356.

Roy, K., Murtie, J. C., El-Khodor, B. F., Edgar, N., Sardi, S. P., Hooks, B. M., Benoit-Marand, M., Chen, C., Moore, H., O'Donnell, P., et al. (2007). Loss of erbB signaling in oligodendrocytes alters myelin and dopaminergic function, a potential mechanism for neuropsychiatric disorders. *Proceedings of the National Academy of Sciences U.S.A.* 104(19): 8131–8136.

Schobel, S. A., Lewandowski, N. M., Corcoran, C. M., Moore, H., Brown, T., Malaspina, D., & Small, S. A. (2009). Differential targeting of the CA1 subfield of the hippocampal formation by schizophrenia and related psychotic disorders. *Archives of General Psychiatry* 66(9): 938–946.

Shelley, A. M., Ward, P. B., Catts, S. V., Michie, P. T., Andrews, S., & McConaghy, N. (1991). Mismatch negativity: An index of a preattentive processing deficit in schizophrenia. *Biological Psychiatry* 30(10): 1059–1062.

Shiota, S., Tochigi, M., Shimada, H., Ohashi, J., Kasai, K., Kato, N., Tokunaga, K., & Sasaki, T. (2008). Association and interaction analyses of NRG1 and ERBB4 genes with schizophrenia in a Japanese population. *Journal of Human Genetics* 53(10): 929–935.

Stefansson, H., Sigurdsson, E., Steinthorsdottir, V., Bjornsdottir, S., Sigmundsson, T., Ghosh, S., Brynjolfsson, J., Gunnarsdottir, S., Ivarsson, O., Chou, T. T., et al. (2002). Neuregulin 1 and susceptibility to schizophrenia. *American Journal of Human Genetics* 71(4): 877–892.

Steiner, H., Blum, M., Kitai, S. T., & Fedi, P. (1999). Differential expression of ErbB3 and ErbB4 neuregulin receptors in dopamine neurons and forebrain areas of the adult rat. *Experimental Neurology* 159(2): 494–503.

Stephens, S. H., Logel, J., Barton, A., Franks, A., Schultz, J., Short, M.,Dickenson, J., James, B., Fingerlin, T. E., Wagner, B., et al. (2009). Association of the 5'-upstream regulatory region of the alpha7 nicotinic acetylcholine receptor subunit gene (CHRNA7) with schizophrenia. *Schizophrenia Research* 109(1–3): 102–112.

Swerdlow, N. R., Braff, D. L., & Geyer, M. A. (2000). Animal models of deficient sensorimotor gating: What we know, what we think we know, and what we hope to know soon. *Behavioural Pharmacology* 11(3–4): 185–204.

Talmage, D. A. (2008). Mechanisms of neuregulin action. *Novartis Foundation Symposium* 289: 74–84; discussion 84–93.

Taveggia, C., Thaker, P., Petrylak, A., Caporaso, G. L., Toews, A., Falls, D. L., Einheber, S., & Salzer, J. L. (2008). Type III neuregulin-1 promotes oligodendrocyte myelination. *Glia* 56(3): 284–293.

Taveggia, C., Zanazzi, G., Petrylak, A., Yano, H., Rosenbluth, J., Einheber, S., Xu, X., Esper, R. M., Loeb, J. A., Shrager, P., et al. (2005). Neuregulin-1 type III determines the ensheathment fate of axons. *Neuron* 47(5): 681–694.

Thuret, S., Alavian, K. N., Gassmann, M., Lloyd, C. K., Smits, S. M., Smidt, M. P., Klein, R., Dyck, R. H., & Simon, H. H. (2004). The neuregulin receptor, ErbB4, is not required for normal development and adult maintenance of the substantia nigra pars compacta. *Journal of Neurochemistry* 91(6): 1302–1311.

Tidcombe, H., Jackson-Fisher, A., Mathers, K., Stern, D. F., Gassmann, M., & Golding, J. P. (2003). Neural and mammary gland defects in ErbB4 knockout mice genetically rescued from embryonic lethality. *Proceedings of the National Academy of Sciences U.S.A.* 100(14): 8281–8286.

Tronche, F., Kellendonk, C., Kretz, O., Gass, P., Anlag, K., Orban, P. C., Bock, R., Klein, R., & Schütz, G. (1999). Disruption of the glucocorticoid receptor gene in the nervous system results in reduced anxiety. *Nature Genetics* 23(1): 99–103.

van den Buuse, M., Wischhof, L., Lee, R. X., Martin, S., & Karl, T. (2009). Neuregulin 1 hypomorphic mutant mice: Enhanced baseline locomotor activity but normal psychotropic drug-induced hyperlocomotion and prepulse inhibition regulation. *International Journal of Neuropsychopharmacology* 12(10): 1383–1393.

Volk, D. W. & Lewis, D. A. (2002). Impaired prefrontal inhibition in schizophrenia: Relevance for cognitive dysfunction. *Physiology and Behavior* 77(4–5): 501–505.

Watanabe, Y., Fukui, N., Nunokawa, A., Muratake, T., Kaneko, N., Kitamura, H., & Someya, T. (2007). No association between the ERBB3 gene and schizophrenia in a Japanese population. *Neuroscience Research* 57(4): 574–578.

Weike, A. I., Bauer, U., & Hamm, A. O. (2000). Effective neuroleptic medication removes prepulse inhibition deficits in schizophrenia patients. *Biological Psychiatry* 47(1): 61–70.

Wen, L., Lu, Y. S., Zhu, X. H., Li, X. M., Woo, R. S., Chen, Y. J., Yin, D. M., Lai, C., Terry, A. V., Jr., Vazdarjanova, A., et al. (2010). Neuregulin 1 regulates pyramidal neuron activity via ErbB4 in parvalbumin-positive interneurons. *Proceedings of the National Academy of Sciences U.S.A.* 107(3): 1211–1216.

Wolpowitz, D., Mason, T. B., Dietrich, P., Mendelsohn, M., Talmage, D. A., & Role, L. W. (2000). Cysteine-rich domain isoforms of the neuregulin-1 gene are required for maintenance of peripheral synapses. *Neuron* 25(1): 79–91.

Woo, R. S., Li, X. M., Tao, Y., Carpenter-Hyland, E., Huang, Y. Z., Weber, J., Neiswender, H., Dong, X. P., Wu, J., Gassmann, M., et al. (2007). Neuregulin-1 enhances depolarization-induced GABA release. *Neuron* 54(4): 599–610.

Yang, X., Kuo, Y., Devay, P., Yu, C., & Role, L. (1998). A cysteine-rich isoform of neuregulin controls the level of expression of neuronal nicotinic receptor channels during synaptogenesis. *Neuron* 20(2): 255–270.

Yurek, D. M., Zhang, L., Fletcher-Turner, A., & Seroogy, K. B. (2004). Supranigral injection of neuregulin1-beta induces striatal dopamine overflow. *Brain Research* 1028(1): 116–119.

Zhong, C., Du, C., Hancock, M., Mertz, M., Talmage, D. A., & Role, L. W. (2008). Presynaptic type III neuregulin 1 is required for sustained enhancement of hippocampal transmission by nicotine and for axonal targeting of alpha7 nicotinic acetylcholine receptors. *Journal of Neuroscience* 28(37): 9111–9116.

Zhuo, L., Theis, M., Alvarez-Maya, I., Brenner, M., Willecke, K., & Messing, A. (2001). hGFAP-cre transgenic mice for manipulation of glial and neuronal function in vivo. *Genesis* 31(2): 85–94.

CONTRIBUTORS

Schahram Akbarian, M.D., Ph.D.
Director
Brudnick Neuropsychiatric Research Institute
Associate Professor
Department of Psychiatry
University of Massachusetts Medical School
Worcester, Mass.

Alan S. Brown, M.D., M.P.H.
Professor of Clinical Psychiatry and Clinical Epidemiology
Department of Psychiatry
Columbia University College of Physicians and Surgeons and
Department of Epidemiology
Mailman School of Public Health of Columbia University
Director, Unit in Birth Cohort Studies
New York State Psychiatric Institute
New York, N.Y.

Thomas H. J. Burne, Ph.D.
Senior Research Fellow
Queensland Brain Institute
University of Queensland
Brisbane, Queensland, Australia

Mary Cannon, M.B., M.Sc., Ph.D., MRCPsych
HRB Clinician Scientist
Associate Professor
Department of Psychiatry
Royal College of Surgeons in Ireland
Education and Research Centre
Consultant Psychiatrist, Beaumont Hospital
Dublin, Ireland

Paola Casadio, M.D.
Consultant Psychiatrist
Faenza Mental Health Centre
Mental Health Department
AUSL
Ravenna, Italy

Yachi Chen, Ph.D.
Research Assistant Professor
Department of Neurobiology and Behavior
State University of New York at Stony Brook
Stony Brook, N.Y.

Iris Cheung, Ph.D.
Brudnick Neuropsychiatric Research Institute
Department of Psychiatry
University of Massachusetts Medical School
Worcester, Mass.

Mary Clarke, M.Sc. (Hons), Ph.D.
Lecturer
Departments of Psychiatry and Psychology
Royal College of Surgeons in Ireland
Dublin, Ireland

Sarah Crystal, B.A.
Doctoral Student
Department of Clinical Psychiatry
Seattle Pacific University
Seattle, Wash.

Xiaoying Cui, M.D., Ph.D.
Research Fellow
Queensland Brain Institute
University of Queensland
Brisbane, Queensland, Australia

Marta Di Forti, M.D., MRCPsych
Clinical Lecturer
Psychosis Center
Department of General Psychiatry
Institute of Psychiatry
London, England

Jubao Duan, Ph.D.
Assistant Professor of Psychiatry
Center for Psychiatric Genetics
University of Chicago
NorthShore University HealthSystem Research Institute
Evanston, Ill.

Lauren M. Ellman, Ph.D.
Assistant Professor
Department of Psychology
Temple University
Philadelphia, Pa.

Darryl W. Eyles, Ph.D.
Senior Lecturer
Queensland Brain Institute
University of Queensland
Brisbane, Queensland, Australia

Pablo V. Gejman, M.D.
Professor of Psychiatry
Center for Psychiatric Genetics
University of Chicago
NorthShore University HealthSystem Research Institute
Evanston, Ill.

Kristin N. Harper, Ph.D.
Robert Wood Johnson Health and Society Scholar
Columbia University
New York, N.Y.

Robin J. Hennessy, Ph.D.
Director of Morphometrics
Molecular and Cellular Therapeutics
Royal College of Surgeons in Ireland
Dublin, Ireland

Mary C. Iampietro, M.A.
Doctoral Student
Department of Psychology
Temple University
Philadelphia, Pa.

Mira Jakovcevski, Ph.D.
Brudnick Neuropsychiatric Research Institute
Department of Psychiatry
University of Massachusetts Medical School
Worcester, Mass.

Maria Karayiorgou, M.D.
Professor, Department of Psychiatry
Columbia University Medical Center
New York State Psychiatric Institute
New York, N.Y.

Karine Kleinhaus, M.D., M.P.H.
Assistant Professor of Psychiatry and Environmental Medicine
NYU School of Medicine
New York, N.Y.

Rebecca J. Levy, B.A., M.Phil.
Doctoral Student in Neurobiology and Behavior
Department of Psychiatry
Columbia University Medical Center
New York, N.Y.

Dolores Malaspina, M.D., M.S.P.H.
Anita Steckler & Joseph Steckler Professor of Psychiatry
NYU School of Medicine
New York, N.Y.

John J. McGrath, A.M., M.B.B.S., M.D., Ph.D., FRANZCP
Director,
Queensland Centre for Mental Health Research
Queensland Brain Institute
University of Queensland
Brisbane, Queensland, Australia

Robin M. Murray, D.Sc., FRS
Professor of Psychiatric Research
Institute of Psychiatry
De Crespigny Park
London, England

Colm M. P. O'Tuathaigh, Ph.D.
Senior Research Fellow
Molecular and Cellular Therapeutics
Royal College of Surgeons in Ireland
Dublin, Ireland

Olabisi Owoeye, MRCPsych
Registrar in Psychiatry
Cavan-Monaghan Mental Health Service
Cavan General Hospital
Cavan, and St. Davnet's Hospital
Monaghan, Ireland
Clinical Research Fellow
Molecular and Cellular Therapeutics
Royal College of Surgeons in Ireland
Dublin, Ireland

Abraham A. Palmer, Ph.D.
Assistant Professor of Human Genetics
University of Chicago
Chicago, Ill.

Paul H. Patterson, Ph.D.
Professor of Biology and Anne P. and
Benjamin F. Biaggini Professor of Biological Sciences
California Institute of Technology
Pasadena, Calif.

Mary Perrin, Dr.P.H., M.P.H.
Assistant Professor of Psychiatry & Environmental Medicine
NYU School of Medicine
New York, N.Y.

David Porteous, Ph.D.
Professor of Human Molecular Genetics & Medicine
Medical Genetics Section
Molecular Medicine Centre
Institute of Genetics and Molecular Medicine
University of Edinburgh
Edinburgh, Scotland

Teresa M. Reyes, Ph.D.
Research Assistant Professor
Department of Pharmacology
Institute for Translational Medicine and Therapeutics
School of Medicine, University of Pennsylvania
Philadelphia, Pa.

Sarah Roddy, Ph.D.
Postdoctoral researcher
Department of Psychiatry
Royal College of Surgeons in Ireland
Dublin, Ireland

Lorna W. Role, Ph.D.
Professor and Chair
Department of Neurobiology and Behavior
Member, Center for Nervous System Disorders
Stony Brook University
Stony Brook, N.Y.
Adjunct Professor of Neuroscience in Psychiatry
College of Physicians and Surgeons of Columbia University
New York, N.Y.

Vincent Russell, F.R.C.Psych.
Consultant Psychiatrist
Cavan-Monaghan Mental Health Service
Cavan General Hospital
Cavan, Ireland
Honorary Senior Lecturer in Psychiatry
Department of Psychiatry
Royal College of Surgeons in Ireland, Beaumont Hospital
Dublin, Ireland

Alan R. Sanders, M.D.
Clinical Associate Professor of Psychiatry
Center for Psychiatric Genetics
University of Chicago
NorthShore University HealthSystem Research Institute
Evanston, Ill.

David A. Talmage, Ph.D.
Associate Professor
Department of Pharmacological Sciences
Member, Center for Nervous System Disorders
Stony Brook University
Stony Brook, N.Y.

Lisa M. Tarantino, Ph.D.
Assistant Professor
Department of Psychiatry
School of Medicine
University of North Carolina
Chapel Hill, N.C.

John L. Waddington, Ph.D., D.Sc., MRIA
Professor of Neuroscience
Molecular and Cellular Therapeutics
Royal College of Surgeons in Ireland
Dublin, Ireland

Bin Xu, Ph.D.
Assistant Professor of Clinical Neurobiology (in Psychiatry)
Department of Psychiatry
Columbia University Medical Center
New York, N.Y.

INDEX

Note: Page numbers followed by *f* or *t* indicate figures or tables.